Cardiovascular Medicine

Series Editor

James T. Willerson
MC 3-116
Texas Heart Institute
Houston, Texas, USA

Cardiovascular Medicine will offer today's most up-to-date, user-friendly guidance on the evaluation, diagnosis, and medical and surgical treatment of heart and vascular disease and will be on the wish list for every trainee and practising cardiologist, cardiac surgeon, vascular surgeon, diabetologist, cardiac radiologist and any physician who manages cardiac patients. The book and online package is dedicated to providing comprehensive coverage of every aspect of cardiovascular medicine from cardiac signs and symptoms through peripheral vascular disease and the genetic basis for cardiovascular disease to preventive cardiology. The Editors – and over 150 world authorities – will offer their decades of scientific and clinical experience. A major selling point will be the consistent chapter organization, clear design, and engaging text that includes user-friendly features such as tables, lists and treatment boxes. The reader will have all the guidance to diagnose and manage a full range of conditions in a series of textbook resources, while also having access to additional video material. More than 1600 illustrations over the eight volumes – including a wealth of color Doppler, nuclear imaging, surgical and pathological images – clarify complex principles and help in the understanding of the subtleties of technique and their application, so that they can be implemented in your practice. The eight volumes of Cardiovascular Medicine, 4th Edition will be the premier resource of its kind, which will advance readers' knowledge and stimulate further study in cardiovascular medicine. Each volume is designed as firstly as a standalone reference in its subject, breaking the field of cardiology down into logical learning modules.

More information about this series at http://www.springer.com/series/10474

David S. Feldman • Paul Mohacsi
Editors

Heart Failure

Springer

Editors
David S. Feldman
Division of Cardiology
Department of Medicine
University of Cincinnati
Cincinnati, OH
USA

Paul Mohacsi
Clinic im Park
Cardiovascular Center Zürich
Hirslanden Zurich
Switzerland

ISSN 2363-5053 ISSN 2363-5061 (electronic)
Cardiovascular Medicine
ISBN 978-3-319-98182-6 ISBN 978-3-319-98184-0 (eBook)
https://doi.org/10.1007/978-3-319-98184-0

Library of Congress Control Number: 2018967000

This Springer imprint is published by the registered company Springer Nature Switzerland AG
The registered company address is: Gewerbestrasse 11, 6330 Cham, Switzerland

Preface

Cardiology has evolved dramatically within the past two decades due to major advances in the treatment of heart disease. At the same time, such progress has required specialization, as knowledge gains and new technological possibilities demand special focus. The European Society of Cardiology (ESC) has stayed abreast with these changes by authoring comprehensive guidelines that define an evidence-based approach not only for interventional cardiology, rhythmology, and heart failure but also for many other subfields of cardiology. Various national research groups have stated recommendations in "curricula," defining the required specialist knowledge and technical skills for subspecialties. This handbook is the first one that summarizes requested knowledge for the curricula in heart failure in Europe and the USA.

We therefore asked in a balanced manner worldwide acknowledged heart failure experts from the USA, Canada, and Europe to summarize their respective and updated knowledge.

We hope you will enjoy reading the book. Please give us your feedback, since this book is the first issue and we like to improve it at the second edition.

With best regards,

Zurich, Switzerland — Paul Mohacsi
Cincinnati, OH, USA — David S. Feldman

Contents

Part I

Definition, Epidemiology & Etiology

Table 1.1 Definition of heart failure with preserved (HFpEF), mid-range (HFmrEF) and reduced ejection fraction (HFrEF)

Type of HF		HFrEF	HFmrEF	HFpEF
Criteria	1	Symptoms ± signs[a]	Symptoms ± signs[a]	Symptoms ± signs[a]
	2	LVEF <40%	LVEF 40–49%	LVEF ≥50%
	3	–	1. Elevated levels of natriuretic peptides[b]; 2. At least one additional criterion: (a) Relevant structural heart disease (LVH and/or LAE), (b) Diastolic dysfunction,	1. Elevated levels of natriuretic peptides[b]; 2. At least one additional criterion: (a) Relevant structural heart disease (LVH and/or LAE), (b) Diastolic dysfunction,

BNP B-type natriuretic peptide, *HF* heart failure, *HFmrEF* heart failure with mid-range ejection fraction, *HFpEF* heart failure with preserved ejection fraction, *HFrEF* heart failure with reduced ejection fraction, *LAE* left atrial enlargement, *LVEF* left ventricular ejection fraction, *LVH* left ventricular hypertrophy, *NT-proBNP* N-terminal pro-B type natriuretic peptide

[a]Signs may not be present in the early stages of HF (especially in HFpEF) and in patients treated with diuretics

[b]BNP > 35 pg/ml and/or NT-proBNP>125 pg/mL

NYHA class I is a HF patient with ordinary functional capacity and no symptoms and class IV is a patient with onset of symptoms at any physical activity [13]. In the ACCF/AHA guidelines the severity of the HF is divided into four stages A-D dependent if there is any existing structural heart disease or not and if so dependent on symptoms or not. In Stage A there are no structural abnormalities and in stage B there is an existent structural heart disease without symptoms, similar to NYHA class I in the ESC guidelines (asymptomatic LV dysfunction). In stage C the severity of HF is dependent on the severity of the symptoms which are progressive and compared to the ESC guidelines similar as NYHA class II and III. Finally there is more refractory HF in stage D and in NYHA class IV. These types of classifications are also in agreement with the guidelines recommended therapy for HF. The different stages A-D selected in the ACCF/AHA guidelines are chosen regarding the difference in mortality and blood concentration of the natriuretic peptides in many studies shown to be prognostic markers [14]. The different classifications are shown in Table 1.2 [5].

Table 1.2 Comparison of ACCF/AHA stages of HF and NYHA functional classifications

ACCF/AHA stages of HF		NYHA functional classification	
A	At high risk for HF but without structural heart disease or symptoms of HF	None	
B	Structural heart disease but without signs or symptoms of HF	I	No limitation of physical activity. Ordinary physical activity does not cause symptoms of HF.
C	Structural heart disease with prior or current symptoms of HF	I	No limitation of physical activity. Ordinary physical activity does not cause symptoms of HF.
		II	Slight limitation of physical activity. Comfortable at rest, but ordinary physical activity results in symptoms of HF.
		III	Marked limitation of physical activity. Comfortable at rest, but less than ordinary activity causes symptoms of HF.
		IV	Unable to carry on any physical activity without symptoms of HF, or symptoms of HF at rest.
D	Refractory HF requiring specialized interventions	IV	Unable to carry on any physical activity without symptoms of HF, or symptoms of HF at rest.

ACCF indicates American College of Cardiology Foundation, *AHA* American Heart Association, *HF* heart failure, *NYHA* New York Heart Association

1.4 Epidemiology

1.4.1 Prevalence of Heart Failure

When talking about prevalence of HF different figures were seen in different studies, which are explained by different definitions of HF used, different study populations (community based vs population based) and different age groups studied. Moreover today there are very few data regarding prevalence on patients with borderline HFpEF or HFmrEF since this is a totally new group of patients. What we know so far is that it is a mix of patients, some have systolic dysfunction and some have diastolic dysfunction and the definition is based on diastolic dysfunction as mentioned before.

Initial studies evaluating the prevalence in HF were often community-based and performed in primary health care. In many of these the diagnosis was based on clinical symptoms and signs and not on an objective evaluation of cardiac function and we know from many studies that clinical symptoms and signs are not reliable for establishing the diagnosis of HF. From a Swedish study performed in random primary health care centers, where records were carefully scrutinized in order to find how the diagnosis of HF was assessed it was found that about only 30% of the patients had performed an echocardiographic investigation evaluating the cardiac function more objectively. In about 70% the diagnosis was set on clinical symptoms and signs, chest X-ray and electrocardiogram [15]. Recently a large Swedish study including more than 88,000 patients estimated the prevalence in Sweden to be 2.2% after adjustment for demographic composition. This was a cross-sectional investigation including all patients in the Stockholm region (population > 2.1 million inhabitants, more than 20% of the whole population in Sweden at this time) who were recorded with a primary or secondary diagnosis of HF on at least one consultation in primary health care (2003–2010) and secondary care (1997–2010) or during hospitalization [16]. The mean age for the prevalent patients in 2010 was 77± 13 years (women 80 ± 12 and men 74 ± 13). In Fig. 1.1 mortality, incidence and prevalence over time (2006–2010) are shown. How reliable are these data? The diagnosis was obtained from patients records and relies on the judgment from the responsible physician. Most of the included patients also visited secondary care or were hospitalized (83%) and there the diagnosis was confirmed by a specialist and should therefore be reliable. The validity of the Swedish National Patient Registry has been evaluated and have shown to have a high validity (82% and if primary diagnosis 95% [17]. Interesting in this study was also that it was found a weak reduction in prevalence compared with similar data from 2006 in contrast to data from Medicare beneficiaries between 1994 and 2003, where there was a slight increase in the number of HF patients suggested to be explained by improved survival [18].

Next we are focusing on population-based studies where the cardiac function has been assessed by means of an echocardiographic investigation. In one study in England including 3960 patients aged 45 years or older coming from 16 randomly selected primary care units LV systolic dysfunction was defined as an EF <40% similar to our definition of HFrEF patients. The prevalence in this study was estimated to vary between 1.8% to 3.5% and 50% of the patients were found to be asymptomatic [19]. A large cross-sectional study was performed in Portugal, the EPICA study, investigating 5434 patients evaluated by 365 general practitioners. The overall prevalence of HF in mainland Portugal was 4.36%, rising from 1.36% in the younger (25–49 years) to 16.14% in the elderly patients older than 80 years and the prevalence due to systolic dysfunction was 1.3% [20].

What we have seen so far is that the prevalence seems to increase with age and therefore it is interesting to search for studies focusing on patients with high age. One of these is The Helsinki Ageing study investigating patients aged 75–86 years and including 501 individuals. The overall prevalence in this study was 8.2%. Interesting was that most individuals (72%) had a normal ventricular function and only 2.3% had a LV systolic dysfunction [21]. Another study worth to mention is the Rotterdam study where in 7983 patients (aged ≥55 years) the prevalence was 0.9% in younger patients (55–64 years of age) increasing to 17.4% in

Fig. 1.1 Temporal trends in prevalence, incidence, and all-cause mortality from 2006 to 2010. The demographic composition in 2006 was used as a reference for adjustment for all values

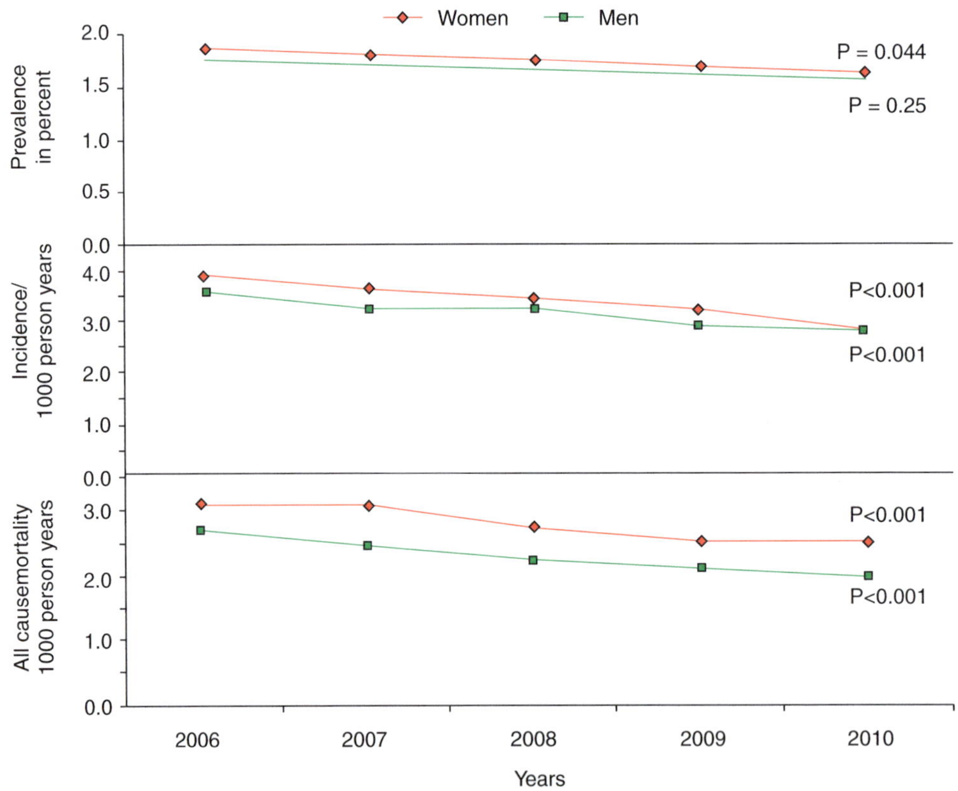

patients older than 85 years [22]. Recently a study from Belgium investigated patients aged 80 years and older, with a mean age of 85 years and where the majority of the patients were women (63%), 567 patients were included and severe cardiac dysfunction was found in 19.3%, with systolic dysfunction in 5.8%, valvular heart disease (mostly aortic stenosis) in 10.4% and severe diastolic dysfunction in 3.1% [23]. From these studies in the elderly we see that more and more of the HF patients were having a HF with a normal EF and most of them are women.

Most of the previous studies regarding prevalence were focused on patients with systolic dysfunction, e.g. patients with HFrEF, who we know from large controlled studies how to treat. However during recent years there has been a growing interest in patients with HFpEF since it has been shown that this type of HF is very common especially in the elderly. In a review by Hogg and coworkers published 2004 a prevalence of HFpEF was found ranging from 1.5% to 4.8% with higher values in the elderly patients [24]. It was also found that the proportion of HFpEF among all HF cases lies somewhere between 40% and 71% (with a mean of 56%) and that there was an increase in the proportion of HFpEF cases in recent studies. The difference in figures is probably due to different definitions of HFpEF, study type (epidemiological study vs observational registry), practice setting (inpatients vs outpatients), and geographic location. The big differences in different studies are here shown with two studies. In the ECHOES study [19] of the general population only 1.1% had definitive HFpEF defined as a LVEF >50%, whereas in Helsinki ageing study [21] 72% had normal EF. In the Rochester study in U.S. Forty-three percent of the patients had HFpEF defined as EF > 50% [25]. In a more recent review by Lam et al. the prevalence of patients with HFpEF was found to variate between 40% and 71% (on an average 54%), thus very similar to the results found by Hogg and coworkers [12]. All this studies confirm that the prevalence increases with age. We also know from these studies that patients with HFpEF are older, more often females, and have more frequently a background of HT and DM.

In a large population based study in Olmsted county in USA it was found that the proportion of patients with HFpEF increased from 38% 1987 to 54% 2001 and this increase was only due to an increase in the number of patients with HFpEF admitted and not because of an reduction of the number of patients with HFrEF. In this study it was found that the prevalence of HFpEF relative to HFrEF is increasing at a rate of 1% per year [11]. During the same time period the number of patients with HF having HT, DM or atrial fibrillation (AF) increased in consequence with the global increase of these diseases, further pointing at the importance of HFpEF as a growing health problem and underscoring the importance of understanding the pathophysiology behind in order to find an appropriate treatment for these patients. The overall prevalence of HFpEF in the community is estimated to be 1.1–5.5% of the general population [26].

Several factors contribute to the increase of HFpEF. These factors are increased life expectancy, aging of the population, concomitant diseases cardiovascular as well as non-cardiovascular and finally better recognition (guidelines definition and improved imaging techniques). In U.S. the number of inhabitants older than 65 years have increased from 9% 1960 to 13% 2013 and projected to increase to 20% 2050, heavily contributing to the so called HF epidemic [5].

1.4.2 Incidence of Heart Failure

What about the incidence of HF. The incidence was investigated in the Hillingdon study. All incident cases were detected in a population of 151,000 covered by 82 general practices, and 99% of the patients were having an echocardiographic investigation. All the results were judged by a panel of three cardiologists making the final diagnosis. The incidence rose from 0.02/1000 per year in those aged 25–34 to 11.6/1000 in those over 85 years. The median age of investigated patients was 76 year. The study confirmed that HF is a disease of elderly [27].

In the Cardiovascular Health study, a population-based study of 5888 elderly people (mean age 73 ± 5 years), performed in USA the incidence rate was 19.3/1000 person years. The incidence of HF increased progressively across age groups and was greater in men than in women [28].

Data of incidence from primary health care are available from the UK general practice database, 696,884 individuals over age of 45 years were selected for the study and 6478 (based on records and medication) were found to have definitive HF and 14,050 with possible HF. The overall incidence of definitive HF was 9.3/1000 per year and the mean age of included patients was 77 years. The incidence was higher in men and increased with age [29]. Data from the Scottish continuous morbidity recording data set showed an overall incidence of 2/1000 per year and 22/1000 in the age over 85 [30]. In the large cross-sectional study from Stockholm, Sweden the incidence of HF was 3.7/1000 person years in women and 3.9 in men (Fig. 1.1). The mean age in this study was 77 ± 13 years [16]. According to the ACCHF guidelines the incidence of HF has been rather stable over the years with >650,000 new cases annually of HF. The incidence rate increases with age from 20/1000 in patients aged 65–69 years to >80/1000 in those over 85 years. In a recently published study, however, with data from Olmsted county in Minnesota (population about 144.248 inhabitants) evaluating incidental HF between the year 2000–2010 it was found that the age and sex adjusted incidence fell from 316/100,000 in 2000 to 219/100,000 in 2010 and the fall was greater for patients with HFrEF (−45%) than HFpEF (−27%) [31].

In summary, despite the rather stable incidence rates of HF reported in many studies and now recently a study evaluating patients up to 2010 reporting a decline in incidental HF we can still expect that the number of cases with HF will increase due to the ageing population and improved survival following better management and use of modern treatment especially in patients with HFrEF where we have seen some decrease. In HFpEF patients do we not today have any recommended treatment and we can also from studies see that the prevalence of patients with HFpEF is increasing.

Also worth to mention is that HF is heavily underdiagnosed at least in the primary health care and a study evaluating patients with shortness of breath at exertion found that 16% of them were having HF, 2.9% had HFrEF and the dominating part (12%) had HFpEF [32].

1.4.3 Risk Factors

HF is associated with many traditional risk factors as cardiovascular comorbidities as well as non-cardiovascular comorbidities and these risk factors may vary in prevalence when looking at HF patients with reduced EF and patients with preserved EF. Patients at high risk for developing HF are patients with HT, DM, atherosclerotic disease including CAD and vascular disease, obesity, AF and those with a metabolic syndrome including any three of the following five; abdominal adiposity, hypertriglyceridemia, low high density lipoprotein, HT and fasting hyperglycemia. According to this definition (established by the National Cholesterol Education Program (NCEP) the prevalence of the metabolic syndrome currently exceeds 20% of individuals who are at least 20 years of age and 40% of the population older than 40 years of age. However the definition has been criticized since many experts think that also inflammatory or hemostatic variables should be included. In studies it has been shown that the predictive power of the metabolic syndrome for CAD and new-onset DM is enhanced by the presence of an elevated C-reactive protein level [33].

Besides these more traditional risk factors we also have more non-cardiac comorbidities as chronic kidney disease, anemia, chronic obstructive pulmonary disease, sleep disordered breathing and depression. In a study from the European Heart Failure Pilot survey evaluating 3226 patients it was found that the majority of the chronic HF patients had at least one comorbidity, of which the most common were chronic kidney disease (41%), anemia (29%) and DM (29%). Furthermore it was demonstrated that comorbidities were independently associated with higher age, higher NYHA functional class, ischemic etiology, higher heart rate, history of HT and AF [34]. Studies have also shown that in HFpEF patients the most common risk factors are HT, high age, female sex and AF. Due to the higher age of HFpEF patients many of the other risk factors are also prevalent as reduced kidney function, anemia, and chronic obstructive pulmonary disease. Regarding CAD most studies are reporting this disease more prevalent in patients with HFrEF. In conclusion HF is associated with a number of different risk factors which are very prevalent and related to the severity of HF.

1.4.4 Prevention of HF

Is it possible to prevent HF? We know from many studies that HF is characterized by high morbidity and mortality and a poor quality of life resulting in high costs for the society [4]. From a number of controlled randomized trials we know how to treat patients with HFrEF and many of those trials have demonstrated improved survival and reduced need for hospital care with drugs as beta-blockers, ACE i:s, angiotensin receptor blockers, mineralocorticoid receptor antagonists, implantable cardioverter defibrillator (ICD) and cardiac resynchronization therapy (CRT) [4]. On the other hand so far no controlled randomized study has shown any therapeutic effect in patients with HFpEF, probably explained in some studies by selecting patients with less disease [35]. There are however observational studies including a large number of patients showing beneficial effects of renin-angiotensin blockers [36] and beta-blockers [37]. These studies show the effect in real world patients and not in selected patients (due to inclusion and exclusion criteria used in controlled randomized trials). However even if sophisticated statistical methods are used in observational studies to eliminate differences between included patients we must be careful when interpretating the results. However by using guidelines recommended drugs it is not prevention of HF we do, since the treatment is started when HF is established and despite these beneficial results using these drugs the death rate in HF and the number of hospitalizations are still unacceptably high and therefore our next step is to move on to how to prevent HF. Patients at high risk for developing HF are patients with HT, DM, atherosclerotic disease including CAD and vascular disease, obesity, AF and those with a metabolic syndrome and many of these risk factors are modifiable and have in studies been shown to prevent HF.

Another step in order to prevent HF is to try to have an early diagnosis of HF by using biomarkers as a screening tool. As far as I know this has just been done in one large controlled study, namely the STOP-HF randomized trial. This study included 1374 participants with one or more cardiovascular risk factor (HT, dyslipidemia, obesity, vascular disease, DM, AF and moderate to severe heart valve disease). Among these patients at risk for developing HF, brain natriuretic peptide (BNP) based screening and collaborative care (collaboration between primary care physician and specialist cardiovascular service) reduced the number of patients developing LV systolic dysfunction both symptomatic as well as asymptomatic, diastolic dysfunction and HF [38]. Still early diagnosis is a challenge to achieve, but the promising results from the STOP-HF trial give us at least some hope. However the strategy used and the results obtained must be confirmed in a larger population to see if this is the right way to decrease the expected epidemic of HF.

What about modifiable lifestyle risk factors. In the Physicians' health study, a prospective cohort study including data from 20,900 apparently healthy men with a mean age of 54 years six modifiable life style factors were assessed. The main outcome was lifetime risk of HF. Overall the lifetime risk of HF was 14% at age 40 years and remained constant through age 70 years. Healthy life style habits (normal body weight with a body mass index <25 kg/m^2, never smoking, regular exercise at least five times per week, moderate alcohol intake with at least five drinks per week, consumption of breakfast cereals at least one serving per week and consumption of fruit and vegetables with at least four servings per day) were associated with a lower lifetime risk of HF, with the highest risk in men adhering to none of the six lifestyle factors (21%) and the lowest risk in men adhering to four or more of the factors (10%) [39].

In a Swedish observational study of 36,019 women the relationship of the DASH diet (dietary approaches to stop hypertension) and the incidence of HF over 7 years were evaluated. The DASH diet has been shown to effectively reduce HT and low density lipoprotein cholesterol and the diet features high intake of fruit and vegetables, low fat dairy products and whole grains resulting in high potassium, magnesium, calcium, and fiber, moderately high protein, and low total and saturated fat consumption. Diet was measured by using food-frequency questionnaires. The included females were of age 48–83 years old without baseline HF, DM or MI. During the study 443 patients developed HF (1.2%). Women adhering best to the diet had a 37% lower rate of HF after adjusting for a number of confounders [40].

These two studies show that HF might to this extent be prevented by living a healthy lifestyle.

HT is an important cause of chronic HF in the western world and the most common cause in the developing countries and more common in patients with HFpEF. HT is very frequent in the United States, it is estimated that 33% of U.S. adults older than 20 years have HT, and about 78% know that they have it but only 64% have a good blood pressure control [41].

HT leads to an increase in afterload, which leads to a concentric or eccentric hypertrophy and initially the systolic function is intact. LV hypertrophy is an increase in the cardiomyocyte mass in response to increased load that often leads to increased wall thickness. It has been described that this condition is an intermediate step between HT and a clinical manifestation of HF. However with progressing hypertrophy the compliance of the left ventricle is reduced and a so called "stiff heart" is generated leading to increased LV filling pressures and reduced end-diastolic volumes and then progression continues to a dilatation of the left ventricle and a systolic dysfunction and finally we have a hypertensive HF with normalized blood pressure.

Malignant HT is an important cause of acute HF with a sudden development of severe high blood pressure and especially high diastolic measurements. This condition frequently presents with acute onset of symptoms as severe headache, confusion, seizures and coma and alarming signs as papilledema, retinal hemorrhages and exsudates and a development of an acute pulmonary edema in patients with a normal or preserved EF. Kidney function is mostly impaired with development of oliguria and uremia. The causes behind may be several but renal artery stenosis as well as phaeochromocytoma and Conn's syndrome are regarded as more frequent occurring [42].

It has been shown that treatment of HT is the most effective strategy for preventing HF as studies have shown that every 5 mm reduction in systolic blood pressure reduces the risk of HF by 24% [43]. Many controlled trials in patients with HT have shown that HF has been reduced. One of the first was the SHEP trial randomizing patients to chlortalidone or placebo, where it was demonstrated after a mean follow-up of 4.5 years that the incidence of stroke was reduced by 36% and HF with 54%. In another trial (HYVET; hypertension in the very elderly) more focusing on elderly individuals (age over 80 years) with HT it was found after a follow-up of 2.1 years in the treatment group receiving indapamide and perindopril that the incidence of fatal and non-fatal HF was reduced by 64% and all-cause mortality was reduced by 21% [44]. A number of meta-analyses have over the years evaluated the effect of different hypertensive medications on cardiovascular outcomes including HF. First we have the meta-analysis published by Sciaretta et al. comparing different classes of antihypertensive drugs in patients with HT or high cardiovascular risk. Here it was clearly shown that diuretics were the most effective drugs of all hypertensive medications in preventing HF followed by renin-angiotensin antagonists [45]. In another meta-analysis by Roush et al. comparing hydrochlorothiazide and chlortalidone on mortality or at least one cardiovascular event, chlortalidone reduced the incidence of HF by 23% and cardiovascular events by 21% [46]. All these studies confirm the importance of blood pressure control in order to reduce or prevent HF. Moreover it has been shown that first-line drugs should be diuretics and especially chlortalidone in order to prevent HF and next in line should be renin-angiotensin antagonists. In summary blood pressure control seems to be important in preventing HF.

DM is a very common comorbidity in patients with HF and the prevalence in different studies are variating between

20% and 40% with no significant differences between patients with HFrEF or HFpEF. The problem we can see in the future with regard to the global health is that the prevalence of DM is continuously increasing. Several epidemiologic studies have shown that DM and insulin resistance is a known predictor of HF [47]. DM is associated with development of myocardial dysfunction even in the absence of CAD or HT and this condition has been called "diabetic cardiomyopathy" [48]. Insulin resistance and hyperglycemia induce the myocardial dysfunction through mechanisms including free fatty acid concentration, mitochondrial dysfunction, abnormal calcium homeostasis, activation of the RAAS, oxidative stress and advanced glycation endproducts [49]. The development of systolic dysfunction may have been preceded by cardiac fibrosis and collagen deposition resulting in a diastolic dysfunction caused by relaxation abnormalities similar to the situation found in HT [50, 51]. In a population-based study from U.S. it was found that diabetic cardiomyopathy is relatively common in the community with a prevalence of 1.1% and was associated with a 1.9 fold increase in risk of developing any LV dysfunction (systolic or diastolic). Among patients with diabetic cardiomyopathy 22% developed HF and development of death or HF was 31% after 9 years [52].

DM is associated with increased morbidity and mortality in patients with HF but its influence as a predictor of long-term outcomes after HF hospitalization is less well-defined [53]. In the OPTIMIZE-HF registry, however, DM patients were at increased short-term risk for rehospitalization, but similar risk for in-hospital and short-term mortality. In patients with HFpEF and DM no increased risk for short-term mortality or rehospitalization were demonstrated in contrast to the findings in patients with HFrEF [54]. Thus the impact of DM on outcomes is not well defined but may be more related to rehospitalization than mortality. No studies have shown that a tight glucose control prevents HF except for the UK prospective DM study (UKPDS) which revealed that reduction in glycemia is associated with a decreased incidence of MI and the development of HF when compared to higher levels [55]. In contrast in the ACCORD study (Action to control cardiovascular risk in diabetes) it was found that intensive clucose control (glycated hemoglobin level (HbA1c) < 6%) compared with standard therapy (HbA1c 7–7.9%) increased mortality and did not significantly reduce major cardiovascular events including HF [56]. A large meta-analysis including 37,229 patients in eight different trials with type 2 DM found similar results [57]. Based on these results the beneficial effects of intensive glucose control with HF prevention are unclear and could also potentially be harmful. Today we do not know how to treat patients with DM and HF, many of the newer drugs have been associated with increased HF risk. A new drug, empagliflozin (an inhibitor of sodium-glucose cotransporter 2), new on the market has in preliminary studies shown promising results with reduction of hospitalization for HF and mortality [58, 59]. Recently published is a large observational trial (including 36,274 patients with HF) studying risk factors, treatment and prognosis in men and women with and without DM. This study confirms that type 2 DM is a strong mortality predictor in men (increased mortality risk by 50%) and women (increased mortality risk by 70%) with HF. The shorter survival found in women was related to comorbidities rather than sex [60]. In summary by modifying the risk factor DM in order to prevent HF does not seem to be beneficial even if DM type 2 is a strong predictor of mortality.

In conclusion the best way to prevent HF is to have a good blood pressure control and also live a healthy life.

1.5 Morbidity and Mortality

1.5.1 Morbidity (Hospitalizations)

Management of HF is associated with a cost about 1–2% of the health care budget in most countries, and about 70% of this cost is caused by frequent, prolonged and repeat hospitalizations for primary diagnosis of HF as well as secondary diagnosis. We know that chronic HF is characterized by a number of exacerbations demanding care in hospital or management in out-patients clinics or specialized HF clinics. We also know that HF today still is the single most frequent cause of hospitalizations in patients 65 years and above. Since many are talking about a future epidemic of HF how is this associated with data collected. Scottish data evaluating hospitalization rates for all patients with HF in Scotland between 1986 and 2003 found that the rates of the first hospitalization for HF increased between 1986 and 1994 and then declined, in parallel with the increase of prescription of more modern HF drugs [61]. Similar findings were found from Sweden evaluating hospital discharges for HF between 1988 and the year 2000. The explanation given besides introduction of modern new drugs is also establishment of HF units and home care programmes [62]. In a study from The Netherlands it was found that the number of HF hospitalizations were increased by 72% between 1980 and 1999, partly explained by the increase in mean age of hospitalized patients [63]. Chen et al. reported similar findings from the United States by looking at Medicare beneficiaries between1998 and 2007 and found that age adjusted HF hospitalization rates declined for all race-sex categories. Black men were found to have the lowest rate of declined [64]. However in another analysis from the same database it was found that the readmission rate within 30 days were higher and included 25% of the HF patients and that 35% of the readmissions were in connection with HF and regardless of age, sex, race, or time after discharge [65]. These results were surprising and indicate that even if the number of unique patients hospitalized for HF has declined in most studies, the number of readmissions have increased. One conclusion to draw is that if a patient has been hospitalized for HF the risk of readmission over time has not been reduced. In the United States this has led to that hospital readmissions are now a quality indicator under the Hospital Readmissions Reduction Program of the Patient Protection and Affordable Care Act with downward adjustment of Medicare payment for hospitals with "excess" 30-day readmission rates. The problem with this program is that most readmissions of HF patients are not caused by HF but instead of many of the concomitant comorbidities these patients have and also by frailty due to elderly patients. Also how the diagnosis of HF has been set is discussed since discharge diagnoses are not validated and also sensitive to changes in the payment system. In order to have more information in HF and especially in "real world" patients large registries have been established in The United States. One of the largest is the American Heart Association Get with the Guidelines (GTWG) program, which includes 558 hospitals and more than 530,000 hospitalized patients with HF [66]. Another important registry is the commercial funded ADHERE registry including patients with acute HF and includes more than 150,000 patients [67]. In Europe we have also several registries and in Sweden we have the Swedish Heart Failure Registry, which has included close to 70,000 unique patients at the end of 2015 [68]. The problem with registries are that all are voluntary to participate in, creating unavoidable selection biases, and most of them are not covering the incidental HF and also many have only one registration without any follow-up. All these factors limit their importance and are important to consider when interpreting the data.

In summary the number of unique patients hospitalized for HF seem to decline in the Western World, but the number of readmissions in HF patients seem to increase not really in patients with the primary diagnosis of HF but instead in those with the secondary diagnoses of HF, explained by more and more elderly patients with a number of non-cardiac comorbidities and also frailty in these patients [69]. This is clearly confirmed in the recently published study from the Olmsted County in Minnesota evaluating incidental HF between the year 2000 and 2010 where it was found that most hospitalizations (63%) were due to non-cardiovascular causes, and with no difference in cardiovascular hospitalizations but instead a significant increase in non-cardiovascular hospitalizations over the years [31]. This is also clearly shown in the study by van Deursen et al. from the European Pilot HF registry [34]. In a paper from U.S. by Collins et al. the controversial question about the necessity of hospitalizing patients with a worsening HF is discussed. They mean that since many of patients admitted with worsening HF do not have pulmonary edema, myocardial ischemia or cardiogenic shock demanding acute intervention or intense monitoring, and therefore after a short period of observation safely could be discharged to their homes with intensified medication and do not need to be hospitalized [70].

1.5.2 Mortality of Heart Failure

There is no doubt that the prognosis of HF patients is poor even if we today have effective drugs and also effective non-pharmacological interventions and studies have shown that the mortality is higher than that find in a number of common malignant diseases [71]. However there is some light in the tunnel since large studies have shown slight improvement in survival over years. One of these are the Scottish trial evaluating mortality in patients hospitalized with a first episode of HF between 1986 and 2003 and find improvement in adjusted 1- and 5-year survival. Median survival increased from 1.33 to 2.34 years in men and from 1.32 to 1.79 years in women [61]. In a study examining changes in HF hospitalization and 1-year mortality rate from Medicare beneficiaries in the United States it was found that there was a slight decline in the 1-year mortality from 31.7% 1999 to 29.6% in 2008 [65]. In a large cross-sectional study in Sweden including more than 88,000 patients the mortality was after adjustment for demographic composition 3.2/1000 person-years in women and 3.0/1000 person-years in men and the 5-year mortality was 48% (Fig. 1.1). In comparancy with similar data from 2006 the mortality was decreased by 0.5/1000 person years demonstrating a slight survival improvement in line with other studies [16]. In contrast the recently mentioned Olmsted County study evaluating incidental HF from year 2000 to 2010 found no decline in the mortality over time. The 5 year mortality found was 24.4% at age 60 and 54.4% at age 80. Interesting was that mortality due to non-cardiovascular causes was dominating (54.3%), again highlighting the importance of comorbidities [31, 34].

Since the HF patients are becoming older and the proportion of HF with preserved EF will increase it is of great interest to see if there are any differences regarding mortality between HFrEF and HFpEF patients. The survey study by Owan et al. from the Olmsted county found that the mortality rates of HFpEF patients did not improve between 1987 and 2001 [11]. It has been suggested by many researchers that the most common cause of death in HFpEF is due to non-cardiovascular causes supporting the belief that HFpEF is something you "die with" and not "die of". It was found that the majority of deaths were cardiovascular (51–60% in epidemiological studies and more than 70% in clinical randomized trials). Among cardiovascular deaths, sudden cardiac death (SCD) and HF death were most frequent, but lower than found in HFrEF patients and the number of deaths due to non-cardiovascular causes was higher especially in the epidemiological studies. In this study the annual mortality were ranging from 10% to 30% [72]. However there is a big variation in mortality rates found in different studies probably explaining that there have been differences in diagnostic criteria and clinical settings. The Maggic group have recently evaluated mortality in 41.972 patients, of which 10,347 (24.7%) had HFpEF from observational and clinical trial studies. It was found that HFpEF patients had a lower mortality (121 deaths per 1000 person years) than patients with HFrEF (141 deaths per 1000 person years) regardless of age, gender and etiology of HF. When excluding randomized clinical trials the mortality rates in HFpEF and HFrEF patients were very similar, 146 versus 159 deaths per 1000 person years [73]. Similar results have been found in other studies. In contrast one meta-analysis based on prospective observational studies have shown a much lower mortality rate for HFpEF patients compared to HFrEF (only 50% of that of HFrEF). One explanation might be that once patients have been hospitalized, the mortality between HFrEF and HFpEF patients is more similar [74].

In summary: Over the years there has been a slight improvement in survival in HF patients. Patients with HFrEF and patients with HFpEF have both a similar and substantial mortality, at least if they have been hospitalized for their HF, even if their characteristics are quite different. The big difference is also that today we know how to treat patients with HFrEF but not with HFpEF and the slight survival improvement found was more evident in HFrEF patients.

1.5.3 Cause of Death

In many years it has been known that HF patients die from a SCD or from a pump failure death and the mode of death depends upon the severity of the HF. It has also been known that the risk of dying suddenly is greater in patients with mild HF and with more severe HF the risk of dying from a pump failure death is much higher. Many believe that SCD is an arrhythmic death but autopsy studies in patients having died suddenly have shown that ischemic events also may be present, demonstrating how difficult it is from the clinical picture to decide the cause of death if autopsy is not performed. In a study it was find an acute MI at autopsy in 55% of the cases, which had been classified as due to an arrhythmia and in 81% of those classified as pump failure death [75]. Today we believe that 50% of the HF patients die from a SCD due to ventricular tachyarrhytmias as well as brady-arrhythmias and the remaining die from a progressive pump failure death. However taken into consideration that we do not perform autopsies in the majority of our HF patients and thereby apparently underestimate the occurrence of CAD leading to an acute MI perhabs this is not true at all.

1.5.4 Asymptomatic Left Ventricular Dysfunction

The prevalence of asymptomatic dysfunction LV systolic or diastolic dysfunction ranges from 6% to 21% and increases with age [76–78]. In the LV dysfunction prevention study, participants with untreated asymptomatic LV dysfunction had a 10% risk for developing HF symptoms and an 8% risk of death or HF hospitalization annually [79]. In a community based population, asymptomatic mild LV diastolic dysfunction was seen in 21% and moderate or severe diastolic dysfunction in 7% and both were associated with an increased risk of symptomatic HF and mortality [78]. In the MONICA study it was shown that ALVSD (asymptomatic left ventricular systolic dysfunction) is an important clinical entity, 21% of the cohort were dead at 4 years [80]. ALVSD is graded in the ACCHF classification as Grade B and in the ESC classification as NYHA class I [4, 5].

1.6 Specific Conditions

1.6.1 Aging – Elderly Patients

According to U.S. population statistics the total population in USA increased by 9.7% between 2000 and 2010, and those older than 65 years of age increased with 15.1%. Furthermore the greatest increases over this 10 years period occurred in the oldest age groups with a 29.9% increase in those 85–94 years of age and a 25% increase in those older than 95 years of age. Based on the aging the prevalence of HF will probably exceed that of other cardiovascular diseases over the next 20 years [81, 82]. As of 2012, an estimated 2.4% of the U.S. population had HF, with prevalence increasing with age such that, among those 80 years and older, almost 12% of both men and women had HF [83] and this was followed by a similar increase in death due to HF. The growing population of older adults with HF and a high incidence of co-morbidity will likely contribute to the increasing costs and hospitalizations accounted for by individuals with HF. In a study of Medicare Beneficiaries with HF patients older than 65 years of age, the annual likelihood for hospitalization was 35%, but among patients with 5 co-morbidities, the likelihood increased to 72%, and among patients with more than 10 comorbidities the likelihood was 94%. Therefore, with increasing prevalence of HF in older populations with multimorbidity, it is likely that annual hospitalization rates will continue to rise affecting the costs attributed to the management of patients with HF since 70% of the cost is related to the cost for hospitalization [84]. In 2010, the direct costs attributed to HF were 24.7 billions in USA [82].

HF is really a disease of the elderly. In different studies it has been found that the mean age at first diagnosis of HF increased over the years and in community studies and registries the mean age of HF patients is between 75 and 80 years and higher in women [85]. It has also been shown that the proportion of hospitalizations with a diagnosis of HF, as well as the prevalence of HF in the general population is much higher in older patients [86]. The epidemic of HF among elderly may in part be explained by improved management of acute conditions and co-morbidities with patients living longer and progressing to clinical HF. Longer exposure to risk factors and age related changes may also make the elderly more prone to develop HF [87]. Although overall survival after HF onset has substantially improved with modern drugs this benefit is less evident in older age groups [88, 89], where advanced age remains a strong predictor for poor outcome in patients with chronic [90] or acute HF [91].

Elderly patients hospitalized for acute HF are more likely to be women and to have a higher prevalence of HFpEF compared with younger patients. They have an increased prevalence of co-morbidities including AF, HT, cerebrovascular disease, anemia, malignancy and chronic kidney disease [92, 93]. Influence of CAD and DM are less common in the very elderly [92]. This may be explained by the longer survival of people not suffering from these diseases.

In contrast to younger patients with systolic HF elderly patients with acute decompensated HF (ADHF) more often present with acute pulmonary edema and HT, consistent with a vascular contribution to the underlying pathophysiology [94]. Several co-morbid conditions, such as osteoarthritis and problems with mobility may act as cofounders and prevent an early detection of HF either by the patient or the physician [95]. Elderly patients are less likely to be referred to specialist care. Adherence to guidelines differ between cardiologists and General practitioners, who are less likely to use echo [15] and natriuretic peptides for diagnosis [96], key elements for diagnosis especially in the elderly where symptoms may be masked by co-morbidities such as pulmonary disease [97]. Elderly patients with acute HF are also less likely to be evaluated by a cardiologist when hospitalized [98]. Prognostic models have shown that low EF may lose its prognostic importance in elderly compared to younger and therefore the presence of HFpEF in the elderly should not be considered benign [92, 99]. Risk assessment in the elderly should also consider the importance of conditions not strictly related to cardiovascular disease which reflect greater frailty and impaired functional status [100, 101]. The risk classification in the elderly with HF improves with the inclusion of the total number of co-morbidities and conditions such as disability and dementia [95, 101]. Elderly patients are less likely to be referred to a cardiologist during hospitalization for acute HF [102], less likely to receive specialist counseling for outpatient care [96] which may prevent their enrolment in trials and registries. Many exclusion criteria in clinical trials as comorbidities common in elderly as renal dysfunction, life expectancy and cancer exclude elderly patients. Finally most trials have been focused on HFrEF and therefore elderly patients who have co-morbidities or HFpEF are more likely to fail trial screening. All these are factors explaining why elderly patients not have been included in clinical trials. Elderly patients represent the majority of those with HF and have distinct features compared with younger patients commonly included in trials. The elderly HF patient is characterized by an increased prevalence of HFpEF, with a greater burden of cardiac and non-cardiac co-morbidities. Despite elderly patients represent the majority of the HF population and have a worse prognosis compared with the younger cohort, targeted treatment strategies have been insufficiently developed for them. Present knowledge of elderly is limited by the enrolment of patients with HFrEF in most trials, with the exclusion of those with increased frailty.

Frailty, common in elderly patients, is associated with worse outcome in elderly patients with HF. According to Fried a person is considered frail if three or more of the following criteria are present, weight loss of more than 10 lbs. in 1 year, physical exhaustion by self-report, weakness as measured by grip strength, decline in walking speed, and low physical activity [103]. Based on these criteria 6.9% of older community dwelling adults are frail. This prevalence increases sharply with age, from 3.2% among persons 65–70 years old to 23.1% among persons 90 years and older. In the Cardiovascular Health study (CHS) the prevalence of HF increased from 1.8% in the non-frail to 4.6% in the intermediate group to 14% in the frail group [104]. A substudy from CHS found that frail persons have significantly higher levels of C-reactive protein, Factor VIII and D-dimers even after adjusting so there seem to be a relationship with common inflammatory, metabolic and autonomic abnormalities [105].

Frailty and multiple comorbidities are two distinct characteristics and are often coexisting and are very common in elderly patients with HF. Elderly HF patients who are frail and have multiple comorbidities are much more likely to be hospitalized, rehospitalized, become disabled, be institutionalized, and ultimately die [106].

Summary: HF in the elderly will continue to be an increasing health burden as this population represents the majority of HF patients and demonstrates worse outcomes compared with younger. Sparse evidence exists for disease management in these patients due to i.e. underrepresentation in clinical trials and less frequent referral to specialist attention. Elderly patients with HF commonly have a complex profile characterized by multiple co-morbidities, and treatment with a number of drugs (polypharmacy), requiring a targeted and multidisciplinary approach, which usually do not exist. In order to improve the prognosis as well as resource allocation in the elderly HF population, distinct strategies for assessment, care, therapy, risk stratification, education and follow-up should be developed for this population [94]. Moreover frailty together with multiple comorbidities, common in these elderly HF patients are associated with an even more worsened prognosis.

1.6.2 Gender Differences

Most of the literature has demonstrated that women are at increased risk of HF complicating acute MI. However as more men than women have acute MI the absolute number of patients with HF complicating an acute MI may still be greater in men. However in the National Registry of acute MI including more than 600,000 cases from 1994 to 2000 women were more likely than men to have HF at the time of acute MI presentation or complicating their MI hospitalization. In total 48% of those developing HF were women compared with 36% of those without HF [107]. In the global registry of acute coronary events (GRACE) among patients admitted with acute MI, women were more likely to present with or develop HF during the hospitalization [108]. However a study from Canada examining acute MI patients found that women were less likely than men to develop HF during hospitalization for acute MI [109]. Sex differences in remodeling may contribute to an increased risk of cardiogenic shock and HF complicating MI in women versus men. Since women had been underrepresented in clinical trials the Metaanalysis of MAGGIC [73], putting together data from 31 studies (33% women), found that women were older, more frequently had HFpEF and after 3 years follow-up with adjustment for confounders such as age and EF, men were at increased risk of death not women. The sex difference was not specific to those with HFrEF, men with HFpEF did also worse than women. The survival benefit was slightly more marked in patients with a non-ischemic etiology for their HF but is attenuated by concomitant DM [110].

While women may have a survival advantage after HF diagnosis they experience increased morbidity. Women with HF experience worse quality of life (QoL) [111] and are more likely to develop depression [112]. It appears also that NYHA class correlates with the incidence of depression or anxiety only in women and not in men [113]. Moreover some of the high risk of hospitalization in women with HF seems to be mediated by the older age of women with HF, and after adjustment it was found that women were at a similar risk or even lower risk than men for hospitalization after HF diagnosis.

Women develop ischemic heart disease at an older age, have less atherosclerotic burden when presenting with acute coronary syndrome (ACS). The female heart is rather protected from apoptosis in response to acute coronary ischemia, and remodels differently, with a tendency to maintain normal LV size and preserved EF, probably related to the occurrence of sex hormones, estrogens and testosterone [114]. HT is a higher risk factor for women than men, who are more likely to suffer from CAD.

1.6.3 Ethnic Differences

Are there any racial or ethnic differences between patients with HF? In order to study this a cohort study (MESA) of 6814 individuals of 4 ethnicities were performed. The study included white patients (38.5%), African Americans (27.8%), Hispanic (21.9%) and finally Chinese American (11.8%). African Americans were find to have the highest risk for developing HF and also the highest proportion of incident HF not preceded by clinical MI. The higher risk of incident HF among African Americans was related to differences in the prevalence of HT and DM as well as socioeconomic status. The mechanisms of HF also differed by ethnicity; interim MI had the least influence among African Americans, and LV mass increase had the greatest effect among Hispanic and white participants [115]. In the ARIC study it was found that HF in non-hispanic black males and females had a prevalence of 4.5% and 3.8% respectively versus 2.7% and 1.8% in non-hispanic white males and females and a higher 5-year mortality than whites [116]. One study investigating elderly people in Memphis and Pittsburg (mean age 74 years) found an incidence rate in African Americans of 1.6% and in white 1.2. More of modifiable risk factors attributed to HF were found in the black participants as smoking, uncontrolled blood pressure to mention the most accessible [117]. From these studies we can see that there are ethnic differences and the highest risk to develop HF seems to be in African Americans and this is not related to CAD but instead HT and DM and poorer socioeconomic status. Lower socioeconomic status may contribute to delaying in seeking care for symptoms associated with heart failure and also contribute to poor adherence to diet and medication recommendations. In studies it was also found that African Americans rarely had a cardiologist as their responsible physician [118]. Based on these different observations it looks like that better blood pressure control with good compliance as well as stop smoking in these patients may decrease the development of HF.

1.7 Etiology of Heart Failure Related to Coronary Artery Disease and Acute Heart Failure

The classical causes of HF include CAD and HT as the most common. However non-ischemic dilated cardiomyopathy and arrhythmias are also important but less frequently occurring. Many times it is difficult for the clinician to decide what is the primary cause of HF since many patients may have co-existing diseases as long-standing HT, previous MI and atrial arrhythmias, which may contribute to the development of HF. To confirm that CAD is the primary cause of HF a MI must have occurred or a coronary angiography evidenced that, otherwise it is not confirmed.

1.7.1 Coronary Artery Disease

Along with HT, CAD is responsible for the largest proportion of the 770,000 newly diagnosed cases of HF in the U.S. In Olmsted County HT and CAD were equally responsible for the highest proportion of new cases though HT played a greater role in women and CAD in men [119]. Despite advances in the treatment of acute MI, HF following an acute MI remains frequent. After a MI initially protective compensatory mechanisms are activated as activation of the sympathetic nervous system (causing an increase in heart rate and cardiac output) and the RAAS (increasing circulatory volume and maintaining preload). Chronic activation of these compensatory systems may lead to development of HF. Long-term activation of the sympathetic nervous system promotes myocyte hypertrophy and interstitial fibrosis and long-term activation of the RAAS system may lead to increased development of myocardial fibrosis due to collagen deposition and also apoptosis and a necrosis of myocytes [120]. Thus the initial protective compensatory mechanisms may lead to altered cardiac structure and function and then to ventricular dilatation, increased preload and finally HF.

Acute HF may also be caused by an acute MI having acute complications as acute mitral regurgitation (MR) due to papillary muscle rupture, ventricular septal rupture, a rupture to the free ventricular wall or development of cardiogenic shock. Other more transient acute complications are stunning (following an ischemic episode) or hibernation (failed normal contraction without any structured alteration of the cardiomyocytes). Both conditions remain during a short period of time and may return to normal when appropriately treated [121].

1.7.2 Acute Heart Failure

Acute HF or acute decompensated HF (ADHF) are the terms used to describe the rapid onset of, or acute worsening of symptoms and signs of HF associated with elevated plasma levels of natriuretic peptides. It is a life-threatening condition that requires immediate medical attention and usually leads to urgent hospital admission. ADHF increases in prevalence and is associated with substantial mortality and morbidity. The clinical presentation of ADHF ranges from moderate volume overload to overt cardiogenic shock. The great majority of the patients have congestion, some present with low perfusion and low cardiac output with or without congestion. Patients can be classified as wet (congested) or cold (low output). Most of the patients (80%) [122] have a worsening of a chronic HF, either HFrEF or HFpEF and about 15% have new onset HF (de novo) [123].

Differential diagnosis of ADHF includes ACS, exacerbation of chronic obstructive pulmonary disease, pneumonia, acute renal failure, and pulmonary embolism. There is always some precipitating factor or trigger in a patient with an ADHF (e.g. an arrhythmia – atrial fibrillation in a patient with a stiff heart and HFpEF resulting in loss of sinus rhythm and development of an acute pulmonary edema or discontinuation of diuretic therapy in a patient with HFrEF with volume overload or a severe HT in patients with HFpEF). The acuteness may vary, many patients are describing it from period of days or weeks of deterioration (increasing shortness of breath or edema) but others are developing HF within hours to minutes, e.g. in association with an acute MI with a spectrum of conditions ranging from life-threatening pulmonary edema or cardiogenic shock to a condition, characterized, predominantly by worsening peripheral edema.

ACS is an important cause of worsening or new-onset HF. Although acute ST elevation MI can be readily apparent on an electrocardiography (ECG) other cases of ACS may be more challenging to diagnose. Complicating the clinical picture is that many patients with ADHF with or without CAD have serum troponin levels that are elevated [124]. In a patient

Table 1.3 Factors triggering acute heart failure

Acute coronary syndrome.
Tachyarrhythmia (e.g. atrial fibrillation, ventricular tachycardia).
Excessive rise in blood pressure.
Infection (e.g. pneumonia, infective endocarditis, sepsis).
Non-adherence with salt/fluid intake or medications.
Bradyarrhythmia.
Toxic substances (alcohol, recreational drugs).
Drugs (e.g. NSAIDs. corticosteroids, negative inotropic substances, cardiotoxic chemotherapeutics).
Exacerbation of chronic obstructive pulmonary disease.
Pulmonary embolism.
Surgery and perioperative complications.
Increased sympathetic drive, stress-related cardiomyopathy.
Metabolic/hormonal derangements (e.g. thyroid dysfunction, diabetic ketosis, adrenal dysfunction, pregnancy and peripartum related abnormalities).
Cerebrovascular insult.
Acute mechanical cause: myocardial rupture complicating ACS (free wall rupture, ventricular septal defect, acute mitral regurgitation), chest trauma or cardiac intervention, acute native or prosthetic valve incompetence secondary to endocarditis, aortic dissection or thrombosis.

ACS acute coronary syndromes, *NSAIDs* non-steroidal anti-inflammatory drugs with a new-onset HF the possibility that CAD is an underlying cause of HF should always be considered [125]. Common factors triggering ADHF are shown in Table 1.3 [4].

1.8 Etiology of Heart Failure Related to Cardiomyopathies

Heart failure is frequently accompanied by cardiomyopathy (CM), defined as a morphologically abnormal heart. Echocardiography provides us with information about chamber dimensions and function and magnetic resonance imaging provides as with visualization of myocardial tissue composition. Major forms of CM are hypertrophic, dilated, restrictive and arrhythmogenic CMs. Each of these forms of CMs has a major heritable component and genetic testing is used in their evaluation [126]. More than 20 genes are implicated in hypertrophic CM (HCM), while fewer genes are linked to arrhythmogenic right ventricular CM (ARVC). Dilated CM (DCM) is the most genetically heterogenous with mutations encoding cytoskeletal, nucleoskeletal, mitochondrial, and calcium handling proteins. The large number of genes responsible for CM, as well as the great number of mutations within each of these genes, produces remarkable heterogeneity for this complex disorder. Genetic variation remains a strong predictor of risk for developing CM, particularly within families where a primary gene mutation has been identified.

Since a lot of terms are used when describing genetics in CMs I will try to give some overview below. Genetic variants occurring with a frequency more than 1% are called polymorphisms and those below are called mutations. Mostly we use something we call Mendelian inheritance that means that we can assess relatives at risk for a familial disease by directly testing other family members. We also use the term autosomal dominant inheritance. That means that a gene located on one of the 22 chromosomes is defined as autosomal and it is called dominant if only one altered copy of the two is needed to induce the disease. We also use the terms penetrance and that means if completed there is a high chance for each individual, which inherit a mutation to also have a manifest disease. Mostly we have reduced penetrance or incompleted instead. We also talk about variable expressivity that means that both genetic and environmental factors are involved. We also have the term autosomal recessive inheritance meaning that a single working copy of a gene is sufficient for full normal function. Finally we have the expression X-linked inheritance meaning that genetic disorders linked to genes on the X-chromosome have unique characteristics. An X-linked recessive disorder is only manifest in men and women and are thus carriers [127].

1.8.1 Hypertrophic Cardiomyopathy

HCM is characterized by a myocardial hypertrophy in the absence of clinically important loading conditions or primary valve diseases. HCM is a primary disease of the myocardium in which a portion of the myocardium is hypertrophied (thickened) without any cause limiting the cardiac output through impaired filling and outflow (Fig. 1.2). In HCM the myocytes in the heart increase in size resulting in thickening. In addition the normal alignment of the cells is disrupted (myocardial disarray) as well as there are also disruptions of the electrical functions of the heart. Moreover

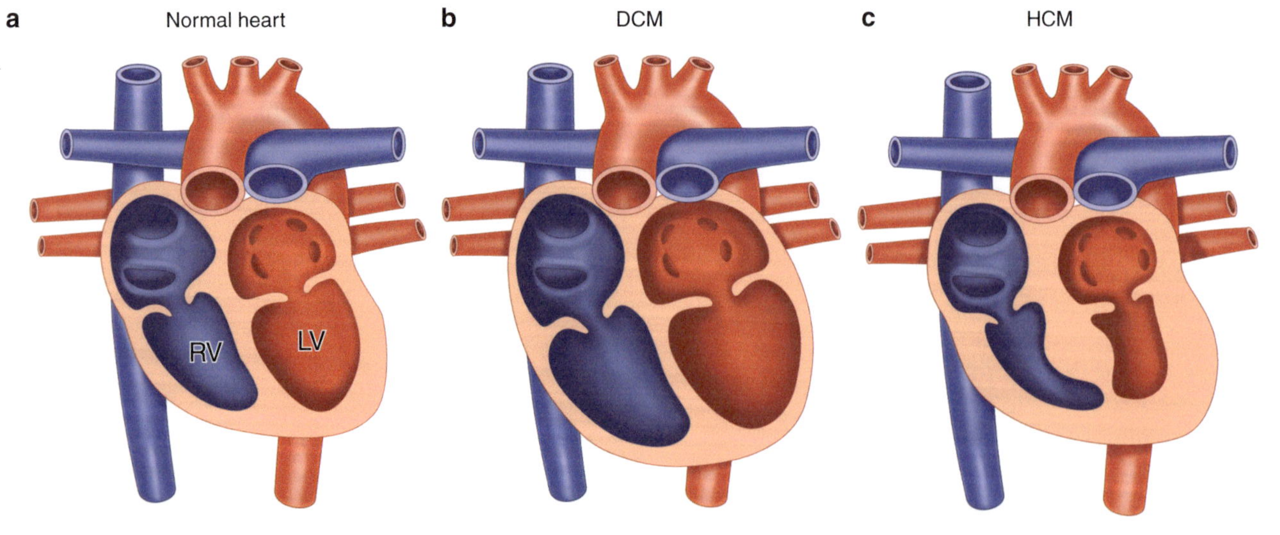

Fig. 1.2 Morphological changes to the heart in cardiomyopathy. (**a**) Normal heart. (**b**) In DCM, the heart enlarges with increased diameter and reduced function. (**c**) In HCM, the myocardium – especially in the LV – becomes thickened, leading to impaired filling and emptying

there are interstitial and replacement fibrosis and medial hypertrophy of intramyocardial small vessels [128, 129]. Familial forms of HCM exhibit an autosomal dominant inheritance pattern. Most mutations are found in sarcomeric protein genes [130].

Diagnosis relies on detection of ECG evidence of LV hypertrophy confirmed by echocardiography or CMR. Screening for HCM is usually recommended for families with imaging tests (echocardiography or CMR) and electrocardiography (ECG). Starting in adolescence the time usually HCM is detected, continued annually up to adult age 18–20 years and thereafter every fifth year. All HCM patients and relatives should have access to genetic counseling. Clinical diagnosis of HCM requires confirmation with cardiac imaging of phenotypic expression, meaning an unexplained increase in LV wall thickness (>15 mm in adults) associated with a non-dilated left ventricular chamber. Wall thickness of 13–14 mm may be diagnostic for HCM especially in family members [131]. Recently CMR has emerged as a complimentary tool, since it provide us with better characterization of the HCM phenotype, more précised LV wall thickness measurements and improved risk stratification by imaging myocardial scars. Thus CMR provide us with a more complete interrogation of HCM morphology, including right ventricular (RV) hypertrophy, differentiation of apical hypertrophy vs LV non-compaction and more. Maximal wall thickening can be found at any location but most frequent at the confluence of the anterior septum and contiguous anterior free wall [132, 133].

Many patients with HCM are having mild symptoms or are asymptomatic and their survival is not effected by the disease. Clinically, HCM is often characterized by a hyperdynamic state in which there is an increase in LVEF from 60% to 70% or more. Absence of hyperdynamic systolic function, systolic anterior motion of the mitral valve (SAM), or myocardial scarring on CMR does not exclude a HCM diagnosis. The most common symptoms of HCM is dyspnea (due to stiffening and decreased cardiac output, which may lead to increased filling pressures and congestion), exertional chest pain (due to reduced blood to the coronary arteries), palpitations and arrhythmias (due to disruption of electrical functions), a sense of fainting, syncope and most serious SCD. Clinical concerns include development of dynamic obstruction of the LV outflow tract (usually due to SAM), occurrence of arrhythmias, atrial or ventricular, development of stroke or SCD (the risk about 1% per years for adults), and progression to a HF of type HFrEF or HFpEF (2–5%). Major risk factors for SCD are prior history of ventricular arrhythmias or cardiac arrest, prior unexplained syncope, and family history of sudden death.

The prevalence is estimated to be in the range of 0.02–0.23% in adults and it is known to occur in a variety of races and ethnic groups and with a generally similar clinical, phenotypic, and genetic expression. Most studies have reported that HCM is a little more common in males [130, 134, 135]. HCM is inherited with an autosomal dominant Mendelian pattern, variable expressivity, and age related penetrance. A number of studies have concluded that HCM is caused by mutations in 11 or more genes encoding thick and thin contractile myofilament protein components of the sarcomere or adjacent Z.-disc, which are expressed in the heart (Fig. 1.3) [136, 137]. About 70–80% of successfully genotyped patients are found to have mutations in the two most common genes, beta-myosin heavy chain and myosin-binding protein C. These genes encode the sarcomere thick filament proteins-myosin heavy chain (MYH7 about 40%) and cardiac myosin binding protein -C (cMyBP-C about 40%). The second major thick filament protein implicated in HCM is MYBPC3, which encodes cardiac myosin binding protein (cMyBP-C). HCM has a vast genetic heterogeneity limiting the role of mutational analysis in predicting prognosis for individual patients (>1500 individual mutations). Studies have shown that genetic testing cannot predict outcome in individual patients or divide patients into high (benefitting from ICD implantation) or low risk patients, and are therefore not reliable. The only reason to use genetic testing is to identify family members at risk to develop HCM but with ECG evidence of left ventricular hypertrophy. However the likelihood to find a pathogenic mutation in the proband is only 35%, if occurrence of a positive family history a little higher [136]. Genetic testing may clarify diagnosis in some patients with metabolic storage diseases (PRKAG2 (mutations in the genes encoding the gamma-2 regulatory subunit of AMP activated protein kinase), Fabry's disease, LAMP2 cardiomyopathy (Danon disease, mutations in the genes encoding the lysosome associated membrane protein 2), which differ from sarcomeric HCM by different pathophysiology, natural history and management but share similar clinical expression and the pattern of LVH. LAMP 2 needs early recognition since it is a lethal disease, survival exceeding the age of 25 is rare, demanding transplantation [138, 139]. Other glycogen storage diseases presenting with an idiopathic hypertrophy and difficult to distinguish on a clinical base alone are Pompes disease and Noonan's syndrome as well as the protein deposition disease (amyloidosis). Most of these phenocopies are seen in a sizeable minority [139, 140].

Subgroups of patients have shown to be at high risk for dying suddenly, developing progressive HF with dyspnea and functional limitations (with or without chest pain) or developing paroxysmal or chronic AF. By using contemporary and aggressive treatment interventions (ICD implant and cardiac transplantation) the death rate has decreased to 0.5% per year. SCD events are more common in younger patients (<30 years of age) and rare in elderly patients [141]. HCM is the most common cause of SCD in young, including

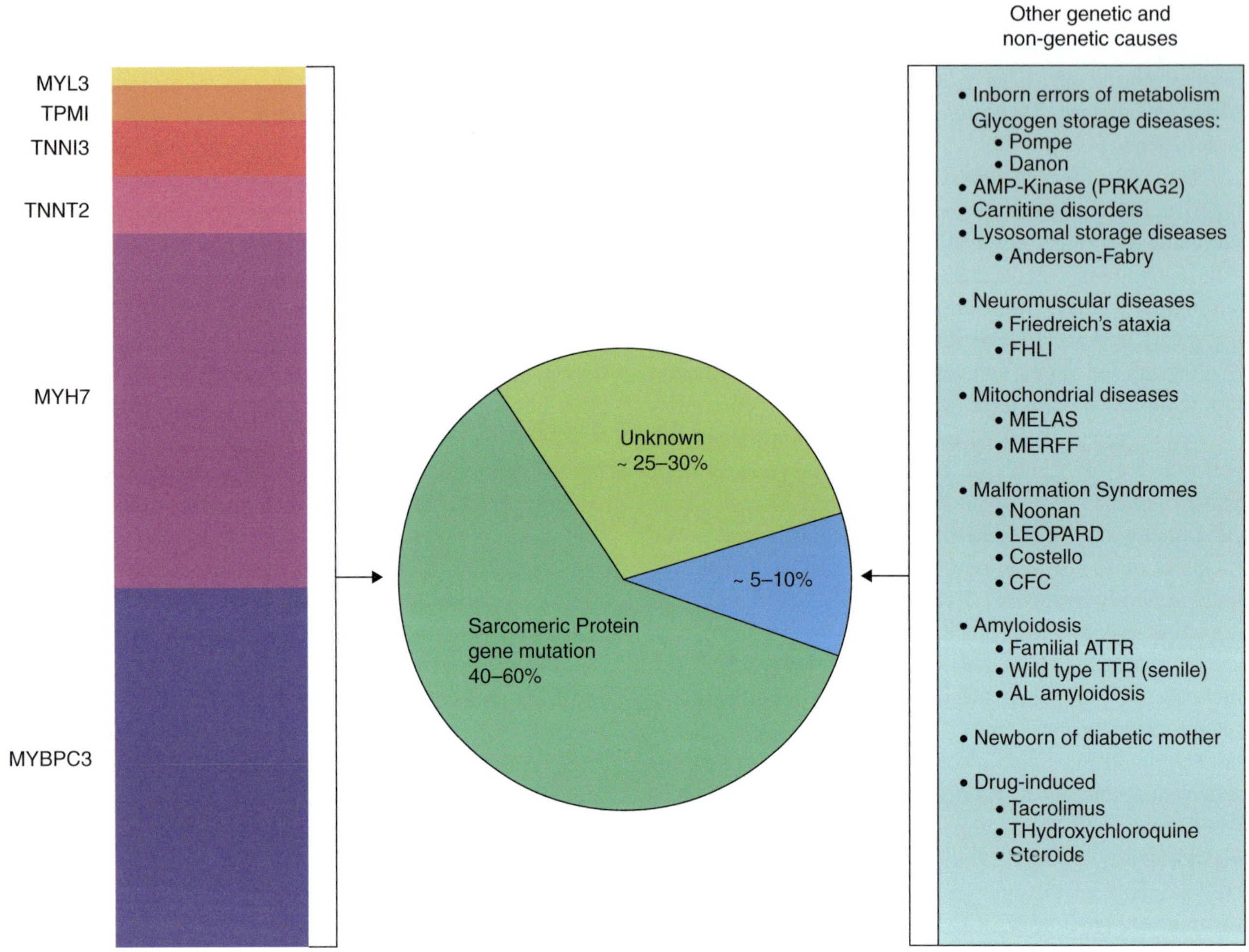

Fig. 1.3 Diverse aetiology of hypertrophic cardiomyopathy. The majority of cases in adolescents and adults are caused by mutations in sarcomere protein gene. AL amyloid light chain; ATTR amyloidosis, transthyretin type; CFC Cardiofaciocutaneous; FHL-I Four and a half LIM domains protein l; LEOPARD lentigines, *ECG* abnormalities, ocular hypertelorism, pulmonary stenosis, abnormal genitalia, retardation of growth and sensorineural deafness; MELAS mitochondrial encephalomyopathy, lactic acidosis, and stroke-like episodes; MERFF myoclonic epilepsy with ragged red fibres; MYL3 myosin light chain 3; MYBPC3 myosin-binding protein C. cardiac-type; MYH7 myosin heavy chain 7; TNNI3 troponin I, cardiac; TNNT2 troponin T, cardiac; TPMI tropomyosin I alpha chain, TTR transthyretin

competitive athletes. One third of athletic field deaths in U.S. are due to HCM (15/year) occurring predominantly in men without previous suspicion of disease and most commonly in African Americans [142, 143]. Recently it was reported promising long-term mortality results from a cohort of young HCM patients, age between 7 and 29 years, when high-risk patients were reliable identified and had an implantation of an ICD [144]. SCD is presumed to be caused by a ventricular tachycardia or ventricular fibrillation, frequently occurring during intense physical activity [145]. Targeting candidates for prophylactic ICD therapy is not easy. Marked degree of LV hypertrophy or syncope is a strong marker. Other markers are intraventricular apical aneurysms with regional scarring or end-stage LV systolic dysfunction. Marked LV outflow obstruction at rest or diffuse LV wall thickness approaching 30 mm can serve as grey zone modifiers [146, 147]. Engagement in intense competitive sports is a modifiable marker. Absence of all risk factors does not convey immunity to SCD [148]. New marker is the substrate of presumed myocardial fibrosis found in CMR by late gadolinium enhancement (LGE). Extensive LGE is a marker of SCD risk and identify patients who will develop adverse LV remodeling and progress to the end-stage with LV systolic dysfunction [131]. Therefore CMR has emerged as a powerful addition to the HCM armamentarium.

Some degree of HF occurs in approximately 50% of HCM patients, expressed clinically as exertional dyspnea in the presence of preserved systolic function. Rarely there are symptoms as chest pain likely related to some extent of microvascular ischemia [149]. The most important cause of limiting HF symptoms is mechanical impedance to LV outflow, usually due to SAM with gradients of ≥30 mm Hg, an independent determinant of progressive HF symptoms and HF or stroke death. For patients without obstruction at rest, exercise echocardiography is the best method to provoke outflow gradients (≥30 mm) identifying patients at greater risk for future symptomatic progression and thereby the possibility of septal reduction intervention [150]. One third of HCM patients have the non-obstructive form of HF without obstruction. Most of them have stable clinical course and only a minority progress to HF with symptom limiting HF symptoms predominantly due to diastolic dysfunction [141]. The most advanced form of HF within the HCM spectrum is the end-stage (or burned out) phase occurring in a subset of patients with non-obstructive HCM (prevalence 3%). HF progression is associated with conversion to systolic dysfunction (EF < 50%) and adverse LV remodeling with extensive myocardial scarring, often resulting in regression of hypertrophy and/or cavity enlargement. Initial treatments are diuretics, beta-blockers and afterload reducing agents as well as prophylactic ICD. In some patients there are a rapid progression of symptoms leading to cardiac transplantation. The only known predictor in those patients is a family history. A small subset of patients with non-obstructive HCM with preserved systolic function develops refractory HF symptoms due to diastolic dysfunction and can also be candidates for cardiac transplantation [151, 152].

There is no evidence that drugs such as beta-blockers or verapamil prevent SCD in HCM. The ICD is the only way to prolong life in HCM by interrupt life-threatening ventricular arrhythmias and prevent SCD. In HCM the ICD is effective despite substantial LV hypertrophy, outflow obstruction, diastolic dysfunction [153, 154]. The successful treatment with ICD comes from a multicenter registry of >500 HCM patients, terminating ventricular fibrillation/ventricular tachycardia was 4%/year for primary prevention and 11%/year for secondary prevention after cardiac arrest and similar results have been found in Europe [155, 156]. Single-chambers ICD most appropriate in younger ages and dual chamber ICDs are reserved for those with paroxysmal AF and/or LV outflow obstruction [157]. The importance of device-related complications (5%/year), including inappropriate shocks, lead defects and psychosocial consequences cannot be underestimated in HCM [154, 158] particularly with implantations in early life. However, in the near future new drugs as myocardial metabolic modulators, late sodium current inhibitors and allosteric myosin inhibitors are coming to the market since they have shown very promising beneficial effects in preclinical research, and human studies are soon going to be started [159].

In patients with HF and obstructive outflow beta-adrenergic blockers together with disopyramide are the most reliable drugs for reducing outflow gradients at risk especially disopyramide. However during long-term use there is a risk of developing parasympathetic side-effects [160, 161]. Surgical septal myectomy is the preferred treatment for patients with advanced limiting HF symptoms due to outflow gradients of ≥50 mm at rest or during provocation in patients refractory to medical treatment. Surgical myectomy reverses HF symptoms by permanently abolishing obstruction, restoring normal LV pressures and reducing or abolishing MR, and with an operative mortality less than 1% [162]. Percutaneous alcohol septal ablation (ASA) is an alternative method, factors influencing the decision is advanced age, significant comorbidity increasing surgical risk and strong desire of patients to avoid surgery [128]. ASA reduces LV outflow gradient by creating a large basal ventricular septal infarction (10% of the left ventricular wall, 30% of the septum) by infusion of absolute alcohol into a major septal perforator coronary artery [163]. Short-term mortality has been shown to be low and similar as surgery. Surgery, however, are providing better symptom relief and gradient improvement in younger patients [164]. In contrast ASA is associated with permanent pacemaker in 10–15% of the cases due to complete heart block and repeat procedures due to persistent obstruction in 12% of the patients. There is also an incompletely defined risk for life threatening arrhythmias and SCD due to the potentially arrhythmogenic septal scar [165, 166]. Recently promising long-term results from 1275 patients undergoing ASA was published. This large registry study (The Euro-ASA study) show durable relief of symptoms and LV outflow tract obstruction. The study had a follow-up up to 10 years and at the end 89% reported dyspnea less than NYHA class II [167].

AF is a very common arrhythmia in HCM patients [168, 169]. AF is linked to increasing age, greater left atrial volume/or impaired left atrial EF. AF is common in patients with HCM and systolic dysfunction and advanced HF. Infrequent AF episodes may be reversed by electrical or pharmacologically cardioversion. Low-dose amiodarone is the most effective agent. To prevent stroke in those patients anticoagulant treatment is recommended with newer oral agents NOAC or warfarin. Risk for thromboembolic stroke is 0.8%/year. When QoL is significantly affected, catheter-based ablation (radiofrequency or cryoablation) have shown promising results [170, 171].

1.8.2 Dilated Cardiomyopathy

DCM is characterized by the presence of LV or biventricular dilatation and systolic dysfunction, when occurring in the absence of an identifiable cause of the disease, as abnormal loading conditions (HT and valve disease) or CAD of enough severity to cause a global systolic depression of hemodynamic importance, and is then referred to as an idiopathic dilated CM (Fig. 1.2). Long-term serial evaluations suggest that DCM is an insidious, slowly progressive inflammatory disease that is familial in the majority of the patients [172, 173] and therefore the causes of DCM can be classified as genetic or nongenetic [4]. Recently there was a proposal from the ESC (European Society of Cardiology) working group on myocardial and pericardial diseases for a revised definition of DCM. They proposed to include in the definition also a group called hypokinetic non-dilated CM (HNDC), patients with LV or biventricular global systolic dysfunction without dilatation (defined as EF < 45%), not explained by abnormal loading conditions or CAD. The reason for this is that many genetic diseases may have delayed or incomplete cardiac expression, with mild symptoms despite the presence of a clinically significant myocardial disease on CMR and sometimes verified by an endomyocardial biopsy (EMB) [174, 175].

Different etiologies can lead to DCM including inherited, infectious and inflammatory diseases. However the majority of cases remain unexplained after a thorough review for secondary cause. Recent studies have suggested that up to 40% of DCM may be inherited [176]. Clinical manifestations can vary tremendously, even within individual families, where a proportion develop end-stage HF as infants while others may survive to the seventh decade with mild subclinical DCM. Most patients are unaware of the diagnosis until HF symptoms or arrhythmia develops or abnormalities are detected during routine evaluation.

Myocardial ischemia remains a common cause of DCM, accounting for approximately half of DCM. Toxic, metabolic and immunologic causes have been linked to DCM, as well as HT and valvular disease. Genetic CM which runs in families, are now more commonly diagnosed. Non-ischemic DCM defined as DCM not from myocardial ischemia or infarct is familial in 25–50% of cases, with estimates that vary based how family members were screened [177]. Familial DCM refers to DCM that is inherited as a single gene disorder in a Mendelian pattern. The primary mode of inheritance for familial DCM is autosomal dominant, with reduced penetrance and variability expressivity but some families also present by an autosomal recessive or X-linked recessive trait. Mitochondrial mutations also contribute to DCM with the expected matrilinear inheritance. At least 50 single genes have been identified as linked to familial DCM and the majority of these elicit disease as dominant mutations. Because mutations in many individual single genes lead to DCM, genetic testing commonly employs multi-genes panels, in which more than 50 genes can be tested simultaneously.

DCM is far more genetically heterogenous than HCM, with mutations in genes encoding cytoskeletal, nucleoskeletal, mitochondrial and calcium handling proteins. Dominant mutations are found in the genes encoding sarcomere proteins (beta myosin heavy chain encoded by MYH7 and myosin binding protein C encoded by MYBPC3 and the giant protein titin encoded by TTN, the later responsible for 25% of DCM) [174, 178]. A comprehensive review of confirmed and putative disease genes has been described [179]. Studies suggest that mutations in sarcomeric genes, including TTN, TNNT2 (cardiac troponin T), MYH7 (myosin heavy chain), and TPMI (alfa-tropomyosin) are the most common reported together with mutations in lamin A/C, accounting for about 20–30% of the cases [178]. Familial DCM with conduction disease secondary to disruption in the nuclear cytoskeleton by mutations in lamin A/C (LMNA) deserves special attention. Nuclear lamins A and C are highly conserved proteins critical in nuclear cytoskeletal integrity. In those affected by LMNA associated CM, conduction disease can precede development of DCM in some families, while in others DCM comes first. The practical significance of this is that individuals who may have mild DCM caused by LMNA may be at risk for SCD, while this scenario is highly unlikely in most sarcomere and all cytoskeletal abnormalities. Therefore when SCD is seen in a family with mild DCM, testing for LMNA mutations may be helpful and lead to early consideration for ICD therapy. Highly competitive sports should be discouraged in patients with LMNA mutations. Reports of increased arrythmogenicity in desmosomal associated DCM indicate that a similar approach may be taken when these mutations are identified [180]. With the advent of high-throughput low-cost sequencing technologies, analysis of many more genes, including large genes as titin encoded by TTN, it has been possible to suggest that mutations in TTN are frequent in DCM, although it remains to be confirmed that truncating mutations in TTN are always pathogenic [181]. There are also studies reporting that more than one gene has potentially causative mutations in patients with DCM [182].

HF, SCD or thromboembolism may be the presenting manifestation of DCM. TTN associated DCM typically does not present until adulthood [177], but mutations in the sarcomere genes can present at any age. The identification of LV chamber dilation and systolic dysfunction with echocardiography is diagnostic of DCM and can allow consideration of secondary causes (e.g. regional wall motion abnormalities in CAD). CMR provides accurate measurement of ventricular chamber size, wall thickness and systolic function. Clinical benefit has been associated with treatment with ACEi, Angiotensin II receptor antagonists, beta receptor blockers and aldosterone antagonists (MRA) in different studies [79, 183, 184]. The prevention of SCD is a primary concern in patients with inherited CMs [185]. ICD therapy can offer incremental prevention of SCD and is advised in selected patients [186]. The indication for primary prevention of SCD with ICD therapy in DCM is largely based on the severity of systolic dysfunction. Consensus guidelines recommend primary prevention ICD placement in patients who have severe systolic dysfunction (EF ≤ 35%), are receiving optimal medical treatment and have reasonable 1 year survival. Recommendations are strongest in those with symptomatic DCM HF (NYHA class II-III) and those with haemodynamically not tolerable ventricular arrhythmias. They also suggest ICD placement for patients with DCM and a confirmed disease-causing MNA mutation and clinical risk factors

[187]. However, guidelines do not advise the use of genetic testing for SCD risk stratification in patients with DCM. Recognition that a patient has a familial disease or genetic CM is accompanied with the responsibility to consider the risk of disease in the patient's family. Prior to offering predictive genetic testing to clinically unaffected family members, the risks of genetic testing should be explained, including implications for the procurement of life insurance. Family members should also be counseled to the limitations of genetic testing and the possibility that current interpretations of variant pathogenicity are subject to change which could lead to reassessment of their risk. Genetically counseling is a recommended component of the management of families with DCM [179].

From a clinical perspective, careful phenotypic evaluation of patients and their families is crucial for correct interpretation of genetic results. With improved DNA sequencing, it is now possible to identify combinations of gene mutations that contribute to CM. A better understanding of the molecular subtypes of CM will help more precisely apply existing and evolving therapies. The use of clinical testing in clinical practice has begun, however the cost of sequencing and relative insensitivity of clinical assays has limited widespread acceptance.

Familial DCM is an important cause of HF and SCD. An important minority of patients with familial DCM will present with associated clinical features, including conduction disease, arrhythmia and skeletal myopathy. When there is a strong family history of important ventricular arrhythmias, heart block or SCD, early prophylactic ICD implantation for genotype-positive relatives even in the presence of mild or no phenotype is recommended.

How prevalent is DCM? In studies it has been estimated to occur in 1 in 2500 adults and be more common in men than in women, and the annual incidence rate is about 7–8/100,000 individuals [187]. Although the overall prognosis in patients with symptomatic HF and DCM is relatively poor, with 25% mortality at 1 year and 50% mortality at 5 years about 25% of DCM patients with recent onset of HF have a relatively benign clinical course with spontaneously improvement in symptoms and partial or in some cases complete recovery of LV function [188]. Three major etiologies of DCM are associated with spontaneous recovery of LV function and reverse LV remodeling, including abnormal energetics, toxic insults and inflammation.

1.8.2.1 Abnormal Energetics

In patients without structural heart disease atrial and less commonly ventricular tachyarrythmias may be the primary cause of a tachycardia-induced cardiomyopathy (TIC). The degree of dysfunction is connected to the duration and rate of the arrhythmia. AF with rapid ventricular response and atrial tachycardia are the most common causes of TIC. With TIC effective antiarrythmic treatment with rate control not necessary maintenance of sinus rhythm, cardioversion and/or radiofrequency ablation can result in improvement and often, but not always full recovery of LV function [189].

Stress cardiomyopathy also called takotsubo CM (first described in Japan) or apical ballooning syndrome is an acute cardiac syndrome characterized by transient apical and mid ventricular wall motion abnormality, electrocardiographic changes that mimic acute MI, and modest cardiac enzyme release in the absence of obstructive CAD [190, 191]. Postmenopausal women between the ages of 60 and 80, who suffer an acute emotional or physical stress, account for the majority of cases. Practically all recover fully although recurrence rates has been reported (5–10%) [192]. The predominant underlying mechanism appears to be acute sympathetic activation leading to "metabolic" myocardial stunning, which argues in favor of comprehensive adrenergic blockade and helps to explain the reversible nature of the LV injury [193]. However recent studies demonstrate that physical triggers are also important and also that takotsubo syndrome may occur without an evident trigger [192, 194]. However still the pathophysiological mechanism behind is unclear and primarily is based on assumptions [195]. Recently an observational study from Sweden concluded that takotsubo CM is a serious condition and affects long-term prognosis [196]. There is also controversy about how good it is to treat patients with beta blockers [194]. In conclusion prospective studies are needed to find out more about this type of CM.

1.8.2.2 Toxins

Alcoholic CM is often overlooked and is in studies suggested to account for 21–32% of DCM [197]. Alcohol causes LV systolic dysfunction in a dose-related manner. Interesting is that alcohol has also been shown to have protective effects on CAD, but is also a known cardiotoxin associated with arrhythmias, HF and LV dysfunction [198]. Alcoholic CM is a complication of long-standing alcohol abuse and related to a patient's total lifetime dose of ethanol. The clinical diagnosis must be suspected in heavy drinkers presenting with LV systolic dysfunction and dilatation, most commonly in middle-aged men being heavy consumers during a number of years. Not so frequent in women (14%) but much more vulnerable despite lower life-time dosages [199, 200]. Frequent co-morbidities include atrial arrhythmias, HT, malnutrition and cirrhosis. In developed countries, up to one third of chronic alcoholics have asymptomatic LV dysfunction [201]. During the course of cardiac remodeling, reduced EF is often preceded by LV dilation, an increase in LV mass and diastolic dysfunction [202]. The risk is increased with consumptions of about 7–8 standard drinks (about 90 g of alcohol) each day during long time. Abstinence can result in full recovery of LV function. Patients who continue to drink heavily demonstrate either no change in EF or further reduction associated with excess cardiac mortality. A minority of patients, who abstain from drinking have no improvement in EF. The understanding behind this CM is not known but there appears to be individual susceptibility that relates to genetic and non-genetic mechanisms.

Trastuzumab related cardiotoxicity. Trastuzumab is a monoclonal antibody that selectively target epidermal growth factor receptor 2 (HER2). For patients with early stage breast cancer that overexpresses HER2, trastuzumab significantly increases response rates and disease-free and overall survival. Cardiotoxicity has been reported in up to 7% of patients treated with trastuzumab alone and is increased to 27% when trastuzumab is combined with an anthracycline. Unlike anthracycline-induced CM, the cardiotoxicity of trastuzumab occurs rapidly and is potentially reversible [203]. The absence of ultrastructural changes on EMB, typically seen with anthracycline, may explain the reversibility of trastuzumab cardiotoxicity [204].

1.8.2.3 Inflammation

Inflammation of the heart may cause HF in about 10% of patients with CM and myocarditis is a recognized cause of DCM [205]. However due to the many different clinical presentations and the lack of performed EMB:s, the gold standard for diagnosis, it is hard to estimate how frequent myocarditis is. Myocarditis is usually defined as an inflammation of the heart muscle as a result of exposure to either external antigens (such as viruses, bacteria, parasites, toxins or drugs) or internal triggers such as autoimmune activation against self-antigens. Although viral infection remains the most commonly identified cause of myocarditis, drug hypersensitivity and toxic drug reactions, and other infections, can also lead to myocarditis. Most common occurring are viral infections with enterovirus, adenovirus, influenza virus, herpes virus, Ebstein-Barr virus, cytomegalovirus and parvovirus B19. Lymphocytic and giant cell myocarditis has been found to be idiopathic or autoimmune if no virus are found [206]. Clinically myocarditis may present with a variety of symptoms of different severity. From very mild symptoms with a prodromal viral illness with fever, myalgia, fatigue and respiratory or gastrointestinal symptoms, and transient ST-T changes on ECG to very severe cardiac dysfunction and sometimes life threatening shock and severe ventricular arrhythmias as seen in fulminant acute myocarditis. Symptoms as chest pain and palpitations are frequently occurring and may mimic a MI. On echocardiography there are both pictures with diastolic dysfunction and a preserved EF, and a general global systolic dysfunction with or without regional abnormalities. Current CMR imaging cannot today differ safely between the three major subtypes of myocarditis, the subacute virus myocarditis, the fulminant acute myocarditis and finally the giant cell myocarditis. With time we hope for better precision and a higher degree of reliability so we in future can avoid patients from an invasive procedure as EMB [207, 208]. The diagnosis of myocarditis is based on a suspicious clinical presentation combined with EMB confirmation (by histology, immunohistology, and molecular evidence for infection). Today EMB is not routine in patients with mild symptoms and a subacute myocarditis, and is not recommended in guidelines, only in selected clinical cases [209]. For documented viral myocarditis, studies have shown a complete resolution of symptoms and recovery of LV function in 40–100% of patients, and complete recovery of LV function in 40–80% of patients [208]. Biopsy-proven myocarditis may be reversible if the acute inflammatory process heals and the cause (for example viral infection) resolves. Twenty to twenty-five percent have a remaining cardiac dysfunction and the remaining may deteriorate to a DCM or progress to an end-stage DCM with need for ventricular assist device as a bridge to cardiac transplantation [210]. Giant cell myocarditis is a rare form of myocarditis but is associated with malignant ventricular arrhythmias and a poor prognosis. Histological findings in EMB may in this form of myocarditis reveal myocardial necrosis and so called multinucleated giant cells. Many patients with this form need intensified HF treatment, LV assist device implantation as a bridge to transplantation. The pathogenetic mechanisms are very well described in a position statement paper from the ESC working group on myocardial and pericardial diseases [210]. In patients with remaining symptoms recommended HF therapy and control of arrhythmia are recommended. Specific treatment using anti-viral agents, high dosages of intravenous immunoglobulin, immunoadsorption or immunosuppressive therapy have in clinically controlled studies of sufficient size not shown beneficial results and are therefore not recommended in guidelines [210]. Until the myocarditis has been completely resolved physical activity is not recommended.

1.8.3 Restrictive Cardiomyopathy (RCM)

RCM is most elusive, in part because the heart may appear morphologically close to normal, with only minor increased wall thickness or modestly decreased EF. The infiltrative process underlying RCM is often not readily detectable in vivo with even the most sensitive imaging technique. RCM is characterized by impaired filling of the heart, known as diastolic dysfunction, which reduces cardiac output. Cardinal clinical features include atrial enlargement with normal sized ventricles with a high burden of atrial arrhythmias, progression to advanced HF, and death either related to ventricular arrhythmias or HF [211]. Familial RCM is increasingly recognized as a specific phenotype within the HCM spectrum in association with sarcomere mutations and is the rarest of the primary myocardial diseases [212]. Desmin gene defects may also cause RCM usually associated with a skeletal myopathy and high degree atrioventricular block [213] or secondary to other diseases, such as storage or infiltrative disorders. Definition is based on anatomic, histological and physiological criteria, namely the presence of abnormal LV diastolic filling associated with interstitial infiltration/fibrosis in the absence of LV dilatation. Many infiltrative myocardial disorders may manifest as either restrictive or DCM.

Common features in patients with RCM is a presentation with symptoms as dyspnea and fatigue. Physical examination may include elevated jugular venous pressure, third or fourth heart sound, pulmonary rales, and peripheral edema. AF and ECG abnormalities are common. Patients may have normal or increased LV wall thickness and normal or reduced LV cavity and frequently even atrial enlargement are seen. Impaired relaxation may be an early sign and decreased LV chamber compliance a late sign. It will be a steep increase of LV filling pressure with small changes in volume. Echocardiography and CMR are diagnostic examinations used. EF is usually preserved [214].

Primary RCM is a rare condition presented in both children and adults with increased myofilament sensitivity to calcium, as well as increased accumulation of desmin, which has been implicated in the pathophysiology. Both familial and sporadic cases have been reported [215]. Familial cases are inherited as autosomal dominant with incomplete penetrance. Mutations in genes encoding sarcomeric proteins similar to HCM have been described [216]. Cardiac transplantation is an effective treatment for patients with endstage RCM [217].

Secondary RCM are subclassified as infiltrative, noninfiltrative and storage disorders. In infiltrative disorders abnormal deposits occur in the interstitial space, whereas in storage disorders, deposits occur within the cell.

Endomyocardial fibrosis (EMF) is the most common cause of RCM affecting 12 million people worldwide and is endemic in tropical and subtropical areas. Parasitic infections, autoimmune disorders and hematological malignancies lead to an initial, acute inflammatory phase with fever, pancarditis eosinophilia, facial and periorbital swelling, urticaria known as Loefflers endocarditis, then an intermediate phase with LV and RV thrombus formation and finally the final state with EMF [218]. Echo and CMR may reveal typical features [219].

1.8.4 Cardiac Amyloidosis (CA)

CA is an iniltrative disorder caused by deposition of insoluble fibrillar protein in the interstitial space. It is a systemic disorder with infiltration in the liver, kidney, bowel, nerves, skin and the tongue. Five major types of CA are recognized., each associated with a different precursor protein.

Primary or amyloid light chain A is the most common and is associated with monoclonal gammopathy or plasma cell dyscrasias such as multiple myeloma. Cardiac involvement is associated with a poor prognosis with a median survival from diagnosis of one year [220].

Wild type transthyretin (wt-TTR) amyloidosis (senile amyloidosis) is seen in 25–36% of patients over 80 years and is caused by the interstitial deposition of normal wt-TTR. Eighty different mutations encoding transthyretin are known [221].

An ECG finding of increased LV wall thickness should race the suspicion of RCM. LV wall thickness >15 mm, restrictive filling on Doppler echocardiography, early mitral inflow (E) deceleration time <150 mm and reduced EF have been associated with a poor prognosis [222]. Up to 50% of the patients die suddenly [223]. However modern treatment has improved survival in light chain amyloidosis [224] as well as treatment with ICD [225, 226]. Diagnosis may be attempted with rectal or abdominal fat pad biopsy the later has replaced the rectal due to fewer complications and higher sensitivity. A positive noncardiac biopsy supports the diagnosis and if cardiac involvement a positive EMB in at least four samples are 100% sensitive.

1.8.5 Hemochromatosis

Defined as an increased iron deposition in the sarcoplasmatic reticulum of cells in a variety of organs, liver, pancreas, heart and gonads. Primary or hereditary Hemochromatosis is a relatively common autosomal recessive disorder affecting up to 0.8% caucasians and results in increased intestinal absorption of iron [227]. Secondary Hemochromatosis results from multiple blood transfusions. Fifteen percent of the patients have cardiac involvement [228]. Clinical features involve liver disease (leading to cirrhosis and also later to development of a hepatocellular malignancy), DM and hypogonadism and also some skin changes (pigmentations). The only treatment shown some effect has been venesection or chelation therapy [229]. In some patients there are a refractory cardiac dysfunction necessitating cardiac and sometimes also a combined cardiac and liver transplantation.

1.8.6 Friedrich's Ataxia

Friedrich's ataxia is an autosomal recessive neurodegenerative disorder caused by a mutation of the fraxatin gene that manifests in the second to third decade of life with DM, ataxia and HF. Estimated prevalence is 1 in 50,000, exclusively in caucasians. No specific treatment is found [230].

1.8.7 Arrhythmogenic Right Ventricular Cardiomyopathy

ARVC or arrythmogenic CM is a progressive heart muscle disorder defined by replacement of cardiomyocytes by fat and fibrosis and is associated with structural and functional abnormalities of the right ventricle that can be seen on CMR. It is usually inherited in more than 50% of the patients as an autosomal dominant trait with reduced penetration caused by mutations in genes encoding for desmosomal proteins (desmoplakin, plakoglobin, plakophilin 2, desmoglein and desmocollin), There are also mutations in extradesmosomal genes as transforming growth factor beta3, transmembrane protein 43, and cardiac ryanodine receptor (this linked to a juvenile form of ARVC and effort-induced polymorphic ventricular tachycardia). While RV disease defines the condition, there are a number of features that can overlap with DCM since some patients may also present with a LV dominant disease with a picture ranging from scars on CMR to systolic dysfunction with a severe LV dilatation and desmosomal gene mutations are also relatively common in patients with a clinical diagnosis of DCM. Presence of RV abnormalities such as dilatation and ventricular ectopy of RV origin in relatives of patients with DCM may be a diagnostic red flag [174].

The clinical spectrum of arrythmogenic right ventricular cardiomyopathy (ARVC) is variable but typified by electroanatomical abnormalities, ventricular arrhythmia and in some cases HF or SCD [231]. It is hard to diagnose. No single test is sufficient to exclude or verify the diagnosis. By performing an EMB the presence of myocytes in various stages of cell death with evidence of fibrous or fibrofatty replacement can be seen. Mostly more fatty replacement can be seen in the elderly in contrast to the younger. However studies have shown that normal elderly in more than 50% have a fatty infiltration so where is the border between a normal heart or a cardiomyopathy [232]. However a negative EMB do not exclude the occurrence of an ARVC since the disease is segmental. There are four subtypes of the disease. There can be a concealed phase I with subtle structural abnormalities and minor ventricular arrhythmias, which may be associated with SCD, indicating the importance of disease identification in this early stage since the mild disease picture mask the risk of having a SCD [233, 234]. Stage II is overt electrical disorder with symptomatic ventricular arrhythmia of left bundle branch block (LBBB), configuration indicating its RV origin, regional structural abnormalities located to RV. Then the disease may progress to stage III with a more isolated RV HF, with regional to global RV dysfunction but still a well-preserved LV function. Finally we have stage IV with a biventricular pump failure with RV as well as LV dysfunction and this is an endstage complication and frequently age-dependent. In more than 50% of the cases a familial disease has been detected with desmosomal gene mutations identified in association with all subtypes leading to an appreciation for the broad spectrum of desmosomal gene expression. Prevalence of ARVC is thought to be 1/1000 in a community-based population, however it is difficult to estimate a true prevalence and the numbers are probably underestimated [235]. ARVC is the most important cause behind SCD in patients younger than 35 years and is responsible for about 10% of the SCD:s occurring in patients below 65 years of age [233]. A number of factors limit the use of clinical genetic testing for ARVC [232].

1.8.8 Mitochondrial Cardiomyopathy (MCM)

Because the heart is a muscle with high energy demands most patients with mitochondrial disease are susceptible to cardiac involvement. MCM is a myocardial disorder characterized by abnormal heart-muscle structure, function or both secondary to genetic defects involving the mitochondrial respiratory chain in the absence of HT, CAD or valvular disease. The presentation of MCM includes hypertrophic, dilated and LV noncompaction CM [236]. The severity can vary from no symptoms to devastating multisystemic disease. Severe cardiac manifestations include HF and ventricular arrhythmias, which can worsen acutely during a metabolic crisis and result in a SCD. Mitochondrial mutations are the typical cause of LV myocardial noncompaction disease.

1.8.9 Left Ventricular Noncompaction Cardiomyopathy (LVNC)

LVNC is defined by three markers: prominent LV trabeculae, deep intertrabecular recesses and the thin compacted layer [237]. LVNC occurs in infants (0.81/100,000 infants per year) and adults (prevalence 0.014%) but with improvements in diagnostic imaging the prevalence seem to increase [238]. Whether LVNC is a distinct cardiomyopathy or a morphologic trait shared by different types of cardiomyopathies is still debated [239]. The LVNC trait may be inherited in 20–50% in adults with an autosomal dominant pattern of inheritance and most familial cases identified are associated with mutations in the same genes that cause other types of cardiomyopathies (HCM, RCM and DCM) as genes encoding sarcomere proteins, LMNA and Taffazin [240]. It has also been demonstrated that some highly trained athletes demonstrate features diagnostic of LVNC [241]. However severe forms of LV apex non-compaction are seen in children with Barth syndrome (an inherited disease with mutations in gene TAZ/G4.5 located on the X-chromosome) and in these patients LVNC is associated with LV dilation and dysfunction [242]. There are also mutations in genes in the Notch 1 pathway leading to hypertrabeculation and non-compaction [243]. Complications associated with LVNC are HF, arrhythmias including SCD and systemic embolic events. However currently there are no specific treatment for LVNC [244].

1.9 Adult Congenital Heart Disease

It is estimated that the expanding population of adults with congenital heart disease is about 1.2 millions in Europe [245] and 1.0 million in U.S. These large numbers are the results from successful cardiothoracic surgery in the childhood and improved cardiac care. Eight out of 1000 live births are diagnosed with a congenital heart defect and about 85% of them reach adulthood and particularly those with more complex disease [246]. In a population-based cohort study from Canada it was shown that the number of deaths from congenital heart diseases (CHD) in infants and childhood markedly have declined from 1987 to 2005, with a reduction in mortality (about 31%), which was higher than in the general population. The mortality was more reduced in infants and especially in those with the most severe forms of CHD. That means that deaths have shifted away from infant to adults in CHD [247]. Most patients with CHD, however, have residual lesions and need life-long care in order to prevent development of further complications. However we know that with increasing survival, complications as HF may develop in patients corrected in early childhood for their CHD. To describe it simply, patients with incomplete or palliative correction of a lesion in the childhood develop a chronic state of hemodynamic stress and later on a HF. Studies have shown that the development of HF depends on age and RV function and the type of CHD [248]. The risk for developing HF was significantly greater in patients with a tetralogy of Fallot (TOF) and for patients with congenitally corrected transposition of the great arteries (ccTGA) after the Mustard procedure (atrial switch). The highest risk, not surprisingly was found in patients with single ventricles after a Fontan procedure (traditionally a surgical separation of the systemic and pulmonary venous returns without a subpulmonary ventricle, restoring them to be in series). These adult patients have also comorbidities (cancer, DM) and especially CAD and due to that they are similar to other patients with chronic HF. To provide this growing population with optimal care it is important that more cardiologists are being trained to take care about these patients since we know that lapse of care is associated with significant morbidity and mortality.

The most common occurring adult CHD found in a large Dutch registry including 8600 patients are shunt lesions (atrial septal defect (ASD) (17.1%), ventricular septal defect (15.8%), and atrioventricular septal defect (1.5%)), aortic stenosis (AS) and/or bicuspid aortic valve (BAV) (13.7%), aortic coarctation (10.1%), TOF (10.1%), pulmonary stenosis (PS) (7.3%) TGA (4.8%), Marfan syndrome (4.8%), Pulmonary atresia (1.8%), Ebstein's anomaly (1.6%), ccTGA (1.3%), univentricular heart/double inlet left ventricle (1.2%), tricuspid atresia (0.8%), double outlet right ventricle (0.7%). Besides that there are other congenital defects estimated to 7.4% [249].

Studies from two large registries, one in Canada [250] and the other in The Netherlands [249] have shown that about 50% of the deaths in patients with adult CHDs are due to cardiovascular causes as HF and SCD. Surprisingly many patients with an ASD (30%) and TOF (40%) and ccTGA (60%) in the Dutch material died from HF. Corresponding figures from Canada were 20, 35% and 40%, respectively. Worth to mention was that more than 50% of the patients with an ASD were older than 75 years and had a number of other concomitant diseases as CAD, valvular heart diseases and atrial arrhythmias and one fourth of them had no correction of their ASD. The TOF patients were somewhat younger than those with ASD but they also had many comorbidities. Interesting from this material is also that patients with aortic diseases and especially those with a BAV had a very low mean age (<50 years of age) and a large number of them died from a SCD (supposed to be ventricular arrhythmias, however not proven) before the age of 35.

In a retrospective cohort study adult CHD patients older than 60 years were studied in order to evaluate the burden of the disease and predictors for outcome. It was found that the number of interventions, hospitalizations, days in hospital and outpatient clinical visits were much higher than in those with CHD aged 20–60 years. Prognostic factors found were CAD, reduction in LV systolic function and symptoms of HF [251]. This study tell us what we can expect in future with more patients with CHD surviving up to higher ages, they need to use healthcare resources much more than younger patients, again telling how important it is that cardiologists are trained to take care about these patients.

As mentioned above certain diseases have a higher risk than others to develop HF in adult age and in the following we are going to look more closely at those.

1.9.1 Atrial Septal Defect (ASD)

An ASD results in a left to right shunt because of the higher compliance of the RV compared to the left and causes thereby a volume overload in the RV. Most patients with an ASD are asymptomatic and develop first symptoms in adult age as exertional dyspnea, palpitations, reduced physical capacity and sometimes also RV HF. Surgical repair with device closure is the recommended treatment. Post-operative complications as arrhythmias (mostly atrial tachyarrhythmias) are common.

1.9.2 Valvular Aortic Stenosis

The most common cause for congenital valvular aortic stenosis is BAV. Prevalence at birth estimated to 1–2%. It is more common in males than in females. The pathophysiological background in most cases is a fusion of the left coronary cusp and the right coronary cusp. As mentioned above many of these adult patients die before the age of 35 and mostly of a SCD and very few develop HF. Mutations in the NOTCH 1 gene has been linked to BAV. Abnormalities in the aortic wall associated with BAV can lead to dilation, rupture or dissection. Many patients are asymptomatic during many years but as soon they have onset of symptoms (chest pain, dyspnea or syncope) there is a rapid deterioration in prognosis [252].

1.9.3 Tetralogy of Fallot

This is the most common cyanotic heart defect and the most common cause of blue baby syndrome in childhood. TOF is caused by a deviation of the outlet septum and is characterized by four specific features. (1) a pulmonary infundibular stenosis often described as a sub-pulmonary stenosis or a subpulmonary obstruction, (2) an overriding aorta, (3) a ventricular septal defect with a right to left shunt, where higher resistance to RV outflow results in more severe cyanosis and (4) RV hypertrophy. About 15% of the patients have chromosome 22 deletions (22q11) called a DiGeorge syndrome with autosomal dominant inheritance. Corrective surgery is often performed within the first year of life but later it is common with problems as arrhythmias, pulmonary regurgitation (PR) and LV systolic dysfunction leading to HF and ventricular arrhythmias, demanding an ICD.

1.9.4 Congenitally Corrected Transposition of the Great Arteries

This is a rare heart defect where both ventricles are reversed as well as the arteries. That means that the heart actually corrects the abnormal development. ccTGA may cause problems particularly for the RV, which must work much harder than it was meant to. Associated intracardiac anomalies are a ventricular septal defect in up to 70% of the patients, PS in about 40% and sometimes also abnormal leakage in the tricuspid valve (Ebstein's malformation). This is a strange syndrome where newborns can have low oxygen level and present with symptoms of refractory HF, especially if they have a large ventricular septal defect, and need urgent surgery, while others have no symptoms and remain undiagnosed and live a normal life in many years. ccTGA is often not diagnosed until adulthood, where problems may arise with HF.

1.9.5 Univentricular Heart

This is one of the most complex congenital heart malformations where either the left ventricle or the right ventricle is missing or, if present, is hypoplastic and is unable to function in a normal way [253, 254]. These patients frequently present with cyanosis, low cardiac output and early symptoms of acute HF, demanding urgent surgery when they are newborn. Some patients may survive after multiple corrective operations using Fontan-type procedures and survival until the seventh decade has been reported in rare cases.

1.9.6 Treatment of Patients with HF and Adult Congenital Heart Defects

How to treat these adult CHD patients when they have HF. As already mentioned these patients are in many ways similar to our conventional patients with chronic HF and should therefore be treated with guideline drugs as renin-angiotensin blockers, beta blockers and aldosterone antagonists. However since HF predominantly depends on age and RV function we do not know if similar beneficial effects can be obtained with guidelines treatment. Studies are needed to evaluate this [255]. Another treatment used in selected patients with HF is CRT. So far only small and short-term studies have been performed with CRT in patients with adult CHD, and they have not been conclusive. Again we need well designed large randomized studies with sufficient long follow up, preferable multi-center studies in order to include enough with patients to reach sufficient statistical power. Following that perhabs there can be some decision how to treat adult patients with CHD and HF and who should have device therapy with CRT.

Moreover arrhythmias are very frequent occurring, both atrial arrhythmias as well as ventricular and studies have shown that death caused by a SCD is common and therefore it is important to find out how to detect high-risk patients in need of ICD therapy [256]. SCD has been shown to be especially common in adult patients with congenital heart diseases as TOF, TGA, ccTGA, AS and univentricular heart. Also it has been found that conduction abnormalities are common (broad QRS complex on ECG, dysssynchrony), risk factors for SCD especially in patients with TOF [257]. Today a high rate of ICD implantations are performed in patients with CHD both as in primary as well as in secondary prevention. The duration of the ICD in those younger patients should be for many years and thereby also the rate of complications as inappropriate shocks and lead-complications will increase indicating a careful selection of patients candidates for this therapy, also taking into consideration costs and benefits. This is discussed more in detail in a position paper recently published in European Heart Journal [258, 259].

1.10 Valvular Heart Diseases

Valvular dysfunction is a wellknown cause of HF, either as a primary cause of HF or a secondary effect of other diseases. Rheumatic fever as a cause of HF is rare in industrialized countries but still very common in developing countries because of less use of modern treatment with antibiotics and poor compliance due to many reasons.

1.10.1 Aortic Valve Disease

Aortic stenosis is the most common valvular heart disease in developed countries. In older adults it is a degenerative disease with abnormalities in the aortic valves with common features as calcification and thickening of the valves without significant obstruction. In the Cardiovascular Health study examining older individuals (>65 years old), abnormalities in the aortic valves were found in 26% of the subjects but only 2% had an important aortic stenosis [260]. With aging the prevalence of abnormalities were increased from 20% to 48% in those very elderly (>85 years) and 1–4% had a real AS. The pathophysiology behind is judged to be an inflammatory process with deposition of lipids followed by calcification of the annulus of the valves thereby obstructing the circulatory flow to the body [261]. Thus the process is similar to that of atherosclerosis and the initial plaque of AS is alike that of CAD. Risk factors are also very similar with age, hyperlipidemia and evidence of inflammation. Controversial is if treatment with statins may retard the progression of AS [262].

Another type of aortic stenosis is the congenital AS common in childhood and attributable to a BAV and this disease is described in the section of CHD.

In developing countries the rheumatic AS is the most common and in this disease it is common with a commissural fusion due to inflammation in contrast to the degenerative calcified AS.

Obstruction of the circulatory flow across the valves lead to a pressure overload hypertrophy and still many researchers think this is a compensatory mechanism in order to offset the pressure overload. Pressure overload by itself increases LV afterload and impair the ejection performance. However hypertrophy may be beneficial in some respects and deleterious in others since it impairs the coronary blood flow and result in a diastolic dysfunction. This augmented diastolic pressure leads to dyspnea and pulmonary congestion [263]. Onset of severe symptoms as angina, syncope and HF is an indication for evaluation of the valve orifice area by use of echocardiography with Doppler interrogation of the aortic valve to decide if the time has come to perform replacement valve surgery with insertion of mechanical valves or biological valves or in selected patients perform a transcatheter aortic valve implantation, thereby repairing the old damaged valve by delivering a fully collapsible replacement valve to the valve site through a catheter. This procedure is most suitable in high risk patients not suitable for conventional replacement surgery [264, 265].

1.10.2 Aortic Regurgitation (AR)

AR is characterized by diastolic reflux of blood from aorta into the left ventricle and is due to malcoaptation of the aortic cusps because of leaflet pathology or aortic root disease. It usually occurs because of a congenital BAV, often resulting from leaflet prolapse, and from calcific aortic valve disease. Infective endocarditis involving the aortic valve may result in AR because of loss of coaptation, leaflet retraction or perforation [266]. In developing countries AR due to rheumatic heart disease is still common. Other diseases causing AR are connective tissue or inflammatory diseases, antiphospholipid syndrome, and use of anorectic drugs. Trauma (chest wall or deceleration injury) may also affect the leaflets [267].

Chronic AR results in volume overloading of the left ventricle and also some component of pressure overload. Chronic AR may be well tolerated for many years with minimal symptoms. The hemodynamic importance of AR reflect the severity of the diastolic leak slowly progressing from volume overload and ventricular hypertrophy to LV dilation and contractile dysfunction. The EF is usually preserved until the late stages of the disease. Surgical intervention is indicated, even in asymptomatic individuals when LV dilation reaches critical dimensions or ventricular dysfunction occur. If surgery is performed directly after that, the LV dysfunction is potentially reversible [267]. In theory patients with chronic AR should benefit from long-term treatment with vasodilating drugs in order to augment forward cardiac output. However studies have shown that they do not change the natural history of the asymptomatic patient. However they may be considered in patients with symptomatic AR not suitable for surgery [268].

On the other hand an acute AR may occur due to acute or a subacute infective endocarditis, aortic dissection and aortic valve damage caused by trauma. This disease is, if untreated, potentially life-threatening by causing high LV filling pressures, low cardiac output and severe advanced HF with pulmonary edema and leading to an early death. Appropriately medical and surgical management are urgent in order to prevent death [269].

1.10.3 Mitral Valve Disease

Mitral valve disease consists of three different types of disease, mitral stenosis, mitral regurgitation and mitral valve prolapse.

1.10.3.1 Mitral Stenosis (MS)

MS is a primary valve disease with a narrowing of the mitral valve orifice resulting in impairment of filling of the left ventricle in diastole. It is usually caused by rheumatic heart disease and persistent inflammatory valve disease and is common in developing countries. In developed countries it is mostly caused by a degenerative disease with severe calcification of the mitral annulus. MS may be asymptomatic during long time but may also progress slowly or more acutely during certain circumstances (onset of AF, infection, emotional stress) leading to a rise in left atrial pressure with dilatation of left atrium and later development of pulmonary hypertension. MS may present with symptoms as exertional dyspnea, atrial arrhythmias, embolic events, hemoptysis or even right sided HF indicating surgical treatment as percutaneous mitral balloon commisurotomy and surgical commisurotomy proving excellent short-term as well as long-term results and delay the need for mitral valve replacement [270, 271].

1.10.3.2 Mitral Regurgitation (MR)

MR may be caused by primary or secondary (functional) valve disease. In primary MR there is a structural or degenerative abnormality of the mitral valve causing backflow of the blood into the left ventricle resulting in volume overload and if severe enough causing left ventricular dysfunction, pulmonary hypertension and HF. Common diseases behind are rheumatic heart disease, mitral valve prolapse, and infective endocarditis. Many patients may tolerate MR for a long time and in others progression to HF with left ventricular dysfunction may be more rapid indicating surgery. However, long-term treatment with vasodilating drugs may reduce the regurgitant flow and delay the time when surgery is the preferred treatment [272].

Secondary MR occurs in the absence of primary valve abnormalities, usually from LV dysfunction caused by global or regional changes in LV geometry due to a myocardial damage or a dilated cardiomyopathy resulting in papillary muscle displacement as well as an annular dilation. Sometimes in connection with an acute MI, an acute MR can develop caused by rupture or stretching of the papillary muscle and this type of MR is categorized as a post MI complication. The prognosis of secondary MR with HF is poor. Recommended treatment is standard guideline recommended treatment for HF. Studies have shown limited benefits of mitral valve surgery [273].

1.10.3.3 Mitral Valve Prolapse (MVP)

MVP is a very common valve disorder in U.S. affecting about 2–3% of the general population. Many patients with MVP have normal mitral leaflets, with little or no MR and thus a benign prognosis and with survival rates similarly as healthy individuals. Patients with MVP due to myxomatous valve disease are at increased risk for cardiovascular complications especially in connection with LV dysfunction. If progressive MR develops, surgery with mitral valve repair or replacement is indicated [274].

1.10.4 Tricuspid Valve Disease

Tricuspid valve dysfunction can result from structural alterations (congenital or acquired) of the valve or from abnormal function of a structurally normal valve and is divided into stenosis or regurgitant diseases. In many papers tricuspid valve has been referred to as "the forgotten valve". However increased understanding about the prognosis of severe TR in patients with RV HF and cardiac remodeling and new surgical techniques has led to an increased interest with more aggressive treatment recommendations.

1.10.4.1 Tricuspid Stenosis

TS is caused by at least four conditions, rheumatic heart disease (more common in developing countries), congenital abnormalities, infective endocarditis and carcinoid heart disease. Rheumatic TS differ from rheumatic MS and is defined as fibrous thickening of the leaflets with no calcific deposits with fusion of two to three commisures but chordal fusion not severely affected. The occurrence of a TS may obstruct right atrial masses such as prolapsing myxoma or obstruct a mechanical valve dysfunction. About 50% of patients with widespread lesions of carcinoid tumor develop various combinations of right-sided valvular lesions TS or pure TR or PS or PR [275]. Clinical signs of HF in TS are those of right HF. Surgical correction is sometimes performed in connection with left heart surgery. Tricuspid valve balloon valvuloplasty is so far of limited value. Fibrinolytic therapy for prosthetic tricuspid valve thrombosis is first line therapy [276].

1.10.4.2 Tricuspid Regurgitation

TR is defined as a leaky valve or a valve, which does not close enough, causing blood to leak backwards across the valve. Pure TR may be caused by rheumatic heart disease, infective endocarditis, Ebstein's anomaly, carcinoid heart disease, Marfan's syndrome and papillary muscle dysfunction. However the most common etiology of pure TR is not associated with intrinsic valve disease but instead dilation of the right ventricle cavity and tricuspid annulus from any cause of RV dysfunction, left-sided valvular disease causing pulmonary hypertension, LV dysfunction and chronic pulmonary diseases. More than 80% of TR found in patients are secondary and related to tricuspid annular dilatation and leaflet tethering [277]. Based on that volume overload or pressure overload of the RV can impair tricuspid function, leading to a dilatation or RV hypertrophy in order to maintain ejection fraction. Advanced tricuspid valve dysfunction may lead to right HF [278]. Interesting is that older patients developing an AF also can develop an important TR in association with abnormalities of RV compliance [278]. The prognosis of TR is not so good and associated with less survival [279]. Medical treatment is limited to diuretics if HF and management of AF. Surgical treatment may be indicated at the time of left-sided heart valve surgery and is intended to improve leaflet coaptation by correcting annular dilatation by performing a tricuspid valve repair. Several transcatheter therapies have emerged on the market but must first be clinically tested before this technique is recommended, many of them have so far only being tested in animals.

1.10.5 Pulmonary Valve Disease

Pulmonary stenosis (PS) and pulmonary regurgitation (PR) are rare. The causes of PS are limited to a few conditions; rheumatic heart disease, congenital heart disease (most common), carcinoid and infective endocarditis. Carcinoid heart disease is the most common of the acquired forms of PS. Pure PR is also a very rare condition and are caused by the same diseases as PS. As with pure TR, the most common cause of pure PR is not intrinsic valve disease but instead dilation of the pulmonary trunk and pulmonic valve annulus secondary to other diseases as diseases causing pulmonary artery hypertension or connective tissue disorders [280]. Pulmonary valve replacement has mostly been performed in patients with CHD mostly after correction of a TOF with few side-effects as thromboembolisms and bleeding events [281].

References

1. Saba MM, Ventura HO, Saleh M, Mehra MR. Ancient Egyptian medicine and the concept of heart failure. J Card Fail. 2006;12:416–21.
2. Katz AM. The "modern" view of heart failure – how did we get here? Circ Heart Fail. 2008;1:63–71.
3. The CONSENSUS Trial Study Group. Effects of enalapril on mortality in severe congestive heart failure. Results of the cooperative North Scandinavian enalapril survival study (CONSENSUS). N Engl J Med. 1987;316:1429–35.
4. Ponikowski P, Voors AA, Anker SD, Bueno H, Cleland JG, Coats AJS, et al. 2016 ESC guidelines for the diagnosis and treatment of acute and chronic heart failure. Eur Heart J. 2016;37:2129–200. https://doi.org/10.1093/eurhartj/ehw128.
5. ACCH/AHA Practice Guidelines, Yancy CW, Jessup M, Bozkurt B, Butler J, Casey DE, Drazner MH, et al. 2013 ACCF/AHA guideline for the management of heart failure. Circulation. 2013;128:e240–327.
6. Lang RM, Bierig M, Devereux RB, Flaschkampf FA, Foster E, Pellikka PA. Recommendations for chamber quantification. Eur J Echocardiogr. 2006;7:79–108.
7. Ho JE, Lyass A, Lee DS, Vasan RS, Kannel WB, Larson MG, et al. Predictors of new-onset heart failure: differences in preserved versus reduced ejection farction. Circ Heart Fail. 2013;6:279–86.
8. Lewis EF, Solomon SD, Jablonski KA, Rice MM, Clemenza F, Hsia J, et al. Predictors of heart failure in patients with stable coronary artery disease: a PEACE study. Circ Heart Fail. 2009;2:209–16.
9. Lee DS, Gona P, Vasan RS, Larson MG, Benjamin EJ, Wang TJ, et al. Relation of disease pathogenesis and risk factors to heart failure with preserved or reduced ejection fraction: insights from the Framingham heart study of the national heart, lung, and blood institute. Circulation. 2009;119:3070–7.
10. Brouwers FP, de Boer RA, van der Harst P, Voors AA, Gansevoort RT, Bakker SJ, et al. Incidence and epidemiology of new onset heart failure with preserved vs. reduced ejection faction in a community-based cohort: 11-year follow-up of PREVEND. Eur Heart J. 2013;34:1424–31.
11. Owan TE, Hodge DO, Herges RM, Jacobsen SJ, Roger VL, Redfield MM. Trends in prevalence and outcome of heart failure with preserved ejection fraction. N Engl J Med. 2006;355:251–9.
12. Lam CSP, Donal E, Kraigher-Krainer E, Vasan RS. Epidemiology and clinical course of heart failure with preserved ejection fraction. Eur J Heart Fail. 2011;13:18–28.
13. The Criteria Committee of the New York Heart Association. Nomenclature and criteria for diagnosis of diseases of the heart and great vessels. 9th ed. Boston: Little & Brown; 1994.
14. Ammar KA, Jacobsen SJ, Mahoney DW, Kors JA, Redfield MM, Burnett JC Jr, et al. Prevalence and prognostic significance of heart failure stages: application of the American College of Cardiology/American Heart Association heart failure staging criteria in the community. Circulation. 2007;115:1563–70.
15. Dahlstrom U, Hakansson J, Swedberg K, Waldenstrom A. Adequacy of diagnosis and treatment of chronic heart failure in primary health care in Sweden. Eur J Heart Fail. 2009;11:92–8.
16. Zarrinkoub R, Wettermark B, Wändell P, Mejhert M, Szulkin R, Ljunggren G, et al. The epidemiology of heart failure, based on data for 2.1 million inhabitants in Sweden. Eur J Heart Fail. 2013;15:995–1002.
17. Ingelsson E, Arnlöv J, Sundström J, Lind L. The validity of a diagnosis of heart failure in a hospital discharge register. Eur J Heart Fail. 2005;7:787–91.
18. Curtis LH, Whellan DJ, Hammill BG, Hernandez AF, Anstrom KJ, Shea AM, et al. Incidence and prevalence of heart failure in elderly persons, 1994-2003. Arch Intern Med. 2008;168:418–24.
19. Davies M, Hobbs F, Davis R, Kenkre J, Roaffe AK, Hare R, et al. Prevalence of left-ventricular systolic dysfunction and heart failure in the echocardiographic heart of England screening study: a population based study. Lancet. 2001;358:439–44.
20. Ceia F, Fonseca C, Mota T, Morais H, Matias F, de Sousa A, et al. Prevalence of chronic heart failure in Southwestern Europe: the EPICA study. Eur J Heart Fail. 2002;4:531–9.
21. Kupari M, Lindroos M, Iivanainen AM, Heikkilä J, Tilvis R. Congestive heart failure in old age: prevalence, mechanisms and 4-year prognosis in the Helsinki Ageing Study. J Intern Med. 1997;241:387–94.
22. Bleumink GS, Knetsch AM, Sturkenboom MC, Straus SM, Hofman A, Deckers JW, et al. Quantifying the heart failure epidemic: prevalence, incidence rate, lifetime risk and prognosis of heart failure The Rotterdam Study. Eur Heart J. 2004;25:1614–9.
23. Vaes B, Rezzoug N, Pasquet A, Wallemacq P, Van Pottelbergh G, Mathei C, et al. The prevalence of cardiac dysfunction and the correlation with poor functioning among the elderly. Int J Cardiol. 2012;155:134–43.
24. Hogg K, Swedberg K, McMurray J. Heart failure with preserved left ventricular systolic function; epidemiology, clinical characteristics, and prognosis. J Am Coll Cardiol. 2004;43:317–27.
25. Senni M, Tribouilloy CM, Rodeheffer RJ, Jacobsen SJ, Evans JM, Bailey KR, et al. Congestive heart failure in the community: a study of all incident cases in Olmsted County, Minnesota, in 1991. Circulation. 1998;98:2282–9.
26. Owan TE, Redfield MM. Epidemiology of diastolic heart failure. Prog Cardiovasc Dis. 2005;47:320–32.

27. Cowie MR, Wood DA, Coats AJ, Thompson SG, Poole-Wilson PA, Suresh V, et al. Incidence and aetiology of heart failure; a population-based study. Eur Heart J. 1999;20:421–8.
28. Gottdiener JS, Arnold AM, Aurigemma GP, Polak JF, Tracy RP, Kitzman DW, et al. Predictors of congestive heart failure in the elderly: The Cardiovascular Health Study. J Am Coll Cardiol. 2000;35:1628–37.
29. De Giuli F, Khaw KT, Cowie MR, Sutton GC, Ferrari R, Poole-Wilson PA. Incidence and outcome of persons with clinical diagnosis of heart failure in a general practice population of 696,884 in the United Kingdom. Eur J Heart Fail. 2005;7:295–302.
30. Murphy NF, Simpson CR, McAlister FA, Stewart S, MacIntyre K, Kirkpatrick M, et al. National survey of the prevalence, incidence, primary care burden, and treatment of heart failure in Scotland. Heart. 2004;90:1129–36.
31. Gerber Y, Weston SA, Redfield MM, Chamberlain AM, Manemann SM, Jiang R, et al. A contemporary appraisal of the heart failure epidemic in Olmsted County, Minnesota, 2000-2010. JAMA Intern Med. 2015;175:996–1004.
32. Van Riet EE, Hoes AW, Limburg A, Landman MA, van der Hoeven H, Rutten FH. Prevalence of unrecognized heart failure in older persons with shortness of breath on exertion. Eur J Heart Fail. 2014;16:772–7.
33. Kereiakes DJ. The fire that burns within: C-reactive protein. Circulation. 2003;107:373–4.
34. Van Deursen VM, Urso R, Laroche C, Damman K, Dahlström U, Tavazzi L, et al. Co-morbidities in patients with heart failure: an analysis of the European Heart Failure Pilot Survey. Eur J Heart Fail. 2014;16:103–11.
35. Pfeffer MA, Glaggett B, Assmann SF, Boineau R, Anand IS, Clausell N, et al. Regional variation in patients and outcomes in the treatment of preserved cardiac function heart failure with an aldosterone antagonist (TOPCAT) trial. Circulation. 2015;131:34–42.
36. Lund LH, Benson L, Dahlström U, Edner M. Association between use of renin-angiotensin system antagonists and mortality in patients with heart failure and preserved ejection fraction. JAMA. 2012;308:2108–17.
37. Lund LH, Benson L, Dahlström U, Edner M, Friberg L. Association between use of beta-blockers and outcomes in patients with heart failure and preserved ejection fraction. JAMA. 2014;312:2008–18.
38. Ledwidge M, Gallagher J, Conion C, Tallon E, O'Connell E, Dawkins I, et al. Natriuretic peptide-based screening and collaborative care for heart failure: the STOP-HF randomized trial. JAMA. 2013;310:66–74.
39. Djoussé L, Driver JA, Gaziano JM. Relation between modifiable lifestyle factors and lifetime risk of heart failure. JAMA. 2009;302:394–400.
40. Levitan EB, Wolk A, Mittleman MA. Consistency with the DASH diet and incidence of heart failure. Arch Intern Med. 2009;169:851–7.
41. Go AS, Mozaffarian D, Roger VL, Benjamin EJ, Berry JD, Borden WB, et al. Heart disease and stroke statistics – 2013 update: a report from the American Heart Association. Circulation. 2013;127:e6–e245.
42. Kitiyakara C, Guzman NJ. Malignant hypertension and hypertensive emergencies. J Am Soc Nephrol. 1998;9:133–42.
43. Verdechia P, Angeli F, Cavallini C, Gattobigio R, Gentile G, Staessen JA, et al. Blood pressure reduction and renin-angiotensin system inhibition for prevention of congestive heart failure: a meta-analysis. Eur Heart J. 2009;30:679–88.
44. Beckett NS, Peters R, Fletcher AE, Staessen JA, Liu L, Dumitrascu D, et al. Treatment of hypertension in patients 80 years of age or older. N Engl J Med. 2008;358:1887–98.
45. Sciaretta S, Palano F, Tocci G, Baldini R, Volpe M. Antihypertensive treatment and development of heart failure in hypertension: a Bayesian network meta-analysis of studies in patients with hypertension and high cardiovascular risk. Arch Intern Med. 2011;171:384–94.
46. Roush GC, Holford TR, Guddati AK. Chlortalidone compared with hydrochlorothiazide in reducing cardiovascular events: a systematic review and network meta-analyses. Hypertension. 2012;59:1110–7.
47. Ingelsson E, Sundström J, Arnlöv J, Zethelius B, Lind L. Insulin resistance and risk of congestive heart failure. JAMA. 2005;294:334–41.
48. Boudina S, Abel ED. Diabetic cardiomyopathy revisited. Circulation. 2007;115:3213–23.
49. Aneja A, Tang WH, Bansilal S, Garcia MJ, Farkouh ME. Diabetic cardiomyopathy: insights into pathogenesis, diagnostic challenges, and therapeutic options. Am J Med. 2008;121:748–57.
50. Liu JE, Palmieri V, Roman MJ, Bella JN, Fabsitz R, Howard BV, et al. The impact of diabetes on left ventricular filling pattern in normotensive and hyptertensive adults: The Strong Heart Study. J Am Coll Cardiol. 2001;37:1943–9.
51. Schannwell CM, Schneppenheim M, Perings S, Plehn G, Strauer BE. Left ventricular diastolic dysfunction as an early manifestation of diabetic cardiomyopathy. Cardiology. 2002;98:33–9.
52. Dandamudi S, Slusser J, Mahoney DVV, Redfield MM, Rodeheffer RJ, Chen HH. The prevalence of diabetic cardiomyopathy: a population-based study in Olmsted County, Minnesota. J Card Fail. 2014;20:304–9.
53. De Groote P, Lamblin N, Mouquet F, Plichon D, McFadden E, Van Belle E, et al. Impact of diabetes mellitus on long-term survival in patients with congestive heart failure. Eur Heart J. 2004;25:656–62.
54. Greenberg BH, Abraham WT, Albert NM, Chiswell K, Clare R, Stough WG, et al. Influence of diabetes on characteristics and outcomes in patients hospitalized with heart failure: a report from the Organized Program to Initiate Lifesaving Treatment in Hospitalized Patients with Heart Failure (OPTIMIZE-HF). Am Heart J. 2007;154:e1–8.
55. Stratton IM, Adler AI, Neil HA, Matthews DR, Manley SE, Cull CA, et al. Association of glycaemia with macrovascular and microvascular complications of type 2 diabetes (UKPDS 35): prospective observational study. BMJ. 2000;321:405–12.
56. Miller ME, Williamson JD, Gerstein HC, Byington RP, Cushman WC, Ginsberg HN, et al. Effects of randomization to intensive glucose control on adverse events, cardiovascular disease, and mortality in older versus younger adults in the ACCORD trial. Diabetes Care. 2014;37:634–43.
57. Gastagno D, Baird-Gunning J, Jhund PS, Biondi-Zoccai G, MacDonald MR, Petrie MC, et al. Intensive glycemic control has no impact on the risk of heart failure in type 2 diabetic patients: evidence from a 37,229 patient meta-analysis. Am Heart J. 2011;162:938–48.
58. Zinmanand B, Wanner C, Lachin JM, Fitchett D, Bluhmki E, Hantel S, et al. Empagliflozin, cardiovascular outcomes, and mortality in type 2 diabetes. N Engl J Med. 2015;373(22):2117–28.
59. Fitchett D, Zinman B, Wanner C, Lachin JM, Hantel S, Salsali A, et al. Heart failure outcomes with empagliflozin in patients with type II diabetes at high cardiovascular risk: results of the EMPA-REG OUTCOME trial. Eur Heart J. 2016;37:1526–34.
60. Johansson I, Dahlström U, Edner M, Näsman P, Rydén L, Norhammar A. Riskfactors, treatment, prognosis in men and women with heart failure with and without diabetes. Heart. 2015;101:1139–48.
61. Jhund PS, Macintyre K, Simpson CR, Lewsey JD, Stewart S, Redpath A, et al. Longterm trends in first hospitalization for heart failure and subsequent survival between 1986 and 2003: a population study of 5.1 million people. Circulation. 2009;119:515–23.
62. Schaufelberger M, Swedberg K, Köster M, Rosen M, Rosengren A. Decreasing one-year mortality and hospitalization rates for heart failure in Sweden. Eur Heart J. 2004;25:300–7.

63. Mosterd A, Hoes AW. Clinical epidemiology of heart failure. Heart. 2007;93:1137–46.
64. Chen J, Normand SL, Wang Y, Krumholz HM. National and regional trends in heart failure hospitalization and mortality rates for Medicare beneficiaries, 1998-2008. JAMA. 2011;306:1669–78.
65. Dharmarajan K, Hsieh AF, Lin Z, Bueno H, Ross JS, Horwitz LI, et al. Diagnoses and timing of 30-day readmissions after hospitalization for heart failure, acute myocardial infarction, or pneumonia. JAMA. 2013;309:355–63.
66. Hong Y, LaBresh KA. Overview of the American Heart Association "Get with the guidelines" programs; coronary heart disease, stroke and heart failure. Crit Pathw Cardiol. 2006;5:179–86.
67. West R, Liang L, Fonarow GC, Kociol R, Mills RM, O'Connor CM, et al. Characterization of heart failure patients with preserved ejection fraction: a comparison between ADHERE-US registry and ADHERE international registry. Eur J Heart Fail. 2011;13:945–52.
68. Jonsson A, Edner M, Alehagen U, Dahlström U. Heart failure registry: a valuable tool for improving the management of patients with heart failure. Eur J Heart Fail. 2010;12:25–31.
69. Blecker S, Paul M, Taksier G, Ogedegbe G, Katz S. Heart failure-associated hospitalizations in the United States. J Am Coll Cardiol. 2013;61:1259–67.
70. Collins SP, Pang PS, Fonarow GC, Yancy CW, Bonow RO, Gheorghiade M. Is hospital admission for heart failure really necessary? The role of ED and observation unit in preventing hospitalization and rehospitalization. J Am Coll Cardiol. 2013;61:121–6.
71. Stewart S, MacIntyre K, Hole DJ, Capewell S, McMurray JJV. More 'Malignant' than cancer? Five-year survival following a first admission for heart failure. Eur J Heart Fail. 2001;3:315–22.
72. Chan MMY, Lam CSP. How do patients with heart failure with preserved ejection fraction die? Eur J Heart Fail. 2013;15:604–13.
73. Meta-analysis Global Group in Chronic Heart Failure (MAGGIC). The survival of patients with heart failure with preserved or reduced left ventricular ejection fraction: an individual patient data meta-analysis. Eur Heart J. 2012;33:1750–7.
74. Somaratne JB, Berry C, McMurray JJ, Poppe KK, Doughty RN, Whalley GA. The prognostic significance of heart failure with preserved left ventricular ejection fraction: a literature-based meta-analysis. Eur J Heart Fail. 2009;11:855–62.
75. Orn S, Cleland JG, Romo M, Kjekshus J, Dickstein K. Recurrent infarction causes the most deaths following myocardial infarction with left ventricular dysfunction. Am J Med. 2005;118:752–8.
76. McDonagh TA, Morrison CE, Lawrence A, Ford J, Tunstall-Pedoe H, McMurray JJ, et al. Symptomatic and asymptomatic left-ventricular systolic dysfunction in an urban population. Lancet. 1997;350:829–33.
77. Mosterd A, Hoes AW, de Bruyne MC, Deckers JW, Linker DT, Hofman A, et al. Prevalence of heart failure and left ventricular dysfunction in the general population: the Rotterdam study. Eur Heart J. 1999;20:447–55.
78. Redfield MM, Jacobsen SJ, Burnett JC Jr, Mahoney DW, Bailey KR, Rodeheffer RJ. Burden of systolic and diastolic ventricular dysfunction in the community: appreciating the scope of the heart failure epidemic. JAMA. 2003;289:194–202.
79. Jong P, Yusef S, Rousseau MF, Ahn SA, Bangdwala SI. Effect of enalapril on 12 year survival and life expectancy in patients with left ventricular systolic dysfunction: a follow-up study. Lancet. 2003;361:1843–8.
80. McDonagh TA, Cunningham AD, Morrison CE, McMurray JJ, Ford I, Morton JJ, et al. Left ventricular dysfunction, natriuretic peptides, and mortality in an urban population. Heart. 2001;86:21–6.
81. Vigen R, Maddox TM, Allen LA. Aging of the United States population: impact on heart failure. Curr Heart Fail Rep. 2012;9:369–74.
82. Heidenreich PA, Trogdon JG, Khavjou OA, Butler J, Dracup K, Ezekowitz MD, et al. Forecasting the future of cardiovascular disease in the United States: a policy statement from the American Heart Association. Circulation. 2011;123:933–44.
83. Roger VL, Go AS, Lloyd-Jones DM, Benjamin EJ, Berry JD, Borden WB, et al. Executive summary: heart disease and stroke statistics – 2012 update: a report from the American Heart Association. Circulation. 2012;125:188–97.
84. Braunstein JB, Anderson GF, Gerstenblith G, Weller VV, Niefeld M, Herbert R, et al. Noncardiac comorbidity increases preventable hospitalizations and mortality among Medicare beneficiaries with chronic heart failure. J Am Coll Cardiol. 2003;42:1226–33.
85. Levy D, Kenchaiah S, Larson MG, Benjamin EJ, Kupka MJ, Ho KK, et al. Long-term trends in the incidence of and survival with heart failure. N Engl J Med. 2002;347:1397–402.
86. Fang J, Mensah GA, Croft JB, Keenan NL. Heart failure-related hospitalization in the U.S., 1979 to 2004. J Am Coll Cardiol. 2008;52:428–34.
87. Jugdutt BI. The continuing saga of aging and heart failure. Heart Fail Rev. 2012;17:529–30.
88. Roger VL, Weston SA, Redfield MM, Hellermann-Homan JP, Killian J, Yawn BP, et al. Trends in heart failure incidence and survival in a community-based population. JAMA. 2004;292:344–50.
89. Goldberg RJ, Glatfelter K, Burbank-Schmidt E, Farmer C, Spencer FA, Meyer T. Trends in mortality attributed to heart failure in Worcester, Massachusetts, 1992 to 2001. Am J Cardiol. 2005;95:1324–8.
90. Pocock SJ, Wang D, Pfeffer MA, Yusuf S, McMurray JJ, Swedberg KB, et al. Predictors of mortality and morbidity in patients with chronic heart failure. Eur Heart J. 2006;27:65–75.
91. Abraham WT, Fonarow GC, Albert NM, Stough WG, Gheorghiade M, Greenberg BH, et al. Predictors of in-hospital mortality in patients hospitalized for heart failure: insights from the Organized Program to Initiate Lifesaving Treatment in Hospitalized patients with Heart Failure (OPTIMIZE-HF). J Am Coll Cardiol. 2008;52:347–56.
92. Mogensen UM, Ersboll M, Andersen M, Andersson C, Hassager C, Torp-Pedersen C, et al. Clinical characteristics and major comorbidities in heart failure patients more than 85 years of age compared with younger age groups. Eur J Heart Fail. 2011;13:1216–23.
93. Komajda M, Hanon O, Hochadel M, Lopez-Sendon JL, Follath F, Ponikowski P, et al. Contemporary management of octogenarians hospitalized for heart failure in Europe: Euro Heart Failure Survey II. Eur Heart J. 2009;30:478–86.
94. Lazzarini V, Mentz RJ, Fiuzat M, Metra M, O'Connor CM. Heart failure in elderly patients: distinctive features and unresolved issues. Eur J Heart Fail. 2013;15:717–23.
95. Chaudhry SI, Wang Y, Gill TM, Krumholz HM. Geriatric conditions and subsequent mortality in older patients with heart failure. J Am Coll Cardiol. 2010;55:309–16.
96. Rutten FH, Grobbee DE, Hoes AW. Differences between general practitioners and cardiologists in diagnosis and management of heart failure: a survey in every-day practice. Eur J Heart Fail. 2003;5:337–44.
97. Manzano L, Escobar C, Cleland JG, Flather M. Diagnosis of elderly patients with heart failure. Eur J Heart Fail. 2012;14:1097–103.
98. Barseshet A, Shotan A, Cohen E, Garty M, Goldenberg I, Sandach A, et al. Predictors of long-term (4-year) mortality in elderly and young patients with acute heart failure. Eur J Heart Fail. 2010;12:833–40.
99. Satomura H, Wada H, Sakakura K, Kubo N, Ikeda N, Sugawara Y, et al. Congestive heart failure in the elderly: comparison between reduced ejection fraction and preserved ejection fraction. J Cardiol. 2012;59:215–9.
100. Oudejans I, Mosterd A, Bloemen JA, Valj MJ, van Velzen E, Wielders JP, et al. Clinical evaluation of geriatric outpatients with suspected heart failure: value of symptoms, signs, and additional tests. Eur J Heart Fail. 2011;13:518–27.

101. Oudejans I, Mosterd A, Zuithoff NP, Hoes AW. Comorbidity drives mortality in newly diagnosed heart failure: a study among geriatric outpatients. J Card Fail. 2012;18:47–52.
102. Boom NK, Lee DS, Tu JV. Comparison of processes of care and clinical outcomes for patients newly hospitalized for heart failure attended by different physician specialists. Am Heart J. 2012;163:252–9.
103. Fried LP, Tangen CM, Walston J, Newman AB, Hirsch C, Gottdiener J, et al. Frailty in older adults: evidence for a phenotype. J Gerontol A Biol Sci Med Sci. 2001;56:M146–56.
104. Newman AB, Gottdiener JS, McBurnie MA, Hirsch CH, Kop WJ, Tracy R, et al. Associations of clinical cardiovascular disease with frailty. J Gerontol A Biol Sci Med Sci. 2001;56:M 158–66.
105. Walston J, McBurnie MA, Newman A, Tracy RP, Kop WJ, Hirsch CH, et al. Frailty and activation of the inflammation and coagulation systems with and without clinical comorbidities: results from the Cardiovascular Health Study. Arch Intern Med. 2002;162:2333–41.
106. Murad K, Kitzman DW. Frailty and multiple comorbidities in the elderly patient with heart failure: implications for management. Heart Fail Rev. 2012;17:581–8.
107. Spencer FA, Meyer TE, Gore JM, Goldberg RJ. Heterogeneity in the management and outcomes of patients with acute myocardial infarction complicated with heart failure: the National Registry of Myocardial Infarction. Circulation. 2002;105:2605–10.
108. Steg PG, Dabbous OH, Feldman LJ, Cohen-Solal A, Aumont MC, Lopez-Sendón J, et al. Determinants and prognostic impact of heart failure complicating acute coronary syndromes: observations from the Global Registry of Acute Coronary Events (GRACE). Circulation. 2004;109:494–9.
109. Ezekowitz JA, Kaul P, Bakal JA, Armstrong PW, Welsh RC, McAlister FA. Declining in-hospital mortality and increasing heart failure incidence in elderly patients with first myocardial infarction. J Am Coll Cardiol. 2009;53:13–20.
110. Martinez-Sellés M, Doughty RN, Poppe K, Whalley GA, Earle N, Tribouilloy C, et al. Gender and survival in patients with heart failure: interactions with diabetes and aetiology. Results from the MAGGIC individual patient-analysis. Eur J Heart Fail. 2012;14:473–9.
111. Riedinger MS, Dracup KA, Brecht ML, SOLVD Investigators. Studies of left ventricular dysfunction. Am J Crit Care. 2002;11:211–9.
112. Gottlieb SS, Khatta M, Friedmann E, Einbinder L, Katzen S, Baker B, et al. The influence of age, gender, and race on the prevalence of depression in heart failure patients. J Am Coll Cardiol. 2004;43:1542–9.
113. Heo S, Moser DK, Wiedener J. Gender differences in the effects of physical and emotional symptoms on health-related quality of life in patients with heart failure. Eur J Cardiovasc Nurs. 2007;6:146–52.
114. Dunlay SM, Roger VL. Gender differences in the pathophysiology, clinical presentation, and outcomes of ischemic heart failure. Curr Heart Fail Rep. 2012;9:267–76.
115. Bahrami H, Kronmal R, Bluemke DA, Olson J, Shea S, Liu K, et al. Differences in the incidence of congestive heart failure by ethnicity: the multi-ethnic study of atherosclerosis. Arch Intern Med. 2008;168:2138–45.
116. Loehr LR, Rosamond WD, Chang PP, Folsom AR, Chambless LE. Heart failure incidence and survival (from the atherosclerosis risk in communities study). Am J Cardiol. 2008;101:1016–22.
117. Kalogeropoulos A, Georgiopoulou V, Kritchevsky SB, Psaty BM, Smith NL, Newman AB, et al. Epidemiology of incident heart failure in contemporary elderly cohort: the health, aging, and body composition study. Arch Intern Med. 2009;169:708–15.
118. Cuyjet AB, Akinboboye O. Acute heart failure in the African American patient. J Card Fail. 2014;20:533–40.
119. Dunlay SM, Weston SA, Jacobsen SJ, Roger VL. Risk factors for heart failure: a population-based case-control study. Am J Med. 2009;122:1023–8.
120. Bristow MR. Beta-adrenergic receptor blockade in chronic heart failure. Circulation. 2000;101:558–69.
121. Dutka DP, Camici PG. Hibernation and congestive heart failure. Heart Fail Rev. 2003;8:167–73.
122. Gheorghiade M, Vaduganathan M, Fonarow GC, Bonow RO. Rehospitalization for heart failure: problems and perspectives. J Am Coll Cardiol. 2013;61:391–403.
123. Teerlink JR, Alburikan K, Metra M, Rodgers JE. Acute decompensated heart failure update. Curr Cardiol Rev. 2015;11: 53–62.
124. Kociol RD, Pang PS, Gheorghiade M, Fonarow GC, O'Connor CM, Felker GM. Troponin elevation in heart failure prevalence, mechanisms, and clinical implications. J Am Coll Cardiol. 2010;56:1071–8.
125. Flaherty JD, Bax JJ, De Luca L, Rossi JS, Davidson CJ, Filippatos G, et al. Acute heart failure syndromes in patients with coronary artery disease, early assessment and treatment. J Am Coll Cardiol. 2009;53:254–63.
126. Arndt AK, MacRae CA. Genetic testing in cardiovascular diseases. Curr Opin Cardiol. 2014;29:235–40.
127. Skrzynia C, Berg JS, Willis MS, Jensen BC. Genetics and heart failure: a concise guide for the clinician. Curr Cardiol Rev. 2015;11:10–7.
128. Maron BJ, Ommen SR, Semsarian C, Spirito P, Olivotto I, Maron MS. Hypertrophic cardiomyopathy. Present and future, with translation into contemporary cardiovascular medicine. J Am Coll Cardiol. 2014;64:83–99.
129. Varnava AM, Elliott PM, Sharma S, McKenna WJ, Davies MJ. Hypertrophic cardiomyopathy: the interrelation of dissarray, fibrosis, and small vessel disease. Heart. 2000;84: 476–82.
130. The Task Force for the Diagnosis and Management of Hypertrophic Cardiomyopathy of the European Society of Cardiology (ESC), Elliott PM, Anastasakis A, Borger MA, Borggrefe M, Cecchi F, Charron P, et al. 2014 ESC guidelines on diagnosis and management of hypertrophic cardiomyopathy. Eur Heart J. 2014;35:2733–79.
131. Maron BJ, Maron MS. Hypertrophic cardiomyopathy. Lancet. 2013;381:242–55.
132. Chan RH, Maron BJ, Olivotto I, Pencina MJ, Assenza GE, Haas T, et al. Prognostic value of quantitative contrast-enhanced cardiovascular magnetic resonance for the evaluation of sudden death risk in patients with hypertrophic cardiomyopathy. Circulation. 2014;130:484–95.
133. Maron MS, Maron BJ, Harrigan C, Buros J, Gibson CM, Olivotto I, et al. Hypertrophic cardiomyopathy phenotype revisited after 50 years with cardiovascular magnetic resonance. J Am Coll Cardiol. 2009;54:220–8.
134. Maron BJ, Gardin JM, Flack JM, Gidding SS, Kurosaki TT, Bild DE. Prevalence of hypertrophic cardiomyopathy in a general population of young adults. Echocardiographic analysis of 4111 subjects in the CARDIA study. Coronary Artery Risk Development in (Young) Adults. Circulation. 1995;92:785–9.
135. Olivotti I, Maron MS, Adabaq AS, Casey SA, Vargiu D, Link MS, et al. Gender-related differences in the clinical presentation and outcome of hypertrophic cardiomyopathy. J Am Coll Cardiol. 2005;46:480–7.
136. Maron BJ, Maron MS, Semsarian C. Genetics of hypertrophic cardiomyopathy after 20 years: clinical perspectives. J Am Coll Cardiol. 2012;60:705–15.
137. Ingles J, Sarina T, Yeates L, Hunt L, Macchiocca I, McCormack L, et al. Clinical predictors of genetic testing outcomes in hypertrophic cardiomyopathy. Genet Med. 2013;15:972–9.

138. Maron BJ, Roberts WC, Arad M, Haas TS, Spirito P, Wright GB, et al. Clinical outcome and phenotypic expression in LAMP2 cardiomyopathy. JAMA. 2009;301:1253–9.
139. Arad M, Benson DW, Perez-Atayde AR, McKenna WJ, Sparks EA, Kanter RJ, et al. Constitutively active AMP kinase mutations cause glycogen storage disease mimicking hypertrophic cardiomyopathy. J Clin Invest. 2002;109:357–62.
140. Arad M, Moskowitz IP, Patel VV, Ahmad F, Perez-Atayde AR, Sawyer DB, et al. Transgenic mice overexpressing mutant PRKAG2 define the cause of Wolff-Parkinson-White syndrome in glycogen storage cardiomyopathy. Circulation. 2003;107: 2850–6.
141. Maron BJ, Rowin EJ, Casey SA, Haas TS, Chan RH, Udelson JE, et al. Risk stratification and outcome of patients with hypertrophic cardiomyopathy >= 60 years of age. Circulation. 2013;127:585–93.
142. Maron BJ, Carney KP, Lever HM, Lewis JF, Barac I, Casey SA, et al. Relationship of race to sudden death in competitive athletes with hypertrophic cardiomyopathy. J Am Coll Cardiol. 2003;41:974–80.
143. Maron BJ, Doerer JJ, Haas TS, Tierney DM, Mueller FO. Sudden deaths in young competitive athletes: analysis of 1866 deaths in the United States, 1980-2006. Circulation. 2009;119:1085–92.
144. Maron BJ, Rowin EJ, Casey SA, Lesser JR, Garberich RF, McGriff DM, et al. Hypertrophic cardiomyopathy in children, adolescents, and young adults associated with low cardiovascular mortality with contemporary management strategies. Circulation. 2016;133:62–73.
145. Maron BJ. The paradox of exercise. N Engl J Med. 2000;343:1409–11.
146. O'Mahony C, Jichi F, Pavlou M, Monserrat L, Anastasakis A, Rapezzi C, et al. A novel clinical risk prediction model for sudden cardiac death in hypertrophic cardiomyopathy. Eur Heart J. 2014;35:2010–20.
147. O'Mahony C, Tome-Esteban M, Lambiase PD, Pantazis A, Dickie S, McKenna WJ, et al. A validation study of the 2003 American College of Cardiology/European Society of Cardiology and 2011 American College of Cardiology Foundation/American Heart Association risk stratification and treatment algorithms for sudden cardiac death in patients with hypertrophic cardiomyopathy. Heart. 2013;99:534–41.
148. Spirito P, Autore C, Formisano F, Assenza GE, Biagini E, Haas TS. Risk of sudden death and outcome in patients with hypertrophic cardiomyopathy with benign presentation and without risk factors. Am J Cardiol. 2014;113:1550–5.
149. Maron BJ, Olivotto I, Zenovich AG, Link MS, Pandian NG, Kuvin JT, et al. Hypertrophic cardiomyopathy is predominantly a disease of left ventricular outflow tract obstruction. Circulation. 2006;114:2232–9.
150. Melacini P, Basso C, Angelini A, Calore C, Bobbo F, Tokajuk B, et al. Clinicopathological profiles of progressive heart failure in hypertrophic cardiomyopathy. Eur Heart J. 2010;31:2111–23.
151. Harris KM, Spirito P, Maron MS, Zenovich AG, Formisano F, Lesser JR, et al. Prevalence, clinical profile, and significance of left ventricular remodeling in the end-stage phase of hypertrophic cardiomyopathy. Circulation. 2006;114:216–25.
152. Maron MS, Kaismith BM, Udelson JE, Li W, DeNofrio D. Survival after cardiac transplantation in patients with hypertrophic cardiomyopathy. Circ Heart Fail. 2010;3:574–9.
153. Schinkel AF, Vriesendorp PA, Sijbrands EJ, Jordaens LJ, ten Cate FJ, Michels M. Outcome and complications after implantable cardioverter defibrillator therapy in hypertrophic cardiomyopathy: systematic review and metaanalysis. Circ Heart Fail. 2012;5:552–9.
154. Maron BJ, Shen WK, Link MS, Epstein AE, Almquist AK, Daubert JP, et al. Efficacy of implantable cardioverter-defibrillators for the prevention of sudden death in patients with hypertrophic cardiomyopathy. N Engl J Med. 2000;342:365–73.
155. Maron BJ, Spirito P, Shen WK, Haas TS, Formisano F, Link MS, et al. Implantable cardioverter-defibrillators and prevention of sudden cardiac death in hypertrophic cardiomyopathy. JAMA. 2007;298:405–12.
156. Christiaans I, van Engelen K, van Langen IM, Birnie E, Bonsel GJ, Elliott PM, et al. Risk stratification for sudden cardiac death in hypertrophic cardiomyopathy: systematic review of clinical risk markers. Europace. 2010;12:313–21.
157. Boriani G, Maron BJ, Shen WK, Spirito P. Prevention of sudden death in hypertrophic cardiomyopathy: but which defibrillator for which patient? Circulation. 2004;110:e438–42.
158. Lin G, Nishimura RA, Gersh BJ, Phil D, Ommen SR, Ackerman MJ, Brady PA. Device complications and inappropriate cardioverter defibrillator shocks in patients with hypertrophic cardiomyopathy. Heart. 2009;95:709–14.
159. Ammirati E, Contri R, Coppini R, Cecchi F, Frigerio M, Olivotto I. Pharmacological treatment of hypertrophic cardiomyopathy: current practice and novel perspectives. Eur J Heart Fail. 2016;18:1106–18. https://doi.org/10.1002/ejhf.541.
160. Nistri S, Olivotto I, Maron MS, Ferrantini C, Coppini R, Grifoni C, et al. Beta blockers for prevention of exercise-induced left ventricular outflow tract obstruction in patients with hypertrophic cardiomyopathy. Am J Cardiol. 2012;110:715–9.
161. Sherrid MV, Barac I, McKenna WJ, Elliott PM, Dickie S, Chojnowska L, et al. Multicenter study of the efficacy and safety of disopyramide in obstructive hypertrophic cardiomyopathy. J Am Coll Cardiol. 2005;45:1251–8.
162. Ommen SR, Maron BJ, Olivotto I, Maron MS, Cecchi F, Betocchi S, et al. Long-term effects of surgical septal myectomy on survival in patients with obstructive hypertrophic cardiomyopathy. J Am Coll Cardiol. 2005;46:470–6.
163. Valeti US, Nishimura RA, Holmes DR, Araoz PA, Glockner JF, Breen JF, et al. Comparison of surgical septal myectomy and alcohol septal ablation with cardiac magnetic resonance imaging in patients with hypertrophic obstructive cardiomyopathy. J Am Coll Cardiol. 2007;49:350–7.
164. Soraija P, Ommen SR, Holmes DR Jr, Dearani JA, Rihai CS, Gersh BJ, et al. Survival after alcohol septal ablation for obstructive hypertrophic cardiomyopathy. Circulation. 2012;126:2374–80
165. Agarwal S, Tuzcu EM, Desai MY, Smedira N, Lever HM, Lytle BW, et al. Updated meta-analysis of septal alcohol ablation versus myectomy for hypertrophic cardiomyopathy. J Am Coll Cardiol. 2010;55:823–34.
166. Noseworthy PA, Rosenberg MA, Fifer MA, Palacios IF, Lowry PA, Ruskin JN, et al. Ventricular arrhythmia following alcohol septal ablation for obstructive hypertrophic cardiomyopathy. Am J Cardiol. 2009;104:128–32.
167. Veselka J, Kvistholm-Jensen M, Liebregts M, Januska J, Krejci J, Bartel T, et al. Long-term clinical outcome after alcohol septal ablation for obstructive hypertrophic cardiomyopathy: results from the euro-ASA registry. Eur Heart J. 2016;37:1517–23.
168. Di Donna P, Olivotto I, Delcré SD, Caponi D, Scaglione M, Nault I, et al. Efficacy of catheter ablation or atrial fibrillation in hypertrophic cardiomyopathy: impact of age, atrial remodeling, and disease progression. Europace. 2010;12:347–55.
169. Kubo T, Kitaoka H, Okawa M, Hirota T, Hayato K, Yamasaki N, et al. Clinical impact of atrial fibrillation in patients with hypertrophic cardiomyopathy. Results from Kochi RYOMA study. Circ J. 2009;73:1599–605.
170. Maron BJ, Olivotto I, Bellone P, Conte MR, Cecchi F, Flygenring BP, et al. Clinical profile of stroke in 900 patients with hypertrophic cardiomyopathy. J Am Coll Cardiol. 2002;39:301–7.
171. Santangeli P, Di Biase L, Themistoclakis S, Ravieli A, Schweikert RA, Lakkireddy D, et al. Catheter ablation of atrial fibrillation

in hypertrophic cardiomyopathy: long-term outcomes and mechanisms of arrhythmia recurrence. Circ Arrythm Electrophysiol. 2013;6:1089–94.
172. Caforio AL, Mahon NG, Baig MK, Tona F, Murphy RT, Elliott PM, et al. Prospective familial assessment in dilated cardiomyopathy: cardiac autoantibodies predict disease development in asymptomatic relatives. Circulation. 2007;115:76–83.
173. McNally EM, Golbus JR, Puckelwartz MJ. Genetic mutations and mechanisms in dilated cardiomyopathy. J Clin Invest. 2013;123:19–26.
174. Pinto YM, Elliott PM, Arbustini E, Adler Y, Anastasakis A, Böhm M, et al. Proposal for a revised definition of dilated cardiomyopathy, hypokinetic non-dilated cardiomyopathy, and its implications for clinical practice: a position statement of the ESC working group on myocardial and pericardial diseases. Eur Heart J. 2016;37:1850–8. https://doi.org/10.1093/eurheartj/ehv727.
175. Mahon NG, Madden BP, Caforio ALP, Elliott PM, Haven AJ, Keogh BE, et al. Immunohistologic evidence of myocardial disease in apparently healthy relatives of patients with dilated cardiomyopathy. J Am Coll Cardiol. 2002;39:455–62.
176. Burkett EL, Hershberger RE. Clinical and genetic issues in familial dilated cardiomyopathy. J Am Coll Cardiol. 2005;45:969–81.
177. Petretta M, Pirozzi F, Sasso L, Paglia A, Bonaduce D. Review and metaanalysis of the frequency of familial dilated cardiomyopathy. Am J Cardiol. 2011;108:1171–6.
178. Herman DS, Lam L, Taylor MR, Teekakirikul P, Christodoulou D, Conner L, et al. Truncations of titin causing dilated cardiomyopathy. N Engl J Med. 2012;366:619–28.
179. Hershberger RE, Siegfried JD. Update 2011; clinical and genetic issues in familial dilated cardiomyopathy. J Am Coll Cardiol. 2011;57:1641–9.
180. Elliott P, O'Mahoney C, Syrris P, Evans A, Rivera Sorensen C, Sheppard MN, et al. Prevalence of desmosomal protein gene mutations in patients with dilated cardiomyopathy. Circ Cardiovasc Genet. 2010;3:314–22.
181. Akinrinade O, Ollila L, Vattulainen S, Tallila J, Gentile M, Salmenperä P, et al. Genetics and genotype-phenotype correlations in Finnish patients with dilated cardiomyopathy. Eur Heart J. 2015;36:2327–37.
182. Haas J, Frese KS, Peil B, Kloos W, Keller A, Nietsch R. Atlas of the clinical genetics of human dilated cardiomyopathy. Eur Heart J. 2015;36:1123–35.
183. Colucci WS, Kolias TJ, Adams KF, Armstrong WF, Ghali JK, Gottlieb SS, et al. Metoprolol reverses left ventricular remodeling in patients with asymptomatic systolic dysfunction: the reversal of ventricular remodeling with Toprol-XL (REVERT) trial. Circulation. 2007;116:49–56.
184. Zannad F, McMurray JJ, Krum H, van Veldhuisen DJ, Swedberg K, Shi H, et al. Eplerenone in patients with systolic heart failure and mild symptoms. N Engl J Med. 2011;364:11–21.
185. Pitt B, Zannad F, Remme WJ, Cody R, Castaigne A, Perez A, et al. The effect of spironolactone on morbidity and mortality in patients with severe heart failure. Randomized Aldactone Evaluation Study Investigators. N Engl J Med. 1999;341: 709–17.
186. Epstein AE. Benefits of the implantable cardioverter-defibrillator. J Am Coll Cardiol. 2008;52:1122–7.
187. The Task Force for the Management of Patients with Ventricular Arrhythmias and the Prevention of Sudden Cardiac Death of the European Society of Cardiology (ESC), Priori SG, Blomström-Lundqvist C, Mazzanti A, Blom N, Borggrefe M, Camm J, et al. 2015 ESC guidelines for the management of patients with ventricular arrhythmias and the prevention of sudden cardiac death. Eur Heart J. 2015;36:2793–867.
188. Dec GW, Fuster V. Idiopathic dilated cardiomyopathy. N Engl J Med. 1994;331:1564–75.
189. Gopinathannair R, Sullivan R, Olshansky B. Tachycardia-mediated cardiomyopathy: recognition and management. Curr Heart Fail Rep. 2009;6:257–64.
190. Gianni M, Dentali F, Grandi AM, Sumner G, Hiralal R, Lonn E. Apical ballooning syndrome or takotsubo cardiomyopathy: a systematic review. Eur Heart J. 2006;27:1523–9.
191. Bybee KA, Prasad A. Stress-related cardiomyopathy syndromes. Circulation. 2008;118:397–409.
192. Sharkey SW, Windenburg DC, Lesser JR, Maron MS, Hauser RG, Lesser JN, et al. Natural history and expansive clinical profile of stress (tako-tsubo) cardiomyopathy. J Am Coll Cardiol. 2010;55:333–41.
193. Booysen HL, Norton GR, Opie LH, Woodiwiss AJ. Reverse chamber remodeling following adrenergic-induced advanced cardiac dilatation and pump dysfunction. Basic Res Cardiol. 2012;107:238. https://doi.org/10.1007/s00395-011-0200.
194. Templin C, Napp C, Ghadri JR. Takotsubo syndrome. Underdiagnosed, underestimated, but understood? J Am Coll Cardiol. 2016;67:1937–40.
195. Ghadri JR, Ruschitzka F, Luscher TF, Templin C. Takotsubo cardiomyopathy: still much more to learn. Heart. 2014;100:1804–12.
196. Tornvall P, Collste O, Ehrenborg E, Järnbert-Pettersson H. A case-control study of risk markers and mortality in Takotsubo stress cardiomyopathy. J Am Coll Cardiol. 2016;67:1931–6.
197. George A, Figueredo VM. Alcoholic cardiomyopathy: a review. J Cardiac Fail. 2011;17:844–9.
198. Laonigro J, Correale M, Di Biase M, Altomare E. Alcohol abuse and heart failure. Eur J Heart Fail. 2009;11:453–62.
199. Piano MR. Alcoholic cardiomyopathy: incidence, clinical characteristics, and pathophysiology. Chest. 2002;121:1638–50.
200. Faris RF, Henein MY, Coats AJ. Influence of gender and reported alcohol intake on mortality in nonischemic dilated cardiomyopathy. Heart Dis. 2003;5:89–94.
201. Urbano-Marquez A, Estruch R, Navarro-Lopez F, Grau JM, Mont L, Rubin E. The effects of alcoholism on skeletal and cardiac muscle. N Engl J Med. 1989;320:409–15.
202. Lazarevic AM, Nakatani S, Neskovic AN, Marinkovic J, Yasumura Y, Stojicic D, et al. Early changes in left ventricular function in chronic asymptomatic alcoholics: relation to the duration of heavy drinking. J Am Coll Cardiol. 2000;35:1599–606.
203. Telli ML, Hunt SA, Carlson RW, Guardino AE. Trastuzumab-related cardiotoxicity: calling into question the concept of reversibility. J Clin Oncol. 2007;25:3525–33.
204. Ewer MS, Vootietich MT, Durand JB, Woods ML, Davis JR, Valero VL, et al. Reversibility of trastuzumab-related cardiotoxicity: new insights based on clinical course and response to medical treatment. J Clin Oncol. 2009;23:7820–6.
205. Kindermann I, Barth C, Mahfoud F, Ukena C, Lenski M, Yilmaz A, et al. Update on myocarditis. J Am Coll Cardiol. 2012;59:779–92.
206. Rose NR. Myocarditis: infection versus autoimmunity. J Clin Immunol. 2009;29:730–7.
207. Lurz P, Luecke C, Eitel I, Föhrenbach F, Frank C, Grothoff M, et al. Comprehensive cardiac magnetic resonance imaging in patients with suspected myocarditis. J Am Coll Cardiol. 2016;67:1800–11.
208. Dec GW. How should we diagnose myocarditis and is its recognition really clinically relevant? J. Am Coll Cardiol. 2016;67:1812–4.
209. Cooper LT, Baughman KL, Feldman AM, Frustaci A, Jessup M, Kuhl U, et al. The role of endomyocardial biopsy in the management of cardiovascular disease: a scientific statement from the American Heart Association, The American College of Cardiology, and the European Society of Cardiology. Endorsed by the Heart Failure Society of America and the heart failure Association of the European Society of Cardiology. J Am Coll Cardiol. 2007;50:1914–31.
210. Caforie ALP, Pankuweit S, Arbustini E, Basso C, Gimeno-Blanes J, Felix SB, et al. Current state of knowledge on aetiology,

diagnosis, management, and therapy of myocarditis: a position statement of the European Society of Cardiology Working Group on Myocardial and Pericardial diseases. Eur Heart J. 2013;34:2636–48.
211. Ammash NM, Seward JB, Bailey KR, Edwards WD, Tajik AJ. Clinical profile and outcome of idiopathic restrictive cardiomyopathy. Circulation. 2000;101:2490–6.
212. Sen-Chowdhry S, Syrris P, McKenna WJ. Genetics of restrictive cardiomyopathy. Heart Fail Clin. 2010;6:179–86.
213. Dalakas MC, Park KY, Semino-Mora C, Lee HS, Sivakumar K, Goldfarb LG. Desmin myopathy, a skeletal myopathy with cardiomyopathy caused by mutations in the desmin gene. N Engl J Med. 2000;342:770–80.
214. Garcia MJ. Constrictive pericarditis versus restrictive cardiomyopathy. J Am Coll Cardiol. 2016;67:2061–76.
215. Angelini A, Calzolari V, Thiene G, Boffa GM, Valente M, Dallento L, et al. Morphologic spectrum of primary restrictive cardiomyopathy. Am J Cardiol. 1997;80:1046–50.
216. Ware SM, Quinn ME, Ballard ET, Miller E, Uzark K, Spicer RL. Pediatric restrictive cardiomyopathy associated with a mutation in beta-myosin heavy chain. Clin Genet. 2008;73:165–70.
217. Bograd AJ, Mital S, Schwarzenberger JC, Mosca RS, Quaegebeur JM, Addonizio LJ, et al. Twenty-year experience with heart transplantation for infants and children with restrictive cardiomyopathy: 1986-2006. Am J Transplant. 2008;8:201–7.
218. Yacoub S, Kotit S, Mocumbi AO, Yacoub MH. Neglected diseases in cardiology: a call for urgent action. Nat Clin Pract Cardiovasc Med. 2009;5:176–7.
219. Syed IS, Martinez MW, Feng DL, Glockner JF. Cardiac magnetic resonance imaging of eosinophilic endomyocardial disease. Int J Cardiol. 2008;126:e50–2.
220. Dubrey SW, Cha K, Anderson J, Chamarthi B, Reisinger J, Skinner M, et al. The clinical features of immunoglobulin light-chain (AL) amyloidosis with heart involvement. QJM. 1998;91:141–57.
221. Gertz MA, Benson MD, Dyck PJ, Grogan M, Coelho T, Cruz M, et al. Diagnosis, prognosis, and therapy of transthyretin amyloidosis. J Am Coll Cardiol. 2015;66:2451–66.
222. Quarta CC, Solomon SD, Uraizee I, Kruger J, Longhi S, Ferlito M, et al. Left ventricular structure and function in transthyretin-related versus light-chain cardiac amyloidosis. Circulation. 2014;129:1840–9.
223. Dubrey SW. Amyloid heart disease: a brief review of treatment options. Postgrad Med J. 2012;88:700–5.
224. Jaccard A, Comenzo RL, Hari P, Hawkins PN, Roussel M, Morel P, et al. Efficacy of bortezomib, cyclophosphamide and dexamethasone in treatment-naïve patients with high-risk cardiac AL amyloidosis (Mayo Clinic Stage III). Haematologica. 2014;99:1479–85.
225. Kristen AV, Dengler TJ, Hagenbart U, Schonland SO, Goldschmidt H, Sack FU, et al. Prophylactic implantation of cardioverter-defibrillator in patients with severe cardiac amyloidosis and high risk for sudden cardiac death. Heart Rhythm. 2008;5:235–40.
226. Varr BC, Zarafshar S, Coakley T, Liedtke M, Lafavette RA, Arai S, et al. Implantable cardioverter-defibrillator placement in patients with cardiac amyloidosis. Heart Rhythm. 2014;11:158–62.
227. Cechetti G, Binda A, Piperno A, Nador F, Fargion S, Fiorelli G. Cardiac alterations in 36 consecutive patients with idiopathic haemochromatosis: polygraphic and echocardiographic evaluation. Eur Heart J. 1991;12:224–30.
228. Alexander J, Kowdley KV. Hereditary hemochromatosis: genetics, pathogenesis, and clinical management. Ann Hepatol. 2005;4:240–7.
229. Brissot P. Optimizing the diagnosis and the treatment of iron overload diseases. Expert Rev Gastroenterol Hepatol. 2016;10:359–70.
230. Durr A, Cossee M, Agid Y, Campuzano V, Mignard C, Penet C, et al. Clinical and genetic abnormalities in patients with Friedreich's ataxia. N Engl J Med. 1996;335:1169–75.
231. Marcus FI, McKenna WJ, Sherrill D, Basso C, Bauce C, Bluemke A, et al. Diagnosis of arrhythmogenic right ventricular cardiomyopathy/dysplasia: proposed modification of the task force criteria. Eur Heart J. 2010;31:806–14.
232. Sen-Chowdhry S, Morgan RD, Chambers JC, McKenna WJ. Arrhytmogenic cardiomyopathy: etiology, diagnosis, and treatment. Annu Rev Med. 2010;61:233–53.
233. Tabib A, Loire R, Chalabreysse L, Meyronnet D, Miras A, Malicier D, et al. Circumstances of death and gross and microscopic observations in a series of 200 cases of sudden death associated with arrhythmogenic right ventricular cardiomyopathy and/or dysplasia. Circulation. 2003;108:3000–5.
234. Sen-Chowdhry S, Syrris P, Ward D, Asimaki A, Sevdalis E, McKenna WJ. Clinical and genetic characterization of families with arrhythmogenic right ventricular dysplasia/cardiomyopathy provides novel insights into patterns of disease expression. Circulation. 2007;115:1710–20.
235. Peters S, Trummel M, Denecke S, Koehler B. Results of ajmaline testing in patients with arrhythmogenic right ventricular dysplasia-cardiomyopathy. Int J Cardiol. 2004;95:499–501.
236. Meyers DE, Basha HI, Koenig HK. Mitochondrial cardiomyopathy. Pathophysiology, diagnosis and management. Tex Heart Inst J. 2013;40:385–94.
237. Jenni R, Oechslin EN, van der Loo B. Isolated ventricular non-compaction of the myocardium in adults. Heart. 2007;93:11–5.
238. Oechslin EN, Attenhofer JCH, Rojas JR, Kaufmann PA, Jenni R. Long-term follow-up of 34 adults with isolated left ventricular non-compaction: a distinct cardiomyopathy with poor prognosis. J Am Coll Cardiol. 2000;36:493–500.
239. Arbustini E, Weidemann F, Hall JL. Left ventricular noncompaction. A distinct cardiomyopathy or a trait shared by different cardiac diseases. J Am Coll Cardiol. 2014;64:1840–50.
240. Oechslin E, Jenni R. Left ventricular non-compaction revisited: a distinct phenotype with genetic heterogeneity? Eur Heart J. 2011;32:1446–56.
241. Gati S, Chandra N, Bennett RL, Reed M, Kervio G, Panoulas VF, et al. Increased left ventricular trabeculation in highly trained athletes: do we need more stringent criteria for the diagnosis of left ventricular non-compaction in athletes? Heart. 2013;99:401–8.
242. Clarke SL, Bowron A, Gonzalez IL, Groves SJ, Newbury-Ecob R, Clayton N, et al. Barth syndrome. Orphanet J Rare Dis. 2013;8:23. https://doi.org/10.1186/1750-1172-8-23.
243. Luxan G, Casanova JC, Martinez-Poveda B, Prados B, D'Amaton G, MacGrogan D, et al. Mutations in the NOTCH pathway regulator MIB 1 cause left ventricular non-compaction cardiomyopathy. Nat Med. 2013;19:193–201.
244. Udeoli DU, Philip KJ, Morrissey RP, Phan A, Schwarz ER. Left-ventricular non-compaction cardiomyopathy: updated review. Ther Adv Cardiovasc Dis. 2013;7:260–73.
245. Moons P, Engelfriet P, Kaemmerer H, Meijboom FJ, Oechslin E, Mulder BJ, et al. Delivery of care for adult patients with congenital heart disease in Europe: results from the Euro Heart Survey. Eur Heart J. 2006;27:1324–30.
246. Warnes CA, Williams RG, Bashore TM, Child JS, Connolly HM, Dearani JA, et al. ACC/AHA 2008 guidelines for the management of adults with congenital heart disease: a report of the American college of cardiology/American Heart Association Task Force on Practice Guidelines (writing committee to develop guidelines on the management of adults with congenital heart disease). Circulation. 2008;118:e714–833.
247. Khairy P, Ionescu-Ittu R, Mackie AS, Abrahamowicz M, Pilote L, Marelli AJ. Changing mortality in congenital heart disease. J Am Coll Cardiol. 2010;56:1149–57.

248. Norozi K, Wessel A, Alpers V, Arnhold JO, Gever S, Zoege M, et al. Incidence and risk distribution of heart failure in adolescents and adults with congenital heart disease after cardiac surgery. Am J Cardiol. 2006;97:1238–43.
249. Zomer AC, Vaartjes I, Uiterwaal CS, van der Velde ET, van der Merkhof LF, Baur LH, et al. Circumstances of death in adult congenital heart diseases. Int J Cardiol. 2012;154:168–72.
250. Oechslin EN, Harrison DA, Connelly MS, Webb GD, Siu SC. Mode of death in adults with congenital heart disease. Am J Cardiol. 2000;86:1111–6.
251. Tutarel O, Kempny A, Alonso-Gonzalez R, Jabbour R, Li W, Uebing A, et al. Congenital heart disease beyond the age of 60: emergence of a new population with high resource utilization, high morbidity, and high mortality. Eur Heart J. 2014;35:725–32.
252. Tzemos N, Therrien J, Yip J, Thanassoulis G, Tremblay S, Jamorski MT, et al. Outcomes in adults with bicuspid aortic valves. JAMA. 2008;300:1317–25.
253. Khairy P, Poirier N, Mercier LA. Univentricular heart. Circulation. 2007;115:800–12.
254. Khairy P, Fernandes SM, Mayer JE Jr, Triedman JK, Walsh EP, Lock JE, et al. Long-term survival, modes of death, and predictors of mortality in patients with Fontan surgery. Circulation. 2008;117:85–92.
255. Van der Bom T, Winter MM, Bouma BJ, Groenink M, Vliegen HW, Pieper PG, et al. Rationale and design of a trial on the effect of angiotensin II receptor blockers on the function of the systemic right ventricle. Am Heart J. 2010;160:812–8.
256. Koyak Z, de Groot JR, van Velder IC, Bouma BJ, van Dessel PF, Budts W, et al. Implantable cardioverter defibrillator therapy in adults with congenital heart disease: who is at risk at shocks. Circ Arrhythm Electrophysiol. 2012;5:101–10.
257. Ghai A, Silversides C, Harris L, Webb GD, Siu SC, Therrien J. Left ventricular dysfunction is a risk factor for sudden cardiac death in adults late after repair of tetralogy of Fallot. J Am Coll Cardiol. 2002;40:1675–80.
258. Vehmeijer JT, Brouwe TF, Limpens J, Knops RE, Bouma BJ, Mulder BJ. Implantable cardioverter-defibrillators in adults with congenital heart disease: a systematic review and meta-analysis. Eur Heart J. 2016;37:1439–48.
259. Budts W, Roos-Hesselink J, Rädle-Hurst T, Eicken A, McDonagh TA, Lambrinou E, et al. Treatment of heart failure in adult congenital heart disease: a position paper of the Working Group of Grown-Up Congenital Heart Disease and the Heart Failure Association of the European Society of Cardiology. Eur Heart J. 2016;37:1419–27.
260. Supino PG, Borer JS, Preibisz J, Bornstein A. The epidemiology of valvular heart disease: a growing public health problem. Heart Fail Clin. 2006;2:379–93.
261. Otto CM, Kuusisto J, Reichenbach DD, Gown AM, O'Brien KD. Characterization of the early lesion of 'degenerative' valvular aortic stenosis. Histological and immunohistochemical studies. Circulation. 1994;90:844–53.
262. Rajamannan NM, Otto CM. Targeted therapy to prevent progression of calcific aortic stenosis. Circulation. 2004;110:1180–2.
263. Rajappan K, Rimoldi OE, Camici PG, Bellenger NM, Pennell DJ, Sheridan DJ. Functional changes in coronary microcirculation after valve replacement in patients with aortic stenosis. Circulation. 2003;107:3170–5.
264. Bax JJ, Delgado V, Bapat V, Baumgartner H, Collet JP, Erbel R, et al. Open issues in transcatheter aortic valve implantation. Part 1: patient selection and treatment strategy for transcatheter aortic valve implantation. Eur Heart J. 2014;35:2627–38.
265. Bax JJ, Delgado V, Bapat V, Baumgartner H, Collet JP, Erbel R, et al. Open issues in transcatheter aortic valve implantation. Part 2: procedural issues and outcomes after transcatheter aortic valve implantation. Eur Heart J. 2014;35:2639–54.
266. Enriquez-Sarano M, Talik AJ. Clinical practice. Aortic regurgitation. N Engl J Med. 2004;35:1539–46.
267. Bekeredjian R, Grayburn PA. Valvular heart disease: aortic regurgitation. Circulation. 2005;112:125–34.
268. Elder DH, Szwejkowski BR, Libianto R, Nadir A, Pauriah M, Rekhrajv S, et al. The impact of renin-angiotensin-aldosterone system blockade on heart failure outcomes and mortality in patients identified to have aortic regurgitation: a large population cohort study. J Am Coll Cardiol. 2011;58:2084–91.
269. Hamirani YS, Dieti CA, Voyies VV, Peralta M, Begay D, Raizada V. Acute aortic regurgitation. Circulation. 2012;126:1121–6.
270. Nishimura RA, Otto CM, Bonow RO, Carabello BA, Erwin JP 3rd, Guyton RA, et al. 2014 AHA/ACC guideline for the management of patients with valvular heart disease: executive summary: a report of the American College of Cardiology/American Heart Association Task Force on Practice Guidelines. J Am Coll Cardiol. 2014;63:2438–88.
271. Joint Task Force on the Management of Valvular Heart Disease of the European Society of Cardiology (ESC), European Association for Cardio-Thoracic Surgery (EACTS), Vahanian A, Alfieri O, Andreotti F, Antunes MJ, Baron-Esquivas G, Baumgartner H, et al. Guidelines on the management of valvular heart disease (version 2012). Eur Heart J. 2012;33:2451–99.
272. Carabello BA. The current therapy for mitral regurgitation. J Am Coll Cardiol. 2008,52:319–26.
273. Asgar AW, Mack MJ, Stone GW. Secondary mitral regurgitation in heart failure: pathophysiology, prognosis, and therapeutic considerations. J Am Coll Cardiol. 2015;65:1231–48.
274. Avierinos JV, Gerah BJ, Melton LJ 3rd, Bailey KR, Shub C, Nishimura RA, et al. Natural history of asymptomatic mitral valve prolapse in the community. Circulation. 2002;106:1355–61.
275. Gustafsson BI, Hauso O, Drozdov I, Kidd M, Modlin IM. Carcinoid heart disease. Int J Cardiol. 2008;129:318–24.
276. Taramasso M, Vanermen H, Maisano F, Guidott A, La Canna G, Alfieri O. The growing clinical importance of secondary tricuspid regurgitation. J Am Coll Cardiol. 2012;59:703–10.
277. Shah PM, Raney AA. Tricuspid valve disease. Curr Probl Cardiol. 2008;33:47–84.
278. Rodes-Cabau J, Taramasso M, O'Gara PT. Diagnosis and treatment of tricuspid valve disease: current and future perspectives. Lancet. 2016;38:2431–42. https://doi.org/10.1016/50140-6736(16)00740-6.
279. Nath J, Foster E, Heidenreich PA. Impact of tricuspid regurgitation on long-term survival. J Am Coll Cardiol. 2004;43:405–9.
280. Waller BF, Howard J, Fess S. Pathology of pulmonic valve stenosis and pure regurgitation. Clin Cardiol. 1995;18:45–50.
281. Shin HJ, Kim YH, Ko JK, Park IS, Seo DM. Outcomes of mechanical valves in the pulmonic position in patients with congenital heart diseases over a 20-year period. Ann Thorac Surg. 2013;95(4):1367–71.

Part II

Pathophysiology

Inter- and Intracellular Mechanisms of Cardiac Remodeling, Hypertrophy and Dysfunction

2

Joerg Heineke, Tibor Kempf, and Johann Bauersachs

2.1 Patterns of Cardiac Remodeling and Growth as Underlying Mechanism of Heart Failure

The heart maintains the capability to change its size and shape throughout live. While the postnatal growth towards adulthood entails a several fold increase in heart size after birth, even in adulthood the myocardium responds to environmental stimulation by a change in its size, i.e. by growing in response to an increased demand, or shrinking after unloading (Fig. 2.1). In this regard it was estimated that the adult heart is able to exert a growth range of at least 100% [1]. The postnatal growth of the heart is mainly the result of hypertrophy, i.e. an increase in size of cardiac myocytes, which largely lose their ability to divide within the first week after birth [2]. Cardiac hypertrophy during physiological states such as postnatal growth, pregnancy or regular strenuous exercise such as in professional athletes is termed physiological hypertrophy. In contrast, hypertrophy occurring in response to pathological stimulation like for example chronic arterial hypertension, aortic stenosis or myocardial infarction is labelled as pathological hypertrophy [2]. While physiological hypertrophy in adulthood is not associated with cardiac dysfunction and is fully reversible, pathological hypertrophy is often coupled with diastolic or systolic ventricular dysfunction and is only partially reversible. On the microscopic and molecular level beside cardiomyocyte enlargement, pathological hypertrophy is associated with cell death, interstitial and perivascular fibrosis, abnormalities in cardiac excitation contraction coupling and a change in cellular metabolism, neither of which is found in physiological myocardial growth [2, 3]. Cardiomyocyte hypertrophy is an integral part of a process called cardiac remodeling, a term originally used to describe the ventricular alterations after myocardial infarction (including for example the formation and extension of the scar region as well as hypertrophy and fibrosis of the remaining myocardium), but is now used more broadly to describe the changes of cardiac size and shape in response to a range of pathological stimuli (like cardiac valve disease, arterial hypertension or genetic mutations).

2.1.1 Concentric Versus Eccentric Ventricular Remodeling

Ventricular remodeling during pathological stimulation follows either a concentric pattern (called concentric hypertrophy, if associated with an overall increased heart weight) or an eccentric pattern (again termed eccentric hypertrophy if associated with a heart weight increase) [4]. Concentric cardiac remodeling occurs as response to cardiac pressure overload (like aortic stenosis or arterial hypertension) or as consequence of a hypertrophic cardiomyopathy (HCM) producing gene mutation. Its characteristic feature is a decrease in cardiac chamber volume and an increase in wall thickness (i.e. a decreased chamber size/wall thickness ratio). At the cellular level the cardiac myocytes become thickened by adding new sarcomere units in parallel to the pre-existing ones. Eccentric hypertrophy, in contrast, leads to an increased chamber volume, thinning of ventricular walls (i.e. increased chamber size/wall thickness ratio), cardiomyocyte elongation and addition of new sarcomeres in series at both ends of the rod shaped cardiomyocytes. Interestingly, in patients with concentric hypertrophy due to aortic stenosis or HCM, disease progression often triggers transition towards eccentric remodeling and cardiac dilation. Whether progression to eccentric remodeling occurs in concentric hypertrophy due to chronic arterial hypertension is still a matter of debate, since adequate longitudinal studies are lacking [5]. Concentric cardiac hypertrophy is the predominant type of remodeling in patients suffering from heart failure with preserved ejection fraction (EF > 50% and predominant

J. Heineke (✉) · T. Kempf · J. Bauersachs (✉)
Medizinische Hochschule Hannover, Klinik für Kardiologie und Angiologie, Hannover, Germany
e-mail: Heineke.Joerg@Mh-Hannover.de; Joerg.Heineke@medma.uni-heidelberg.de
Bauersachs.Johann@Mh-Hannover.de

D. S. Feldman, P. Mohacsi (eds.), *Heart Failure*, Cardiovascular Medicine, https://doi.org/10.1007/978-3-319-98184-0_2

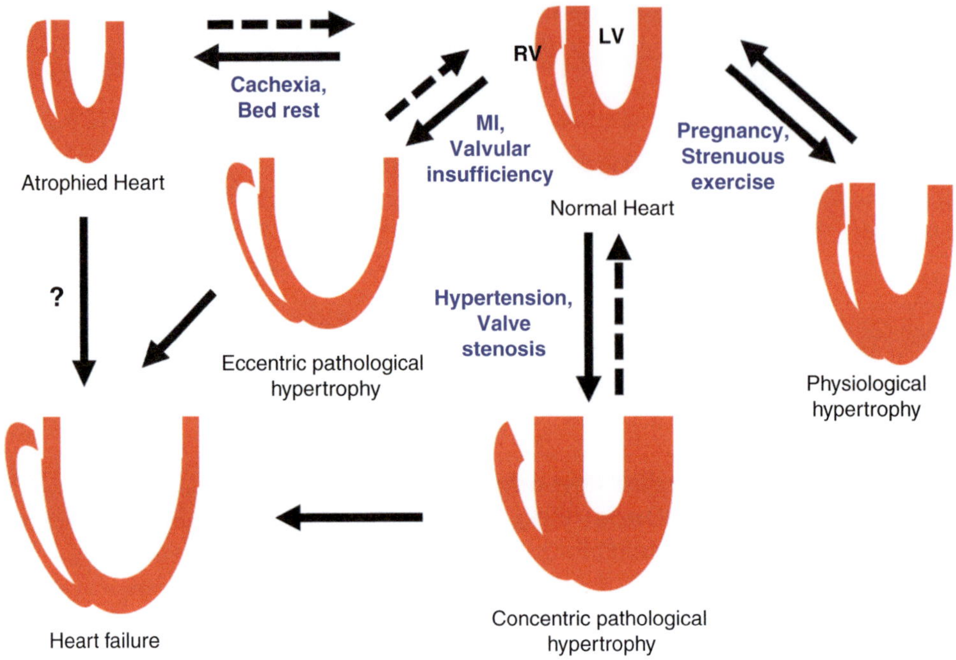

Fig. 2.1 Patterns of cardiac remodeling as induced by distinct physiological or pathological stimuli (in blue letters). Details are described in the text

diastolic dysfunction), although up to 12% of these patients exert an eccentric type of ventricular remodeling [6]. Heart failure patients with preserved ejection fraction and eccentric remodeling tended to have a lower EF and therefore might constitute a different subset of patients in this group that are pathophysiologically more similar to heart failure patients with reduced ejection fraction, which typically show eccentric ventricular remodeling [6].

Beside the difference in sarcomeric assembly pattern, subcellular mechanisms of eccentric and concentric cardiac remodeling remain poorly defined. A recent landmark paper by Jeff Molkentin and his group suggested that at least in patients with genetic cardiomyopathy the form of ventricular remodeling might be determined by the extent of internally generated tension by the contractile apparatus: In this comprehensive model, gene mutations that for example increase the calcium sensitivity (i.e. the calcium binding) of troponin C (like the L48Q mutation) and thereby lead to prolonged generation of tension trigger concentric hypertrophy, while mutations leading to reduced tension, like for example the I61Q troponin C mutation (associated with reduced calcium sensitivity) induce eccentric remodeling [7]. A specific algorithm was developed allowing the prediction of concentric or eccentric remodeling based on integrated tension values and was successfully tested for 11 different mouse genotypes as well as 4 human mutations using iPS cell technology. In terms of signal transduction, it was suggested that the MAP Kinase ERK1/2 triggers concentric while ERK5 and cardiotrophin/gp130 induce eccentric remodeling [7].

2.1.2 Reverse Remodeling

Reverse remodeling is defined as partial or full recovery of ventricular geometry and function upon reversal of pathological stimulation and/or upon initiation of (medical) treatment [8]. For example, replacement of the aortic valve in patients with aortic stenosis leads to an improvement of left ventricular function and a reduction in cardiac hypertrophy to a degree that depends mainly on the stage of disease before surgery [9, 10]. Similarly, abstinence from alcohol or heart rate control lead to a significant increase (but not normalization) of left ventricular function in alcoholic or tachycardia induced cardiomyopathy, respectively [8].

Medical treatment to alleviate the action of neurohormones (such as angiotensin II, epinephrine, norepinephrine or aldosterone) on the heart also partially reverses the remodeling processes during heart failure: Angiotensin receptor blockade by candesartan, for example was associated with a significant increase in left ventricular ejection fraction in echocardiography (by +24% in the candesartan group compared to +8% in the placebo group) within only 6 months. Beta-receptor blockers are viewed as having the strongest potency to induce reverse remodeling, as Metoprolol Succinate for instance reduced enddiastolic cardiac dilation by 16% and improved the ejection fraction by 27% in a MRI substudy of the double-blind, randomized, placebo controlled MERIT-HF trial of heart failure patients with an ejection fraction ≤40%.

The advent of left ventricular assist devices (LVADs) enabled ventricular unloading of the LV chamber well beyond what is possible through pharmacological interventions. LVADs are implanted in patients with endstage heart failure as bridge to heart transplant, but also as destination therapy, when patients live with the device for multiple years a rather normal life. Rarely (reportedly in 4–18.5% of the cases), the ventricle even recovers to such an extent that the LVAD can be explanted. The severely ill patients that receive an LVAD exert a strongly reduced mortality rate versus pure medical treatment [11]. In addition, LVAD therapy may go along with markedly improved (but most often not normalized) left ventricular function and reduced dilatation [12]. Because left ventricular myocardial tissue becomes available during LVAD implantation and during its later explantation due to cardiac transplant or myocardial recovery, reverse remodeling could be studied for the first time on the histological and molecular level in paired cardiac patients samples (before and after LVAD therapy) [13]. These studies revealed a marked reduction (but again no normalization) of cardiomyocyte hypertrophy, as revealed by a reduced cardiomyocyte thickness, length and volume in isolated human cardiomyocytes after LVAD explantation [12]. According to a recent study, no cardiomyocyte atrophy develops [14]. In addition, an increase in cardiomyocyte proliferation and cardiac angiogenesis was noted in response to LVAD therapy [15, 16]. On the more cellular level an increase in autophagy, an improvement of metabolic function (with increased substrate oxidation and ATP production), more effective excitation-contraction coupling (with enhanced expression of the sarcoplasmatic calcium pump SERCA2a and restoration of T-tubule architecture) as well as an elevated abundance of contractile sarcomeric proteins has been observed [13]. Paradoxically, although still somewhat controversial, there appears to be an increase in interstitial myocardial fibrosis during LVAD therapy [16]. Clearly, more needs to be learned about the molecular mechanisms of reverse remodeling with the aim to develop novel therapeutic strategies fostering complete myocardial recovery in patients suffering from heart failure.

2.1.3 Cardiac Atrophy

Decrease in heart weight and cardiac myocyte size below the values observed in healthy individuals is termed cardiac or cardiomyocyte atrophy, respectively. Cardiac atrophy occurs for example in space during weightlessness or during prolonged bed rest. Twelve weeks of bed rest led to a decrease in left ventricular mass index by 15% in healthy individuals [1]. Cardiac atrophy also occurs during cachexia as consequence of advanced cancer [17]. Indeed, patients who died as a result of cancer cachexia exerted strongly reduced heart weight (−25%) versus healthy individuals [18]. Remarkably, cachexia is a major contributor of cancer related mortality, as therapeutic amelioration of cachexia strongly improves cancer survival in mouse models [19]. To this end, cardiac cachexia might in fact be the main trigger of cachexia associated mortality, because in experimental animal models (patient data are currently not available) cardiac atrophy in cancer is associated with systolic and diastolic cardiac dysfunction and in severe cases heart failure [17]. Cardiac cachexia is triggered by neurohumoral factors like aldosterone, inflammatory mediators like interleukin-6, but also by factors secreted by tumor cells such as ataxin-10 [18, 20]. Cancer induced cardiac atrophy is associated with cardiac fibrosis in patients as well as in experimental animal models, such as Colon-26 tumor-bearing mice or Yoshida-130 tumor-bearing rats [17]. Loss of cardiac mass during atrophy is associated with reduced intracellular abundance of contractile proteins (such as myosin heavy chain) and is induced on one hand by reduced intracellular growth signaling, as evident by decreased phosphorylation (i.e. decreased activation) of the protein synthesis promoting kinase mTOR and on the other hand through specific protein degrading mechanisms such as autophagy and enhanced proteasomal activity [21]. Autophagy is a conserved process that leads to bulk degradation and recycling of cytoplasmatic components like long-lived proteins and organelles, which are encircled by a double membrane (called the autophagosome) and then fused to lysosomes to form autolysosomes [22]. Lysosomal hydrolases then degrade the content of the autolysosome and release amino acids and lipids into the cytoplasm for cellular reuse. The ubiquitin proteasome system degrades intact monomeric intracellular proteins, which are covalently linked and thereby labelled for proteasomal degradation with ubiquitin by so called E3 ubiquitin ligases such as atrogin-1 or Murf-1 [22]. To which extent both processes (i.e. autophagy and ubiquitin/proteasome) are involved in cardiac atrophy is still a subject of debate and needs to be clarified in the future [23].

2.2 Intercellular Mechanisms of Cardiac Remodeling and Hypertrophy

The heart is a multicellular organ consisting of endothelial cells, cardiomyocytes, fibroblasts, smooth muscle cells, inflammatory cells, stem cells and other perhaps currently unknown cell types. Virtually all of these cell types contribute in different ways to the remodeling processes described above. On one hand each cell type fulfills a specific function as cardiomyocytes mediate the contractile function of the heart, large part of the hypertrophy response and propagation of excitation, while for example fibroblasts entail changes in the extracellular matrix. On the other hand rich communication between all cell types exists, which under many instances is crucial for adaptive remodeling in response to overload.

Although especially about the mode of intercellular communication during cardiac overload and its impact on remodeling a lot still needs to be deciphered, we summarize here some key aspects of this emerging field.

2.2.1 Communication Between Cardiomyocytes

Although in terms of cell number cardiomyocytes represent only 30–45% (depending on species) of all heart cells, because of their size they contribute to more than 90% of myocardial volume. Rich communication takes place among cardiomyocytes. Importantly, cardiac myocytes are directly coupled via gap junction at the intercalated disk (Fig. 2.2) [24]. Mainly ions (Ca^{++}) and small solutes pass through gap junction to promote impulse conduction in the cardiac conduction system and the working myocardium. The gap junctions in adult mice are constituted by connexin40 in myocytes of the conduction system, but by connexin43 in the working myocardium. Besides impulse conduction, the connexins are important for cardiac morphogenesis, since heterozygous and homozygous deletion of connexin40 leads to developmental abnormalities of the heart, including double-outlet right ventricle, tetralogy of Fallot and endocardial cushion defects [25]. Cardiomyocyte specific deletion of connexin43 results in outflow tract abnormalities and cardiac hypertrophy after birth.

Cardiomyocytes also secrete various growth factors, which either act in an autocrine fashion on the secreting cell, a neighbouring cardiomyocyte or on non-cardiomyocytes. Among the myocyte derived factors with functional autocrine effects are endothelin-1, ANP and BNP as well as multiple TGFβ family members, including TGFβ, growth differentiation factor (GDF) 15 and myostatin (GDF8). TGFβ is released from cardiac fibroblasts, but also from cardiomyocytes. Ablation of the TGFβ receptor (R)2 specifically in cardiac myocytes strongly reduced cardiac hypertrophy, fibrosis and improved cardiac function during experimental pressure overload in mice by transverse aortic constriction (TAC) [26]. In this procedure, which often is used as a model of human disease in mice, a ligature is placed between the left common carotid artery and the right innominate artery around the ascending aortic arch. This leads to a robust mechanical pressure overloading of the left ventricle with cardiac hypertrophy (+30–60% in heart weight) within 2 weeks and reduced cardiac function within 4–8 weeks after surgery. The data from cardiomyocyte specific Tgfβr2 knock-out mice indicate that intrinsic cardiomyocyte TGFβ signaling is a strong promoter of pathological hypertrophy and dysfunction under these circumstances. In contrast, cardiomyocyte GDF15 inhibits hypertrophy and death in these cells. Similarly, ANP and BNP, which act via the GC-A receptor, mediate local antihypertrophic, antifibrotic and positive inotropic effects in the heart [27]. Intracellular mediators of these effects are cGMP and the antihypertrophic cGMP-activated protein kinase 1. Positive inotropic effects are due to increased cAMP levels. Systemic actions include natriuretic and vasodilatory effects as well as favourable metabolic consequences. Although ANP and BNP levels rise during heart failure, this cannot sufficiently alleviate disease progression, which might be due to impaired ANP, BNP function under these circumstances. ANP and BNP resistance is believed to be the cause of their increased internalization through the NPR-C receptor, desensitization of the GC-A receptor as well as increased degradation of intracellular cGMP by the phosphodiesterase PDE9. Interestingly, the new drug LCZ696 combines angiotensin/AT1 receptor blockade with inhibition of neprilysin – a degrading enzyme of ANP and BNP. Therefore LCZ696 acts in part via elevation of ANP and BNP levels to improve the outcome of patients suffering from heart failure.

Myocardial Myostatin is crucial for the maintenance of cardiac homeostasis, as its selective induced genetic ablation under baseline conditions resulted in hypertrophy, heart failure and death associated with metabolic imbalance and

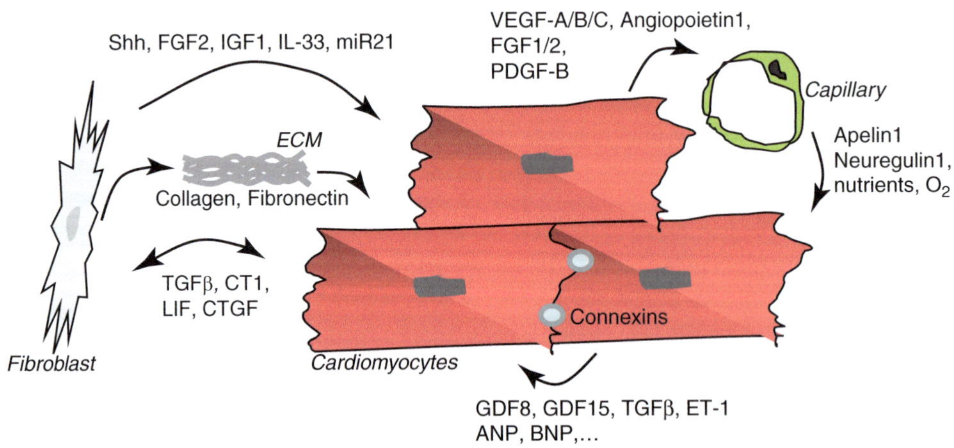

Fig. 2.2 Intercellular communication in the adult myocardium as it occurs during hemodynamic overload. Details are described in the text

over-activation of the AMP-activated kinase (AMPK), which is typically activated in low energy states in the cell [28].

2.2.2 Fibroblasts and Fibrosis

Cardiac fibroblasts are spindle shaped cells that specifically express the PDGF receptor α as well as vimentin. They arise through EMT from the epicardium as well as the endocardium during embryonic development [21]. The primary function of cardiac fibroblasts is to synthesize (and degrade) extracellular matrix, which forms a three dimensional structural network that supports cohesion of myocardial cells, cardiac shape and function. Extracellular matrix (ECM) in the heart consists mainly of collagen I and III, fibronectin, proteoglycans and glycoproteins [29]. In addition, fibroblasts communicate with cardiomyocytes via the release of specific growth factors, through extracellular matrix and even more directly by forming connexin containing gap-junction between these two different cell types.

In the embryonic heart, release of fibronectin, EGF-like growth factor and collagen by fibroblasts promotes cardiac myocyte proliferation, by stimulating β1-integrin dependent signaling in these cells [30]. In the healthy adult heart, fibroblasts are mainly quiescent, but become activated in response to mechanical overload and pro-fibrotic molecules like TGF-β and connective tissue growth factor (CTGF), which are expressed in fibroblasts as well as cardiomyocytes (Fig. 2.2). Activation leads to a dramatic increase in fibro blast proliferation, secretion of extracellular matrix proteins and growth factors. In addition, a fraction of fibroblasts (around 15% in murine pressure overload) become myofibroblasts, which is a contractile cell type, characterized by the expression of α-smooth-muscle actin.

Co-culture with adult heart fibroblasts leads to hypertrophy in cardiomyocytes [30]. One of the growth factor responsible for this effect could be TGFβ1, which is released abundantly from myocytes as well as fibroblasts and which induces hypertrophy and dysfunction in cardiomyocytes and extracellular matrix production in fibroblasts. Interestingly, the endogenous pro-hypertrophic agonist Angiotensin II primarily acts on the Angiotensin type 1 receptor on cardiac fibroblasts and triggers cardiomyocyte growth indirectly through the induction of TGFβ1 and FGF2. FGF2 is mainly produced in myocardial fibroblasts and induces hypertrophy of adjacent cardiomyocytes. In support of this, FGF2 knock-out mice showed reduced hypertrophy during pressure overload. Cardiac IGF1 is predominantly derived from fibroblasts, where its expression is induced by the transcription factor Krüppel-like-factor 5 (KLF5) [31]. Fibroblast IGF1 promotes cardiomyocyte hypertrophy and myocardial fibrosis, but is also essential for preventing heart failure and mortality during pressure overload in mice. Members of the IL-6 family like cardiotrophin-1 and leukemia inhibitory factor (LIF) are synthesized by cardiac fibroblasts and myocytes and signal through the transmembrane gp130 receptor to induce cardiomyocyte hypertrophy. In addition, CT-1 also promotes fibroblast migration, while LIF inhibits myofibroblast transition and collagen synthesis.

Fibroblasts do not only release factors that induce growth in cardiac myocytes. Interleukin-33 (IL-33), which is expressed by cardiac fibroblast in response to mechanical load, inhibits cardiomyocyte hypertrophy in a paracrine and dose-dependent manner by binding to its receptor STL2.

It is currently emerging that cardiomyocyte–fibroblast crosstalk is not only regulated by proteins, but also by non-coding RNA molecules such as micro-RNAs (miRs) [32]. MiRs are short (17–25 nucleotides) noncoding RNAs that function mainly to inhibit gene-expression and protein synthesis of specific mRNAs. They are processed from 60–70 nucleotides pre-miRs, which are exported to the cytosol where they are cleaved by the enzyme dicer to produce the mature duplex miR, consisting of a guide strand and a passenger strand. Mainly the guide strand targets cellular mRNA for silencing. miR133a is predominantly expressed in cardiomyocytes, where it blocks the expression of the profibrotic factor CTGF. As a result, miR133 knock-out mice develop heart failure with massive myocardial fibrosis, while cardiomyocyte specific overexpression protected the mice from cardiac fibrosis after pressure-overload. miR21, in contrast, was found to be specifically upregulated in fibroblasts of failing hearts, where it targets intracellular signaling and the paracrine influence on cardiomyocytes [33]. Inhibition of miR21 by an antagomiR (small, chemically modified RNA) reduces cardiac fibrosis and hypertrophy after pressure overload. Fibroblasts also release the passenger strand of miR21 in exosomes (small vesicles), which are taken up by cardiomyocytes, and thereby induce hypertrophy in these cells [34].

2.2.3 Endothelial Cells and Angiogenesis

As an organ highly dependent on oxidative energy production, the capillary density in the heart is high, and each cardiomyocyte is supplied roughly by one capillary [35]. Recent evidence even suggests that endothelial cells (in terms of their number) are the most abundant cell type in the heart [36]. Capillary endothelial cells are closely associated with cardiomyocytes in an ideal diffusion range for capillary derived nutrients and oxygen, but also for reciprocal paracrine signals between these cells. It has been demonstrated that cardiomyocytes regulate the formation and adaptation of the myocardial capillary network and that angiogenesis (i.e the formation of capillaries from pre-existing endothelial cells) is enhanced during increased hemodynamic load and cardiac hypertrophy in multiple different species (mice, sheep, humans). In fact, this increase in myocardial capillaries (by about 30–50%) is important for the preservation of cardiac function during hypertrophy.

How is myocardial angiogenesis regulated, especially during pathological overload? Around 85% of the VEGF-A within the heart is produced by cardiac myocytes [37]. Similarly, high expression of pro-angiogenic growth factors like VEGF-B, VEGF-C, Angiopoietin1, FGF1, FGF2, EGF, matrix metallo-proteinase (MMP) 9 as well as PDGF-B has been reported in these cells (Fig. 2.2). Expression of these molecules is triggered by central signaling molecules, transcription factors and transcriptional co-regulators in cardiomyocytes. In this regard, the transcription factor GATA4, which is activated by mechanical overload in cardiomyocytes, directly binds and activates the *Vegfa* promoter [38]. Consequently, cardiomyocyte specific GATA4 overexpression induces VEGF-A and capillary angiogenesis in the myocardium of mice, while in turn, genetic deletion of GATA4 in cardiac myocytes reduces myocardial angiogenesis and also leads to heart failure. In parallel, the hypoxia sensitive transcription factor HIF1-α, which is a known direct regulator of VEGF-A and other angiogenic growth factors, becomes activated early in the course of cardiac pressure-overload, when cardiomyocyte growth exceeds the ability of the existing capillary network to deliver enough oxygen for the muscle cells and hypoxia emerges [23]. Other cardiomyocyte based regulators with positive effects on myocardial capillary growth include the transcriptional co-regulator peroxisome proliferator-activated receptor gamma, coactivator 1 alpha (PGC1α), the transcription factor signal transducer and activator of transcription 3 (STAT3) and protein kinase B/Akt. Although capillary growth in the heart is enhanced during the initial compensatory phase of cardiac overload, capillary density decreases with disease progression and capillary rarefaction is ultimately present in terminal heart failure [10]. This might, at least in part, be due to the fact that cardiomyocyte GATA4 activation decreases and Hif1-α becomes inhibited by p53 in persisting pressure overload. Restitution of capillary density under these conditions, for example by the delivery of angiogenic growth factors like VEGF-A and Angiopoietin1, improves cardiac function, indicating that sufficient angiogenesis is crucial for the maintenance of heart function under pathological stress. Cardiac angiogenesis is inhibited by endothelial microRNAs such as miR-92a and miR-24. Inhibition of these microRNAs by antagomir based approaches increases myocardial vascularization and thereby improves functional recovery of the heart after myocardial infarction [39, 40].

How do endothelial cells influence cardiomyocytes to maintain their function? First and foremost, they deliver oxygen and nutrients (i.e. amino acids, glucose and fatty acids) to enable the production of ATP by myocytes. Second, paracrine factors released by the endothelial cells play an important role for cardiac homeostasis and survival. In a co-culture system of cardiomyocytes and endothelial cells, in which oxygen and nutrient delivery by capillaries naturally do not play a role, endothelial cells are essential for the survival of myocytes and also trigger their spacial organization and rhythmic contraction. As endothelial-derived paracrine factors, Neuregulin1, which acts on ErbB2 and ErbB4 receptors on cardiomyocytes and which promotes myocyte survival and hypertrophy, as well as Apelin1, which induces a strong positive inotropic response via its G-protein coupled receptor APJ, have been identified [24, 41]. Of note, endothelial cells also exert maladaptive influences on cardiomyocytes, as it was demonstrated that during peripartum cardiomyopathy (PPCM) they release exosomes containing miR-146, which are taken up by cardiomyocytes, where miR-146 suppresses ErbB4 abundance [42]. Inhibition of miR-146 by an antagomir, in turn, attenuates PPCM in a mouse model.

Interestingly, both Neuregulin1 and Apelin1 are being evaluated as therapy in patients with heart failure, indicating that the understanding of intercellular communication in the heart might be a valuable approach to identify potential novel therapeutic targets.

2.3 Cardiomyocyte Intracellular Signaling Regulators

Although multiple cell types exert essential contributions to the myocardial response to stress (see above), cardiomyocytes are still the main substrate of cardiac growth and function. Thus, in the following sections, we will highlight intracellular mechanisms of signaling (this chapter), calcium handling and regulation of contractility (this chapter and Chap. 4).

2.3.1 Signaling from the Cell Membrane to the Nucleus

During pathological overload of the heart, both biomechanical stretch and neurohormonal factors act on cardiomyocytes and induce intracellular signaling. It remains unclear, how mechanical stretch is translated into biochemical signals in these cells, although stretch sensitive ion channels and structural proteins in proximity to the cell membrane like integrins or the muscle lim protein might be involved [1, 2, 43]. Mechanical stretch also triggers autocrine and paracrine release of neurohormones such as Angiotensin II, Endothelin-1 and α-adrenergic catecholamines, which bind to seven-transmembrane-spanning receptors that are coupled to heterotrimeric G proteins of the $G\alpha q/\alpha 11$ subclass and activate phospholipase Cβ (PLCβ, Fig. 2.3) [2]. Interestingly,

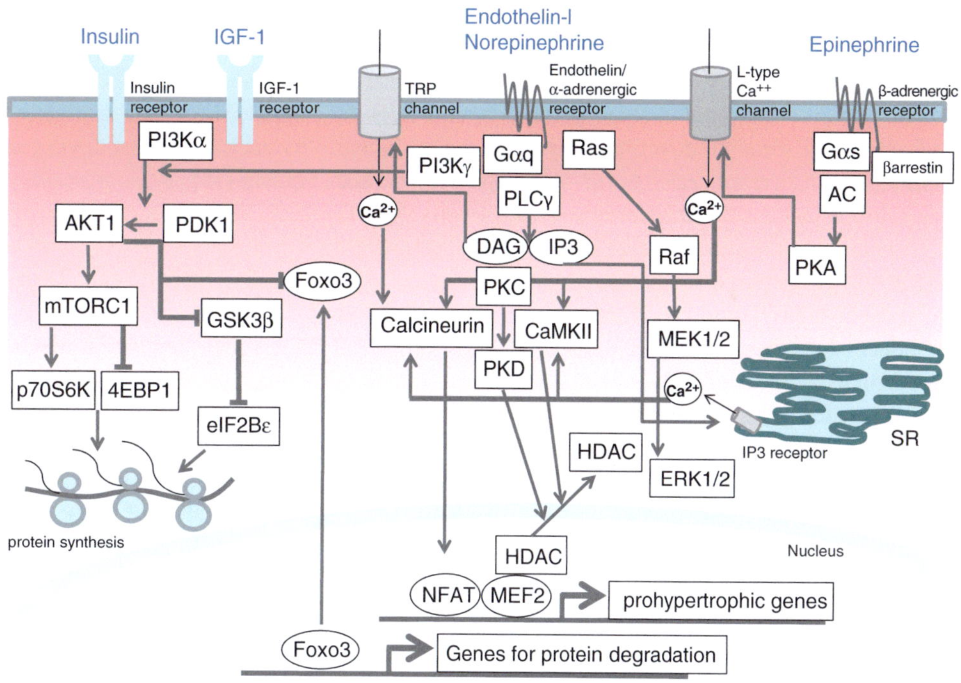

Fig. 2.3 Prohypertrophic intracellular signal transduction in cardiac myocytes. Details are described in the text. Abbreviations not mentioned in the text: AC, adenylat cyclase; p70S6K, p70 S6 kinase

the angiotensin II type 1 receptor can also be activated directly by mechanical stress (without the involvement of angiotensin II) [44]. PLCβ induces the generation of diacyglycerol (DAG), which functions as an intracellular ligand for protein kinase C (PKC), leading to PKC activation and induction of inositol-1,4,5-triphosphate (IP3). IP3 triggers the mobilization of internal calcium by direct binding to the IP3 receptor at the sarcoplasmatic reticulum or the nuclear envelope. DAG and IP3 also induce opening of transient receptor potential (TRPC) channels, which leads to influx of sodium and mainly calcium into cardiac myocytes. Increase in this signaling associated calcium occurs in cellular microdomains associated with specialized lipid rafts (termed caveolae) or in proximity to plasma membrane invaginations, called T-tubules [45]. Signaling associated calcium is shielded from the highly abundant and mainly sarcoplasmatic reticulum based calcium that activates cardiomyocyte contraction by binding to contractile filaments ("contractile calcium"). Signaling calcium binds to calmodulin and subsequently activates prohypertrophic downstream signaling by the calmodulin dependent kinase (CaMK)II and the phosphatase calcineurin. In addition, Gαq triggered signaling leads to activation of MAPK (exact mechanisms not known) and AKT through the PI3Kγ. The β-adrenergic receptor also initiates prohypertrophic signaling: it is associated with Gαs dependent activation of the adenylate cyclase and subsequent activation of protein kinase A (PKA). PKA induces calcium influx from the extracellular space through the L-type calcium channel, thereby also contributing to signaling calcium to activate CaMKII and calcineurin. In addition, the scaffold protein β-arrestin associates with the intracellular portion of β-receptor to activate CaMKII as well as MAPkinase signaling [46].

CaMKII is induced in expression and becomes activated in response to pressure overload in the myocardium [47]. Among its different isoforms, CaMKIIδ is the most abundant in the heart, although CaMKIIγ is also expressed there. CaMKII is a serine/threonine kinase that is directly activated by calcium/calmodulin binding and by reactive oxygen species. The splice variant CaMKIIδB is localized to the nucleus, while CaMKIIδC is found in the cytosol. Genetic ablation of CaMKIIδ reduced cardiac hypertrophy, fibrosis and dysfunction in mice. Cardiomyocyte specific overexpression of CaMKII, in turn, leads to cardiac hypertrophy (in the case of CaMKIIδB) or dilated cardiomyopathy (CaMKIIδC). CaMKII directly phosphorylates the histone deacetylase (HDAC) 4 and thereby promotes binding of the chaperone 14-3-3 to cause export of HDAC4 from the nucleus. Reduction of nuclear HDAC4 leads to enhanced activation of the prohypertrophic transcription factor MEF2, which usually is directly repressed by class II HDACs. Indeed, class IIa HDACs (HDACS 4, 5, 7, 9) are known to inhibit cardiac hypertrophy and mice lacking HDAC5 or HDAC9 show spontaneous myocardial hypertrophy with aging or exaggerated hypertrophy in response to pressure overload. Nuclear export of class IIa HDACs can also be induced through phosphorylation by protein kinase D. In contrast, class I HDACs like HDAC 1, 2 and 3, which are constitutively present in the nucleus, are not regulated by kinases, and promote cardiac hypertrophy and failure, as demonstrated with specific pharmacological inhibitors like apicidin that improve adverse remodeling in mice.

The calcium dependent serine/threonine protein-phosphatase calcineurin consists of a catalytic subunit (CnA) and a 19-kDa regulatory subunit (CnB) [2, 45]. The dimeric protein becomes activated in response to increased calcium concentrations through direct binding of calcium bound calmodulin. Activated calcineurin dephosphorylates the transcription factor nuclear factor of activated T-cells (NFAT) in proximity to the cardiomyocyte plasma-membrane, where calcineurin is anchored by the small adaptor protein CIB1. Upon dephosphorylation, NFAT translocates into the nucleus to induce the expression of hypertrophy inducing genes. Myocardial calcineurin/NFAT signaling appears to be selectively activated in pathological hypertrophy and heart failure, but not under conditions of physiological hypertrophy. Genetic ablation of the CnAβ isoform in mice, which is upregulated in the heart during pressure overload, blunts pathological hypertrophy, as does genetic elimination of NFATc3 and NFATc2 [48, 49, 50].

Among the MAP kinases mainly the activation of ERK1/2 contributes to the development of cardiac hypertrophy. Activation of ERK kinases occurs downstream of G-protein coupled receptors, receptor tyrosine kinases (e.g. IGF1 and FGF receptors), receptor serine/threonine kinases (TGFβ receptors), gp130 receptors as well as integrins in response to mechanical stretch [37]. Downstream of these receptors the small G protein Ras is activated, which then recruits the MAP kinase (MAP 3 K) Raf-1 to the plasma-membrane. Raf-1 then activates the dual-specificity kinases MEK1 and MEK2 (MAP 2 K) that finally phosphorylate and activate ERK1/2. Constitutive expression of an activated MEK1 mutant in cardiomyocytes results in a concentric from of hypertrophy with increased myocyte width, but lack of cardiac fibrosis or dysfunction. Genetic elimination of cardiomyocyte ERK1 and ERK2, in turn, leads to spontaneous eccentric cardiac hypertrophy (i.e. cardiac dilation with cardiomyocyte elongation at the microscopic level) and ventricular dysfunction [51]. Thus, ERK1/2 promotes a compensated form of concentric cardiac hypertrophy. The other MAP kinases p38 and JNK, which are also activated in response to pathological stress, appear to inhibit cardiomyocyte hypertrophy by re-phosphorylating NFAT and thereby promoting its export from the nucleus. Casein kinase 2α, in contrast, is a kinase that promotes cardiac hypertrophy through phosphorylation of the tumor suppressor protein p27, which is degraded in response, as well as the through the activation of HDAC2 [52, 53].

Beside NFAT and MEF2, other transcription factors with prohypertrophic effects in cardiomyocyte include GATA4, GATA6, serum response factor (SRF) and nuclear factor (NF)-κB. In addition, nuclear receptors such as estrogen, androgen and mineralocorticoid receptor in cardiomyocytes are essentially involved in myocardial remodeling. Cell-specific deletion of the mineralocorticoid receptor in cardiomyocytes markedly improved healing and remodeling processes after myocardial infarction [54]. These results indicate that the well-proven beneficial effects of mineralocorticoid receptor antagonists in heart failure are to a large extent mediated by direct modification of cardiomyocyte signaling [55].

2.3.2 Epigenetic Regulation

Epigenetic regulation mediates changes in the activity of a certain set of genes without alterations of the DNA sequence. It typically involves covalent modifications of the DNA, such as methylation or hydroxymethylation of cytosine residues or covalent modification of histone proteins (e.g. acetylation or methylation of lysine residues), around which the DNA is wrapped. In general, these modifications lead to changes in the state of the chromatin – either highly condensed and inaccessible for transcription factors or in a relaxed mode allowing for active gene transcription [56].

In this regard, DNA methylation is associated with transcriptional suppression. Methylated cytosines are preferentially found on cytosine-(phosphate)-guanine dinucleotides (CpG), which tends to cluster in regions of CpG islands, mainly at the 5′ end but also throughout the entire gene body. DNA methylation is mediated by one of three so far identified DNA methyltransferases (DNMTs): DNMT1, DNMT3A and DNMT3B. It directly inhibits binding of transcription factor to the DNA, or it recruits methyl-binding proteins (for example methyl-CpG-binding protein 2, MECP2) that in turn attract co-repressor complexes. In human endstage heart failure, immunoprecipitation of methylated DNA from cardiac biopsies and subsequent sequencing showed that DNA methylation differed significantly at CpGs of promoters and gene bodies in cardiomyopathic versus healthy hearts [57]. Remarkable, demethylation of DNA in gene-promoters was associated with increased gene-expression, while hypermethylation did not correlate with reduced expression [57]. A study in isolated cardiomyocytes from neonatal versus adult healthy hearts and versus adult hypertrophic hearts uncovered strong changes in the DNA methylation pattern between neonatal and adult healthy cardiomyocytes, which correlated well with changes in gene expression (i.e. demethylation was associated with increased gene expression, while methylation was related to decreased expression). Interestingly, the hypertrophy induced changes in gene methylation were overall less pronounced, but partially resembled the neonatal pattern [58].

Covalent modification of histone H3 occurs at a site specific manner. High levels of monoacetylated (ac) Lys-9 and Lys-14 (H3K9ac and H3K14ac) and trimethylated (me3) Lys-4 (H3K4me3) at the promoter or trimethylated Lys-36 (H3K36me3) and dimethylated Lys-79 (H3K79m2) in the gene body are found in transcriptionally active regions [59]. High levels of trimethylated histone H3 on Lys-9 (H3K9m3) and Lys-27 (H3K27me3), in contrast, are detected in inactive regions [59]. In isolated cardiomyocytes from mice with compensated cardiac hypertrophy (after 1 week of pressure overload) 9.1% of the genome in comparison to sham operated healthy mice exerted a change in at least one of these histone marks mainly around the transcriptional start side of genes related to epigenetic regulation of gene expression, heart function, organization of sarcomere structure and a mouse hypertrophic phenotype. Importantly, the expression of 1109 genes that were regulated by pressure overload correlated well with the abundance of the aforementioned 7 histone marks. The same study also examined the presence of active or inactive enhancers decorated by the H3K27ac or H3K27me3 histone marks, respectively [59]. In contrast to typical promoter elements directly adjacent to the gene they regulate, enhancers are DNA elements that modulate expression of genes from a more distant site in the genome. From the 9.207 differentially activated enhancers, a lot changed toward the more activated (H3K27ac labelled) class, while only 34 were inactive (H3K27me3 labelled). A transcription factor binding analysis revealed that motifs for the prohypertrophic transcription factors MEF2C and MEF2A were enriched and also bound to these enhancer elements.

Histone acetylation to promote transcriptionally active chromatin is mediated by acetyltransferases such as p300, which has previously been shown to be involved in cardiac development and heart failure through transcription controlled by MEF2 and GATA4 [56]. In turn, and as addressed already in detail in the previous section, HDACs are mediating histone deacetylation to induce chromatin condensation. In addition to its effect on chromatin remodeling, HDAC class 2 molecules inhibit cardiac hypertrophy by directly binding and suppressing transcriptional activation by MEF2. Class 1 HDACs, in turn, exert a prohypertrophic effect (see above for details) and inhibition of these molecules mediates beneficial effects in mouse models of hypertrophy and heart failure [60].

Histone methylation occurs at lysine and arginine residues on histones H3 and H4 through histone methyltransferases and can lead to activation or repression of transcription depending on location and degree of the modification [56]. Histone demethylases remove the methyl residues. Of note, HDACs can also modulate histone methylation: for upregulation of ANP as embryonic gene in failing human hearts, HDAC4 export out of the nucleus decreased di- and trimethylation of the H3K9 residue [61].

Histone modifications are identified by reader proteins. For example the binding of acetylated histone residues is mediated by members of the bromodomain and extraterminal (BET) family of reader proteins, which mediates transcriptional activation by recruiting co-regulatory complexes and in the heart aggravates hypertrophy and heart failure. BET inhibition by the component JQ-1 prevented pathological hypertrophy and heart failure during pressure overload through broad, but specific effects on the cardiac transcriptome [62].

Another family of epigenetic regulators is constituted by the ATP-dependent chromatin remodeling complexes, which use the energy from ATP hydrolysis to modulate the distribution of histones and the packaging state of chromatin. The Brg1/Brm-associated-factor (BAF) complex, consisting of 12 subunits, is an important ATP-dependent remodeling complex in vertebrates, whereby Brg1 is the essential ATPase subunit of this complex. Brg1, by interacting with HDAC and PARP1 represses expression of Myh6 (α-MHC) and facilitates Myh7 (β-MHC) expression and therefore maintains the cardiomyocytes in an embryonic state. Brg1 is highly expressed during embryonic heart development and is inactivated in the adult organ. During adult heart disease, Brg1 becomes re-expressed and promotes an increased Myh7/Myh6 ratio, hypertrophy and cardiac dysfunction [63].

2.3.3 Non-coding RNAs (miRNAs, lncRNAs)

New sequencing technology has revealed the unexpected fact that more than 80% of the genome is transcribed into RNA. Strikingly, however, only 3% of the whole genome encodes for proteins. As a consequence, the vast majority of RNA species is non-coding. Noncoding RNA can be divided into small (<200bp) RNAs, for example microRNAs, tRNAs and small nucleolar RNAs and long RNAs (>200bp), including ribosomal RNAs and long non-coding RNAs (lncRNAs) [64].

As already alluded to above, microRNAs are single-stranded RNAs, about 22 nucleotides in length that repress protein expression by binding to a complementary sequence in the 3′untranslated region of target mRNAs within the RNA-induced silencing complex (RISC). Within the human genome, around 2000 microRNAs have been identified so far [65]. In the adult organism, microRNAs mainly function to modulate cellular stress responses, as revealed for example by microRNA knock-out mice, which often show a phenotype only under conditions of stress [66]. Each microRNA typically modulates the expression of dozens or even hundreds of mRNAs. Often microRNAs target multiple mRNAs encoding for proteins with similar functional annotation. As an example, the miR-29 targets multiple proteins involved in fibrosis, including multiple collagens, fibrillins and elastin. In fact, miR-29 is downregulated in a variety of fibrotic disorders (for example also in the border zone of a myocardial infarction) and thereby promotes tissue fibrosis.

One of the first microRNAs discovered to promote cardiac hypertrophy and heart failure was the miR-208, which is encoded within the myosin heavy chain (MHC) gene and belongs to a family referred to as MyomiRs. MyomiRs regulate a collection of transcriptional repressors and signaling proteins that control MHC expression. Genetic ablation of miR-208 blunts activation of the fetal β-MHC gene during pressure overload and also protects the heart from hypertrophic cardiac remodeling [67]. Another example of a pro-hypertrophic cardiomyocyte derived microRNA is the miR212/132 family. MiR-212 and miR-132 are both upregulated in cardiomyocytes upon hypertrophic stimulation [68]. They target the anti-hypertrophic and pro-autophagic transcription factor FOXO3 and also trigger exaggerated calcineurin/NFAT signaling. Accordingly, miR212/132 knock-out mice are protected from cardiac hypertrophy and dysfunction, while cardiac transgenic overexpression triggers cardiomyopathy and death. Examples for anti-hypertrophic cardiac microRNAs include the miR-1, which targets insulin-like growth factor 1 signaling, miR-133, as well as miR-378 that suppresses the MAP kinase signaling pathway [69–71]. Of note, these 3 microRNAs decreased in cardiac hypertrophy and it was demonstrated that restoration of miR-378 levels by an adeno-associated virus improved cardiac remodeling during pressure overload. MicroRNAs are also involved in the re-expression of fetal genes observed in the failing myocardium in animals as well as in patients [72].

Although the field is still in its infancy, based on what is currently known, lncRNAs appear to be even more versatile regulators than microRNAs, because they represent a very heterogeneous group. For example, when divided by their structure or location in the genome, they can be either polyadenylated (like mRNAs) or not, they can be located between genes (intergenic, also called lincRNAs for long intergenic non-coding RNA), within introns of genes, they can overlap with genes (while being transcribed either in sense or antisense direction), or they are associated with enhancers. LncRNAs can bind complementary to DNA or RNA in a sequence specific manner and on the other hand are also able to interact with proteins through a distinct secondary structure [64, 65, 73]. Therefore, as mechanism of action, lncRNAs can function in multiple different ways: (1) by imprinting genes (like for example the lncRNAs XIST, which covers one of the two female X chromosomes) to shut down expression; (2) by acting as scaffold for recruiting transcription factors or epigenetic regulators, like for instance the lincRNA HOTAIR that binds the polycomb repressor complex 2 (PRC2) and the LSD1/REST complex to tether these to the HOXC locus or select genes on other chromosomes to induce epigenetic silencing; (3) by acting as "sponge" to sequester microRNAs (like for example *CHRF* that binds miR-489, see below); (4) by functioning as natural antisense transcripts, whereby it is estimated that for around 70% of mouse genes anti-sense transcription exists, which function by regulating transcription, stability and splicing of the associated mRNA; (5) as enhancer RNAs, which are around 2-kb long and regulate the expression of surrounding mRNAs. Importantly, since it was recently shown that putative lncRNAs do get translated into micropeptides (consisting of 30–40 amino acids) in some cases, this possibility needs to be ruled out by proteomic or ribosomal binding analysis before an RNA sequence can be truly assigned as non-coding [74, 75].

In terms of potential function in heart failure various expression screens have been conducted from diseased versus healthy mouse or human heart tissue. In human failing myocardium, 18,480 lncRNA were detected and 679 and 570 were differentially expressed in ischemic versus non-ischemic heart failure, respectively [76]. One study noted that although a marked difference between fetal and adult mouse hearts was found in lncRNAs expression, only 17 lncRNAs were regulated in transverse aortic constriction based pressure overload. It is unclear, why only this few lncRNAs were found to be regulated in this study in hypertrophy, but the number of regulated cardiac lncRNAs might rise strongly in more advanced disease, i.e. in heart failure. A similar study interrogating angiotensin II-regulated lncRNAs identified the lncRNAs hypertrophy related factor (*CHRF*) as induced by angiotensin II as well as in in murine pressure overload and in human heart failure samples [77]. *CHRF* triggered cardiac hypertrophy in isolated cardiomyocytes by acting as sponge and thus sequestering the anti-hypertrophic miR-489. A recent study identified another cardiomyocyte derived pro-hypertrophic lncRNA, which was termed *Chast* and was upregulated in transverse aortic constriction in mice as well as in human hypertrophic heart tissue [78]. Mechanistically, *Chast* negatively regulates expression of Pleckstrin homology domain-containing protein family M member 1 (Plekhm1), which was found to inhibit hypertrophy. Downregulation of *Chast* expression in mice by short antisense molecules termed GapmeRs (sold by the company Exiqon) reduces pathological remodeling after pressure overload. In contrast, the lncRNAs *Mhrt* (Myheart) was reported as protective lncRNAs in the heart [79]. *Mhrt* RNAs are alternatively spliced anti-sense transcripts of the *Myh7* locus, which encodes for the β-MHC gene that is expressed in the embryonic heart and under pathological stress conditions in the adult heart. *Mhrt* expression, in contrast, is very low in the embryonic heart, strongly increases towards adulthood, but then becomes repressed by about 70% in pathological pressure overload. This repression is mediated by the chromatin remodeling factor Brg1 (see above). Interestingly, as negative feedback, Brg1 becomes sequestered by the lncRNAs *Mhrt* and thereby prevents it to activate *Myh7* or osteopontin (another Brg1 target gene that promotes cardiac fibrosis) expression. Accordingly, mild inducible transgenic overexpression of *Mhrt* to reconstitute endogenously repressed *Mhrt* rescues cardiac hypertrophy, fibrosis and dysfunction and reduces *Myh7* expression. Remarkably (because sometimes lncRNAs are not well conserved) *Mhrt* is also present in the human genome and is also repressed in myocardium from patients with left ventricular hypertrophy or ischemic or dilated cardiomyopathy.

By a comprehensive deep sequencing effort to define the regulation of lncRNAs in the heart during myocardial infarction and during differentiation of cardiomyocytes Pedrazzini et al. demonstrated that the poly-A based cardiac transcriptome consists mainly of mRNAs (15,075, 85.7%), followed by newly discovered lncRNAs (1521, 8.7%) and then known lncRNAs (988, 5.6%) [80, 81]. After myocardial infarction 67 known and 86 novel lncRNAs were upregulated, while 66 known and 225 novel lncRNAs were downregulated. Importantly, 73% of the novel lncRNAs also mapped to the human genome, thus suggesting conservation between species. Expression of the lncRNAs correlated with cardiac dimensions and function. The vast majority of the identified lncRNAs were associated with active cardiac specific enhancers. As an example, the lncRNAs *Novlnc6* is mainly downregulated in the border zone after myocardial infarction. As possible functional consequence and as revealed by experimental GapmeR mediated downregulation of *Novlnc6* in isolated mouse cardiomyocytes, the suppression of this lncRNA entails the downregulation of important known regulatory genes like Nkx2.5 and BMP10.

Interestingly, lncRNAs are also expressed in blood cells and have been detected in plasma, where they likely exist within exosomes. This makes their use as biomarker possible, which is in fact also the case for microRNAs. Indeed, Thum et al. identified a circulating, mitochondrial lincRNA, termed LIPCAR. LIPCAR levels identified patients after myocardial infarction that develop cardiac remodeling and were associated with future cardiovascular death independent of other risk markers [82].

2.4 Regulation of Cardiac Contractility

Beside its function as second messenger in signal transduction the main role of calcium in cardiomyocytes is undoubtedly the initiation of cellular contraction.

2.4.1 Excitation-Contraction Coupling in Healthy Hearts

During systole, an action potential leads to depolarization of the plasma membrane in cardiac myocytes, which triggers opening of the L-type calcium channel (LTCC) [83, 84]. This calcium binds the sarcoplasmic calcium release channel, termed the ryanodine receptor (RyR2), and thereby induces a massive release of calcium from the SR into the cytosol. This leads to a ten-fold increase in cytosolic calcium concentrations from 100 nM in diastole to about 1 μM in systole (this phenomenon is also termed "calcium induced calcium release"). The released calcium binds troponin C at the myofilaments and initiates muscle contraction. Relaxation is initiated by pumping back about 70% of the cytosolic calcium into the SR via the SR calcium ATPase (SERCA2a). Approximately 30% is transported outside the cell across the plasma membrane mainly by the sodium-calcium exchanger (NCX) and the plasma membrane calcium ATPase (PMCA). Adrenalin, for example during exercise, enhances cardiac contractility by modulating excitation-contraction coupling through binding to the β-adrenergic receptor, thereby triggering the production of cAMP and activating the protein kinase A (PKA). PKA phosphorylates the LTCC (to increase the influx of calcium) as well as the SERCA2A-inhibitory protein phospholamban (PLB), leading to reduced PLB mediated inhibition of the SERCA2a pump. Both together results in an increased SR calcium content and therefore an increased systolic calcium release (i.e. and an increased calcium transient) and enhanced contractility.

2.4.2 Abnormalities of Excitation-Contraction Coupling in Heart Failure

Cardiomyocytes in the failing heart are characterized by reduced contractile function. To a large extent these changes are the consequence of defective excitation-contraction coupling [83, 84]. These defects manifest in changes in the calcium transient: reduced amplitude, increased duration, prolonged decay and increased cytosolic calcium concentration in diastole. Furthermore, the reduced SR calcium content is an important characteristic in the failing cardiomyocyte. What are the reasons for these changes? The depletion of SR calcium load on one hand is the result of reduced SERCA2a activity. This is brought about by reduced protein levels of SERCA2a in the failing heart, but unchanged levels of its inhibitor protein PLB. Moreover, a reduced phosphorylation of PLB, which occurs at Serine16 by PKA and at Threonine17 by CamKII, is detectable in the failing myocardium. This leads to increased inhibitory potency of PLB towards SERCA2a and is in part due to increased activity of protein phosphatase 1 (PP1), which dephosphorylates PLB at these residues. In addition, there is decreased expression and phosphorylation of protein phosphatase inhibitor-1 (I-1), a PP-1 specific inhibitor. This all culminates in decreased SERCA2a activity in heart failure, which leads to slower and incomplete pumping of calcium into the SR at the end of systole. On the other hand, as second reason for decreased SR calcium load in heart failure (and at the same time increased diastolic calcium in the cytosol) the sarcoplasmatic calcium release channel RyR2 becomes leaky in failing cardiomyocytes: the huge homotetramer (each monomer has a molecular weight of 565 kDa) becomes hyperphosphorylated by PKA and CamKII leading to reduced binding of calstablin (FKBP12.6) to RyR2 and thereby triggering spontaneous calcium release into the cytosol, because calstablin stabilizes the RyR2 channel in the closed state. The decreased SR calcium load in heart failure entails a reduced calcium release from the SR in systole (as displayed by the diminished amplitude of the calcium transient), and consequently a reduced myofilament contraction. Relaxation of cardiomyocytes is also impaired due to slow removal of calcium from the cytosol, which also triggers delayed after-depolarisations precipitating arrhythmias. Altered calcium transport also occurs at the sarcolemma: the NCX in the failing myocardium, for instance, is less effective in extruding intracellular calcium (and sometimes might even work in the reverse mode, i.e. it transports calcium into the cell) and thereby contributes to increased diastolic calcium abundance. With regard to the LTCC, the availability and open probability of this channel appears to be increased, but the overall density of the channel and its response to β-adrenergic stimulation seem to be decreased under these circumstances. In addition, while in healthy cardiomyocytes the LTCC and the RyR2 are in close proximity to each other in order to enable very efficient excitation-contraction coupling, this assembly becomes disturbed in failing cardiomyocytes, with an increased distance between LTCC and RyR2 or even the appearance of "orphaned" RyR2 receptors that have no adjacent LTCC at all.

Multiple potential treatment approaches are being evaluated to target disturbed excitation-contraction coupling in heart failure: While restoration of SERCA2a levels by AAV1 mediated gene therapy has been effective to improve heart failure in animal models and in an small scale clinical trial [85], the larger double blind, placebo controlled, CUPID 2 trial failed to show a benefit. Along similar lines, modification of SERCA2a with the small ubiquitin-related modifier 1 (SUMO1), enhanced SERCA2a activity and stability. In a porcine MI model treatment with AAV1-SUMO resulted in improved ejection fraction and reduced left ventricular dilatation [83]. Furthermore, treatment with a small molecule (N106) to increase the SUMOylation of SERCA2a improves ventricular function in mice with heart failure, indicating that there might also be also non-gene-therapy based options to restore the function of SERCA2a in failing hearts [86].

Beside increasing SERCA function, other approaches targeting excitation-contraction coupling are based on the prevention of SR calcium leak [83]. In this regard, the overexpression of calstablin or different pharmacological approaches are under investigation. A further potential therapeutic approach involves the small calcium binding protein S100A, a calcium sensing protein downregulated in heart failure, which upon overexpression can improve contractile function, calcium handling and cardiac energetics.

2.5 Cardiac Metabolism in Heart Failure

2.5.1 Cardiac Metabolism in Heart Failure

The heart requires large amounts of high-energy phosphates to maintain contractile function und structural integrity. Most of cardiac ATP is derived from fatty acid oxidation, but approximately one third is derived from glucose, lactate and amino acid oxidation [87]. In heart failure, cardiac metabolism exerts direct effects on cardiac structure, function and remodeling. Metabolic changes depend on the etiology of heart failure and the degree of functional impairment. Metabolic remodeling restricts cardiac ATP availability, but non-ATP producing pathways are now considered equally important for myocardial hypertrophy and failure [88, 89]. ATP and non-ATP producing pathways are interlinked parts of a metabolic network. During the development of heart failure the energy metabolism of the heart reverts to a fetal-like metabolic profile with reduced fatty acid uptake and oxidation. Cardiac glucose uptake and oxidation in heart failure has been reported to be increased, unchanged or decreased. Overall, there is consensus that the failing heart produces less energy from fatty acids, which is not compensated by glucose oxidation [90]. Because metabolites from the Krebs cycle are used for hypertrophic growth, anaplerotic pathways become activated to maintain Krebs cycle activity. For example, glycolysis derived pyruvate is transferred into the Krebs cycle by anaplerotic pathways (carboxylation to oxaloacetat or malat) to compensate for the loss of metabolic intermediates. This further reduces glucose oxidation and aggravates the energetic deficit [88, 91]. Mitochondrial remodeling during heart failure progression leads to reduced mitochondrial biogenesis, energetic enzyme activity, oxidative phosphorylation and reduced ATP production [92]. Together, these structural and metabolic changes are responsible for the consistently reduced ATP availability in the failing heart. However, until now it has not been elucidated whether reduced ATP availability is causative for contractile dysfunction or reflects the reduced ATP demand of the failing heart due to structural remodeling and contractile impairment. Besides reduced ATP abundance, there are also defects in transport of ATP from the mitochondria to the myofibrils, where it is mainly utilized. The energy transfer within cardiomyocytes is carried out by the creatine kinase system: high energy phosphate is transferred by this enzyme to creatine to generate phosphocreatine at the mitochondria and gets then transferred back to ADP at the myofibrils. A defect in ATP transfer capacity in heart failure is mainly the consequence of reduced creatine kinase levels. Interestingly, transgenic replenishment of cardiomyocyte creatine kinase improved cardiac function and decreased mortality in mice during experimental pressure overload, thus rendering intracellular ATP transfer as potential therapeutic target [93]. Other mechanisms of mitochondrial dysfunction may be equally important, for example as enhanced reactive oxygen species released from the electron transfer chain can lead to oxidative damage and augment adverse remodeling. Non-ATP producing pathways of cardiac metabolism also influence cellular homeostasis and hypertrophic growth [88, 89]: Metabolic intermediates, such as fatty acid derivatives, pyruvate, hexosamines and adenosine monophosphate activate specific signaling circuits to regulate ion channel activity, cardiomyocyte growth and apoptosis. Alternative pathways of glucose and fatty acid metabolism like the hexosamine biosynthetic pathway via O-GlcNAc synthesis and protein modification, affect cardiomyocyte hypertrophy [94]. In addition, mitochondrial damage along with energy starvation promotes autophagy in the failing heart and may thereby also affect hypertrophy and inflammation [95]. In conclusion, the failing heart undergoes metabolic remodeling that leads to reduced ATP production as well as activation of non-ATP producing pathways interlinked with oxidative stress, hypertrophic growth, and contractile dysfunction.

2.5.2 Iron Deficiency

Iron deficiency, a frequent comorbidity in heart failure, is associated with higher mortality rates and impaired exercise capacity independent of coexisting anemia [96]. Iron supplementation improves symptoms and exercise capacity and may reduce the number of heart failure hospitalizations [97, 98]. Iron is required in all mammalian cells for fundamental processes including oxygen transport, storage and energy metabolism. Iron–sulphur clusters (ISC) are recognized as essential cofactors of proteins involved in energy production in the Krebs cycle and electron transfer chain [99]. Because the heart has high energy demands, it has been proposed that iron deficiency per se may contribute to energy starvation and cardiac dysfunction in heart failure [100]. Evidence for this came from rat models of severe nutritional iron deficiency that triggered systemic iron deficiency, anemia and cardiac failure; however, these models did not delineate between high-output failure due to anemia and the contribution of iron deficiency for cardiac remodeling [101]. In a recent experimental approach a genetic model of cardiomyocyte-restricted iron regulatory protein 1 and 2 (Irp1/2) ablation was established, which specifically induced cardiomyocyte iron deficiency without affecting systemic iron content [102]. Irp1 and Irp2 redundantly coordinate cellular iron uptake, utilization, and storage to assure the availability of appropriate iron supplies within the cell [103]. Mice with cardiomyocyte restricted iron deficiency showed mitochondrial dysfunction, reduced activity of the electron transfer chain and impaired oxidative phosphorylation. Whereas cardiac function under baseline conditions was not affected, iron deficiency diminished the contractile reserve upon acute β-adrenergic stimulation and increased the vulnerability of the heart to chronic stress after MI. Iron supplementation reversed mitochondrial dysfunction, recovered the positive inotropic response to acute stress, and prevented pathological remodeling after MI in the IRP1/2 ablated mice [102]. Therefore, iron deficiency in the failing heart seems to directly affect cardiomyocyte hypertrophy and cardiac function.

2.6 Translational Strategies to Combat Heart Failure in the Future

Translational strategies to successfully improve the outcome of heart failure patients would need to target either, or, if possible, multiple of the of the following points: (1) structural pathological remodeling such as eccentric or concentric cardiomyocyte hypertrophy, interstitial fibrosis and/or insufficient angiogenesis, (2) decreased cardiac contractility and perturbed excitation/contraction coupling, (3) dearranged myocardial energy metabolism and/or it could (4) alleviate myocardial damage by for example reducing the infarct size after myocardial infraction or by neutralizing a disease specific mechanism. These mechanisms could be tackled by new drugs, including small molecules, by therapy with proteins (including antibodies) or peptides, via gene therapy, by antagomirs or GapmeRs to inhibit microRNAs or lncRNAs, by miR"mimics" to enhance the effect of a certain microRNA or through modified RNA. Some of these strategies (especially gene therapy, but also the GapmeRs and miR"mimics") still need to be refined until they can be routinely used in patients. We addressed different possible strategies that are currently being tested in the previous sections, but we still want to highlight some promising strategies below.

Strategies to prevent or reverse myocardial damage have not been described in this chapter so far. These would mainly involve approaches to minimize myocardial injury after myocardial infarction, which is the main reason for the development of heart failure today. For example, an enhancement of angiogenesis and prevention of cardiomyocyte cell death through Mydgf protein therapy, which is a novel cytokine endogenously produced by inflammatory cells, reduces infarct size and prevents heart failure [104]. Similarly, the cardiac administration of VEGF modified RNA results in an especially favorable pharmacokinetic profile of VEGF expression, promoting angiogenesis and cardiomyogenesis in the infarct region by mobilizing epicardial progenitor cells in mice [105]. In general, approaches to enhance cardiomyocyte proliferation appear promising as well. Indeed, for example the administration of Neuregulin-1 promotes cardiac myocyte cell division and improves the outcome after mouse myocardial infarction [106]. In that manner, also targeting microRNAs might be effective. For example members of the miR-15 family are upregulated in postnatal cardiomyocytes when the proliferative capacity of these cells usually seizes. However, their antagomir based inhibition sustains cardiomyocyte proliferation until adulthood and confers benefit after myocardial infarction [107]. In turn, miR-199a and miR-590 and members of the miR-17~92 cluster enhance cardiac regeneration and therefore miR"mimics" might be a good strategy [108].

With regard to pathological remodeling, especially the epigenetic therapies with the HDAC class 1 inhibitor apicidin or with the BET-bromodomain protein inhibitor JQ-1 appear promising (see above). In addition, we recently described that the anti-androgenic substance Finasteride, which is widely used since many years in patients with prostate disease, reverses pathological hypertrophy and fibrosis and improves cardiac function and mouse mortality in different mouse models of pathological cardiac remodeling by inhibiting the local deleterious effects of the highly active testosterone metabolite dihydrotestosterone [109]. It will also be important to better understand the ANP/BNP system in heart failure and in this regard also the effects of LCZ696 on cardiac remodeling in patients. Inhibiting the cGMP degrading PDE9 by the substance PF-9613 should also be examined further for its beneficial effects on remodeling [110].

Improving excitation contraction coupling in heart failure is an important task, because besides contractility it might also improve the energetic status of the failing heart. SERCA2a targeted therapy appears to be a good concept in principal, although its delivery method in patients needs major improvement. Pharmacological inhibition of PKC-α for example by ruboxistaurin –currently tested in phase 2/3 clinical trials for diabetic retinopathy- is improving cardiac contractility (through enhancement of SERCA activity and calcium cycling) and also cardiac remodeling in mice, rats and pigs with heart failure [111]. The effects on remodeling in PKC-α inhibition likely stems from increased cardiac contractility that secondarily reduces neurohormonal/catecholamine drive.

Important from our perspective is the fact that almost all of these novel translational strategies highlighted in this whole chapter arise from the understanding of basic cellular or subcellular mechanism of disease, highlighting the necessity for promoting basic and translational research in the field of heart failure for the good of our patients.

References

1. Hill JA, Olson EN. Cardiac plasticity. N Engl J Med. 2008;358:1370–80.
2. Heineke J, Molkentin JD. Regulation of cardiac hypertrophy by intracellular signalling pathways. Nat Rev Mol Cell Biol. 2006;7:589–600.
3. Maillet M, van Berlo JH, Molkentin JD. Molecular basis of physiological heart growth: fundamental concepts and new players. Nat Rev Mol Cell Biol. 2013;14:38–48.
4. Kehat I, Molkentin JD. Molecular pathways underlying cardiac remodeling during pathophysiological stimulation. Circulation. 2010;122:2727–35.
5. Drazner MH. The transition from hypertrophy to failure: how certain are we? Circulation. 2005;112:936–8.
6. Katz DH, Beussink L, Sauer AJ, Freed BH, Burke MA, Shah SJ. Prevalence, clinical characteristics, and outcomes associated with eccentric versus concentric left ventricular hypertrophy in heart failure with preserved ejection fraction. Am J Cardiol. 2013;112:1158–64.
7. Davis J, Davis LC, Correll RN, Makarewich CA, Schwanekamp JA, Moussavi-Harami F, Wang D, York AJ, Wu H, Houser SR, Seidman CE, Seidman JG, Regnier M, Metzger JM, Wu JC, Molkentin JD. A tension-based model distinguishes hypertrophic versus dilated cardiomyopathy. Cell. 2016;165:1147–59.
8. Saraon T, Katz SD. Reverse remodeling in systolic heart failure. Cardiol Rev. 2015;23:173–81.
9. Krayenbuehl HP, Hess OM, Monrad ES, Schneider J, Mall G, Turina M. Left ventricular myocardial structure in aortic valve disease before, intermediate, and late after aortic valve replacement. Circulation. 1989;79:744–55.
10. Hein S, Arnon E, Kostin S, Schonburg M, Elsasser A, Polyakova V, Bauer EP, Klovekorn WP, Schaper J. Progression from compensated hypertrophy to failure in the pressure-overloaded human heart: structural deterioration and compensatory mechanisms. Circulation. 2003;107:984–91.
11. Slaughter MS, Rogers JG, Milano CA, Russell SD, Conte JV, Feldman D, Sun B, Tatooles AJ, Delgado RM 3rd, Long JW, Wozniak TC, Ghumman W, Farrar DJ, Frazier OH, HeartMate III. Advanced heart failure treated with continuous-flow left ventricular assist device. N Engl J Med. 2009;361:2241–51.
12. Ambardekar AV, Walker JS, Walker LA, Cleveland JC Jr, Lowes BD, Buttrick PM. Incomplete recovery of myocyte contractile function despite improvement of myocardial architecture with left ventricular assist device support. Circ Heart Fail. 2011;4:425–32.
13. Birks EJ. Molecular changes after left ventricular assist device support for heart failure. Circ Res. 2013;113:777–91.
14. Diakos NA, Selzman CH, Sachse FB, Stehlik J, Kfoury AG, Wever-Pinzon O, Catino A, Alharethi R, Reid BB, Miller DV, Salama M, Zaitsev AV, Shibayama J, Li H, Fang JC, Li DY, Drakos SG. Myocardial atrophy and chronic mechanical unloading of the failing human heart: implications for cardiac assist device-induced myocardial recovery. J Am Coll Cardiol. 2014;64:1602–12.
15. Canseco DC, Kimura W, Garg S, Mukherjee S, Bhattacharya S, Abdisalaam S, Das S, Asaithamby A, Mammen PP, Sadek HA. Human ventricular unloading induces cardiomyocyte proliferation. J Am Coll Cardiol. 2015;65:892–900.
16. Drakos SG, Kfoury AG, Hammond EH, Reid BB, Revelo MP, Rasmusson BY, Whitehead KJ, Salama ME, Selzman CH, Stehlik J, Clayson SE, Bristow MR, Renlund DG, Li DY. Impact of mechanical unloading on microvasculature and associated central remodeling features of the failing human heart. J Am Coll Cardiol. 2010;56:382–91.

17. Murphy KT. The pathogenesis and treatment of cardiac atrophy in cancer cachexia. Am J Physiol Heart Circ Physiol. 2016;310:H466–77.
18. Springer J, Tschirner A, Haghikia A, von Haehling S, Lal H, Grzesiak A, Kaschina E, Palus S, Potsch M, von Websky K, Hocher B, Latouche C, Jaisser F, Morawietz L, Coats AJ, Beadle J, Argiles JM, Thum T, Foldes G, Doehner W, Hilfiker-Kleiner D, Force T, Anker SD. Prevention of liver cancer cachexia-induced cardiac wasting and heart failure. Eur Heart J. 2014;35:932–41.
19. Zhou X, Wang JL, Lu J, Song Y, Kwak KS, Jiao Q, Rosenfeld R, Chen Q, Boone T, Simonet WS, Lacey DL, Goldberg AL, Han HQ. Reversal of cancer cachexia and muscle wasting by actriib antagonism leads to prolonged survival. Cell. 2010;142:531–43.
20. Schafer M, Oeing CU, Rohm M, Baysal-Temel E, Lehmann LH, Bauer R, Volz HC, Boutros M, Sohn D, Sticht C, Gretz N, Eichelbaum K, Werner T, Hirt MN, Eschenhagen T, Muller-Decker K, Strobel O, Hackert T, Krijgsveld J, Katus HA, Berriel Diaz M, Backs J, Herzig S. Ataxin-10 is part of a cachexokine cocktail triggering cardiac metabolic dysfunction in cancer cachexia. Mol Metab. 2016;5:67–78.
21. Moore-Morris T, Guimaraes-Camboa N, Banerjee I, Zambon AC, Kisseleva T, Velayoudon A, Stallcup WB, Gu Y, Dalton ND, Cedenilla M, Gomez-Amaro R, Zhou B, Brenner DA, Peterson KL, Chen J, Evans SM. Resident fibroblast lineages mediate pressure overload-induced cardiac fibrosis. J Clin Invest. 2014;124:2921–34.
22. Nishida K, Yamaguchi O, Otsu K. Degradation systems in heart failure. J Mol Cell Cardiol. 2015;84:212–22.
23. Sano M, Minamino T, Toko H, Miyauchi H, Orimo M, Qin Y, Akazawa H, Tateno K, Kayama Y, Harada M, Shimizu I, Asahara T, Hamada H, Tomita S, Molkentin JD, Zou Y, Komuro I. P53-induced inhibition of hif-1 causes cardiac dysfunction during pressure overload. Nature. 2007;446:444–8.
24. Tirziu D, Giordano FJ, Simons M. Cell communications in the heart. Circulation. 2010;122:928–37.
25. Gu H, Smith FC, Taffet SM, Delmar M. High incidence of cardiac malformations in connexin40-deficient mice. Circ Res. 2003;93:201–6.
26. Koitabashi N, Danner T, Zaiman AL, Pinto YM, Rowell J, Mankowski J, Zhang D, Nakamura T, Takimoto E, Kass DA. Pivotal role of cardiomyocyte tgf-beta signaling in the murine pathological response to sustained pressure overload. J Clin Invest. 2011;121:2301–12.
27. Kuhn M. Molecular physiology of membrane guanylyl cyclase receptors. Physiol Rev. 2016;96:751–804.
28. Biesemann N, Mendler L, Wietelmann A, Hermann S, Schafers M, Kruger M, Boettger T, Borchardt T, Braun T. Myostatin regulates energy homeostasis in the heart and prevents heart failure. Circ Res. 2014;115:296–310.
29. Kakkar R, Lee RT. Intramyocardial fibroblast myocyte communication. Circ Res. 2010;106:47–57.
30. Ieda M, Tsuchihashi T, Ivey KN, Ross RS, Hong TT, Shaw RM, Srivastava D. Cardiac fibroblasts regulate myocardial proliferation through beta1 integrin signaling. Dev Cell. 2009;16:233–44.
31. Takeda N, Manabe I, Uchino Y, Eguchi K, Matsumoto S, Nishimura S, Shindo T, Sano M, Otsu K, Snider P, Conway SJ, Nagai R. Cardiac fibroblasts are essential for the adaptive response of the murine heart to pressure overload. J Clin Invest. 2010;120:254–65.
32. Viereck J, Bang C, Foinquinos A, Thum T. Regulatory rnas and paracrine networks in the heart. Cardiovasc Res. 2014;102:290–301.
33. Thum T, Gross C, Fiedler J, Fischer T, Kissler S, Bussen M, Galuppo P, Just S, Rottbauer W, Frantz S, Castoldi M, Soutschek J, Koteliansky V, Rosenwald A, Basson MA, Licht JD, Pena JT, Rouhanifard SH, Muckenthaler MU, Tuschl T, Martin GR, Bauersachs J, Engelhardt S. Microrna-21 contributes to myocardial disease by stimulating map kinase signalling in fibroblasts. Nature. 2008;456:980–4.
34. Bang C, Batkai S, Dangwal S, Gupta SK, Foinquinos A, Holzmann A, Just A, Remke J, Zimmer K, Zeug A, Ponimaskin E, Schmiedl A, Yin X, Mayr M, Halder R, Fischer A, Engelhardt S, Wei Y, Schober A, Fiedler J, Thum T. Cardiac fibroblast-derived microrna passenger strand-enriched exosomes mediate cardiomyocyte hypertrophy. J Clin Invest. 2014;124:2136–46.
35. Heineke J. Wag the dog: how endothelial cells regulate cardiomyocyte growth. Arterioscler Thromb Vasc Biol. 2012;32:545–7.
36. Pinto AR, Ilinykh A, Ivey MJ, Kuwabara JT, D'Antoni ML, Debuque R, Chandran A, Wang L, Arora K, Rosenthal NA, Tallquist MD. Revisiting cardiac cellular composition. Circ Res. 2016;118:400–9.
37. Giordano FJ, Gerber HP, Williams SP, VanBruggen N, Bunting S, Ruiz-Lozano P, Gu Y, Nath AK, Huang Y, Hickey R, Dalton N, Peterson KL, Ross J Jr, Chien KR, Ferrara N. A cardiac myocyte vascular endothelial growth factor paracrine pathway is required to maintain cardiac function. Proc Natl Acad Sci U S A. 2001;98:5780–5.
38. Heineke J, Auger-Messier M, Xu J, Oka T, Sargent MA, York A, Klevitsky R, Vaikunth S, Duncan SA, Aronow BJ, Robbins J, Crombleholme TM, Molkentin JD. Cardiomyocyte gata4 functions as a stress-responsive regulator of angiogenesis in the murine heart. J Clin Invest. 2007;117:3198–210.
39. Fiedler J, Jazbutyte V, Kirchmaier BC, Gupta SK, Lorenzen J, Hartmann D, Galuppo P, Kneitz S, Pena JT, Sohn-Lee C, Loyer X, Soutschek J, Brand T, Tuschl T, Heineke J, Martin U, Schulte-Merker S, Ertl G, Engelhardt S, Bauersachs J, Thum T. Microrna-24 regulates vascularity after myocardial infarction. Circulation. 2011;124:720–30.
40. Bonauer A, Carmona G, Iwasaki M, Mione M, Koyanagi M, Fischer A, Burchfield J, Fox H, Doebele C, Ohtani K, Chavakis E, Potente M, Tjwa M, Urbich C, Zeiher AM, Dimmeler S. Microrna-92a controls angiogenesis and functional recovery of ischemic tissues in mice. Science. 2009;324:1710–3.
41. Lemmens K, Doggen K, De Keulenaer GW. Role of neuregulin-1/erbb signaling in cardiovascular physiology and disease: implications for therapy of heart failure. Circulation. 2007;116:954–60.
42. Halkein J, Tabruyn SP, Ricke-Hoch M, Haghikia A, Nguyen NQ, Scherr M, Castermans K, Malvaux L, Lambert V, Thiry M, Sliwa K, Noel A, Martial JA, Hilfiker-Kleiner D, Struman I. Microrna-146a is a therapeutic target and biomarker for peripartum cardiomyopathy. J Clin Invest. 2013;123:2143–54.
43. Knoll R, Hoshijima M, Hoffman HM, Person V, Lorenzen-Schmidt I, Bang ML, Hayashi T, Shiga N, Yasukawa H, Schaper W, McKenna W, Yokoyama M, Schork NJ, Omens JH, McCulloch AD, Kimura A, Gregorio CC, Poller W, Schaper J, Schultheiss HP, Chien KR. The cardiac mechanical stretch sensor machinery involves a z disc complex that is defective in a subset of human dilated cardiomyopathy. Cell. 2002;111:943–55.
44. Zou Y, Akazawa H, Qin Y, Sano M, Takano H, Minamino T, Makita N, Iwanaga K, Zhu W, Kudoh S, Toko H, Tamura K, Kihara M, Nagai T, Fukamizu A, Umemura S, Iiri T, Fujita T, Komuro I. Mechanical stress activates angiotensin ii type 1 receptor without the involvement of angiotensin ii. Nat Cell Biol. 2004;6:499–506.
45. Heineke J, Ritter O. Cardiomyocyte calcineurin signaling in subcellular domains: from the sarcolemma to the nucleus and beyond. J Mol Cell Cardiol. 2012;52:62–73.
46. Noor N, Patel CB, Rockman HA. Beta-arrestin: a signaling molecule and potential therapeutic target for heart failure. J Mol Cell Cardiol. 2011;51:534–41.

47. Kreusser MM, Backs J. Integrated mechanisms of camkii-dependent ventricular remodeling. Front Pharmacol. 2014;5:36.
48. Wilkins BJ, De Windt LJ, Bueno OF, Braz JC, Glascock BJ, Kimball TF, Molkentin JD. Targeted disruption of nfatc3, but not nfatc4, reveals an intrinsic defect in calcineurin-mediated cardiac hypertrophic growth. Mol Cell Biol. 2002;22:7603–13.
49. Bourajjaj M, Armand AS, da Costa Martins PA, Weijts B, van der Nagel R, Heeneman S, Wehrens XH, De Windt LJ. Nfatc2 is a necessary mediator of calcineurin-dependent cardiac hypertrophy and heart failure. J Biol Chem. 2008;283:22295–303.
50. Bueno OF, Lips DJ, Kaiser RA, Wilkins BJ, Dai YS, Glascock BJ, Klevitsky R, Hewett TE, Kimball TR, Aronow BJ, Doevendans PA, Molkentin JD. Calcineurin abeta gene targeting predisposes the myocardium to acute ischemia-induced apoptosis and dysfunction. Circ Res. 2004;94:91–9.
51. Kehat I, Davis J, Tiburcy M, Accornero F, Saba-El-Leil MK, Maillet M, York AJ, Lorenz JN, Zimmermann WH, Meloche S, Molkentin JD. Extracellular signal-regulated kinases 1 and 2 regulate the balance between eccentric and concentric cardiac growth. Circ Res. 2011;108:176–83.
52. Eom GH, Cho YK, Ko JH, Shin S, Choe N, Kim Y, Joung H, Kim HS, Nam KI, Kee HJ, Kook H. Casein kinase-2alpha1 induces hypertrophic response by phosphorylation of histone deacetylase 2 s394 and its activation in the heart. Circulation. 2011;123:2392–403.
53. Hauck L, Harms C, An J, Rohne J, Gertz K, Dietz R, Endres M, von Harsdorf R. Protein kinase ck2 links extracellular growth factor signaling with the control of p27(kip1) stability in the heart. Nat Med. 2008;14:315–24.
54. Fraccarollo D, Berger S, Galuppo P, Kneitz S, Hein L, Schutz G, Frantz S, Ertl G, Bauersachs J. Deletion of cardiomyocyte mineralocorticoid receptor ameliorates adverse remodeling after myocardial infarction. Circulation. 2011;123:400–8.
55. Bauersachs J, Jaisser F, Toto R. Mineralocorticoid receptor activation and mineralocorticoid receptor antagonist treatment in cardiac and renal diseases. Hypertension. 2015;65:257–63.
56. Greco CM, Condorelli G. Epigenetic modifications and noncoding rnas in cardiac hypertrophy and failure. Nat Rev Cardiol. 2015;12:488–97.
57. Movassagh M, Choy MK, Knowles DA, Cordeddu L, Haider S, Down T, Siggens L, Vujic A, Simeoni I, Penkett C, Goddard M, Lio P, Bennett MR, Foo RS. Distinct epigenomic features in end-stage failing human hearts. Circulation. 2011;124:2411–22.
58. Gilsbach R, Preissl S, Gruning BA, Schnick T, Burger L, Benes V, Wurch A, Bonisch U, Gunther S, Backofen R, Fleischmann BK, Schubeler D, Hein L. Dynamic DNA methylation orchestrates cardiomyocyte development, maturation and disease. Nat Commun. 2014;5:5288.
59. Papait R, Cattaneo P, Kunderfranco P, Greco C, Carullo P, Guffanti A, Vigano V, Stirparo GG, Latronico MV, Hasenfuss G, Chen J, Condorelli G. Genome-wide analysis of histone marks identifying an epigenetic signature of promoters and enhancers underlying cardiac hypertrophy. Proc Natl Acad Sci U S A. 2013;110:20164–9.
60. Backs J, Olson EN. Control of cardiac growth by histone acetylation/deacetylation. Circ Res. 2006;98:15–24.
61. Hohl M, Wagner M, Reil JC, Muller SA, Tauchnitz M, Zimmer AM, Lehmann LH, Thiel G, Bohm M, Backs J, Maack C. Hdac4 controls histone methylation in response to elevated cardiac load. J Clin Invest. 2013;123:1359–70.
62. Anand P, Brown JD, Lin CY, Qi J, Zhang R, Artero PC, Alaiti MA, Bullard J, Alazem K, Margulies KB, Cappola TP, Lemieux M, Plutzky J, Bradner JE, Haldar SM. Bet bromodomains mediate transcriptional pause release in heart failure. Cell. 2013;154:569–82.
63. Hang CT, Yang J, Han P, Cheng HL, Shang C, Ashley E, Zhou B, Chang CP. Chromatin regulation by brg1 underlies heart muscle development and disease. Nature. 2010;466:62–7.
64. Uchida S, Dimmeler S. Long noncoding rnas in cardiovascular diseases. Circ Res. 2015;116:737–50.
65. Thum T, Condorelli G. Long noncoding rnas and micrornas in cardiovascular pathophysiology. Circ Res. 2015;116:751–62.
66. Small EM, Olson EN. Pervasive roles of micrornas in cardiovascular biology. Nature. 2011;469:336–42.
67. van Rooij E, Sutherland LB, Qi X, Richardson JA, Hill J, Olson EN. Control of stress-dependent cardiac growth and gene expression by a microrna. Science. 2007;316:575–9.
68. Ucar A, Gupta SK, Fiedler J, Erikci E, Kardasinski M, Batkai S, Dangwal S, Kumarswamy R, Bang C, Holzmann A, Remke J, Caprio M, Jentzsch C, Engelhardt S, Geisendorf S, Glas C, Hofmann TG, Nessling M, Richter K, Schiffer M, Carrier L, Napp LC, Bauersachs J, Chowdhury K, Thum T. The mirna-212/132 family regulates both cardiac hypertrophy and cardiomyocyte autophagy. Nat Commun. 2012;3:1078.
69. Elia L, Contu R, Quintavalle M, Varrone F, Chimenti C, Russo MA, Cimino V, De Marinis L, Frustaci A, Catalucci D, Condorelli G. Reciprocal regulation of microrna-1 and insulin-like growth factor-1 signal transduction cascade in cardiac and skeletal muscle in physiological and pathological conditions. Circulation. 2009;120:2377–85.
70. Care A, Catalucci D, Felicetti F, Bonci D, Addario A, Gallo P, Bang ML, Segnalini P, Gu Y, Dalton ND, Elia L, Latronico MV, Hoydal M, Autore C, Russo MA, Dorn GW 2nd, Ellingsen O, Ruiz-Lozano P, Peterson KL, Croce CM, Peschle C, Condorelli G. Microrna-133 controls cardiac hypertrophy. Nat Med. 2007;13:613–8.
71. Ganesan J, Ramanujam D, Sassi Y, Ahles A, Jentzsch C, Werfel S, Leierseder S, Loyer X, Giacca M, Zentilin L, Thum T, Laggerbauer B, Engelhardt S. Mir-378 controls cardiac hypertrophy by combined repression of mitogen-activated protein kinase pathway factors. Circulation. 2013;127:2097–106.
72. Thum T, Galuppo P, Wolf C, Fiedler J, Kneitz S, van Laake LW, Doevendans PA, Mummery CL, Borlak J, Haverich A, Gross C, Engelhardt S, Ertl G, Bauersachs J. Micrornas in the human heart: a clue to fetal gene reprogramming in heart failure. Circulation. 2007;116:258–67.
73. Schonrock N, Harvey RP, Mattick JS. Long noncoding rnas in cardiac development and pathophysiology. Circ Res. 2012;111:1349–62.
74. Nelson BR, Makarewich CA, Anderson DM, Winders BR, Troupes CD, Wu F, Reese AL, McAnally JR, Chen X, Kavalali ET, Cannon SC, Houser SR, Bassel-Duby R, Olson EN. A peptide encoded by a transcript annotated as long noncoding rna enhances serca activity in muscle. Science. 2016;351:271–5.
75. Anderson DM, Anderson KM, Chang CL, Makarewich CA, Nelson BR, McAnally JR, Kasaragod P, Shelton JM, Liou J, Bassel-Duby R, Olson EN. A micropeptide encoded by a putative long noncoding rna regulates muscle performance. Cell. 2015;160:595–606.
76. Yang KC, Yamada KA, Patel AY, Topkara VK, George I, Cheema FH, Ewald GA, Mann DL, Nerbonne JM. Deep rna sequencing reveals dynamic regulation of myocardial noncoding rnas in failing human heart and remodeling with mechanical circulatory support. Circulation. 2014;129:1009–21.
77. Wang K, Liu F, Zhou LY, Long B, Yuan SM, Wang Y, Liu CY, Sun T, Zhang XJ, Li PF. The long noncoding rna chrf regulates cardiac hypertrophy by targeting mir-489. Circ Res. 2014;114:1377–88.
78. Viereck J, Kumarswamy R, Foinquinos A, Xiao K, Avramopoulos P, Kunz M, Dittrich M, Maetzig T, Zimmer K, Remke J, Just A, Fendrich J, Scherf K, Bolesani E, Schambach A, Weidemann F, Zweigerdt R, de Windt LJ, Engelhardt S, Dandekar T, Batkai S,

Thum T. Long noncoding rna chast promotes cardiac remodeling. Sci Transl Med. 2016;8:326ra322.
79. Han P, Li W, Lin CH, Yang J, Shang C, Nurnberg ST, Jin KK, Xu W, Lin CY, Lin CJ, Xiong Y, Chien HC, Zhou B, Ashley E, Bernstein D, Chen PS, Chen HS, Quertermous T, Chang CP. A long noncoding rna protects the heart from pathological hypertrophy. Nature. 2014;514:102–6.
80. Ounzain S, Pezzuto I, Micheletti R, Burdet F, Sheta R, Nemir M, Gonzales C, Sarre A, Alexanian M, Blow MJ, May D, Johnson R, Dauvillier J, Pennacchio LA, Pedrazzini T. Functional importance of cardiac enhancer-associated noncoding rnas in heart development and disease. J Mol Cell Cardiol. 2014;76:55–70.
81. Ounzain S, Micheletti R, Beckmann T, Schroen B, Alexanian M, Pezzuto I, Crippa S, Nemir M, Sarre A, Johnson R, Dauvillier J, Burdet F, Ibberson M, Guigo R, Xenarios I, Heymans S, Pedrazzini T. Genome-wide profiling of the cardiac transcriptome after myocardial infarction identifies novel heart-specific long non-coding rnas. Eur Heart J. 2015;36:353–368a.
82. Kumarswamy R, Bauters C, Volkmann I, Maury F, Fetisch J, Holzmann A, Lemesle G, de Groote P, Pinet F, Thum T. Circulating long noncoding rna, lipcar, predicts survival in patients with heart failure. Circ Res. 2014;114:1569–75.
83. Gorski PA, Ceholski DK, Hajjar RJ. Altered myocardial calcium cycling and energetics in heart failure – a rational approach for disease treatment. Cell Metab. 2015;21:183–94.
84. Yano M, Ikeda Y, Matsuzaki M. Altered intracellular ca2+ handling in heart failure. J Clin Invest. 2005;115:556–64.
85. Jessup M, Greenberg B, Mancini D, Cappola T, Pauly DF, Jaski B, Yaroshinsky A, Zsebo KM, Dittrich H, Hajjar RJ. Calcium upregulation by percutaneous administration of gene therapy in cardiac disease I. Calcium upregulation by percutaneous administration of gene therapy in cardiac disease (cupid): A phase 2 trial of intracoronary gene therapy of sarcoplasmic reticulum ca2+−atpase in patients with advanced heart failure. Circulation. 2011;124:304–13.
86. Kho C, Lee A, Jeong D, Oh JG, Gorski PA, Fish K, Sanchez R, Devita RJ, Christensen G, Dahl R, Hajjar RJ. Small-molecule activation of serca2a sumoylation for the treatment of heart failure. Nat Commun. 2015;6:7229.
87. Gibbs CL. Cardiac energetics. Physiol Rev. 1978;58:174–254.
88. Doenst T, Nguyen TD, Abel ED. Cardiac metabolism in heart failure: implications beyond atp production. Circ Res. 2013;113:709–24.
89. Kolwicz SC Jr, Purohit S, Tian R. Cardiac metabolism and its interactions with contraction, growth, and survival of cardiomyocytes. Circ Res. 2013;113:603–16.
90. Neubauer S. The failing heart – an engine out of fuel. N Engl J Med. 2007;356:1140–51.
91. Sorokina N, O'Donnell JM, McKinney RD, Pound KM, Woldegiorgis G, LaNoue KF, Ballal K, Taegtmeyer H, Buttrick PM, Lewandowski ED. Recruitment of compensatory pathways to sustain oxidative flux with reduced carnitine palmitoyltransferase i activity characterizes inefficiency in energy metabolism in hypertrophied hearts. Circulation. 2007;115:2033–41.
92. Rosca MG, Hoppel CL. Mitochondrial dysfunction in heart failure. Heart Fail Rev. 2013;18:607–22.
93. Gupta A, Akki A, Wang Y, Leppo MK, Chacko VP, Foster DB, Caceres V, Shi S, Kirk JA, Su J, Lai S, Paolocci N, Steenbergen C, Gerstenblith G, Weiss RG. Creatine kinase-mediated improvement of function in failing mouse hearts provides causal evidence the failing heart is energy starved. J Clin Invest. 2012;122:291–302.
94. Facundo HT, Brainard RE, Watson LJ, Ngoh GA, Hamid T, Prabhu SD, Jones SP. O-glcnac signaling is essential for nfat-mediated transcriptional reprogramming during cardiomyocyte hypertrophy. Am J Physiol Heart Circ Physiol. 2012;302:H2122–30.
95. Rabinowitz JD, White E. Autophagy and metabolism. Science. 2010;330:1344–8.
96. Jankowska EA, Kasztura M, Sokolski M, Bronisz M, Nawrocka S, Oleskowska-Florek W, Zymlinski R, Biegus J, Siwolowski P, Banasiak W, Anker SD, Filippatos G, Cleland JG, Ponikowski P. Iron deficiency defined as depleted iron stores accompanied by unmet cellular iron requirements identifies patients at the highest risk of death after an episode of acute heart failure. Eur Heart J. 2014;35:2468–76.
97. Anker SD, Comin Colet J, Filippatos G, Willenheimer R, Dickstein K, Drexler H, Luscher TF, Bart B, Banasiak W, Niegowska J, Kirwan BA, Mori C, von Eisenhart RB, Pocock SJ, Poole-Wilson PA, Ponikowski P, Investigators F-HT. Ferric carboxymaltose in patients with heart failure and iron deficiency. N Engl J Med. 2009;361:2436–48.
98. Ponikowski P, van Veldhuisen DJ, Comin-Colet J, Ertl G, Komajda M, Mareev V, McDonagh T, Parkhomenko A, Tavazzi L, Levesque V, Mori C, Roubert B, Filippatos G, Ruschitzka F, Anker SD, Investigators C-H. Beneficial effects of long-term intravenous iron therapy with ferric carboxymaltose in patients with symptomatic heart failure and iron deficiencydagger. Eur Heart J. 2015;36:657–68.
99. Lill R. Function and biogenesis of iron-sulphur proteins. Nature. 2009;460:831–8.
100. Jankowska EA, von Haehling S, Anker SD, Macdougall IC, Ponikowski P. Iron deficiency and heart failure: diagnostic dilemmas and therapeutic perspectives. Eur Heart J. 2013;34:816–29.
101. Dong F, Zhang X, Culver B, Chew HG Jr, Kelley RO, Ren J. Dietary iron deficiency induces ventricular dilation, mitochondrial ultrastructural aberrations and cytochrome c release: involvement of nitric oxide synthase and protein tyrosine nitration. Clin Sci. 2005;109:277–86.
102. Haddad S, Wang Y, Galy B, Korf-Klingebiel M, Hirsch V, Baru AM, Rostami F, Reboll MR, Heineke J, Flogel U, Groos S, Renner A, Toischer K, Zimmermann F, Engeli S, Jordan J, Bauersachs J, Hentze MW, Wollert KC, Kempf T. Iron-regulatory proteins secure iron availability in cardiomyocytes to prevent heart failure. Eur Heart J. 2016;38(5):362–72.
103. Hentze MW, Muckenthaler MU, Galy B, Camaschella C. Two to tango: regulation of mammalian iron metabolism. Cell. 2010,142:24–38.
104. Korf-Klingebiel M, Reboll MR, Klede S, Brod T, Pich A, Polten F, Napp LC, Bauersachs J, Ganser A, Brinkmann E, Reimann I, Kempf T, Niessen HW, Mizrahi J, Schonfeld HJ, Iglesias A, Bobadilla M, Wang Y, Wollert KC. Myeloid-derived growth factor (c19orf10) mediates cardiac repair following myocardial infarction. Nat Med. 2015;21:140–9.
105. Zangi L, Lui KO, von Gise A, Ma Q, Ebina W, Ptaszek LM, Spater D, Xu H, Tabebordbar M, Gorbatov R, Sena B, Nahrendorf M, Briscoe DM, Li RA, Wagers AJ, Rossi DJ, Pu WT, Chien KR. Modified mrna directs the fate of heart progenitor cells and induces vascular regeneration after myocardial infarction. Nat Biotechnol. 2013;31:898–907.
106. Polizzotti BD, Ganapathy B, Walsh S, Choudhury S, Ammanamanchi N, Bennett DG, Dos Remedios CG, Haubner BJ, Penninger JM, Kuhn B. Neuregulin stimulation of cardiomyocyte regeneration in mice and human myocardium reveals a therapeutic window. Sci Transl Med. 2015;7:281ra245.
107. Porrello ER, Mahmoud AI, Simpson E, Johnson BA, Grinsfelder D, Canseco D, Mammen PP, Rothermel BA, Olson EN, Sadek HA. Regulation of neonatal and adult mammalian heart regeneration by the mir-15 family. Proc Natl Acad Sci U S A. 2013;110:187–92.
108. Olson EN. Micrornas as therapeutic targets and biomarkers of cardiovascular disease. Sci Transl Med. 2014;6:239ps233.

109. Zwadlo C, Schmidtmann E, Szaroszyk M, Kattih B, Froese N, Hinz H, Schmitto JD, Widder J, Batkai S, Bahre H, Kaever V, Thum T, Bauersachs J, Heineke J. Antiandrogenic therapy with finasteride attenuates cardiac hypertrophy and left ventricular dysfunction. Circulation. 2015;131:1071–81.
110. Lee DI, Zhu G, Sasaki T, Cho GS, Hamdani N, Holewinski R, Jo SH, Danner T, Zhang M, Rainer PP, Bedja D, Kirk JA, Ranek MJ, Dostmann WR, Kwon C, Margulies KB, Van Eyk JE, Paulus WJ, Takimoto E, Kass DA. Phosphodiesterase 9a controls nitric-oxide-independent cgmp and hypertrophic heart disease. Nature. 2015;519:472–6.
111. van Berlo JH, Maillet M, Molkentin JD. Signaling effectors underlying pathologic growth and remodeling of the heart. J Clin Invest. 2013;123:37–45.

Inflammation and Innate Immunity

3

Stefan Frantz

In the 1990ies data were generated indicating an upregulation of certain cytokines, especially TNF (tumor necrosis factor alpha), in heart failure (HF) patients [1]. Subsequently it became clear that this phenomenon is not restricted to the cytokine TNF, but that there is an activation of several parts of the immune system in HF with pathophysiologic importance.

Indeed, we find an activation of the immune system in HF analogous to what we see when an infection takes place (see Fig. 3.1). Usually invading pathogens first face the so called innate immune system. The innate immune system is non-specific. It is evolutionary old. Receptors of the innate immune system recognize specific patterns (and not specific epitopes) of pathogens, as for example double-stranded RNA as a marker of a viral infection. They express specific receptors for this purpose, the so-called pattern recognition receptor. Activation of the receptors leads to the production of cytokines and recruitment of inflammatory cells like macrophages and neutrophils that can kill pathogens. Furthermore, the innate immune system is also able to activate the adaptive or specific immune system. The adaptive immune system consists of highly specialized cells (lymphocytes). The reaction targets specific antigens, takes time to be activated (e.g. for antibody production), and generates an immunologic memory.

It might seem rather odd that a disease like HF that is with the exception of a viral myocarditis usually not caused by pathogens, activates an immune system. However, from an evolutionary point of view the immune system has not only been developed to react to pathogens, but to all forms of stress or injury. For example it is well known that healing of a wound, even if the wound is not infected, activates neutrophils and macrophages. Indeed, inflammatory cells are necessary for adequate scar formation. Thus activation of the immune system has to be seen in a broader perspective. To explain the innate immune activation in non-infectious diseases the danger theory has been developed: The danger theory assumes that it is necessary to have so called alarm signals from stressed or injured tissue to activate an innate immune response. Those signals could be factors that are released by dying cells as for example heat shock proteins. Indeed, important innate immune receptors recognize not only pathogens, but also alarm signals.

The components of the immune system are expressed in the heart, upregulated under ischemic conditions, and of pathophysiologic importance. For the innate immune system all cellular components can be found in the heart as e.g. neutrophils and macrophages (see Fig. 3.2). Also pattern recognition receptors in the heart have been described and are of functional importance. The most important innate immune receptors are toll like receptors (TLRs) [2]. TLR4 for example is the receptor for lipopolysaccharides. Most of TLRs have been described to be expressed in the heart and on cardiac myocytes. TLRs are upregulated in the ischemic and failing heart. Mice deficient e.g. in TLR2 or TLR4 have improved left ventricular remodeling after myocardial infarction. NLRs (NOD-like receptors) are another important class of innate immune receptors and cytosolic sensors of alarm signals. They are again expressed in the heart and contribute to the ischemic damage. Also, downstream signaling components of innate immune receptors like the transcription factor nuclear factor kappa B (NF-κB) are pathophysiological important.

Parts of the adaptive immune system contribute to the development of heart failure. T-cells are activated in heart draining lymph nodes after myocardial infarction. Regulatory T-cells interact with macrophages (see below) and are necessary for adequate healing after myocardial infarction. B-cells can directly influence the response to ischemic injury [3]. Later in the disease process autoimmunity may also play a role. Autoimmunity means that in the disease course antibodies are built that are directed against antigens of the heart. Anti-myosin antibodies can generate a cardiomyopathy in

S. Frantz (✉)
Department of Internal Medicine I, Comprehensive Heart Failure Center, University of Würzburg, Würzburg, Germany
e-mail: frantz_s@ukw.de

D. S. Feldman, P. Mohacsi (eds.), *Heart Failure*, Cardiovascular Medicine, https://doi.org/10.1007/978-3-319-98184-0_3

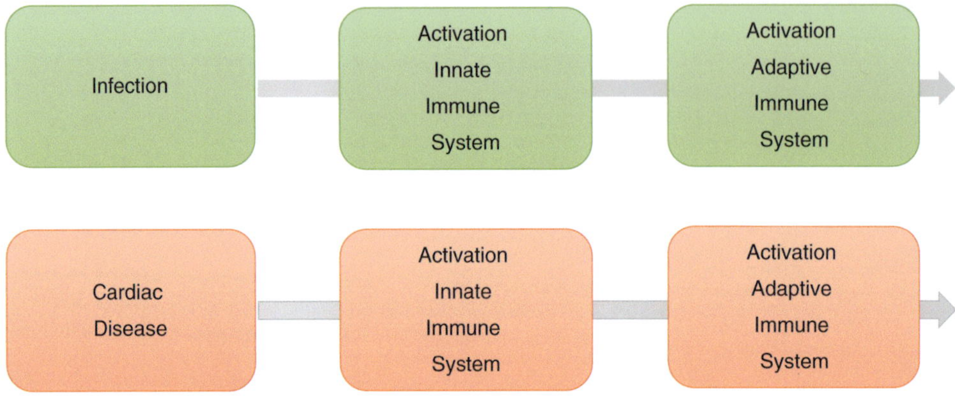

Fig. 3.1 Activation of the immune system in the heart upon injury is analogous to what happens upon infection

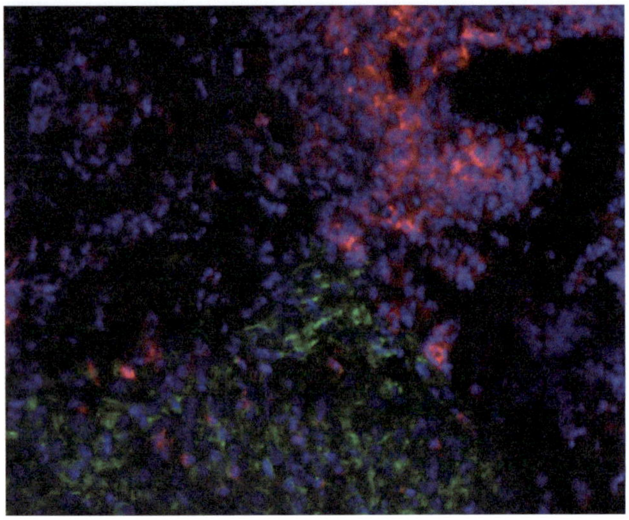

Fig. 3.2 Neutrophils are activated after myocardial infarction. This is an immunohistochemistry of myocardium after experimental myocardial infarction in a mouse (200x magnification). The tissue was stained with Phalloidin-Alexa488 (stains F-actin in green), Ly6G-Alexa-555 (stains neutrophils orange) and Höchst (stains DNA blue)

mice. Different autoantibodies have been measured in patients and animals with heart failure. E.g. a betareceptor stimulating antibody develops in a subpopulation of heart failure patients and is of prognostic significance. This autoantibody can lead to development of heart failure in animals. However, the role of autoimmunity in the pathophysiology is currently under debate, as is which autoantigens could be of importance [4].

To get a better understanding of the role of the immune system it helps to understand activation of the immune system in heart failure after myocardial infarction (see Fig. 3.3). Today we differentiate three different phases [5]: The first phase after a myocardial infarction is called the pro-inflammatory phase. Here, cells dye due to apoptosis and necrosis. Neutrophils and macrophages infiltrate the diseased myocardium and there is a massive production of cytokines. In the second phase, the healing phase, a solid scar has to be built. The dominant immune cells in this phase are macrophages. Ischemic tissue attracts initially proinflammatory Ly6^{high} monocytes that are released by the bone marrow or spleen. Once recruited monocytes may differentiate in macrophages. We differentiate several macrophage subtypes today. Probably most important is initially the pro-inflammatory M1 macrophage, what is followed by a pro-healing phenotype (so-called M2). Monocytes usually infiltrate the heart from outside after development in spleen and bone marrow with fast myocardial turnover times. In the mouse initially proinflammatory Ly6^{high} monocytes can be found, followed by Ly6^{low}. Corresponding monocyte subtypes have been detected in humans. Sedentary macrophages have also been identified; they might have regenerative capacity; however, their number is limited. Macrophages secret cytokines leading to extracellular matrix generation through activation of fibroblast or myofibroblasts as well as neovascularisation. In this phase proinflammatory cytokines are downregulated. T-cells from the adaptive immune system seem to be important in this case. Regulatory T-cells have the ability to switch macrophages from a pro-inflammatory to a healing phenotype [6]. Finally a solid scar has been built and the proinflammatory reaction is terminated leading to the remodeling phase.

Thus, there is a first pro-inflammatory response that has to be terminated for an optimal disease course. An instructive experiment shows that inflammation is absolutely necessary for an adequate response to myocardial infarction: In an experimental setting macrophages were depleted before a myocardial infarction was induced. This led to increased mortality and inadequate healing together with left ventricular

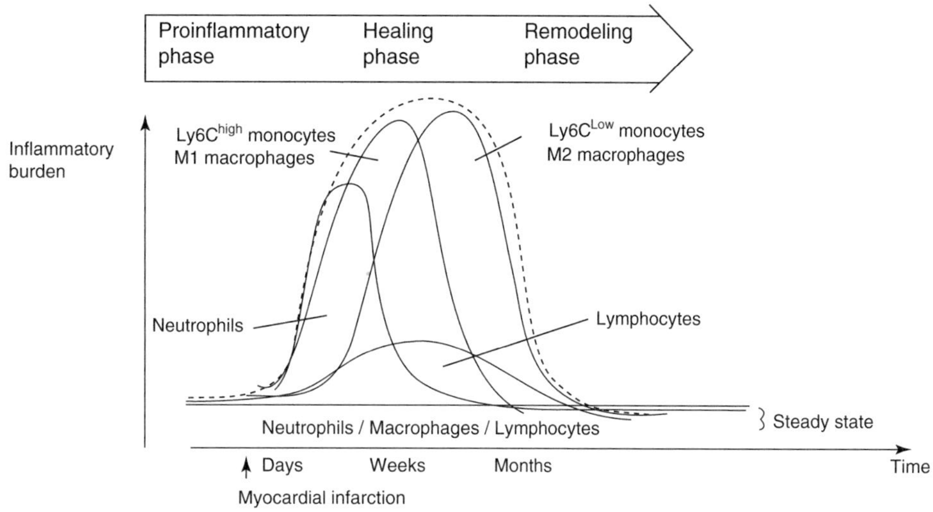

Fig. 3.3 Phases of immune activation after myocardial infarction

thrombus formation [7]. Indeed, macrophages remove dead cells. When macrophages are depleted necrotic tissue cannot be eliminated and healing is hampered. Macrophages are also necessary for a reduction of neutrophil infiltration. This indicates that inflammation is not something "bad" as is often suggested. A timely activation is absolutely necessary for adequate healing.

On the other hand, we know that prolonged inflammatory activation is not useful. TNF is probably the best studied cytokine in heart failure. Overexpression of TNF in the myocardium leads to a heart failure phenotype in mice [8]. Rats treated with TNF doses yielding serum levels that can be measured in heart failure patients, had a decrease in left ventricular function [9]. Animals with an inhibited TNF response had better left ventricular remodeling after myocardial infarction [10]. This indicates that a sustained activation of TNF leads to adverse effects and that a prolonged proinflammatory reaction leads to adverse pathophysiologic reactions.

In conclusion, we know today that the innate as well as the adaptive immune system are present under basal conditions in the heart. They are activated upon injury in different phases that are tightly regulated. Immune activation is necessary for adequate healing. However, chronic immune activation has adverse effects. Right now, we just begin to decipher the various aspects of the immune system and hope to identify adequate targets for a potential pharmacologic intervention.

References

1. Levine B, Kalman J, Mayer L, et al. Elevated circulating levels of tumor necrosis factor in severe chronic heart failure. N Engl J Med. 1990;323:236–41.
2. Hofmann U, Ertl G, Frantz S. Toll-like receptors as potential therapeutic targets in cardiac dysfunction. Expert Opin Ther Targets. 2011;15:753–65.
3. Hofmann U, Frantz S. Role of T-cells in myocardial infarction. Eur Heart J. 2016;37:873–9.
4. Hofmann U, Frantz S. How can we cure a heart "in flame"? A translational view on inflammation in heart failure. Basic Res Cardiol. 2013;108:356.
5. Frantz S, Nahrendorf M. Cardiac macrophages and their role in ischaemic heart disease. Cardiovasc Res. 2014;102:240–8.
6. Hofmann U, Frantz S. Role of lymphocytes in myocardial injury, healing, and remodeling after myocardial infarction. Circulation Res. 2015;116:354–67.
7. Frantz S, Hofmann U, Fraccarollo D, et al. Monocytes/macrophages prevent healing defects and left ventricular thrombus formation after myocardial infarction. FASEB J: Offl Publ Fed Am Soc Exp Biol. 2013;27:871–81.
8. Sivasubramanian N, Coker ML, Kurrelmeyer KM, et al. Left ventricular remodeling in transgenic mice with cardiac restricted overexpression of tumor necrosis factor. Circulation. 2001;104:826–31.
9. Bozkurt B, Kribbs SB, Clubb FJ Jr, et al. Pathophysiologically relevant concentrations of tumor necrosis factor- alpha promote progressive left ventricular dysfunction and remodeling in rats. Circulation. 1998;97:1382–91.
10. Sun M, Dawood F, Wen WH, et al. Excessive tumor necrosis factor activation after infarction contributes to susceptibility of myocardial rupture and left ventricular dysfunction. Circulation. 2004;110:3221–8.

Part III

Special Pathophysiology

Comorbidities and Co-Existing Conditions in Heart Failure Around Pregnancy

4

Denise Hilfiker-Kleiner, Johann Bauersachs, and Karen Sliwa

4.1 Introduction

It is estimated that 0.2 to 4% of all pregnancies in industrialized countries are complicated by cardiovascular diseases (CVD) with increasing number of women who develop cardiac problems during pregnancy [1]. Indeed, pregnancy challenges the cardiovascular system and may lead to disease states such as hypertensive complications with its severe forms preeclampsia and the HELLP syndrome (**H:** hemolysis, **EL:** elevated liver enzymes, **LP:** low platelets counts) [2]. Especially the phase towards the end of pregnancy, during delivery and postpartum is a special challenge for the cardiovascular system since it has to cope with massive hormonal fluctuations, fluid changes and mechanical stress. Alterations in metabolism (subclinical insulin resistance in pregnancy) and immune response (repressed in pregnancy and activated after delivery) take place as well. Moreover, endothelial stress promotes hypertensive disorders and additional enhanced coagulation activity lead to higher risk for myocardial infarction and stroke and cardiomyopathies as outlined below. It is therefore not surprising that acceleration of heart failure towards the end of the second trimester, under delivery or in the early postpartum phase is frequently observed in women with pre-existing cardiomyopathies or pulmonary hypertension and is associated with adverse maternal and perinatal outcome [3]. Moreover, the cardiac stress model "pregnancy" may even unmask unrecognized genetic and non-genetic heart diseases [2, 4, 5].

It is also important to note, that cardiovascular disease around pregnancy provides substantial challenges for the patient and the treating physician because evidence-based clinical data are scarce and even the understanding for normal physiological processes operating on the maternal cardiovascular system during pregnancy are poorly understood. Moreover, medical therapy is limited since many well established medications are contra-indicated during pregnancy and large clinical trials are rarely performed.

In this chapter we summarize the current knowledge on comorbidities and co-existing conditions in heart failure as well as new onset cardiovascular disease around pregnancy. We will discuss state of the art treatment options, prognosis and novel insights in pathophysiological mechanisms behind pregnancy-mediated cardiovascular diseases.

4.2 What Is Known on Normal Physiological Changes of the Cardiovascular System During Pregnancy

The nature of physiological stress factors to the cardiovascular system such as hemodynamic changes, increased cardiac workload and cardiac output around pregnancy are summarized in articles by Hilfiker-Kleiner et al. and by Chung et al. [6, 7]. In brief, marked hemodynamic changes in the maternal circulation occur in the first trimester of pregnancy and cause a profound decline in systemic vascular resistance that, in turn, abets a reciprocal increase in cardiac output of approximately 40% or 2 L/min lasting throughout pregnancy. These circulatory changes are thought to condition the maternal system for the rapid growth phase of the foetus and placenta in the 2nd half of pregnancy, when oxygen and nutrient demands are rising exponentially. At the same time powerful dilatory mechanism(s) are started that counteract

D. Hilfiker-Kleiner (✉) · J. Bauersachs
Department of Cardiology and Angiology, Medical School Hannover, Hannover, Germany
e-mail: hilfiker.denise@mh-hannover.de

K. Sliwa
Hatter Institute for Cardiovascular Research in Africa & IDM, SA MRC Cape Heart Group, University of Cape Town, Cape Town, South Africa

Soweto Cardiovascular Research Unit, University of the Witwatersrand, Johannesburg, South Africa

D. S. Feldman, P. Mohacsi (eds.), *Heart Failure*, Cardiovascular Medicine, https://doi.org/10.1007/978-3-319-98184-0_4

compensatory structural and functional hypertrophy for which pregnancy hormones such as progesterone and relaxin seem to be responsible [6, 8].

The hormonal changes during pregnancy alter also the propensity to blood clotting and haemorrhage thereby increasing the risk for embolic complications such as stroke and myocardial infarction [9].

In addition, a metabolic switch is induced in the mother's system away from glucose towards fatty acids and glycogen since glucose has to be efficiently shuttled to the foetus, a feature that leads to a "physiological" type of insulin resistance in the mother [9].

In summary, pregnancy leads to a system-wide hormonal, hemodynamic and metabolic reprogramming for which our current understanding is limited. Therefore, intensive research in this field is needed to better define what is "normal" and where serious disturbance and disease starts.

4.3 Pregnant or Postpartum Women with Heart Failure

Heart failure in pregnant or postpartum women may arise newly or may have pre-existed already prior pregnancy. Pre-existing conditions can be known to the patient and treating physician or be unknown and unmasked due to the above mentioned stress condition of pregnancy. We therefore suggest a systematic approach in these patients as outlined in Fig. 4.1. Using this scheme, a first classification in patients with pre-existing vs patients with new onset cardiovascular disease can be made.

Fig. 4.1 Scheme to classify heart failure in pregnant and peripartum women

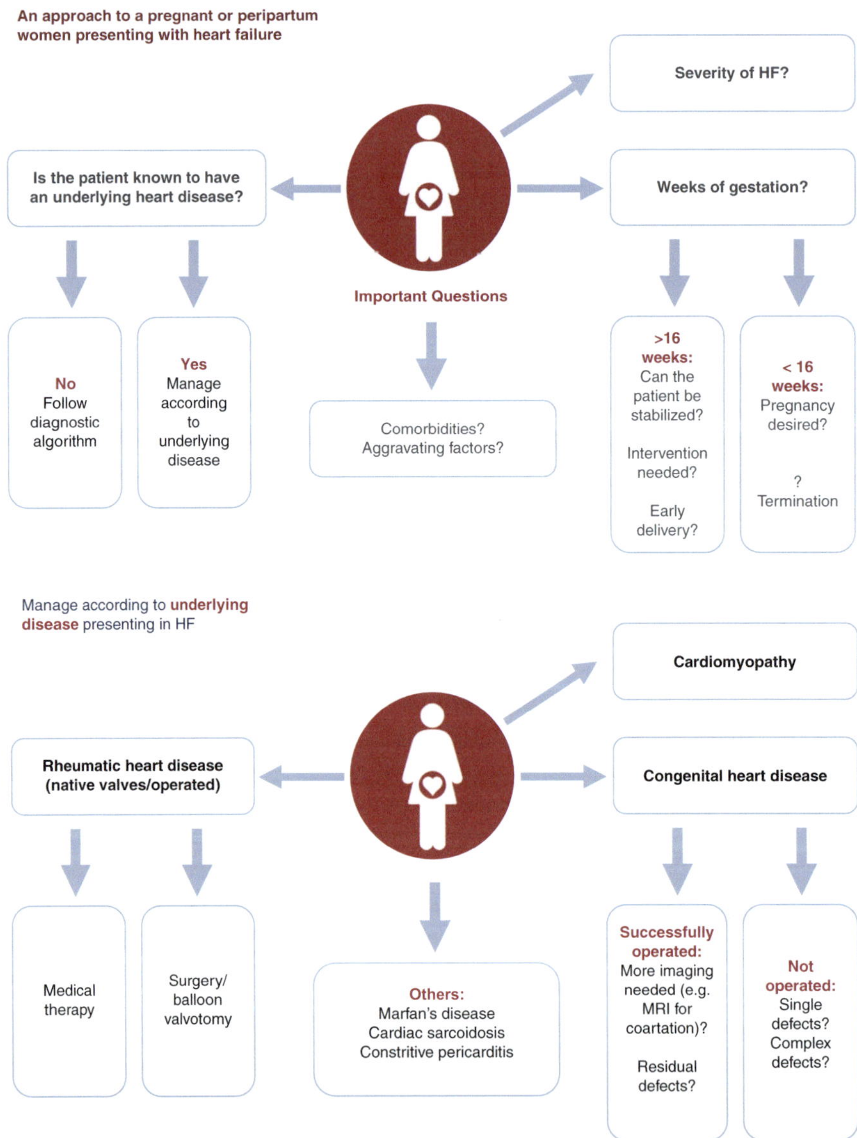

4.4 Pre-Existing Cardiovascular Disease in Pregnant Women

In the world-wide Registration Of Pregnancy And Cardiac disease (ROPAC), 7% of pregnancies in women with cardiovascular diseases involved cardiomyopathies [3, 10–13]. In ROPAC women with cardiomyopathies had a 2.4% mortality compared to women with other underlying heart diseases (0–2.1%).

Women known with cardiomyopathy or mutation carriers of an inheritant cardiomyopathy and their partners need to be counselled before pregnancy addressing maternal risk of complications while pregnant and postpartum and the influence of maternal disease on fetal outcome. The possible influence of pregnancy on cardiac function after pregnancy must be taken into account. Date on longer-term impact of pregnancy on deterioration of cardiac function are unknown and not studied so far. The most common pre-existing cardiomyopathies are dilated cardiomyopathies (DCM) or hypertrophic cardiomyopathy (HCM),

Dilated Cardiomyopathy DCM in women of child-bearing age is commonly idiopathic. Secondary causes for DCM can be myocarditis, hypertensive heart disease (particularly common in Africans) and cardiotoxins such as anti-neoplastic drugs [14]. Currently, more than 30 genes are known to be responsible to DCM [15]. Among 88 pregnancies in women with cardiomyopathies in the ROPAC registry one death occurred in a women with DCM and another in a women with anthracycline related cardiomyopathy [10]. However, 6 months outcome data were not available for all and no date for long-term maternal mortality (≥1 year post partum were recorded). A recent study from South Africa showed that eight out of nine death of women with heart disease occurred later than the standard rate of maternal mortality reporting of 42 days [16]. In a series from Canada studying 36 pregnancies in women with DCM, no death occurred but 39% of women developed heart failure or arrhythmias during pregnancy with moderate to severe LV systolic dysfunction and NYHA functional class III or IV with adverse cardiac event rates of 72% and 83% respectively [17]. Fetal and neonatal complications are also common in pregnancies in women with DCM. In the series from Canada 20% of the pregnancies had adverse fetal or neonatal outcomes [17].

Left Ventricular Noncompaction Cardiomyopathy (LVNCCM) LVNCCM is a condition characterized by thickening of the myocardium, which consists of a thin compacted and thick non-compacted layer of myocardium. LVNCCM has a familial occurrence in a large proportion of patients with several underlying gene mutations being identified. A recent study by **Gati S** [18] showed that increased trabeculations fulfilling the criteria of non-compaction develop in a substantial proportion of healthy pregnant women. Their data suggest that increased preload is associated with LV trabeculations resembling LVNCCM. A new diagnosis of LVCCM should be made with caution in pregnant women, especially when there is no heart failure or familial disease [18]. Only limited data from case reports are available regarding pregnancy in women with LVNCCM [19]. Clinical presentation varied from uneventful pregnancy to arrhythmias and severe heart failure. Increase in thromboembolic events have not been reported.

Hypertrophic Cardiomyopathy (HCM) HCM occurs in the general population in 1:500 individuals (0.2%). Localization and severity of hypertrophy differs between individuals due to heterogeneous expression of sarcomeric genes. Limited data are available on the outcome of pregnancy in women with HCM. Mortality appears rare (0.5%) and has only been reported in high risk patients [20]. A meta-analysis on 408 pregnancies in 237 women reported a maternal complication rate of 29% [21]. These complications included heart failure in up to 30% and arrhythmias in up to 48%. All women with HCM should have risk assessment and counselling before pregnancy according to current guidelines, giving attention to both maternal risk and offspring risk, including the risk of transmission of disease [1].

4.5 Newly Onset Cardiovascular Disease Around Pregnancy

Hypertension in Pregnancy Hypertensive complications in pregnancy occur with an estimated frequency of 8% worldwide and are responsible for substantial maternal and foetal morbidities and mortalities [22–24]. Most recent data from an American study suggest that the frequency of hypertensive complications is even higher and may affect one fifth of all pregnancies [25]. The severity of maternal hypertension ranges from slightly elevated systolic and diastolic blood pressure to severe and life threatening conditions. The study of Coel et al. [25] showed that 23% of women with antepartum hypertension were diagnosed with preeclampsia, 60% with transient hypertension, 9.4% with gestational hypertension, and 7.5% with chronic hypertension. Preeclampsia as a severe form of pregnancy associated hypertension is defined as onset of sustained hypertension (>140 mmHg systolic or > 90 mmHg diastolic blood pressure) with development of proteinuria of at least 1+ on dipstick or > 300 mg per 24 h after 20 weeks of gestation. Critical preeclampsia or HELLP syndrome (H: hemolysis, EL: elevated liver enzymes, **LP:** low platelets counts) are defined as blood pressure > 160 mmHg systolic or > 110 mmHg diastolic, proteinuria >5 g per 24 h, neurological symptoms such as seizures, pulmonary edema, hepatic or renal dysfunction, thrombocytopenia or fetal growth restriction [8]. Preeclampsia and HELLP are leading causes for premature delivery with high risk for maternal, foetal and neonatal morbidity and mortality [8]. Treatment of hypertension in pregnancy is limited since only a few compounds as summarized in the guidelines for treatment of cardiovascular disease in pregnancy [1] are considered safe in pregnancy not harming mother and child. Therefore, the only "cure" for severe hypertensive complications is often (premature) delivery. After delivery acute symptoms and renal damage resolve relatively fast. However, hypertension may take up to 2 years to disappear implying that endothelial injury may be long-lasting. Women with transient left ventricular hypertrophy or preeclampsia appeared more likely to develop postpartum hypertension compared with women with chronic or gestational hypertension [25, 26]. A novel observation is the development of postpartum hypertension in women who had no hypertension during pregnancy [25, 26]. This observation indicates that in general more careful cardiovascular monitoring is required in women not only during pregnancy but also in the first postpartum months. Postpartum women with a specifically high risk for postpartum hypertension had a higher body mass index at delivery and were more likely to have a history of diabetes mellitus [25, 26]. Hypertensive disorders and preeclampsia during pregnancy are associated with additional cardiovascular disorders such as a higher risk for developing PPCM [27]. Indeed, since preeclampsia and PPCM share common pathomechanisms including endothelial damage hypertensive disorders in pregnancy may predispose women to PPCM [4, 28]. Moreover, women with preeclampsia have 3- to eight-fold increased risk for ischemic heart disease, hypertension and stroke as well as obesity, dyslipidemia and end-stage renal disease later in life [29–31].

Finally, hypertensive disorders in pregnancy seem also to impact on the foetus since children resulting from these pregnancies have higher risks for high blood pressure and stroke [24].

Pregnancy as a Stress Test for Underlying Genetic Forms of Heart Failure The physiological impact of pregnancy on the human heart with regard to hormonal and mechanical stress is substantial and is therefore able to unmask unnoticed genetic forms of cardiomyopathies. Indeed, a subset of patients with peripartum heart failure turned out to be carriers of mutations associated with familial forms of dilated cardiomyopathies (DCM), including mutations MYH7, SCN5A, PSEN2, MYH6, TNNT2, cardiac troponin C (TNNC1), and MYBPC3 [32, 33] [5]. The German PPCM registry reports around 16% of patients with a positive family history for cardiomyopathies [27]. A recent study on a large international collective of PPCM patients reported a significantly higher prevalence (15% v.s. 4.7%) of truncating variants of genes whose mutations are associated with cardiomyopathies in PPCM patients compared to normal collectives [5]. Interestingly, two thirds of the identified truncating variants were affecting the Titin gene [5]. Additional genetic factors may also contribute to the susceptibility to peripartum heart failure, a feature that is especially interesting in the light of the higher incidence of the disease observed in patients with African ancestry [34, 35].

However, in general it is not easy to distinguish non-genetic from genetic forms of peripartum heart failure to date. May be the emerging field of next generation sequencing may help to identify disease causing factors and co-factors in patients presenting with new-onset heart failure around pregnancy. Moreover, since the pathophysiology between genetic and non-genetic forms of peripartum heart failure may differ, biomarkers could be developed for a cost saving pre-screening process. This would be important since "true" non-genetic PPCM patients seem to have a higher chance for recovery compared to the genetic forms [27] and family counselling would be recommended if mutations are detected.

Peripartum Cardiomyopathy (PPCM) Among peripartum diseases affecting the heart, PPCM is one of the more severe forms. PPCM is an independent disease that is defined as "an idiopathic cardiomyopathy presenting with heart failure secondary to left ventricular (LV) systolic dysfunction towards the end of pregnancy or in the months following delivery, where no other cause of heart failure is found" as proposed by the Working Group on PPCM from the Heart Failure Association of the ESC [35]. For many years PPCM has been considered a very rare disease in Western countries. Meanwhile, it is recognized as an important condition for women's health worldwide with increasing incidence in the USA and in Europe (from 1 in 4350 in 1990 to 1993 to 1 in 2229 in 2000 to 2002 in the USA [36]. Socio-economic changes in Western societies such as rising maternal age and a substantial increase in multifetal pregnancies due to reproductive techniques may account for the higher prevalence [2, 36, 37]. Additionally, the rising awareness of pregnancy related cardiovascular complications, the EUR*Observational* Research Programme on PPCM (http://www.eorp.org) [38] and other national and international reporting facilities [27, 39–41] may also contribute to the larger number of PPCM cases diagnosed in recent years.

In contrast to the above mentioned hypertensive disorders of the cardiovascular system or the genetic forms of peripartum heart failure, the etiology of PPCM is not known. The clinical presentation of PPCM patients is highly variable ranging from phenotypes similar to dilated cardiomyopathy (DCM), cases with almost normal ventricular dimensions or borderline non-compaction cardiomyopathies [2]. No typical

ECG pattern has been described and to date the diagnosis is only based on reduced ejection fraction (EF nearly always below 45%) and the exclusion of other forms of cardiomyopathies [35, 42].

PPCM can present with acute heart failure needing immediate admission to the intensive care unit, or it may develop subtly over several weeks. Especially in the slow developing PPCM, it is difficult to distinguish between normal peripartum discomfort, i.e. fatigue, mild shortness of breath or mild edema, and pathological symptoms of heart failure. Due to these overlapping symptoms even if accompanied by typical heart failure symptoms (congestion, abdominal discomfort, pleuritic chest pain and/or palpitations) diagnosis is often late and subsequent heart failure treatment delayed [2, 4, 35].

Therefore, biomarkers are needed to identify PPCM patients and refer them to expert physicians for further diagnostic assessment. So far, NT-proBNP, a well established marker for heart failure, turned out to be increased in most PPCM patients [27, 43] and would therefore be an easy marker for any peripartum woman reporting discomfort. In addition, enhanced shedding of endothelial microparticles has been reported in PPCM patients [44]. A long the same line, microRNA-146a (miR-146a), present in endothelial exosomes, has been shown to be specifically upregulated in PPCM patients but not in healthy postpartum women or patients with DCM [27, 45]. Since miR146a is directly associated with the pathophysiology of PPCM (outlined below) it appears to be the first PPCM specific marker.

The etiology of PPCM is still unknown but several pathomechanisms that contribute and/or drive the disease have been identified in recent years. For example low selenium level, various viral infections, stress-activated cytokines, inflammation and autoimmune reaction and a pathologic response to hemodynamic stress are suspected factors [34, 46]. Meanwhile, it is suggested that several factors may induce PPCM but finally all merge into a common pathway, which includes the coincidental presence of unbalanced oxidative stress and high levels of the nursing hormone Prolactin (PRL), which lead to the proteolytically produced angiostatic and pro-apoptotic 16 kDa PRL fragment [45, 47]. The 16 kDa PRL complexes with the fibrinolytic inhibitor plasminogen activator inhibitor-1 (PAI-1), and via binding to the PAI-1-urokinase-type plasminogen activator (uPA)-uPA receptor (uPAR), exerts antiangiogenic effects mainly via activation of NFkappaB and subsequent upregulation of miR-146a [45, 48].

Together with additional anti-angiogenic factors such as soluble fms-like tyrosine kinase-1 (sFlt1) the 16 kDa PRL disturbs the angiogenic balance in the peripartum phase damaging the endothelium, which subsequently induces a metablic shortage leading to heart failure [4, 28]. Indeed, there is evidence that the maternal heart needs protection against these angiogenic dysbalance and up-regulates the expression of pro-angiogenic factors, i.e. vascular endothelial growth factor (VEGF) [28, 47]. However, there is experimental and clinical evidence that pathways responsible for the upregulation of VEGF, i.e. the signal transducer and activator of transcription 3 (STAT3) and peroxisome proliferator-activated receptor gamma coactivator 1-alpha (PGC1α) related signaling, seem to be compromised in PPCM [28, 47, 49]. The same signalling pathways are also required for protection from oxidative stress, which in normal pregnancy rises specifically towards the end of pregnancy [50]. STAT3 and PGC1a play central roles in the anti-oxidative defence of the maternal heart during the peripartum phase because they increase the expression of anti-oxidative enzymes such as manganese superoxide dismutase (MnSOD) [28, 47]. STAT3 is downregulated in cardiac tissue form PPCM patients and cardiomyocyte specific knockout of STAT3 or PGC1a lead to PPCM in mice [28, 47, 49]. Latest data suggest that hyperosmolar stress caused by excessive bleeding during delivery or by ethnic traditions with high salt intake in the postpartum phase may accidently cause a decrease of the protective STAT3 in the heart of peripartum women [49].

Taken together, these data indicate that PPCM may often start as a disease of the endothelium, leading to loss or damage of the vasculature. Moreover, PPCM may be a multifactorial disease caused by the coincidential presence of unbalanced oxidative stress, impaired cardioprotective and pro-angiogenic signalling and high expression of anti-angiogenic factors. Part of these mechanisms may already be initiated during pregnancy for example by preeclampsia. The current understanding of pathomechanisms inducing PPCM is explained in more detail in recent reviews [2, 4].

4.6 Therapeutic Concepts and Management of Peripartum Heart Failure

Currently, peripartum heart failure is treated according to the ESC guidelines for heart failure in pregnancy [1]. In brief, late in pregnancy therapeutic interventions need to consider the health of the mother and the foetus while after delivery standard therapy for heart failure (beta-blockers, ACE-inhibitors/AT1-blockers, diuretics, mineralocorticoid receptor antagonists) is recommended. The more recent insights into the pathophysiology of peripartum heart failure and especially PPCM provide novel and more disease specific therapeutic concepts. In this regard, prolactin blockade with the dopamine D2 receptor agonist bromocriptine to eliminate the prolactin (the full-length nursing hormone and its angiostatic and pro-apoptotic 16 kDa form) has been successfully tested in several experimental models and in small clinical pilot trials and case reports [28, 47, 51, 52]. The concept of bromocriptine treatment is investigated in a larger controlled randomized multicenter trial in Germany evaluated the dosing of bromocriptine (ClinicalTrials.gov, study number: NCT00998556) [53]. This study showed that 2.5 mg bromocriptine and anticoagulation therapy applied daily on top of heart failure medication is sufficient to promote healing in the majority of PPCM patients while severely diseased patients may need longer (6 weeks) and higher doses (5mg per day) of bromocriptine [43, 54–56]. Since at the same time, PPCM patients have a good chance to recover from the disease early implantation of a defibrillator (ICD) is not recommended and ICD therapy might be even unnecessary [57]. In turn, a first study using wearable cardioverter/defibrillator (WCD) in PPCM patients with severely depressed cardiac function and/or ventricular arrhythmias confirmed their high risk for ventricular tachyarrhythmias in the early phase of the disease. In addition, this study showed that WCD provides protection against sudden cardiac death in the vulnerable phase of the first 3–6 months, and ordinates the need for necessary ICD-implantation in patients recovering from reduced LV-function [57]. An additional, recent study shows that the early therapeutic concept might also crucially influence the patient's chance for recovery. In this respect, analyses of data from the German PPCM registry indicated that patients who were treated with the β1-adrenergic receptor (AR) agonist dobutamine developed frequently terminal heart failure needing either heart transplantation and/or ventricular assist devices [2, 49]. Experimental studies confirmed that low cardiac STAT3 levels in PPCM seem to be responsible for cardiomyocyte necrosis and energy deficits induced by β1-AR agonist treatment [49]. It is important to note that bromocriptine treatment is inefficient to prevent these β1-AR agonist induced heart failure progression. These data support the concept of a restricted use of dobutamine during acute heart failure in PPCM patients. One of the most frequently asked question concerns the possibility of future pregnancies in PPCM patients. Interestingly, PPCM patients seem to tolerate the pregnancy state quite well, especially if they enter the subsequent pregnancy with fully recovered cardiac function [35, 58]. However, cardiac dysfunction re-emerges often in the peri- and postpartum phase [35, 58]. Therefore, PPCM patients should carefully be informed about the risk of relapse and should in general be discouraged from having additional pregnancies. They should be informed about contraceptive options (we recommend IUD since hormonal contraceptives may interact with heart failure medication, and counsel them about the risk for relapse in subsequent pregnancies). However, if they get pregnant again, termination of pregnancy may not prevent PPCM as we observe the disease also in pregnancies terminated in the first and second trimester. In turn, since they tolerate pregnancy normally quite well, they should carefully be followed in experienced centres with close collaboration between obstetricians and heart failure cardiologists. This is especially important in PPCM patients who become pregnant without complete recovery of LV function.

4.7 Conclusion

In recent years the awareness for cardiovascular disease around pregnancy has increased for the benefit of women's health in general. Larger clinical data sets are collected and analysed, thus allowing more insight into the pathophysiology of these diseases and providing important information for diagnosis and management of these patients. Large clinical registries as for example the ones of the EURO OBS program (ESC EURO*OBS* program (www.escardio.org) on pregnancy and cardiac disease (ROPAC) [3, 10–13] or on PPCM [38] together with experimental research are needed to further broaden our understanding of pathophysiology, prevention, treatment and management of cardiovascular disease around pregnancy.

References

1. Regitz-Zagrosek V, Blomstrom Lundqvist C, Borghi C, Cifkova R, Ferreira R, Foidart JM, Gibbs JS, Gohlke-Baerwolf C, Gorenek B, Iung B, Kirby M, Maas AH, Morais J, Nihoyannopoulos P, Pieper PG, Presbitero P, Roos-Hesselink JW, Schaufelberger M, Seeland U, Torracca L, Bax J, Auricchio A, Baumgartner H, Ceconi C, Dean V, Deaton C, Fagard R, Funck-Brentano C, Hasdai D, Hoes A, Knuuti J, Kolh P, McDonagh T, Moulin C, Poldermans D, Popescu BA, Reiner Z, Sechtem U, Sirnes PA, Torbicki A, Vahanian A, Windecker S, Aguiar C, Al-Attar N, Garcia AA, Antoniou A, Coman I, Elkayam U, Gomez-Sanchez MA, Gotcheva N, Hilfiker-Kleiner D, Kiss RG, Kitsiou A, Konings KT, Lip GY, Manolis A, Mebaaza A, Mintale I, Morice MC, Mulder BJ, Pasquet A, Price S, Priori SG, Salvador MJ, Shotan A, Silversides CK, Skouby SO, Stein JI, Tornos P, Vejlstrup N, Walker F, Warnes C. ESC Guidelines on the management of cardiovascular diseases during pregnancy: the Task Force on the Management of Cardiovascular Diseases during Pregnancy of the European Society of Cardiology (ESC). Eur Heart J. 2011;32(24):3147–97.
2. Hilfiker-Kleiner D, Haghikia A, Nonhoff J, Bauersachs J. Peripartum cardiomyopathy: current management and future perspectives. Eur Heart J. 2015;36(18):1090–7.
3. Ruys TP, Roos-Hesselink JW, Hall R, Subirana-Domenech MT, Grando-Ting J, Estensen M, Crepaz R, Fesslova V, Gurvitz M, De Backer J, Johnson MR, Pieper PG. Heart failure in pregnant women with cardiac disease: data from the ROPAC. Heart. 2014;100(3):231–8.
4. Hilfiker-Kleiner D, Sliwa K. Pathophysiology and epidemiology of peripartum cardiomyopathy. Nat Rev Cardiol. 2014;11(6):364–70.

5. Ware JS, Li J, Mazaika E, Yasso CM, De-Souza T, Cappola TP, Tsai EJ, Hilfiker-Kleiner D, Kamiya CA, Mazzarotto F, Cook SA, Halder I, Prasad SK, Pisarcik J, Hanley-Yanez K, Alharethi R, Damp J, Hsich E, Elkayam U, Sheppard R, Kealey A, Alexis J, Ramani G, Safirstein J, Boehmer J, Pauly DF, Wittstein IS, Thohan V, Zucker MJ, Liu P, Gorcsan J 3rd, DM MN, Seidman CE, Seidman JG, Arany Z, Imac, Investigators I. Shared Genetic Predisposition in Peripartum and Dilated Cardiomyopathies. N Engl J Med. 2016;374(3):233–41.
6. Hilfiker-Kleiner D, Bauersachs J. Pregnancy associated cardiomyopathies. Cardiovasc Med. 2014;17(9):245–51.
7. Chung E, Leinwand LA. Pregnancy as a cardiac stress model. Cardiovasc Res. 2014;101(4):561–70.
8. Conrad KP, Davison JM. The renal circulation in normal pregnancy and preeclampsia: is there a place for relaxin? Am J Physiol Renal Physiol. 2014;306(10):F1121–35.
9. Liu LX, Arany Z. Maternal cardiac metabolism in pregnancy. Cardiovasc Res. 2014;101(4):545–53.
10. Roos-Hesselink JW, Ruys TP, Stein JI, Thilen U, Webb GD, Niwa K, Kaemmerer H, Baumgartner H, Budts W, Maggioni AP, Tavazzi L, Taha N, Johnson MR, Hall R, Investigators R. Outcome of pregnancy in patients with structural or ischaemic heart disease: results of a registry of the European Society of Cardiology. Eur Heart J. 2013;34(9):657–65.
11. Ruys TP, Maggioni A, Johnson MR, Sliwa K, Tavazzi L, Schwerzmann M, Nihoyannopoulos P, Kozelj M, Marelli A, Elkayam U, Hall R, Roos-Hesselink JW. Cardiac medication during pregnancy, data from the ROPAC. Int J Cardiol. 2014;177(1):124–8.
12. Ruys TP, Roos-Hesselink JW, Pijuan-Domenech A, Vasario E, Gaisin IR, Iung B, Freeman LJ, Gordon EP, Pieper PG, Hall R, Boersma E, Johnson MR, Investigators R. Is a planned caesarean section in women with cardiac disease beneficial? Heart. 2015;101(7):530–6.
13. van Hagen IM, Roos-Hesselink JW, Ruys TP, Merz WM, Goland S, Gabriel H, Lelonek M, Trojnarska O, Al Mahmeed WA, Balint HO, Ashour Z, Baumgartner H, Boersma E, Johnson MR, Hall R, Investigators R, The ERPT. Pregnancy in women with a mechanical heart valve: data of the European Society of Cardiology Registry of Pregnancy and Cardiac Disease (ROPAC). Circulation. 2015;132(2):132–42.
14. Sliwa K, Boehm M. Incidence and prevalence of pregnancy associ ated heart disease. Cardiovasc Res. 2014.
15. Van Tintelen JP, Pieper PG, Van Spaendonck-Zwarts KY, Van Den Berg MP. Pregnancy, cardiomyopathies, and genetics. Cardiovasc Res. 2014;101(4):571–8.
16. Sliwa K, Libhaber E, Elliott C, Momberg Z, Osman A, Zuhlke L, Lachmann T, Nicholson L, Thienemann F, Roos-Hesselink J, Anthony J. Spectrum of cardiac disease in maternity in a low-resource cohort in South Africa. Heart. 2014;100(24):1967–74.
17. Grewal J, Siu SC, Ross HJ, Mason J, Balint OH, Sermer M, Colman JM, Silversides CK. Pregnancy outcomes in women with dilated cardiomyopathy. J Am Coll Cardiol. 2009;55(1):45–52.
18. Gati S, Papadakis M, Papamichael ND, Zaidi A, Sheikh N, Reed M, Sharma R, Thilaganathan B, Sharma S. Reversible de novo left ventricular trabeculations in pregnant women: implications for the diagnosis of left ventricular noncompaction in low-risk populations. Circulation. 2014;130(6):475–83.
19. Krul SP, van der Smagt JJ, van den Berg MP, Sollie KM, Pieper PG, van Spaendonck-Zwarts KY. Systematic review of pregnancy in women with inherited cardiomyopathies. Eur J Heart Fail. 2011;13(6):584–94.
20. Schinkel AF. Pregnancy in women with hypertrophic cardiomyopathy. Cardiol Rev. 2014;22(5):217–22.
21. Ashikhmina E, Farber MK, Mizuguchi KA. Parturients with hypertrophic cardiomyopathy: case series and review of pregnancy outcomes and anesthetic management of labor and delivery. Int J Obstet Anesth. 2015;24(4):344–55.
22. Bello N, Rendon IS, Arany Z. The relationship between preeclampsia and peripartum cardiomyopathy: a systematic review and meta-analysis. J Am Coll Cardiol. 2013;62(18):1715–23.
23. Rana S, Powe CE, Salahuddin S, Verlohren S, Perschel FH, Levine RJ, Lim KH, Wenger JB, Thadhani R, Karumanchi SA. Angiogenic factors and the risk of adverse outcomes in women with suspected preeclampsia. Circulation. 2012;125(7):911–9.
24. Ahmed R, Dunford J, Mehran R, Robson S, Kunadian V. Preeclampsia and future cardiovascular risk among women: a review. J Am Coll Cardiol. 2014;63(18):1815–22.
25. Goel A, Maski MR, Bajracharya S, Wenger JB, Zhang D, Salahuddin S, Shahul SS, Thadhani R, Seely EW, Karumanchi SA, Rana S. Epidemiology and mechanisms of de novo and persistent hypertension in the postpartum period. Circulation. 2015;132(18):1726–33.
26. August P, Malha L. Postpartum hypertension: "It ain't over 'til it's over". Circulation. 2015;132(18):1690–2.
27. Haghikia A, Podewski E, Libhaber E, Labidi S, Fischer D, Roentgen P, Tsikas D, Jordan J, Lichtinghagen R, von Kaisenberg CS, Struman I, Bovy N, Sliwa K, Bauersachs J, Hilfiker-Kleiner D. Phenotyping and outcome on contemporary management in a German cohort of patients with peripartum cardiomyopathy. Basic Res Cardiol. 2013;108(4):366.
28. Patten IS, Rana S, Shahul S, Rowe GC, Jang C, Liu L, Hacker MR, Rhee JS, Mitchell J, Mahmood F, Hess P, Farrell C, Koulisis N, Khankin EV, Burke SD, Tudorache I, Bauersachs J, del Monte F, Hilfiker-Kleiner D, Karumanchi SA, Arany Z. Cardiac angiogenic imbalance leads to peripartum cardiomyopathy. Nature. 2012;485(7398):333–8.
29. Mannisto T, Mendola P, Vaarasmaki M, Jarvelin MR, Hartikainen AL, Pouta A, Suvanto E. Elevated blood pressure in pregnancy and subsequent chronic disease risk. Circulation. 2013;127(6):681–90.
30. Vikse BE. Pre-eclampsia and the risk of kidney disease. Lancet. 2013;382(9887):104–6.
31. Williams D. Long-term complications of preeclampsia. Semin Nephrol. 2011;31(1):111–22.
32. Morales A, Painter T, Li R, Siegfried JD, Li D, Norton N, Hershberger RE. Rare variant mutations in pregnancy-associated or peripartum cardiomyopathy. Circulation. 2010;121(20):2176–82.
33. van Spaendonck-Zwarts KY, van Tintelen JP, van Veldhuisen DJ, van der Werf R, Jongbloed JD, Paulus WJ, Dooijes D, van den Berg MP. Peripartum cardiomyopathy as a part of familial dilated cardiomyopathy. Circulation. 2010;121(20):2169–75.
34. Sliwa K, Fett J, Elkayam U. Peripartum cardiomyopathy. Lancet. 2006;368(9536):687–93.
35. Sliwa K, Hilfiker-Kleiner D, Petrie MC, Mebazaa A, Pieske B, Buchmann E, Regitz-Zagrosek V, Schaufelberger M, Tavazzi L, van Veldhuisen DJ, Watkins H, Shah AJ, Seferovic PM, Elkayam U, Pankuweit S, Papp Z, Mouquet F, JJ MM. Current state of knowledge on aetiology, diagnosis, management, and therapy of peripartum cardiomyopathy: a position statement from the Heart Failure Association of the European Society of Cardiology Working Group on peripartum cardiomyopathy. Eur J Heart Fail. 2010;12(8):767–78.
36. Mielniczuk LM, Williams K, Davis DR, Tang AS, Lemery R, Green MS, Gollob MH, Haddad H, Birnie DH. Frequency of peripartum cardiomyopathy. Am J Cardiol. 2006;97(12):1765–8.
37. Hilfiker-Kleiner D. Social freezing' of women's eggs. Eur Heart J. 2015;36(13):773.
38. Sliwa K, Hilfiker-Kleiner D, Mebazaa A, Petrie MC, Maggioni AP, Regitz-Zagrosek V, Schaufelberger M, Tavazzi L, van Veldhuisen

DJ, Roos-Hesslink JW, Shah AJ, Seferovic PM, Elkayam U, van Spaendonck-Zwarts K, Bachelier-Walenta K, Mouquet F, Kraigher-Krainer E, Hall R, Ponikowski P, JJ MM, Pieske B. EURObservational Research Programme: a worldwide registry on peripartum cardiomyopathy (PPCM) in conjunction with the Heart Failure Association of the European Society of Cardiology Working Group on PPCM. Eur J Heart Fail. 2014;16(5):583–91.
39. Elkayam U. Clinical characteristics of peripartum cardiomyopathy in the United States: diagnosis, prognosis, and management. J Am Coll Cardiol. 2011;58(7):659–70.
40. Safirstein JG, Ro AS, Grandhi S, Wang L, Fett JD, Staniloae C. Predictors of left ventricular recovery in a cohort of peripartum cardiomyopathy patients recruited via the internet. Int J Cardiol. 2012;154(1):27–31.
41. McNamara DM, Elkayam U, Alharethi R, Damp J, Hsich E, Ewald G, Modi K, Alexis JD, Ramani GV, Semigran MJ, Haythe J, Markham DW, Marek J, Gorcsan J 3rd, Wu WC, Lin Y, Halder I, Pisarcik J, Cooper LT, Fett JD, Investigators I. Clinical outcomes for peripartum cardiomyopathy in North America: results of the IPAC study (Investigations of Pregnancy-Associated Cardiomyopathy). J Am Coll Cardiol. 2015;66(8):905–14.
42. Pearson GD, Veille JC, Rahimtoola S, Hsia J, Oakley CM, Hosenpud JD, Ansari A, Baughman KL. Peripartum cardiomyopathy: national heart, lung, and blood institute and office of rare diseases (National Institutes of Health) workshop recommendations and review. JAMA. 2000;283(9):1183–8.
43. Forster O, Hilfiker-Kleiner D, Ansari AA, Sundstrom JB, Libhaber E, Tshani W, Becker A, Yip A, Klein G, Sliwa K. Reversal of IFN-gamma, oxLDL and prolactin serum levels correlate with clinical improvement in patients with peripartum cardiomyopathy. Eur J Heart Fail. 2008;10(9):861–8.
44. Walenta K, Schwarz V, Schirmer SH, Kindermann I, Friedrich EB, Solomayer EF, Sliwa K, Labidi S, Hilfiker-Kleiner D, Bohm M. Circulating microparticles as indicators of peripartum cardiomyopathy. Eur Heart J. 2012;33(12):1469–79.
45. Halkein J, Tabruyn SP, Ricke-Hoch M, Haghikia A, Nguyen NQ, Scherr M, Castermans K, Malvaux L, Lambert V, Thiry M, Sliwa K, Noel A, Martial JA, Hilfiker-Kleiner D, Struman I. MicroRNA-146a is a therapeutic target and biomarker for peripartum cardiomyopathy. J Clin Invest. 2013;123(5):2143–54.
46. Sliwa K, Forster O, Libhaber E, Fett JD, Sundstrom JB, Hilfiker-Kleiner D, Ansari AA. Peripartum cardiomyopathy: inflammatory markers as predictors of outcome in 100 prospectively studied patients. Eur Heart J. 2006;27(4):441–6.
47. Hilfiker-Kleiner D, Kaminski K, Podewski E, Bonda T, Schaefer A, Sliwa K, Forster O, Quint A, Landmesser U, Doerries C, Luchtefeld M, Poli V, Schneider MD, Balligand JL, Desjardins F, Ansari A, Struman I, Nguyen NQ, Zschemisch NH, Klein G, Heusch G, Schulz R, Hilfiker A, Drexler H. A cathepsin D-cleaved 16 kDa form of prolactin mediates postpartum cardiomyopathy. Cell. 2007;128(3):589–600.
48. Bajou K, Herkenne S, Thijssen VL, D'Amico S, Nguyen NQ, Bouche A, Tabruyn S, Srahna M, Carabin JY, Nivelles O, Paques C, Cornelissen I, Lion M, Noel A, Gils A, Vinckier S, Declerck PJ, Griffioen AW, Dewerchin M, Martial JA, Carmeliet P, Struman I. PAI-1 mediates the antiangiogenic and profibrinolytic effects of 16 K prolactin. Nat Med. 2014;20(7):741–7.
49. Stapel B, Kohlhaas M, Ricke-Hoch M, Haghikia A, Erschow S, Knuuti J, Silvola JM, Roivainen A, Saraste A, Nickel AG, Saar JA, Sieve I, Pietzsch S, Muller M, Bogeski I, Kappl R, Jauhiainen M, Thackeray JT, Scherr M, Bengel FM, Hagl C, Tudorache I, Bauersachs J, Maack C, Hilfiker-Kleiner D. Low STAT3 expression sensitizes to toxic effects of beta-adrenergic receptor stimulation in peripartum cardiomyopathy. Eur Heart J. 2017;38(5):349–61.
50. Toescu V, Nuttall SL, Martin U, Kendall MJ, Dunne F. Oxidative stress and normal pregnancy. Clin Endocrinol. 2002;57(5):609–13.
51. Habedank D, Kuhnle Y, Elgeti T, Dudenhausen JW, Haverkamp W, Dietz R. Recovery from peripartum cardiomyopathy after treatment with bromocriptine. Eur J Heart Fail. 2008.
52. Meyer GP, Labidi S, Podewski E, Sliwa K, Drexler H, Hilfiker-Kleiner D. Bromocriptine treatment associated with recovery from peripartum cardiomyopathy in siblings: two case reports. J Med Case Rep. 2010;4:80.
53. Haghikia A, Podewski E, Berliner D, Sonnenschein K, Fischer D, Angermann CE, Bohm M, Rontgen P, Bauersachs J, Hilfiker-Kleiner D. Rationale and design of a randomized, controlled multicentre clinical trial to evaluate the effect of bromocriptine on left ventricular function in women with peripartum cardiomyopathy. Clin Res Cardiol. 2015;104(11):911–7.
54. Arrigo M, Blet A, Mebazaa A. Bromocriptine for the treatment of peripartum cardiomyopathy: welcome on BOARD. Eur Heart J. 2017;38(35):2680–2.
55. Hilfiker-Kleiner D, Haghikia A, Berliner D, Vogel-Claussen J, Schwab J, Franke A, Schwarzkopf M, Ehlermann P, Pfister R, Michels G, Westenfeld R, Stangl V, Kindermann I, Kuhl U, Angermann CE, Schlitt A, Fischer D, Podewski E, Bohm M, Sliwa K, Bauersachs J. Bromocriptine for the treatment of peripartum cardiomyopathy: a multicentre randomized study. Eur Heart J. 2017;38(35):2671–9.
56. Sliwa K, Forster O, Tibazarwa K, Libhaber E, Becker A, Yip A, Hilfiker-Kleiner D. Long-term outcome of peripartum cardiomyopathy in a population with high seropositivity for human immunodeficiency virus. Int J Cardiol. 2011;147(2):202–8.
57. Duncker D, Haghikia A, Konig T, Hohmann S, Gutleben KJ, Westenfeld R, Oswald H, Klein H, Bauersachs J, Hilfiker-Kleiner D, Veltmann C. Risk for ventricular fibrillation in peripartum cardiomyopathy with severely reduced left ventricular function-value of the wearable cardioverter/defibrillator. Eur J Heart Fail. 2014;16(12):1331–6.
58. Elkayam U, Tummala PP, Rao K, Akhter MW, Karaalp IS, Wani OR, Hameed A, Gviazda I, Shotan A. Maternal and fetal outcomes of subsequent pregnancies in women with peripartum cardiomyopathy. N Engl J Med. 2001;344(21):1567–71.

Myocardial Dysfunction Associated with Cancer Therapy

5

Margot K. Davis and Sean A. Virani

5.1 Introduction

An understanding of the effects of cancer therapy on the heart has become increasingly important for cardiologists in recent years. As the efficacy of cancer therapies improves, the population of cancer survivors increases, creating a new population of patients at risk for late toxicity of cancer treatment. Moreover, many targeted cancer therapies are associated with cardiovascular toxicity through on-target or off-target effects, and the rapid expansion of this exciting field has seen a parallel growth in new cardiotoxicities. Cancer therapies may be associated with QT prolongation, atrial fibrillation, myocardial ischemia, hypertension, or the metabolic syndrome, but heart failure and left ventricular (LV) dysfunction still account for a majority of patients seen in many cardio-oncology clinics. An understanding of the indications for various cancer treatments, the mechanisms by which they cause myocardial damage, and appropriate screening and management strategies is essential for general cardiologists and heart failure specialists who provide care to this complex population.

5.2 Epidemiology and Pathophysiology

5.2.1 Anthracyclines

The risk of heart failure with anthracyclines was first recognized in the 1960s [1]. These agents, including doxorubicin (Adriamycin), epirubicin, and daunorubicin, are commonly used in breast cancer, hematologic malignancies, and sarcomas [2]. Decades of advances in cancer therapy, including the introduction of targeted cancer therapy, have not displaced anthracyclines from the backbone of treatment for many malignancies [3, 4]. The mechanism of anthracycline cardiotoxicity remains incompletely understood. Oxygen free radicals are generated via electron exchange between anthracyclines and oxygen molecules and through the formation of anthracycline-iron complexes [5]. More recent evidence supports the role of topoisomerase IIβ (TOPIIβ) in the pathogenesis, whereby inhibition of TOPIIβ leads to DNA strand breaks and cardiomyocyte death [2]. Moreover, inhibition of TOPIIβ promotes the generation of reactive oxygen species, providing a link between these two proposed mechanisms of toxicity [6].

Early data indicated that the risk of cardiotoxicity was low until a cumulative dose of 450 mg/m^2 or doxorubicin was reached, falsely giving rise to a perceived "safe dose" [7]. Subsequent studies with rigorous monitoring of cardiac function have refuted this. At the modest doxorubicin dose of 300 mg/m^2, the risk of clinical heart failure is 1.7% and the risk of left ventricular dysfunction is 16% [8]. The risk of cardiotoxicity continues to rise with increasing cumulative doses, with LV dysfunction occurring in 32% and 65% of patients receiving 400 mg/m^2 and 550 mg/m^2, respectively.

Beyond cumulative dose, additional risk factors have been identified for anthracycline cardiotoxicity. Extremes of age (i.e. young children and the elderly), coronary artery disease, hypertension and other atherosclerotic risk factors, LV dysfunction or other structural heart disease, bolus administration, concomitant or prior thoracic irradiation, and administration of other cardiotoxic therapies (e.g. cyclophosphamide, trastuzumab) are all associated with increased incidence of anthracycline cardiotoxicity [9]. Strategies to mitigate this risk are discussed in depth later in this chapter.

5.2.2 Alkylating Agents

Alkylating agents including cyclophosphamide and ifosfamide have been reported to cause cardiotoxicity in up to 28% of patients [10, 11], but heart failure associated with this class of agents is rarely seen in modern clinical practice

M. K. Davis · S. A. Virani (✉)
Division of Cardiology, University of British Columbia, Vancouver, BC, Canada
e-mail: svirani@telus.net

D. S. Feldman, P. Mohacsi (eds.), *Heart Failure*, Cardiovascular Medicine, https://doi.org/10.1007/978-3-319-98184-0_5

[12]. Cardiac manifestations include myopericarditis, heart failure, and arrhythmia, and generally occur within the first 10 days after administration [10, 13, 14]. Increased risk is associated with advanced age, higher daily and cumulative doses, and concomitant radiation or anthracycline therapy [10]. Autopsy findings in patients with cyclophosphamide-induced heart failure include endothelial injury and hemorrhagic myocarditis [14, 15]. Similarly, autopsy findings in patients with ifosfamide toxicity include petechial and hemorrhagic changes in the myocardium [16].

5.2.3 Other Cytotoxic Chemotherapy

Heart failure and LV dysfunction are uncommonly associated with other classes of cytotoxic chemotherapy, including the antimetabolites decitabine and clofarabine and the taxane docetaxel [16]. Myocardial infarction resulting in HF may occur in association with taxanes and with the fluoropyrimidine agents 5-fluorouracil (5-FU) and capecitabine, mediated by coronary vasospasm and prothrombotic effects [17–19]. This risk is increased among patients with pre-existing coronary artery disease or atherosclerotic risk factors, and in the case of 5-FU, in the setting of continuous infusion (vs. bolus dosing) [20].

5.2.4 HER2-Targeted Therapies

Approximately 25–30% of breast cancers overexpress the human epidermal growth factor receptor-2 (HER2), a marker that is associated with more aggressive disease and shorter survival [21]. The HER2-targeted monoclonal antibody trastuzumab prevents the dimerization of this receptor tyrosine kinase and inhibits downstream signaling. Trastuzumab is approved for use in HER2-overexpressing breast cancer as well as gastric cancer. In the landmark trials of adjuvant trastuzumab, the drug was associated with a 50% reduction in disease recurrence and a 33% improvement in survival [22, 23]. HER2 is also part of important cell survival signaling pathways in the heart and is particularly important under conditions of myocardial stress [24].

In a landmark trial of trastuzumab in patients with metastatic breast cancer, the administration of trastuzumab with paclitaxel following prior anthracycline therapy was associated with a 13% risk of LV dysfunction and a 2% risk of New York Heart Association class III/IV heart failure, while these risks rose to 27% and 16%, respectively, in patients receiving concomitant trastuzumab and anthracycline therapy [25]. Subsequent trials in the adjuvant population demonstrated lower risks when patients with baseline LV dysfunction were excluded, lower doses of anthracyclines were used, no patients received concomitant anthracycline therapy, and all patients underwent rigorous monitoring of LV function during therapy [22, 23].

Concomitant administration of anthracycline, higher doses of anthracycline, and baseline LV dysfunction (or low-normal LV function) are thus accepted risk factors for trastuzumab cardiotoxicity. Additional risk factors include coronary artery disease, hypertension, and advanced age [9]. Importantly, the LV dysfunction associated with trastuzumab (in the absence of anthracycline exposure) is generally reversible upon cessation of therapy.

5.2.5 VEGF Signaling Pathway Inhibitors

The vascular endothelial growth factor (VEGF) signaling pathway (VSP) is an important mediator of tumor angiogenesis, leading to the development of new blood and lymphatic vessels and facilitating tumor growth and metastasis [26]. Bevacizumab is a humanized monoclonal antibody against VEGF; small molecule tyrosine kinase inhibitors including sunitinib, sorafenib, pazopanib, and axitinib disrupt VSP signaling by binding to the intracellular domain of the VEGF receptor [27]. VSP inhibitors are widely used in a variety of malignancies including renal cell carcinoma, hepatocellular carcinoma, colorectal cancers, breast cancer, and non-small cell lung cancer [28]. Cardiovascular toxicities of these agents include heart failure, asymptomatic LV dysfunction, hypertension, and arterial thromboembolic events (myocardial infarction, stroke, peripheral arterial events) [29]. LV dysfunction has been reported in up to 28% of patients receiving sunitinib for metastatic renal cell carcinoma [30].

Disruption of the VSP disturbs normal endothelial cell function; this "on-target" effect is thought to mediate the associated cardiotoxicity through endothelial cell dysfunction, reduced production of vasodilatory and fibrinolytic proteins, capillary rarefaction, and increased vascular tone [31]. There also appears to be a direct toxicity to cardiomyocytes, manifest as cell hypertrophy with vacuolization and mitochondrial damage, and which may be potentiated by concomitant hypertension [30].

The risk of cardiotoxicity with this class of agents is increased among patients with pre-existing hypertension or coronary artery disease [30]. Reduced LV function occurs most commonly during the first treatment cycle and may be reversible with appropriate management, primarily focused on blood pressure control, even with continued drug challenge [32].

5.2.6 Proteasome Inhibitors

The proteasome inhibitors bortezomib, carfilzomib, and ixazomib are widely used in the treatment of multiple myeloma and other plasma cell dyscrasias. They exert their anti-tumour effects by interfering with the ubiquitin-proteasome complex-mediated degradation of misfolded intracellular proteins; malignant plasma cells are particularly susceptible to these agents due to their production of abnormal immunoglobulin chains [33]. While the reversible proteasome inhibitors bortezomib and ixazomib do not appear to increase the risk of LV dysfunction or heart failure, the second-generation agent carfilzomib, which causes irreversible inhibition of the proteasome, has been associated with frequent cardiotoxic effects, including heart failure in up to 20% of patients [34]. The mechanism of cardiotoxicity and the reasons for agent-specific toxicity profiles are incompletely understood, but it is postulated that cardiotoxicity may be dependent on the extent of protease inhibition, the particular proteasome moiety inhibited, and/or off-target effect profiles of specific agents [33].

5.2.7 Immune Checkpoint Inhibitors

Inhibitors of "immune checkpoints" enhance the immune system's anti-tumor activity by interfering with receptor-ligand interactions that prevent autoimmune responses. Agents that target PD-1 (pembrolizumab, nivolumab), PD-L1 (atezolizumab, avelumab, durvalumab), and CTLA-4 (ipilimumab) have proven efficacy in a number of malignancies, including metastatic melanoma, non-small cell lung cancer, bladder cancer, head and neck cancers, and Hodgkin lymphoma [35]. The major toxicities of this drug class are predictably immune-mediated, and include dermatitis, hepatitis, gastroenteritis, pneumonitis, and endocrinopathy [36]. Myocarditis has been reported in several case reports and case series, although routine screening has not been performed in studies to date and the true incidence is therefore unknown. The majority of cases appear to occur within the first 3 months of therapy [37]. One registry-based study reported an incidence of 1.14% at a single institution [37]. When reported, cases are often fulminant and fatal, and may be associated with heart block and/or ventricular arrhythmias [38, 39]. Biopsy specimens reveal a lymphocytic infilatrate with CD8 T cell predominance [40], described as being similar to the pathology seen in cardiac transplant rejection [37]. The risk of myocarditis appears to be greater among patients receiving combination therapy with two checkpoint inhibitors, but other risk factors have not been well described [41]. Ongoing post-marketing surveillance and more rigorous screening for cardiotoxicity in clinical trials of new agents in this class will clarify the incidence, risk factors, and optimal screening and management of cardiotoxicity.

5.2.8 BCR-ABL-Targeted Therapies

Left ventricular dysfunction has not been significant toxicity with first- and second-generation members of this class of agents, used in the treatment of chronic myeloid leukemia (CML) and Philadelphia chromosome-positive acute lymphoblastic leukemia (Ph + ALL). Imatinib, the first-generation BCR-ABL tyrosine kinase inhibitor, is associated with incidence rates of congestive heart failure similar to age-matched population values [42]. Dasatinib, a second-generation TKI, is associated with increased risk of pulmonary artery hypertension, but not left ventricular dysfunction [43]. Nilotinib, another second-generation agent, increases the risk of arterial thrombotic events but does not appear to increase the risk of heart failure [44]. The third-generation TKI ponatinib has the most concerning cardiovascular toxicity profile, with venous and arterial thrombotic events reported in 27% of patients, and heart failure, sometimes fatal, in up to 8% [45]. The mechanisms of myocardial toxicity have not been fully elucidated but may involve inhibition of survival signaling pathways, cytoskeletal and mitochondrial damage, and cell death [46]. The risk of heart failure with ponatinib appears to be dose-related, and increased risk is also associated with history of ischemic heart disease, advanced age, and time from diagnosis to first dose [47].

5.2.9 Radiation

Radiation-induced heart disease (RIHD) represents a spectrum of cardiovascular disease that may include pericardial disease, myocardial disease, valvular pathology, conduction abnormalities, and coronary artery disease (CAD). Radiation therapy (RT) remains a mainstay of treatment for most malignancies, and patients receiving RT to the mediastinum, thorax, or breast (when the heart is included in the radiation field) may be at risk for RIHD. The risks of RT have been best described in Hodgkin lymphoma and breast cancer patients, though it should be noted that much of the available data reflects outcomes of patients treated prior to the modern era [48, 49].

Irradiation of the myocardium results in endothelial damage in small capillaries, leading to capillary loss and subsequent small vessel ischemia [50]. In turn, this causes diffuse myocardial fibrosis and diastolic dysfunction [51, 52], with systolic dysfunction being relatively uncommon in the modern era [53]. Additional mechanisms for heart failure after RT include constrictive pericarditis [54], severe valvular regurgitation and stenosis (typically affecting left-sided valves) [54–56], and RT-induced CAD with myocardial infarction and ischemic LV dysfunction [57].

The risk of RIHD is related to the volume and region of heart that is irradiated, the total RT dose, the dose per fraction, age at time of treatment, time since exposure, concomitant cardiotoxic chemotherapy, and the presence of traditional cardiovascular risk factors [58, 59]. Among adult survivors of childhood cancer in the Childhood Cancer Survivor Study, those who had received >35 Gy of RT had a 4.5-fold increase in risk of HF compared to those who had received no RT [60]. In another analysis of the CCSS focused on adult survivors of childhood Wilms tumour, the hazard ratio for HF among survivors compared to their siblings was 6.6 in the absence of anthracycline treatment, and 18.3 among those who had received >250 mg/m2 of anthracycline in addition to RT [61].

5.3 Screening and Diagnosis

A major limitation to the early detection of cancer treatment related cardiotoxicity is the lack of a consistent definition as to what constitutes myocardial dysfunction in this context. Initial reports relied on the development of overt symptoms of heart failure [62] while more contemporary clinical trials have integrated echocardiographic data to enable sub-clinical detection of left ventricular (LV) dysfunction primarily for the purposes of adverse event reporting [63]. In these studies, an asymptomatic reduction in left ventricular ejection fraction (LVEF) of >10% from baseline to a value below the lower limit of normal was considered diagnostic of cardiotoxicity. Most recently, the Common Terminology Criteria for Adverse Events (CTCAE) has further refined the definition of cardiotoxicity to include advanced imaging techniques such as global longitudinal strain (GLS) and other blood based biomarkers to improve early diagnostic accuracy [64].

Patients experiencing myocardial injury and dysfunction early in their treatment course are at greater risk of developing clinical heart failure and irreversible LV dysfunction over time [65, 66], thus highlighting the need for rigorous screening strategies that can inform on-going cardiac surveillance, treatment and prognosis.

5.3.1 Echocardiography

Echocardiography is the preferred imaging modality for the assessment of cardiotoxicity given that it is widely available, provides data on cardiac structure as well as function, and avoids additional radiation exposure. 2D-Echo is limited however by relative imprecision for detecting small changes in LV function with a reported variability of up to 10 percentage points [67]. Additionally, cancer patients may experience dynamic changes in preload and afterload which further complicates LVEF assessment by echo and undermines the value of comparing studies performed on the same individual at different time points. 3D-Echo is more accurate for the detection of chemotherapy related cardiotoxicity [68] with less variability, as compared to 2D-Echo, in terms of LVEF determination [69]. Regardless of the imaging strategy employed, serial assessments of LV function should use the same modality on a go-forward basis.

There is no consensus with respect to the optimal timing and frequency of cardiac imaging in those receiving potentially cardiotoxic cancer therapies, particularly if they remain asymptomatic. Current recommendations are largely based on expert consensus [70, 71] or adapted from clinical trials. In the real-world setting, imaging protocols are largely driven by local practice and customized based on a given patient's risk profile including the presence of pre-treatment LV dysfunction and the extent to which their cancer therapies may be associated with cardiotoxicity. In the case of anthracyclines, the vast majority of patients who experience myocardial dysfunction will do so within the first year after their last cycle of treatment [72]. However, among those with baseline risk factors [73] or those who acquire additional risk factors, the incidence of developing overt heart failure continues to rise over the individual's lifetime [9], suggesting that surveillance regimens must be tailored based on comprehensive risk assessment.

Given that a decrease in LV systolic function may be a relatively late manifestation of myocardial dysfunction, there is growing interest in developing and applying techniques for the early detection of cardiotoxicity that may influence treatment ahead of a drop in LVEF. Global longitudinal strain (GLS) imaging has emerged as a useful predictive tool for the subsequent development of LV dysfunction. A > 15% relative change in GLS from baseline is an early marker of LV myocardial dysfunction and is highly predictive of later developing cardiotoxicity [74–76]. Beyond the acute phase of treatment, many cancer survivors will continue to have abnormal GLS, even in the presence of normal LVEF, although the relevence of this finding is somewhat unclear at present [65, 77].

5.3.2 Biomarkers

Troponin I is a biomarker released in response to myocyte necrosis and is a well validated tool for the early detection of myocardial injury, regardless of cause. In the case of cancer therapy associated cardiotoxicity, an early and sustained release of troponin I, after the initiation of cancer treatment, is a powerful predictor for the subsequent development of LV dysfunction and heart failure [66, 78, 79]. More importantly, outcomes appear to be improved when cardioprotective therapies such as ACE inhibitors are initiated early in response to a rise in troponin I [72]. The corollary of both these statements is also true; patients who do not experience a rise in troponin I with cancer treatment have a relatively low likelihood of developing LV dysfunction and those who are delayed in the initiation of cardioprotective therapies in response to rising troponin I have worse outcomes [72, 75]. Despite demonstrated predictive accuracy for the development of cardiotoxicity in clinical trials, routine measurement of troponin I has not been consistently integrated into clinical practice largely based on heterogeneity in the performance of commercially available assays as well as inconsistency as to when levels should be drawn in relation to the delivery of chemotherapy and what value constitutes an abnormal result [70]. Major society guidelines however have suggested that biomarkers may "be considered" as a tool for the early detection of cardiotoxicity [9, 70].

In contrast to troponin I, the value of natriuretic peptides (NP) for the early diagnosis of myocardial injury related to cancer treatment is less clear with conflicting results from clinical trials [80]. A more consistent finding is that sustained elevations in NP levels are associated with a worse long term prognosis [81–83] and perhaps the need for heightened surveillance and early initiation of LV enhancement therapies. As with other blood-based biomarkers, interpretation of a given NP result is limited by characteristics of the specific assay used to perform the test as well as patient specific factors include age, sex and comorbidity.

5.4 Treatment and Prognosis

Once ACC/AHA Stage B or Stage C heart failure develops, individuals experiencing cardiotoxicity should be initiated on evidence based and guideline driven LV enhancement therapies as per routine care [84–86]. While major societies have recommended that triple therapy including ACE inhibitors, angiotensin receptor blockers, beta-blockers and mineralocorticoid receptor antagonists be instituted as first line therapies in all comers with heart failure and reduced ejection fraction (LVEF≤40%), there is a paucity of clinical trial data to inform treatment decisions for patients with mid-range and preserved ejection fraction, at this time.

In the case of myocardial dysfunction related to cancer treatment, the development of cardiotoxicity (LVEF≤50% or >10% drop in LVEF to below lower limits of normal) should trigger initiation of standard heart failure therapies to prevent further deterioration in LV function [9, 70] even when LVEF remains greater than 40%. Combination therapy with ACE inhibitors and beta-blockers appears to be a more efficacious strategy for treatment of cardiotoxicity than monotherapy with either agent [72, 87–90] resulting in a net greater improvement of LV function over the near term. Mineralocorticoid receptor antagonists have been less well studied in this patient population but there is a strong pathophysiological postulate for how and why they would be of benefit for the prophylaxis and treatment of cardiotoxicity [91]. Once therapies for myocardial dysfunction are initiated, treatment should be continued indefinitely irrespective of normalization in LV function [70, 92] with the exception of trastuzumab related cardiotoxicity, which appears to be largely reversible upon discontinuation [93].

It is worth restating that early treatment initiation with combination LV enhancement therapies, in individuals demonstrating clinical or subclinical cardiotoxicity, is associated with better outcomes [72]. Beyond just improving prognosis from a heart failure perspective, institution of ACE inhibitors and beta-blockers enable better outcomes from an oncological perspective in so much as they optimize LV function, thereby minimizing the risk of interruption or discontinuation of cancer treatment, which should be avoided at all cost.

Some have proposed cut-points for a drop in LVEF beyond which cardiotoxic cancer therapy should be, at least temporarily, withheld [16]. We believe that the decision to hold potentially life saving cancer treatment should be individualized and informed by the competing risks of cancer and cardiovascular mortality, as well as by a practitioner facile with both the natural history of various cardiotoxic agents and knowledge of the efficacy of heart failure treatments in this patient population. These considerations are particularly relevant in the metastatic setting and/or when limited cancer treatment options exist. In the event that cancer treatment is withheld due to clinically meaningful LV dysfunction or the development of overt heart failure, causality should be established and other potential etiologies for myocardial dysfunction excluded. The decision to re-challenge a patient, who has clinically stabilized or improved, necessitates a firm grasp of the mechanisms by which cardiotoxicity has occurred. For example, while anthracyclines may result in a dose-dependent progressive and irreversible cardiomyopathy if left untreated [94], LV dysfunction associated with trastuzumab is largely reversible and exquisitely responsive to heart failure therapies [93]. Immune checkpoint inhibitors, particularly when used in combination, may result in acute myocarditis, heart failure and cardiogenic shock such that re-challenging patients who have experienced these outcomes would be ill advised [41].

In the presence of persistent LV dysfunction, advanced functional status and refractory heart failure symptomatology despite optimal medical therapy, cancer survivors with cardiotoxicity should be considered for cardiac transplantation or mechanical circulatory support. In the short-term, for those who may still be in the vulnerable period for cancer recurrence, a bridge to candidacy or destination therapy strategy may be well suited while long-term survivors should be considered for cardiac transplantation. Ten-year survival, among those transplanted for a primary indication of anthracycline cardiomyopathy, was superior to those transplanted for all other causes, allaying fears that the risk of recurrent malignancy would limit long term survival in this cohort [95].

Establishing prognosis for those who experience cardiotoxicity is challenging given our evolving understanding of the mechanisms by which cardiotoxicity for various cancer treatments occurs, the extent to which these toxicities may be reversible and the impact of LV enhancement therapies towards mitigating or reversing myocardial dysfunction. The natural history of cardiotoxicity is similarly changing with development of novel screening techniques that allow for early subclinical detection of cardiac injury and with increased adoption of extended surveillance protocols [96] all of which ideally lead to earlier intervention with heart failure therapies. Nonetheless, it is clear that cardiovascular disease is the leading cause for late mortality in some cancer survivors [97] underscoring the need for life long assessment and treatment of cardiovascular risk in this cohort of patients.

References

1. Tan C, Tasaka H, Yu KP, Murphy ML, Karnofsky DA. Daunomycin, an antitumor antibiotic, in the treatment of neoplastic disease. Clinical evaluation with special reference to childhood leukemia. Cancer. 1967;20(3):333–53.
2. Vejpongsa P, Yeh ETH. Prevention of anthracycline-induced cardiotoxicity: challenges and opportunities. J Am Coll Cardiol. 2014;64(9):938–45.
3. Harbeck N, Gluz O. Neoadjuvant therapy for triple negative and HER2-positive early breast cancer. Breast. 2017;34(Suppl 1):S99–S103.
4. Murphy T, Yee KWL. Cytarabine and daunorubicin for the treatment of acute myeloid leukemia. Expert Opin Pharmacother. 2017;18(16):1765–80.
5. Ichikawa Y, Ghanefar M, Bayeva M, Wu R, Khechaduri A, Naga Prasad SV, et al. Cardiotoxicity of doxorubicin is mediated through mitochondrial iron accumulation. J Clin Invest. 2014;124(2):617–30. American Society for Clinical Investigation.
6. Zhang S, Liu X, Bawa-Khalfe T, Lu L-S, Lyu YL, Liu LF, et al. Identification of the molecular basis of doxorubicin-induced cardiotoxicity. Nat Med. 2012;18(11):1639–42.
7. Hoff Von DD, Layard MW, Basa P, Davis HLJ, Hoff Von AL, Rozencweig M, et al. Risk factors for doxorubicin-induced congestive heart failure. Ann Intern Med. 1979;91(5):710–7.
8. Swain SM, Whaley FS, Ewer MS. Congestive heart failure in patients treated with doxorubicin: a retrospective analysis of three trials. Cancer. 2003;97(11):2869–79.
9. Virani SA, Dent S, Brezden-Masley C, Clarke B, Davis MK, Jassal DS, et al. Canadian cardiovascular society guidelines for evaluation and management of cardiovascular complications of cancer therapy. Can J Cardiol. 2016;32:831–41.
10. Yeh ETH, Bickford CL. Cardiovascular complications of cancer therapy: incidence, pathogenesis, diagnosis, and management. J Am Coll Cardiol. 2009;53(24):2231–47.
11. Quezado ZM, Wilson WH, Cunnion RE, Parker MM, Reda D, Bryant G, et al. High-dose ifosfamide is associated with severe, reversible cardiac dysfunction. Ann Intern Med. 1993;118(1):31–6.
12. Mehta LS, Watson KE, Barac A, Beckie TM, Bittner V, Cruz-Flores S, et al. Cardiovascular disease and breast cancer: where these entities intersect: a scientific statement from the American Heart Association. Circulation. 2018;137(8):e30–66. American Heart Association, Inc.
13. Agarwal N, Burkart TA. Transient, high-grade atrioventricular block from high-dose cyclophosphamide. Tex Heart Inst J. 2013;40(5):626–7.
14. Gottdiener JS, Appelbaum FR, Ferrans VJ, Deisseroth A, Ziegler J. Cardiotoxicity associated with high-dose cyclophosphamide therapy. Arch Intern Med. 1981;141(6):758–63.
15. Katayama M, Imai Y, Hashimoto H, Kurata M, Nagai K, Tamita K, et al. Fulminant fatal cardiotoxicity following cyclophosphamide therapy. J Cardiol. 2009;54(2):330–4.
16. Chang H-M, Moudgil R, Scarabelli T, Okwuosa TM, Yeh ETH. Cardiovascular complications of cancer therapy: best practices in diagnosis, prevention, and management: part 1. J Am Coll Cardiol. 2017;70(20):2536–51.
17. Shah K, Gupta S, Ghosh J, Bajpai J, Maheshwari A. Acute non-ST elevation myocardial infarction following paclitaxel administration for ovarian carcinoma: a case report and review of literature. J Cancer Res Ther. 2012;8(3):442–4.
18. Nguyen-Ho P, Kleiman NS, Verani MS. Acute myocardial infarction and cardiac arrest in a patient receiving paclitaxel. Can J Cardiol. 2003;19(3):300–2.
19. Polk A, Vistisen K, Vaage-Nilsen M, Nielsen DL. A systematic review of the pathophysiology of 5-fluorouracil-induced cardiotoxicity. BMC Pharmacol Toxicol. 2014;15(1):47.
20. Sorrentino MF, Kim J, Foderaro AE, Truesdell AG. 5-fluorouracil induced cardiotoxicity: review of the literature. Cardiol J. 2012;19(5):453–8.
21. Slamon DJ, Clark GM, Wong SG, Levin WJ, Ullrich A, McGuire WL. Human breast cancer: correlation of relapse and survival with amplification of the HER-2/neu oncogene. Science. 1987;235(4785):177–82.
22. Piccart-Gebhart MJ, Procter M, Leyland-Jones B, Goldhirsch A, Untch M, Smith I, et al. Trastuzumab after adjuvant chemotherapy in HER2-positive breast cancer. N Engl J Med. 2005;353(16):1659–72.
23. Romond EH, Perez EA, Bryant J, Suman VJ, Geyer CE, Davidson NE, et al. Trastuzumab plus adjuvant chemotherapy for operable HER2-positive breast cancer. N Engl J Med. 2005;353(16):1673–84.
24. Coté GM, Sawyer DB, Chabner BA. ERBB2 inhibition and heart failure. N Engl J Med. 2012;367(22):2150–3.
25. Slamon DJ, Leyland-Jones B, Shak S, Fuchs H, Paton V, Bajamonde A, et al. Use of chemotherapy plus a monoclonal antibody against HER2 for metastatic breast cancer that overexpresses HER2. N Engl J Med. 2001;344(11):783–92.
26. Hicklin DJ, Ellis LM. Role of the vascular endothelial growth factor pathway in tumor growth and angiogenesis. J Clin Oncol. 2005;23(5):1011–27. American Society of Clinical Oncology.
27. Hsieh JJ, Purdue MP, Signoretti S, Swanton C, Albiges L, Schmidinger M, et al. Renal cell carcinoma. Nat Rev Dis Primers. 2017;3:17009. Nature Publishing Group.
28. Vasudev NS, Reynolds AR. Anti-angiogenic therapy for cancer: current progress, unresolved questions and future directions. Angiogenesis. 2014;17(3):471–94. Springer Netherlands.
29. Abdel-Qadir H, Ethier J-L, Lee DS, Thavendiranathan P, Amir E. Cardiovascular toxicity of angiogenesis inhibitors in treatment of malignancy: a systematic review and meta-analysis. Cancer Treat Rev. 2017;53:120–7.

30. Chu TF, Rupnick MA, Kerkela R, Dallabrida SM, Zurakowski D, Nguyen L, et al. Cardiotoxicity associated with tyrosine kinase inhibitor sunitinib. Lancet. 2007;370(9604):2011–9.
31. Chen HX, Cleck JN. Adverse effects of anticancer agents that target the VEGF pathway. Nat Rev Clin Oncol. 2009;6(8):465–77.
32. Narayan V, Keefe S, Haas N, Wang L, Puzanov I, Putt M, et al. Prospective Evaluation of Sunitinib-Induced Cardiotoxicity in Patients with Metastatic Renal cell carcinoma. Clin Cancer Res. 2017;23(14):3601–9. American Association for Cancer Research.
33. Li W, Garcia D, Cornell RF, Gailani D, Laubach J, Maglio ME, Richardson PG, Moslehi J. Cardiovascular and thrombotic complications of novel multiple myeloma therapies: a review. JAMA Oncol. 2017;3(7):980–8.
34. Wang M, Cheng J. Overview and management of cardiac and pulmonary adverse events in patients with relapsed and/or refractory multiple myeloma treated with single-agent carfilzomib. Oncology (Williston Park). 2013;27(Suppl 3):24–30.
35. Puzanov I, Diab A, Abdallah K, Bingham CO, Brogdon C, Dadu R, et al. Managing toxicities associated with immune checkpoint inhibitors: consensus recommendations from the Society for Immunotherapy of Cancer (SITC) Toxicity Management Working Group. J Immunother Cancer. 2017;5(1):95. BioMed Central.
36. Brahmer JR, Lacchetti C, Thompson JA. Management of immune-related adverse events in patients treated with immune checkpoint inhibitor therapy: American Society of Clinical Oncology Clinical Practice Guideline Summary. J Oncol Pract. 2018;14(4):247–9. American Society of Clinical Oncology.
37. Mahmood SS, Fradley MG, Cohen JV, Nohria A, Reynolds KL, Heinzerling LM, et al. Myocarditis in patients treated with immune checkpoint inhibitors. J Am Coll Cardiol. 2018;71(16):1755–64.
38. Gibson R, Delaune J, Szady A, Markham M. Suspected autoimmune myocarditis and cardiac conduction abnormalities with nivolumab therapy for non-small cell lung cancer. BMJ Case Rep. 2016;2016:bcr2016216228. BMJ Publishing Group Ltd.
39. Arangalage D, Delyon J, Lermuzeaux M, Ekpe K, Ederhy S, Pages C, et al. Survival after fulminant myocarditis induced by immune-checkpoint inhibitors. Ann Intern Med. 2017;167(9):683–4.
40. Läubli H, Balmelli C, Bossard M, Pfister O, Glatz K, Zippelius A. Acute heart failure due to autoimmune myocarditis under pembrolizumab treatment for metastatic melanoma. J Immunother Cancer. 2015;3(1):11. BioMed Cent.
41. Johnson DB, Balko JM, Compton ML, Chalkias S, Gorham J, Xu Y, et al. Fulminant myocarditis with combination immune checkpoint blockade. N Engl J Med. 2016;375(18):1749–55.
42. Atallah E, Durand J-B, Kantarjian H, Cortes J. Congestive heart failure is a rare event in patients receiving imatinib therapy. Blood Am Soc Hematol. 2007;110(4):1233–7.
43. Moslehi JJ, Deininger M. Tyrosine kinase inhibitor-associated cardiovascular toxicity in chronic myeloid leukemia. J Clin Oncol. 2015;33(35):4210–8. American Society of Clinical Oncology.
44. Hochhaus A, Saglio G, Hughes TP, Larson RA, Kim D-W, Issaragrisil S, et al. Long-term benefits and risks of frontline nilotinib vs imatinib for chronic myeloid leukemia in chronic phase: 5-year update of the randomized ENESTnd trial. Leukemia. 2016;30(5):1044–54.
45. Hoy SM. Ponatinib: a review of its use in adults with chronic myeloid leukaemia or Philadelphia chromosome-positive acute lymphoblastic leukaemia. Drugs. 2014;74(7):793–806. Springer International Publishing.
46. Talbert DR, Doherty KR, Trusk PB, Moran DM, Shell SA, Bacus S. A multi-parameter in vitro screen in human stem cell-derived cardiomyocytes identifies ponatinib-induced structural and functional cardiac toxicity. Toxicol Sci. 2015;143(1):147–55.
47. Dorer DJ, Knickerbocker RK, Baccarani M, Cortes JE, Hochhaus A, Talpaz M, et al. Impact of dose intensity of ponatinib on selected adverse events: multivariate analyses from a pooled population of clinical trial patients. Leuk Res. 2016;48:84–91.
48. Taylor CW, Povall JM, McGale P, Nisbet A, Dodwell D, Smith JT, et al. Cardiac dose from tangential breast cancer radiotherapy in the year 2006. Int J Radiat Oncol Biol Phys. 2008;72(2):501–7.
49. Maraldo MV, Brodin NP, Aznar MC, Vogelius IR, Munck af Rosenschöld P, Petersen PM, et al. Estimated risk of cardiovascular disease and secondary cancers with modern highly conformal radiotherapy for early-stage mediastinal Hodgkin lymphoma. Ann Oncol. 2013;24(8):2113–8.
50. Seemann I, Gabriels K, Visser NL, Hoving S, Poele Te JA, Pol JF, et al. Irradiation induced modest changes in murine cardiac function despite progressive structural damage to the myocardium and microvasculature. Radiother Oncol. 2012;103(2):143–50.
51. Chello M, Mastroroberto P, Romano R, Zofrea S, Bevacqua I, Marchese AR. Changes in the proportion of types I and III collagen in the left ventricular wall of patients with post-irradiative pericarditis. Cardiovasc Surg. 1996;4(2):222–6.
52. Heidenreich PA, Hancock SL, Vagelos RH, Lee BK, Schnittger I. Diastolic dysfunction after mediastinal irradiation. Am Heart J. 2005;150(5):977–82.
53. Constine LS, Schwartz RG, Savage DE, King V, Muhs A. Cardiac function, perfusion, and morbidity in irradiated long-term survivors of Hodgkin's disease. Int J Radiat Oncol Biol Phys. 1997;39(4):897–906.
54. Veinot JP, Edwards WD. Pathology of radiation-induced heart disease: a surgical and autopsy study of 27 cases. Hum Pathol. 1996;27(8):766–73.
55. Wethal T, Lund M-B, Edvardsen T, Fosså SD, Pripp AH, Holte H, et al. Valvular dysfunction and left ventricular changes in Hodgkin's lymphoma survivors. A longitudinal study. Br J Cancer. 2009;101(4):575–81.
56. Carlson RG, Mayfield WR, Normann S, Alexander JA. Radiation-associated valvular disease. Chest. 1991;99(3):538–45.
57. Applefeld MM, Wiernik PH. Cardiac disease after radiation therapy for Hodgkin's disease: analysis of 48 patients. Am J Cardiol. 1983;51(10):1679–81.
58. Carver JR, Shapiro CL, Ng A, Jacobs L, Schwartz C, Virgo KS, et al. American Society of Clinical Oncology clinical evidence review on the ongoing care of adult cancer survivors: cardiac and pulmonary late effects. J Clin Oncol. 2007;25(25):3991–4008.
59. Hancock SL, Tucker MA, Hoppe RT. Factors affecting late mortality from heart disease after treatment of Hodgkin's disease. JAMA. 1993;270(16):1949–55.
60. Mulrooney DA, Yeazel MW, Kawashima T, Mertens AC, Mitby P, Stovall M, et al. Cardiac outcomes in a cohort of adult survivors of childhood and adolescent cancer: retrospective analysis of the Childhood Cancer Survivor Study cohort. BMJ. 2009;339:b4606.
61. Termuhlen AM, Tersak JM, Liu Q, Yasui Y, Stovall M, Weathers R, et al. Twenty-five year follow-up of childhood Wilms tumor: a report from the Childhood Cancer Survivor Study. Pediatr Blood Cancer. 2011;57(7):1210–6.
62. Hoff Von DD, Layard MW, Basa P, Davis HL, Hoff Von AL, Rozencweig M, et al. Risk factors for doxorubicin-induced congestive heart failure. Ann Intern Med. 1979;91(5):710–7.
63. Seidman A, Hudis C, Pierri MK, Shak S, Paton V, Ashby M, et al. Cardiac dysfunction in the trastuzumab clinical trials experience. J Clin Oncol. 2002;20(5):1215–21.

64. National Cancer Institute. Common Terminology Criteria for Adverse Events (CTCAE). https://ctep.cancer.govprotocoldevelopmentelectronicapplicationsdocsCTCAEvQuickReference.x.pdf. 2017. pp. 1–147.
65. Thavendiranathan P, Poulin F, Lim K-D, Plana JC, Woo A, Marwick TH. Use of myocardial strain imaging by echocardiography for the early detection of cardiotoxicity in patients during and after cancer chemotherapy: a systematic review. J Am Coll Cardiol. 2014;63(25 Pt A):2751–68.
66. Cardinale D, Sandri MT, Colombo A, Colombo N, Boeri M, Lamantia G, et al. Prognostic value of troponin I in cardiac risk stratification of cancer patients undergoing high-dose chemotherapy. Circulation. 2004;109(22):2749–54. Lippincott Williams & Wilkins.
67. Otterstad JE, Froeland G, St John Sutton M, Holme I. Accuracy and reproducibility of biplane two-dimensional echocardiographic measurements of left ventricular dimensions and function. Eur Heart J. 1997;18(3):507–13.
68. Armstrong GT, Plana JC, Zhang N, Srivastava D, Green DM, Ness KK, et al. Screening adult survivors of childhood cancer for cardiomyopathy: comparison of echocardiography and cardiac magnetic resonance imaging. J Clin Oncol. 2012;30(23):2876–84.
69. Plana JC, Galderisi M, Barac A, Ewer MS, Ky B, Scherrer-Crosbie M, et al. Expert consensus for multimodality imaging evaluation of adult patients during and after cancer therapy: a report from the American Society of Echocardiography and the European Association of Cardiovascular Imaging. J Am Soc Echocardiogr. 2014;27(9):911–39.
70. Zamorano JL, Lancellotti P, Rodriguez Muñoz D, Aboyans V, Asteggiano R, Galderisi M, et al. 2016 ESC Position Paper on cancer treatments and cardiovascular toxicity developed under the auspices of the ESC Committee for Practice Guidelines: The Task Force for cancer treatments and cardiovascular toxicity of the European Society of Cardiology (ESC). Eur Heart J. 2016;37(36):2768–801.
71. Curigliano G, Cardinale D, Suter T, Plataniotis G, de Azambuja E, Sandri MT, et al. Cardiovascular toxicity induced by chemotherapy, targeted agents and radiotherapy: ESMO Clinical Practice Guidelines. Ann Oncol. 2012;23(7):vii155–66.
72. Cardinale D, Colombo A, Bacchiani G, Tedeschi I, Meroni CA, Veglia F, et al. Early detection of anthracycline cardiotoxicity and improvement with heart failure therapy. Circulation. 2015; https://doi.org/10.1161/CIRCULATIONAHA.114.013777. Lippincott Williams & Wilkins.
73. Pinder MC, Duan Z, Goodwin JS, Hortobagyi GN, Giordano SH. Congestive heart failure in older women treated with adjuvant anthracycline chemotherapy for breast cancer. J Clin Oncol. 2007;25(25):3808–15.
74. Fallah-Rad N, Walker JR, Wassef A, Lytwyn M, Bohonis S, Fang T, et al. The utility of cardiac biomarkers, tissue velocity and strain imaging, and cardiac magnetic resonance imaging in predicting early left ventricular dysfunction in patients with human epidermal growth factor receptor II-positive breast cancer treated with adjuvant trastuzumab therapy. J Am Coll Cardiol. 2011;57(22):2263–70.
75. Sawaya H, Sebag IA, Plana JC, Januzzi JL, Ky B, Tan TC, et al. Assessment of echocardiography and biomarkers for the extended prediction of cardiotoxicity in patients treated with anthracyclines, taxanes, and trastuzumab. Circ Cardiovasc Imaging. 2012;5(5):596–603.
76. Negishi K, Negishi T, Hare JL, Haluska BA, Plana JC, Marwick TH. Independent and incremental value of deformation indices for prediction of trastuzumab-induced cardiotoxicity. J Am Soc Echocardiogr. 2013;26(5):493–8.
77. Ho E, Brown A, Barrett P, Morgan RB, King G, Kennedy MJ, et al. Subclinical anthracycline- and trastuzumab-induced cardiotoxicity in the long-term follow-up of asymptomatic breast cancer survivors: a speckle tracking echocardiographic study. Heart. 2010;96(9):701–7.
78. Cardinale D, Sandri MT, Martinoni A, Tricca A, Civelli M, Lamantia G, et al. Left ventricular dysfunction predicted by early troponin I release after high-dose chemotherapy. J Am Coll Cardiol. 2000;36(2):517–22.
79. Cardinale D, Sandri MT, Martinoni A, Borghini E, Civelli M, Lamantia G, et al. Myocardial injury revealed by plasma troponin I in breast cancer treated with high-dose chemotherapy. Ann Oncol. 2002;13(5):710–5.
80. Thakur A, Witteles RM. Cancer therapy-induced left ventricular dysfunction: interventions and prognosis. J Card Fail. 2013;20(3):155–8.
81. Suzuki J, Yanagisawa A, Shigeyama T, Tsubota J, Yasumura T, Shimoyama K, et al. Early detection of anthracycline-induced cardiotoxicity by radionuclide angiocardiography. Angiology. 1999;50(1):37–45.
82. Meinardi MT, van Veldhuisen DJ, Gietema JA, Dolsma WV, Boomsma F, van den Berg MP, et al. Prospective evaluation of early cardiac damage induced by epirubicin-containing adjuvant chemotherapy and locoregional radiotherapy in breast cancer patients. J Clin Oncol. 2001;19(10):2746–53.
83. Daugaard G, Lassen U, Bie P, Pedersen EB, Jensen KT, Abildgaard U, et al. Natriuretic peptides in the monitoring of anthracycline induced reduction in left ventricular ejection fraction. Eur J Heart Fail. 2005;7(1):87–93. Wiley-Blackwell.
84. Yancy CW, Jessup M, Bozkurt B, Butler J, Casey DE, Colvin MM, et al. 2017 ACC/AHA/HFSA Focused Update of the 2013 ACCF/AHA guideline for the management of heart failure: a report of the American College of Cardiology/American Heart Association Task Force on Clinical Practice Guidelines and the Heart Failure Society of America. J Am Coll Cardiol. 2017;70(6):776–803.
85. Justin A, Ezekowitz MC, Eileen O'Meara MC-C, Michael McDonald MD, Howard Abrams MD, Michael Chan M, Anıque Ducharme MD, et al. 2017 Comprehensive update of the Canadian Cardiovascular Society guidelines for the management of heart failure. Can J Cardiol. 2017;33(11):1–200. Canadian Cardiovascular Society.
86. Ponikowski P, Voors AA, Anker SD, Bueno H, Cleland JGF, Coats AJS, et al. 2016 ESC Guidelines for the diagnosis and treatment of acute and chronic heart failure: The Task Force for the diagnosis and treatment of acute and chronic heart failure of the European Society of Cardiology (ESC). Developed with the special contribution of the Heart Failure Association (HFA) of the ESC. Eur J Heart Fail. 2016;18:891–975. Wiley-Blackwell.
87. Cardinale D, Colombo A, Lamantia G, Colombo N, Civelli M, De Giacomi G, et al. Anthracycline-induced cardiomyopathy: clinical relevance and response to pharmacologic therapy. J Am Coll Cardiol. 2010;55(3):213–20.
88. Tallaj JA, Franco V, Rayburn BK, Pinderski L, Benza RL, Pamboukian S, et al. Response of doxorubicin-induced cardiomyopathy to the current management strategy of heart failure. J Heart Lung Transplant. 2005;24(12):2196–201.
89. Oliva S, Cioffi G, Frattini S, Simoncini EL, Faggiano P, Boccardi L, et al. Administration of angiotensin-converting enzyme inhibitors and β-blockers during adjuvant trastuzumab chemotherapy for nonmetastatic breast cancer: marker of risk or cardioprotection in the real world? Oncologist. 2012;17(7):917–24. AlphaMed Press.
90. Ewer MS, Vooletich MT, Durand J-B, Woods ML, Davis JR, Valero V, et al. Reversibility of trastuzumab-related cardiotoxicity: new insights based on clinical course and response to medical treatment. J Clin Oncol. 2005;23(31):7820–6. American Society of Clinical Oncology.
91. Akpek M, Ozdogru I, Sahin O, Inanc M, Dogan A, Yazici C, et al. Protective effects of spironolactone against anthracycline-induced

cardiomyopathy. Eur J Heart Fail. 2015;17(1):81–9. John Wiley & Sons, Ltd.
92. Howlett JG, Chan M, Ezekowitz JA, Harkness K, Heckman GA, Kouz S, et al. The Canadian cardiovascular society heart failure companion: bridging guidelines to your practice. Can J Cardiol. 2016;32(3):296–310.
93. Suter TM, Procter M, van Veldhuisen DJ, Muscholl M, Bergh J, Carlomagno C, et al. Trastuzumab-associated cardiac adverse effects in the herceptin adjuvant trial. J Clin Oncol. 2007;25(25):3859–65.
94. Swain SM, Whaley FS, Ewer MS. Congestive heart failure in patients treated with doxorubicin: a retrospective analysis of three trials. Cancer. 2003;97(11):2869–79.
95. Lenneman AJ, Wang L, Wigger M, Frangoul H, Harrell FE, Silverstein C, et al. Heart transplant survival outcomes for adriamycin-dilated cardiomyopathy. Am J Cardiol. 2013;111(4):609–12.
96. Armenian SH, Lacchetti C, Barac A, Carver J, Constine LS, Denduluri N, et al. Prevention and monitoring of cardiac dysfunction in survivors of adult cancers: American society of clinical oncology clinical practice guideline. J Clin Oncol. 2017;35:893–911.
97. Patnaik JL, Byers T, DiGuiseppi C, Dabelea D, Denberg TD. Cardiovascular disease competes with breast cancer as the leading cause of death for older females diagnosed with breast cancer: a retrospective cohort study. Breast Cancer Res. 2011;13(3):R64.

Part IV

Diagnostics

Diagnosis of Heart Failure

6

Kevin J. Clerkin, Donna M. Mancini, and Lars H. Lund

6.1 Patient Evaluation

6.1.1 History

Heart failure can be challenging to diagnose given the spectrum of associated symptoms and the overlap of those symptoms with other diseases (e.g. renal, pulmonary, hepatic) as well as with aging and frailty. Despite advances in modern medicine, the history and physical exam remain the cornerstone of the diagnosis of heart failure, whether acute or chronic. The patient's history is highlighted by symptoms of fluid overload ("backward failure"), decreased cardiac output ("forward failure"), or both.

Dyspnea is one of the more common presenting symptoms in heart failure and is multifactorial. It may result from increased left ventricular end diastolic pressure leading to pulmonary venous hypertension triggering J-receptors to increase vagal stimulation to the brain, pulmonary venous congestion causing ventilation perfusion mismatch in the lung, decreased lung compliance from pulmonary venous congestion, peripheral chemoreceptor hypersensitivity, and/or anxiety. The dyspnea in acute heart failure can be elicited from the patient as shortness of breath on (less than usual) exertion (walking on flat ground or up flights of stairs). Dyspnea may be present at home, where orthopnea (shortness of breath when recumbent) often develops secondary to increased venous return from lower extremities and increased pulmonary venous pressures. A common history is increasing pillow use or the need to sleep in a chair due to shortness of breath. Less frequent, but equally important are complaints of paroxysmal nocturnal dyspnea or episodes of severe shortness of breath and/or coughing at night, waking the patient from sleep. This finding is less sensitive but has has a specificity of 81% for the diagnosis of heart failure [1].

K. J. Clerkin · D. M. Mancini · L. H. Lund (✉)
Karolinska Institutet, Department of Medicine, Stockholm, Sweden
e-mail: lars.lund@alumni.duke.edu

Fatigue is a common symptom among patients with heart failure. Fatigue is the final common pathway of decreased cardiac output, and skeletal muscle dysfunction. Dyspnea and poor cardiac output were initially believed to be responsible for reduced functional capacity in heart failure. However studies have demonstrated that even with an acute increase in cardiac output and decrease in pulmonary capillary wedge pressure exercise capacity does not significantly improve [2–4]. The skeletal muscle wasting and dysfunction in heart failure is likely a combination of chronic hypoperfusion, physical deconditioning, and resultant systemic and skeletal muscle biochemical changes.

Congestion or symptoms of systemic volume overload are common. The most frequent is edema. Edema results when an imbalance between hydrostatic pressure, oncotic pressure, and vascular permeability exists. Traditionally edema in heart failure was attributed to increases in venous hydrostatic pressure resulting to edema in the lungs, abdomen, and periphery. However heart failure is a systemic process that leads to a catabolic state with decreased serum albumin (oncotic pressure) and increased pro-inflammatory cytokines (vessel permeability) [5], adding to extravascular fluid translocation. Edema evident to the patient is present in the form of peripheral edema, manifesting as swelling of the lower extremities due to humans' upright nature and the addition of gravitational forces to the aforementioned alteration in capillary hemodynamics. However, in a patient with severe volume overload thigh, scrotal, and abdominal wall edema may also be present.

Edema also exists in the pleural space and intraperitoneal space, which may not be evident to the patient. Pulmonary vascular congestion may lead to pleural effusions. The traditional teaching is that pleural effusions from heart failure are more common on the right side due to the increased surface area on the right [6]; however recent studies have questioned that [7]. Interestingly, the observation of increased right sided pleural effusions may be due to the right lateral decubitus position being the preferential sleeping position for heart failure patients [8]. Pleural effusions are often

D. S. Feldman, P. Mohacsi (eds.), *Heart Failure*, Cardiovascular Medicine, https://doi.org/10.1007/978-3-319-98184-0_6

absent in chronic heart failure, however, as increased pulmonary lymphatic activity removes pulmonary and pleural fluid. Ascites may also result from chronic venous congestion from heart failure. This often will go unnoticed by the patient unless severe.

Patients that are suffering from right heart or biventricular heart failure will have a varying degree of abdominal symptoms, ranging from diffuse abdominal fullness to right upper quadrant tenderness to anorexia. Abdominal fullness is the result of venous congestion, manifesting through hepatic congestion and in more severe cases ascites. Anorexia in heart failure is likely multifactorial, resulting from bowel wall edema causing decreased absorption in addition to compromised splanchnic blood flow, an unpalatable diet due to sodium restriction, medication side effects, and hormonal changes including ghrelin resistance (levels are increased in CHF) [9], GH resistance [10], and elevated cortisol & TNF-α [11].

The history is important not only to elicit symptoms and their severity, but also to help identify the cause of and contributors to the syndrome. Past medical and family history are central to the diagnosis of heart failure. The presence of chest pain, a past history of rheumatic fever, a family history of heart disease, and substance abuse (alcohol and illicit drugs) are all key areas to be targeted. Heart failure is often accompanied by comorbid conditions including hypertension, renal insufficiency, obesity (or cachexia), risk factors for coronary artery disease (dyslipidemia, diabetes, smoking), tachyarrhythmias, chronic substance abuse (alcohol or cocaine), infection (viral myocarditis), or other systemic diseases (amyloidosis, sarcoidosis, malignancies treated with anthracyclines). Similarly a history of non-ischemic heart failure or sudden cardiac death in a family member before the age of 60 should trigger a multi-generation family pedigree. Sleep history may also suggest a diagnosis of heart failure. Sleep disordered breathing is a common symptom present in as many as half of patients with heart failure [12] and over three-quarters with acute heart failure [13]. Central sleep apnea with Cheyne-Stokes breathing is more common than obstructive sleep apnea. Major life events are important to explore in this setting. Originally described in 1990 in Japan, takotsubo or stress cardiomyopathy is becoming increasingly recognized [14]. In this population 36% are suggested to have a physical trigger, 28% have an emotional trigger, and 8% have both [15]. An additional key piece of history is pregnancy, current or recent. Peripartum cardiomyopathy has a prevalence as high as 1:100 in some African nations [16] and is currently estimated to be 1:2,000–4,000 in the United States. It typically occurs after 36 weeks gestation and within the first few months post-partum.

Lastly, in acute heart failure it is important to attempt to identify the trigger of the current episode. Questions should be tailored to identify medication or dietary non-adherence, acute coronary syndrome, hypertensive urgency or emergency, infection, arrhythmias (atrial and ventricular), substance abuse (alcohol or cocaine), pulmonary embolus, acute kidney injury, hyperthyroidism, and medication use (calcium channel blockers, NSAIDS, glucocorticoids, antiarrhythmics, anti-diabetics).

6.1.2 Physical Exam

The physical exam of the heart failure patient begins with visual inspection; clinical gestalt has been shown to be highly specific (86%) for the diagnosis of heart failure in a dyspneic patient [1]. Basic vital signs are the next step in assessment. Tachycardia is common in heart failure, especially acute, due to sympathetic nervous system activation [17]. The blood pressure is important to note as a proportional pulse pressure $\left(\frac{SBP-DBP}{SBP}\right)$ of less than 25% detects a cardiac index of less than 2.2 L/min/m^2 with high fidelity (91% sensitivity, 83% specificity) [18]. Chronic hypotension is a particularly important negative prognostic sign. Further, malignant hypertension also suggests etiology of hypertensive cardiomyopathy.

Visual inspection continues with assessment of the neck veins to estimate cardiac filling pressures. Patients should first be examined in an upright position so as not to miss severely elevated jugular venous pressures (JVP). The patient is then placed in a recumbent position with the head of the bed elevated 30–45° above horizontal, and the vertical distance (in cm) of the right internal jugular vein pulsation above the angle of Louis is determined. The internal jugular vein is preferred to the external jugular vein as the internal jugular vein is parallel to the SVC. The JVP in cm H_20 is vertical distance plus 5 (the angle of Louis is 5 cm above the right atrium). An elevated JVP (defined as venous pulsation height greater than 4 cm) has been shown to correlate with a pulmonary capillary wedge pressure (PCWP) above 18 mmHg [19–21]. An adjunct to the JVP is the assessment of the hepatojugular reflux (HJR). HJR is assessed by placing firm abdominal pressure (20–30 mmHg) in the center of the abdomen for at least 10 s and inspection of the JVP upon release. Sustained elevation of the JVP during compression with an abrupt decrease of at least 4 cm following release of pressure signifies a positive test, and has been demonstrated to correlate with elevated right atrial pressure and PCWP [19, 22].

The pulmonary examination is neither sensitive nor adequate for the diagnosis of heart failure. Typical findings are those of rales or pulmonary crackles, resulting from the opening of fluid compressed alveoli. While these are pathognomonic with a specificity of 89–100%, they are frequently absent due to lymphatic compensation, resulting in a sensitivity of just 15–24% to detect an elevated PCWP [19, 21]. Additional pulmonary findings include dullness at the lung bases associated with decreased tactile fremitus, whisper pectoriloquy and egophony due to a pleural effusion.

The cardiac exam begins with palpation of the precordium, feeling for a right ventricular heave (RV hypertrophy) and enlargement (>2 cm) and lateral displacement of the apical point of maximal impulse (PMI) suggestive of left ventricular enlargement. Frequently patients with chronic heart failure will have a diffuse PMI or a non-palpable PMI due to the decrease in contractility. A LV heave may be present suggesting LVH. Classically heart failure with a reduced ejection fraction (HFrEF) is associated with a S3 gallop. Occurring in early diastole, the S3 results from "an abnormal relation between the rate of rapid filling and the ventricle's ability to accommodate its increasing diastolic volume" [23]. While this finding is not sensitive, it is specific and when present increases the risk of hospitalization for heart failure or death by 42% [24]. Occasionally an S3 can be palpable. The fourth heart sound or S4 occurs prior to closure of the AV valves and is the result of atrial contraction in the setting of systolic ventricular overload [23]. Additional heart sounds include a prominent P2 or second heart sound over the pulmonic valve, often present in severe pulmonary hypertension. Lastly, regurgitant and stenotic murmurs can aid in the diagnosis of a valvular cardiomyopathy, though frequently functional tricuspid and mitral regurgitation will result secondary to ventricular dilation.

The last component of the heart failure focused physical exam is assessment of the abdomen and periphery. The abdominal examination assesses the liver, palpating for hepatomegaly (venous congestion) and pulsatility (tricuspid regurgitation). Examination of the periphery focuses on edema (venous congestion), skin warmth, and pulses. Edema, as described earlier, may be present in the periphery, most commonly the lower extremities and also more proximally when more severe. The absence of peripheral edema does not rule out heart failure however, as 2+ edema only has a 41% sensitivity to diagnose a PCWP of over 22 mmHg [21]. Cool extremities and pulsus alternans are both markers of systemic hypoperfusion and have been shown to be prognostic in heart failure [25]. Lastly, examination of the extremities for may identify an arteriovenous fistula leading to high output heart failure. This fistula may be iatrogenic (hemodialysis fistula, fistula from arterial puncture), traumatic (knife or bullet wound), or congenital (hereditary hemorrhagic telangiectasia, cutaneous & rarely hepatic hemangiomas).

6.1.3 Emergency Room Assessment of Dyspnea

There is much commonality in the assessment of a patient with heart failure and acute dyspnea. The assessment again begins with a history and physical exam. The history, when the patient is able to provide one, greatly aids in the diagnosis of heart failure. A prior history of heart failure (Likelihood ratio [LR] 5.8, 95% CI 4.1–8.0) and myocardial infarction (LR 3.1, 95% CI 2.0–4.9) are highly valuable for the confirmation of heart failure [1]. Similarly orthopnea, edema, and PND are highly specific for the diagnosis of heart failure (77–84%) [1]. Also useful is a history of worsened dyspnea or exertion, fatigue, and weight gain. A history of substance abuse, palpitations, and anginal chest pain may also help identify heart failure as the precipitant of the dyspnea. Many emergency room algorithms for the diagnosis of CHF employ the Framingham criteria that require two major or one major plus two minor criteria. The major criteria include presence of acute pulmonary edema, cardiomegaly, hepatojugular reflex, paroxysmal nocturnal dyspnea or orthopnea, pulmonary rales or a third heart sound; minor criteria are less specific and include ankle edema, dyspnea on exertion, hepatomegaly, nocturnal cough, pleural effusion, tachycardia (heart rate > 120 beats/min). The sensitivity and specificity of a heart failure diagnosis based on Framingham criteria is 97% and 79% [26].

Physical exam again begins with visual inspection of the patient. The patient's vital signs may be helpful, with hypotension and a narrow proportional pulse pressure signaling a low output state, hypoxia indicating an impairment of pulmonary gas exchange, and an elevations in the heart rate suggesting a compensatory response (CO=HR × SV) or inciting factor (e.g. atrial fibrillation with rapid ventricular response). Visual inspection of the neck veins provides an assessment of volume status, with elevated JVP suggestive of right and/or biventricular failure. As previously discussed an elevated JVP is a sensitive marker of an elevated PCWP but may be absent in acute left-sided heart failure. Pulmonary auscultation will frequently yield crackles or rales and wheezing. Wheezing or cardiac asthma may be present in up to one-third of older patients with acute heart failure [27] and is the result of bronchospasm secondary to elevated pulmonary venous pressure. Cardiac examination of a patient with dyspnea due to heart failure may include a gallop (S3 or S4) and/or a new or worsened murmur (e.g. acute mitral regurgitation, severe aortic stenosis). The exam then moves to the periphery, starting with the abdomen assessing for hepatomegaly or ascites. The lower extremities are examined for edema, though the absence of edema does not preclude heart failure. Lastly a visual and tactile assessment of the skin may demonstrate mottling and coolness, both suggestive of low cardiac output.

The components of the history and physical exam may be used to classify a patient into one of four profiles reflecting congestion and systemic perfusion: dry & warm, wet & warm, cold & wet, or cold & dry [28] (Fig. 6.1). Markers of congestion are orthopnea, PND, elevated JVP, positive HJR, an S3, ascites, and/or peripheral edema. Markers of low

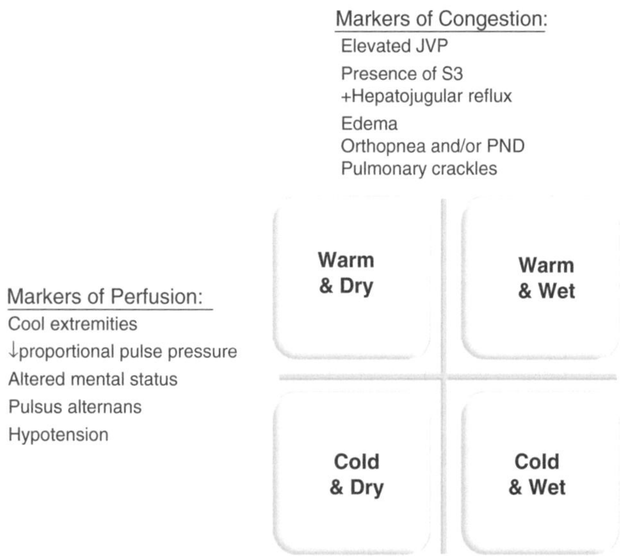

Fig. 6.1 Profiles of acute decompensated heart failure

cardiac output are cool extremities, a narrow proportional pulse pressure, hypotension, pulsus alternans, and/or altered mental status. Classification of patients into these profiles can be used to identify precipitants, tailor therapy and predict outcomes [25]. Close to 50% of the patients are classified into the warm and wet profile which means perfusion is adequate but patients are congested. These patients generally will do well with additional diuresis and vasodilators. Approximately 20% of the patients will have underperfused (cold) profiles which generally require more complex therapy sometimes including inotropic support.

Imaging and laboratory data will supplement the physical exam in the assessment of the patient with dyspnea. An ECG may demonstrate if a tachyarrythmia or ischemia is a precipitant of CHF. A chest x-ray will frequently show pulmonary vascular congestion, interstitial, and/or alveolar edema which are highly specific for a diagnosis of heart failure (96–99%) [1]. Natriuretic peptide levels (B-type natriuretic peptide [BNP] and N-terminal pro-BNP) provide incremental information, as a BNP level over 100 pg/mL has a diagnostic accuracy of 83.4% to distinguish between heart failure and pulmonary causes for dyspnea [29]. Additional laboratory data such as troponin level, hyponatremia, acute or chronic kidney injury, makers of a congestive hepatopathy (elevated transaminases and/or bilirubin), complete blood count (anemia or infection), and an arterial blood gas to quantify the level of hypoxia and acid-base status are useful.

In more difficult cases, echocardiography with Doppler will aid in the diagnosis by demonstrating decreased systolic contractility and/or impaired diastolic relaxation, and estimating cardiac filling pressures and presence and degree of valvular pathology. Routine invasive hemodynamic assessment is discouraged by both the ACC/AHA and ESC guidelines [30, 31], though may be useful in patients where the hemodynamics are uncertain and/or patients refractory to initial interventions (ACC/AHA Class IIa, Level of Evidence [LOE] C; ESC Class IIb, LOE C).

6.2 Quality of Life Assessment

Quality of life is important in the assessment of a patient with heart failure and has served as an endpoint in many clinical studies. Objective tools have been developed and validated in an effort to quantify this metric. The Minnesota Living with Heart Failure Questionnaire (MLHFQ) was developed in 1984 [32] as a patient self-assessment tool to describe how heart failure impacts daily life. The questionnaire contains 21 questions scored on a scale of 0–5, takes patients 5–10 min on average to complete, and increasing scores reflect worse quality of life. It has been demonstrated to be valid and reliable [33] and has been used extensively in research for medical therapy [34–37], mechanical circulatory support [38–41], cardiac resynchronization therapy [42, 43], and gene therapy [44]. Its use has been validated in a number languages and cultures [45–48].

In 2000 the Kansas City Cardiomyopathy Questionnaire (KCCQ) was developed in an effort to improve on the MLFHQ [49]. It is a self-administered "23-item questionnaire that quantifies physical limitations, symptoms, self-efficacy, social interference and quality of life." [49] Similar to the MLHFQ, it has been translated into and demonstrated to be valid in multiple languages [50–53]. The two questionnaires have been used together in research studies as quality of life measures, but there has been little head to head comparison. The study introducing the KCCQ suggested that both are valid and reliable but the KCCQ is more responsive to clinical changes.

6.3 Diagnostic Tests

6.3.1 Electrocardiogram

ECG's carry a Class I, LOE C from both major societies [30, 31] for any patient with heart failure. The ECG of a patient is frequently abnormal (though with non-specific changes), such that a normal ECG has a 98% negative predictive value [54]. The ECG may provide evidence of chamber enlargement, prior infarction, arrhythmia, increased muscle mass (hyptertrophic cardiomyopathy), low-voltage (infiltration e.g. amyloidosis), or conduction system abnormality (e.g. LBBB) that may help to guide therapy.

6.3.2 Imaging

6.3.2.1 Chest X-Ray

Chest radiography is a useful initial test in the evaluation of heart failure, both in the acute and chronic setting (ACC/AHA Class I, LOE C; ESC Class IIa, LOE C) [30, 31] (Fig. 6.2). The first suggestion of heart failure on the x-ray is cardiomegaly, with the cardiac silhouette occupying at least 50% of the thoracic diameter. However cardiomegaly may be absent in heart failure, in particular with preserved ejection fraction. In addition to general cardiomegaly, evidence of specific chamber enlargement or enlargement of the pulmonary arteries may be apparent on x-ray. Inspection of the pulmonary vasculature allows for the diagnosis of cardiogenic pulmonary edema. Increased hydrostatic pressure in the pulmonary veins from increased left ventricular end diastolic and/or left atrial pressure leads to venous dilation. This creates the typical cephalization pattern with vascular prominence. As hydrostatic pressure increases further Kerley B lines (short horizontal lines in the lower lung field periphery representing edematous interlobular septa), peribronchial cuffing (fluid surrounding a bronchus on end), and a bat-wing (peri-hilar) or diffuse pattern of interstitial edema. Another finding in heart failure is pleural effusion, which become evident on the frontal view once 200 mL of fluid accumulates. Lastly, the x-ray may show pericardial calcification (notably in the lateral view), which in the setting of an appropriate history (prior cardiac surgery, pericarditis, mediastinal radiation, or pericardial effusion) is suggestive of constrictive pericarditis.

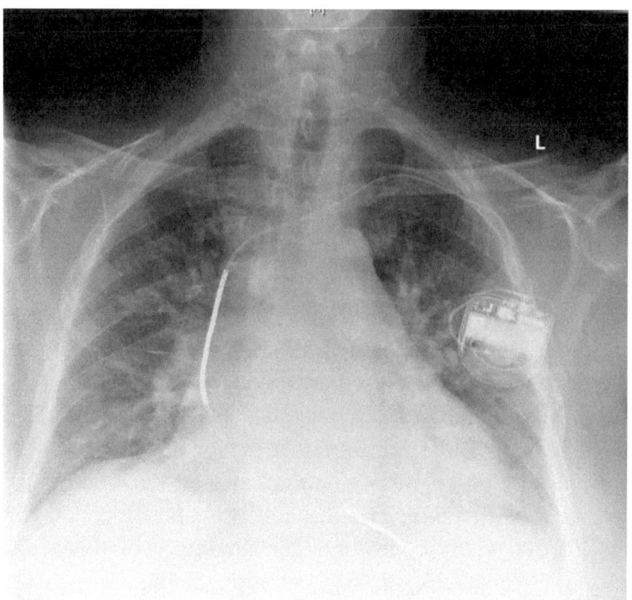

Fig. 6.2 Chest X-ray in heart failure

6.3.2.2 Echocardiography

Transthoracic Echocardiography

Echocardiography is the primary imaging modality for the diagnosis and characterization of HF, carrying a Class I recommendation from both major societies [30, 31]. Echocardiography provides information about cardiac structure and function. Systolic function is most frequently determined by the ejection fraction, using quantitative measurement (biplane method of disks summation) (Fig. 6.3). While ejection fraction has been shown to be predictive of cardiovascular mortality [55], alone it does not always correlate with symptoms. Furthermore it is a volumetric measurement, not a true measure of contractility, which requires tissue Doppler imaging or speckle tracking strain imaging. The echocardiogram provides measurements of chamber walls to evaluate for left ventricular hypertrophy and chamber size to assess left ventricular dilation. The echocardiographic evaluation of the left ventricle also assesses regional wall motion, which may be suggestive of ischemia.

Right ventricular dimensions (including wall thickness) should be measured and if 3D echocardiography is available volumes should be quantified. Function of the right ventricle may be assessed through a variety of quantitative measures (tricuspid annular plane systolic excursion, pulsed tissue Doppler S wave, fractional area change, right ventricular index of myocardial performance, strain imaging), though all are limited for accurate assessment right ventricular function due to its complex, non-ellipsoid shape. Atrial size should also be quantified; the left atrium by body surface area indexed volume and the right atrium by volume. Left atrial enlargement may be a marker of impaired diastolic function as it reflects chronic elevations in left ventricular pressure (in the absence of mitral disease or atrial fibrillation). Imaging of the pericardium is limited in echocardiography, though it is valuable for identification of a pericardial effusion.

Color Doppler echocardiography is used to evaluate cardiac valves. Through both qualitative and quantitative measures, the degree of stenosis or regurgitation can be determined. Further, pressure gradients across stenotic valves, valve areas, and regurgitant volumes can be quantified. Doppler echocardiography also may provide reliable assessment of right and left ventricular hemodynamics in patients with acute heart failure. Right atrial pressure estimation via measurement of the IVC ($r = 0.85$), estimation of the pulmonary artery systolic pressure using the tricuspid regurgitant jet ($r = 0.83$), and detection of a pulmonary capillary wedge pressure greater than 15 mm Hg through measurement of average E/e′ greater than 15 (area under the receiver operating characteristic curve [AUC] 0.92) are all possible non-invasive hemodynamic measurements [56]. Lastly,

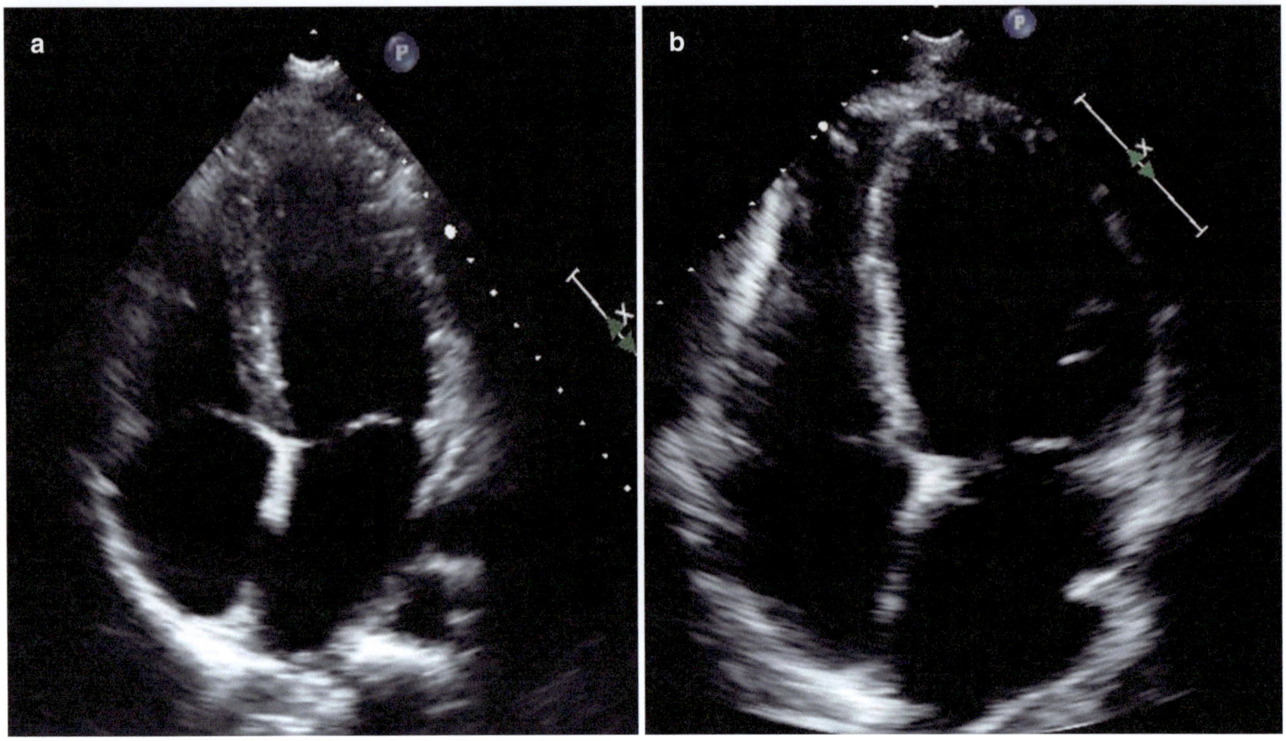

Fig. 6.3 (**a**) Normal apical four chamber transthoracic echocardiogram (**b**) Dilated cardiomyopathy

Doppler echocardiography allows for assessment of diastolic function through assessment of transmitral inflow velocity (E-wave and A-wave velocities in sinus rhythm) and tissue Doppler velocities. Adjunctive parameters for impaired diastolic function include increase left atrial volume index, elevated pulmonary artery systolic pressures (elevated tricuspid regurgitation velocity), and elevated left ventricular filling pressures (E/e' > 15 and/or pulmonary vein peak systolic to peak diastolic velocity <1) [57].

6.3.2.3 Non-invasive Stress Testing

Non-invasive imaging is recommended by both the ACC/AHA (Class IIa, LOE C) [31] and ESC (Class IIb, LOE B) [30] for patients eligible for revascularization who are suspected to have coronary artery disease, but without angina. Multiple modalities are available to the physician to make a non-invasive diagnosis.

Stress Echocardiography

Stress echocardiography may use exercise or pharmacologic agents (dobutamine preferred over vasodilator testing) to increase myocardial oxygen demand. In this procedure baseline rest images are obtained and images are again obtained within 90 s of peak stress. In pooled analyses, stress echocardiography has a sensitivity and specificity of 80% and 86% respectively for the detection of coronary artery stenosis >50% [58]. The benefits of stress echocardiography are the lack of ionizing radiation, short imaging time, low cost (compared to other modalities), supplementary information regarding chamber size and function, and (if exercise is used) a functional assessment is obtained [59]. Limitations include atrial fibrillation, technically difficult imaging windows, an inability to reach an age predicted maximum heart rate, and the ability to detect wall motion abnormalities with an already depressed ejection fraction.

Single Photon Emission Computed Tomography (SPECT)

Myocardial perfusion imaging using SPECT can be performed with a number of modalities including exercise (treadmill or bicycle), dobutamine, or vasodilator (regadenoson, adenosine, dipyridamole). During peak stress a radioisotope, classically thallium-201 though technetium Tc-99 m has become increasingly used, is injected through an intravenous catheter. After a period of time images are acquired. Myocardial perfusion imaging with SPECT has been shown to be 84% sensitive and 77% specific for the detection of coronary artery stenosis >50% [58]. The advantages of this procedure are regional localization of flow limiting ischemia, quantification of left ventricular volumes & function, and the ability to perform delayed myocardial viability testing. The drawback of this technique is exposure to ionizing radiation, attenuation artifact from surrounding structures (breast, chest wall), and the time commitment.

Positron Emission Tomography (PET)

PET stress testing is not as widely available, but is a good alternative to other modalities and capable of performing stress and viability imaging in a short time period. Predominantly performed using vasodilators, PET can reduce radiation as low as 2.4 mSv using certain protocols [60]. In addition to limiting radiation it is a highly accurate test with a sensitivity of 92% and specificity of 81% to detect ≥50% stenosis of any epicardial coronary artery [61]. Limitations of PET are the cost, availability of radiotracers (13 N-ammonia requires an on-site cyclotron, rubidium-82 does not), and radiation exposure.

6.3.2.4 Coronary Angiography

Coronary angiography remains the gold standard to diagnose coronary artery disease (Fig. 6.4). In the diagnosis of heart failure it plays a role in patients who are at risk (family history, diabetes, hypertension, tobacco use, dyslipidemia) of coronary artery disease. Diagnosis of an ischemic cardiomyopathy allows for revascularization and adjustment of pharmacotherapy. The diagnosis of an ischemic cardiomyopathy has also been shown to be an independent predictor of mortality in patients with heart failure [62]. Current societal guidelines differ slightly in whom angiography is recommended. The ACC/AHA provides a Class IIa, LOE C recommendation for coronary angiography among candidates for revascularization when ischemia may be playing a role in their heart failure syndrome [31]. ESC guidelines recommend angiography in patients suitable for revascularization who have angina or a history of cardiac arrest (Class I, LOE C) [30].

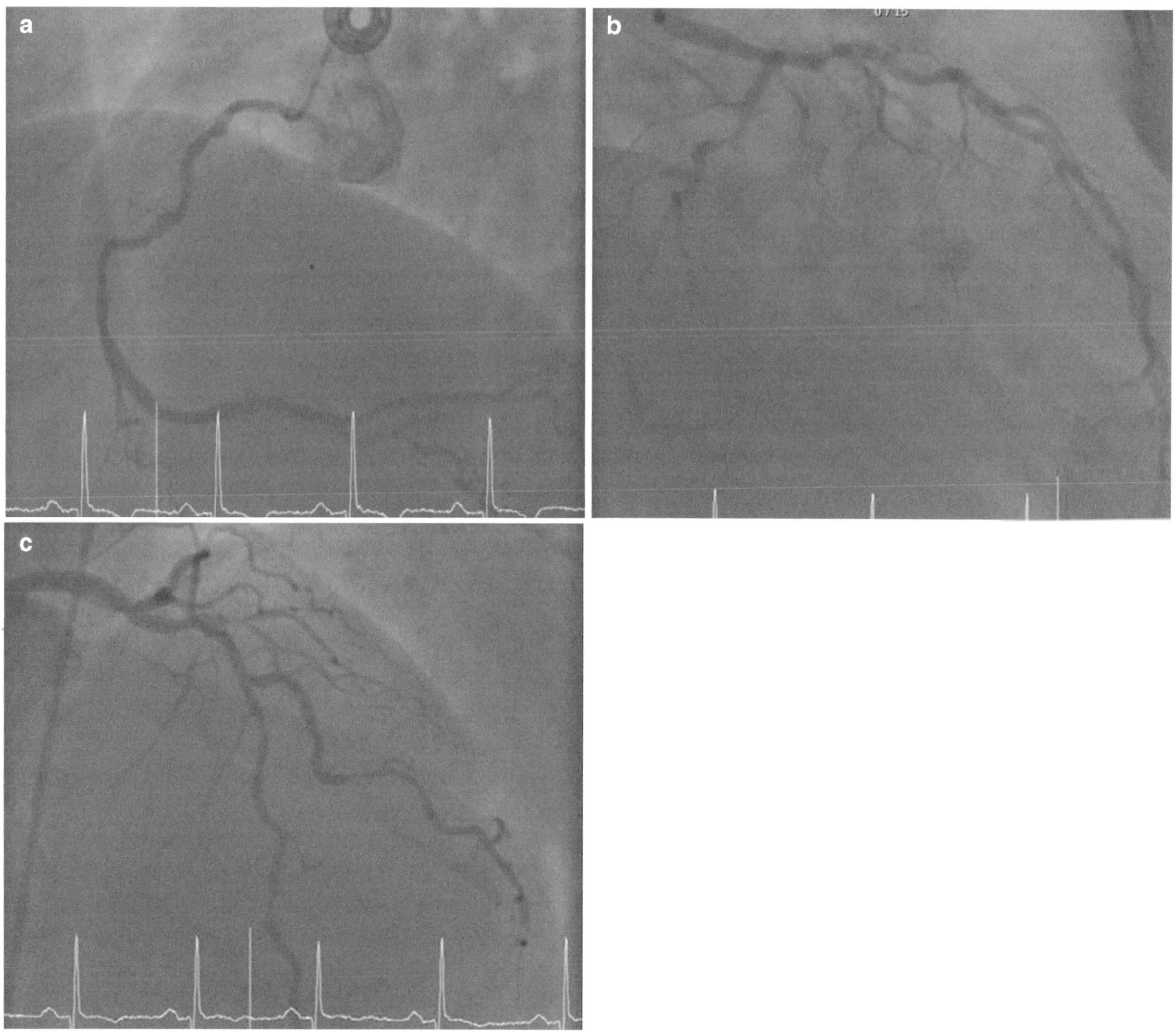

Fig. 6.4 Coronary angiogram (**a**) mild proximal right coronary artery stenosis (**b**) severe mid circumflex artery stenosis (**c**) Severe left anterior descending artery and second diagonal artery stenosis

Coronary Computed Tomography Angiogram (CTA)

Coronary CTA is a technique that has gained popularity for the diagnosis of coronary artery disease and acute coronary syndromes. In order to obtain accurate images a heart rate of 60 or less is typically required, which sometimes necessitates beta blocker administration. The remainder of the test involves injection of 60–120 mL of contrast medium and image acquisition. This modality has good accuracy, shown to have a sensitivity to detect coronary artery stenosis >50% of 85–99% and a specificity of 83–97% in three multicenter trials [63–65]. Advantages are that it is quick (less than 1 min acquisition), accurate, and widely available. Drawbacks are exposure to radiation, need for contrast, need for bradycardia, limited resolution in smaller vessels (<1.5 mm), arrhythmias, poor specificity due to coronary artery calcification and inability to detect ischemia.

6.3.2.5 Magnetic Resonance Imaging

Magnetic resonance imaging is a technique that produces high resolution images without ionizing radiation. Applied to the heart MRI can provide useful functional, structural, and valvular information. Cardiac MRI (CMR) provides accurate and reproducible measurements of volumes, biventricular function, wall motion, and anatomy (especially the pericardium) (Fig. 6.5). Identification of myocardial disease, whether infiltrative (sarcoidosis, hemochromatosis, amyloidosis), hypertrophic (especially variant HCM, e.g. apical), fibrotic (acute and chronic infarction), or ischemic (myocardial viability, stress) is an additional strength of CMR. CMR with gadolinium contrast is a valuable tool to help differentiate acute myocarditis (epicardial and mid-myocardial late gadolinium enhancement) from an ischemic cardiomyopathy (endocardial late gadolinium enhancement with variable extension into the mid-myocardium and epicardium). However, CMR is not sensitive enough (76% sensitivity) to definitively rule out acute myocarditis [66]. Cardiac sarcoidosis not only can be diagnosed using CMR, but CMR can also help differentiate between chronic and active disease, assess the response to treatment with corticosteroids [67–69], and predict mortality [70].

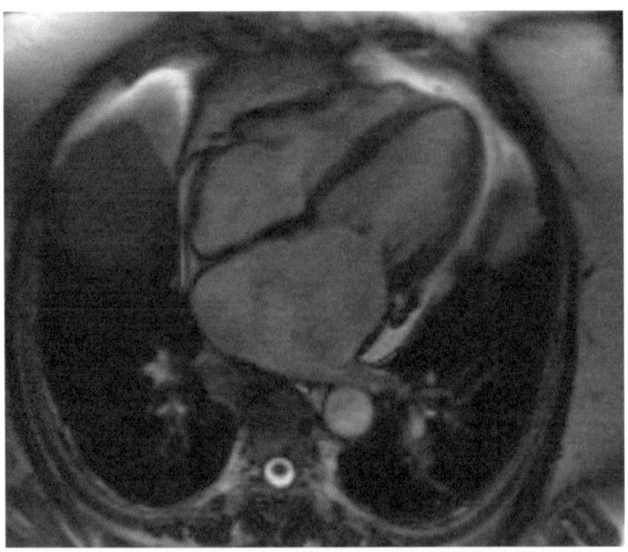

Fig. 6.5 Cardiac MRI of heart failure with a preserved ejection fraction

CMR also provides functional information and is beneficial in the assessment of valvular regurgitation, stenosis, and cardiac output. CMR may provide the greatest benefit in patients with congenital heart disease. The ESC provides a strong recommendation for CMR use (Class I, LOE C) [30], especially when echocardiographic images are limited. The ACC/AHA recommend CMR for assessment of scar or myocardial infiltration (Class IIa, LOE B) [31]. The application of this technology is limited by access to machines, the time required for a study (30–60 min), the use of gadolinium (in selected cases), patient claustrophobia, and presence of implanted metal devices.

6.3.3 Biomarkers

6.3.3.1 BNP and NT-proBNP

Btype natriuretic peptide (BNP) is a hormone primarily secreted by the cardiac ventricle in the setting of increased ventricular pressure. BNP is created by the cleavage of proBNP into BNP and the inert Nterminal proBNP (NTproBNP). Physiologically, BNP secretion is adaptive, promoting natriuresis, diuresis, inhibition of the renin-angiotensin system, a decrease in blood pressure, and inhibition of the sympathetic nervous system. Neprilysin inibitors, such as sacubitril/valsartan, aim to take advantage of those benefits through inhibition of BNP degradation among other effects. As such, BNP is not a useful diagnostic or monitoring tool for heart failure among patients on sacubitril/valsartan therapy. NT-proBNP levels will need to be assessed in these patients.

A BNP level of 100 ng/mL was found to have a diagnostic accuracy for heart failure of 83.4% in one large trial [29]. NT-proBNP levels are on a difference scale and "use of age-related cut-points of 450, 900, and 1800 pg/mL for ages<50, 50–75, and>75 yielded 90% sensitivity and 84% specificity for acute HF." [71] Levels of BNP or NT-proBNP are impacted by co-morbid conditions. Levels are higher in patients with chronic kidney disease, the elderly, women (compared with men), and those with pulmonary hypertension. Obese patients have a lower BNP that those of normal BMI.

BNP and NT-proBNP have both been shown to be prognostic of future mortality in acute heart failure [72, 73]. However the results of using BNP or NT-proBNP to guide therapy, whether acute or chronic, have not been consistently favorable. The ESC provides a Class IIa, LOE C recommendation to use BNP or NT-proBNP to exclude alternate causes or dyspnea or provide prognostic information [30]. The ACC/AHA gives a Class I, LOE A recommendation for the use of these biomarkers for the diagnosis of heart failure and for the prognosis of heart failure. They also provide a Class IIa, LOE B recommendation to use BNP to achieve goal directed medical therapy and caution (Class IIb, LOE C) that BNP guided diuresis in acute heart failure is not well established [31].

6.3.3.2 Troponin

Troponins are a family of proteins (Troponin I, T, C) that are incorporated into the thin filament of the cardiac sarcomere. They play a central role in cardiac contraction by mediating the interaction between actin and myosin. These proteins, when found in the blood, are sensitive markers of myocardial damage. In the setting of heart failure, a serum troponin elevation may be a marker of acute coronary syndrome or simply decompensated heart failure (myocardial strain from pressure and volume overload). An elevated troponin in a patient with heart failure not in the setting of acute coronary syndrome is associated with an increased risk of mortality [74].

6.3.3.3 Genetic Testing

With improvement of genetic testing has come an increased recognition of genetic causes of previously idiopathic causes of heart failure. For instance, as many as 20–35% of patients with an idiopathic dilated cardiomyopathy have familial cardiomyopathy [31]. Genetic causes have been identified for familial dilated cardiomyopathy (DCM), idiopathic restrictive cardiomyopathy (RCM), left ventricular non-compaction cardiomyopathy (LVNC), hypertrophic cardiomyopathy (HCM), arrhythmogenic right ventricular dysplasia/cardiomyopathy (ARVD/C), lysosomal storage disease related cardiomyopathies (Fabry, Pompe, or Danon diseases), muscular dystrophies (Becker, Duchenne, or Emery-Dreifuss muscular dystrophy), or systemic diseases (amyloidosis, sarcoidosis). Evaluation for genetic causes of a cardiomyopathy begins with a detailed family history, allowing for identification of age of onset, penetrance, and the modality of inheritance (autosomal dominant or recessive, X-linked). Once a patient with a potential genetic cause is identified, referral to a center experienced in the diagnosis and care of patients with genetic cardiomyopathies is recommended [75]. Further, asymptomatic first-degree relatives of patients with DCM, RCM, LVNC, HCM, or ARVD/C should have clinical screening for cardiomyopathy [75].

Incorporation of genetic information to the classification of heart failure has been proposed, though remains limited in practice. Nearly two-thirds of patients with HCM have identifiable genetic mutations [76], however classification of HCM by mutations has been limited as there is little genotype-phenotype concordance [77, 78]. The MOGE(S) classification system was proposed in 2013 and classifies patients using the morphofunctional phenotype (M), organ or organs involved (O), genetic inheritance pattern (G), etiological annotation (E) including genetic defect or underlying disease/substrate, and the functional status (S) [79, 80]. However this classification system has yet to achieve widespread use.

6.3.3.4 Laboratory Testing

Serum Sodium

Heart failure is a state of neurohumoral activation with increased levels of renin, anti-diuretic hormone, and norepinephrine. The degree of neurohumoral activation is related to the degree of left ventricular dysfunction and serum sodium level is a readily available biomarker of this activation [81]. Hyponatremia in heart failure has been linked to worse outcomes [82, 83]. This parameter is incorporated into several widely used predictive models in CHF such as the Seattle Heart Failure Model and Heart Failure Survival Score.

Renal Function

Chronic kidney disease (CKD) is a common comorbidity among heart failure patients, with 29–44% of heart failure patients having CKD Stage III or worse [84–87]. Often referred to as the cardiorenal syndrome, the kidney and heart are linked through a number of interactions. The pathophysiology behind this link is multifactorial: neurohumoral activation due to left ventricular dysfunction (increased renin-angiotensin-aldosterone system activity, elevated vasopressin, elevated endothelin-1, and increased sympathetic activity), increased venous pressure (and thereby renal venous pressure), and decreased renal perfusion. Mortality for patients with heart failure increases 7% for every 10 mL/min decrease in glomerular filtration rate [87].

Complete Blood Count

Anemia is present in one of five heart failure patients [88]. Anemia may serve as the cause (high output heart failure) or as a complication and important comorbidity. The mechanism of anemia may be due to iron deficiency [89], increased inflammation [89], hemodilution [90], or renal dysfunction and decreased erythropoietin. Anemia has been shown to be associated with worse functional capacity and worse outcomes [91, 92], though this may be due in part to other comorbidities and not independently prognostic.

Ferritin

Ferritin is a protein synthesized by the liver that is used for iron storage. Serum ferritin serves as a marker of total body iron stores, and useful to identify potential candidates for iron replacement therapy, but is also an acute phase reactant that will be elevated in the setting of inflammation or anemia of chronic disease. Ferritin is an important diagnostic test as heart failure may cause anemia (discussed in prior section) or may be the result of excess iron. Primary hemochromatosis is a genetic disease most commonly found in those of northern European descent that results in excessive iron absorption leading to iron overload. Secondary hemochromatosis may develop in patients who require frequent transfusion of red blood cells. Levels over 200 ng/mL in men and 150 ng/mL in women (along with elevated iron and transferrin saturation above 45%) signal the possibility of hemochromatosis and should prompt genetic testing [93]. Many organs may be affected, but in the heart it will result in a dilated cardiomyopathy.

Thyroid Function Tests

Thyroid stimulating hormone (TSH) should be checked in patients with a diagnosis of heart failure to screen for hypo or hyperthyroidism. Hyperthyroidism causes tachycardia (sinus or atrial fibrillation), increased contractility, and decreased systemic vascular resistance (SVR). As a result cardiac output increases 50–300% and some patients develop symptoms of high output heart failure [94]. Those with long standing untreated hyperthyroidism may develop low-output heart failure, which is likely secondary to tachycardia [95]. In hypothyroidism, a deficiency in thyroid hormone results in both decreased cardiac output (decreased heart rate, contractility, and increased SVR) and impaired diastolic dysfunction [94]. However overt clinical heart failure is not common.

Nutritional Markers

Nutritional deficiencies (selenium, calcium, thiamine) have been linked to the development of heart failure [96]. Cardiac cachexia is a well described syndrome whereby patients with heart failure experience muscle loss, adipose tissue loss, and increased catabolism [97]. This syndrome may be due to increased energy expenditure and/or inadequate nutrition. Hypoalbuminemia, while not truly a marker of nutritional status, has been associated with a marked increased risk of mortality in heart failure [98].

Serologies

There is a limited role for checking viral serologies when a viral cause is suspected as their diagnostic yield has been shown to be limited [98]. If a patients Is from an endemic region, testing for Chagas disease may be warranted. Similarly if an autoimmune disease is suspected, ANA or systemic lupus erythematosus serologies should be checked.

Symptomatic HFrEF occurred in 1–2% of all patients with HIV prior to the current era of anti-retroviral therapy (ART) [99]. While it is less common in the current era, nearly half of patients receiving ART develop echocardiographic evidence of diastolic dysfunction and 8% will have systolic dysfunction [100].

Amyloidosis

When amyloidosis is part of the differential for the etiology of heart failure, cardiac biopsy remains the gold standard diagnostic test. Adjunctive laboratory tests include serum free light chain ratio and 24-h urine and serum immunofixation for the diagnosis of light chain or AL amyloid. Genetic testing is recommended for transthyretin or TTR amyloid to differentiate between hereditary (familial) transthyretin-related amyloid and wild-type or senile systemic amyloidosis [101].

6.4 Functional Assessment

The most commonly used functional assessment for heart disease is the New York Heart Association functional classification of heart failure. Since 1994, NYHA Class I has defined patients with structural or functional cardiac disease but no functional limitations. Class II patients have no symptoms at rest, but ordinary physical activity results in fatigue, dyspnea, palpitations, or angina. Patients with Class III symptoms are free of symptoms at rest however less than ordinary physical activity results in the aforementioned symptoms. Those with Class IV functional status are severely debilitated by their symptoms, experiencing them at rest [102]. One episode of PND classifies a patient as NYHA Class IV. An unofficial but commonly used term is NYHA Class IIIb. The first mention of NYHA Class IIIb in the medical literature was in 1996 [103], though this classification never has been formally codified. It is generally used to describe patients with functional symptoms greater than Class III but not quite Class IV. It is often used to select those NYHA III patients who need expeditious work-up for heart transplantation or mechanical circulatory support and its adoption has been so widespread that the Heartmate II left ventricular assist device received Food and Drug Administration (FDA) approval for both NYHA Class IIIb and Class IV patients [104].

Using the NYHA classification a patients' functional class can change based on their current symptoms. A limitation and criticism of this classification system is the subjectivity, as there are no standardized criteria for each class. This fact is illustrated by one study showing two independent cardiologists agreed on a patient's NYHA class only 54% of the time (though never varying by more than 1 class) [105]. Additionally, patient reporting of symptoms is variable depending on their perceived level of dyspnea and fatigue. Lastly, this method of functional assessment is unable to determine if a limitation is due to heart disease or comorbid conditions such as lung disease, peripheral arterial disease, obesity, or deconditioning. However, the NYHA classification is familiar to broad ranges of clinicians and useful in referral settings, and interestingly discriminates outcomes nearly as well as more complex prognostic tools such as the Heart Failure Survival Score and the Seattle Heart Failure Model [106].

6.4.1 Exercise Testing

6.4.1.1 Cardiopulmonary Exercise Testing

The principal key methodology for objective functional assessment of a patient with heart failure is the cardiopulmonary exercise test (CPET). The CPET is a non-invasive exercise test that can provide important diagnostic and prognostic information about the cause and degree of functional impairment. The test is based on the principle of gas exchange during exercise whereby inspired oxygen diffuses into the blood through the lungs and is transported to muscle where oxygen-carbon dioxide exchange occurs, and ultimately carbon dioxide is eliminated through expiration. During exercise muscles require increased amounts of oxygen and this need is met though increased oxygen delivery (cardiac output) and extraction by the muscles.

Exercise capacity is decreased in all heart failure patients, with increasing impairment correlating with disease severity. The reason for this decreased exercise capacity is partly attributable to a decreased cardiac output response to exercise and increased filling pressures (pulmonary capillary wedge pressures reaching as high as 50–60 mm Hg). However, use of inotropes or vasodilators to control PCWP and cardiac output fail to normalize exercise capacity [2–4]. Skeletal muscle has been identified as the other source of decreased exercise capacity, as chronic hypoperfusion in heart failure leads to muscle loss [107] and intrinsic changes. Vascular changes with altered endothelial function also leads to peripheral abnormalities exacerbating skeletal muscle hypoperfusion and development of intramuscular lactic acidosis [108].

The CPET incorporates ventilatory gas measurements. Patients use a mouthpiece that is connected to a metabolic cart equipped with rapidly responding O2 and CO2 sensors, capable of on line measurement of oxygen uptake and carbon dioxide production. Pneumotachs measure minute ventilation. Exercise may be performed using a treadmill or stationary bicycle. With either modality patient workload incrementally increases until exhaustion. As exercise progresses the VO_2 increases and will begin to plateau. Prior to peak VO2 the patient will achieve a ventilatory anaerobic threshold (point at which the rate of VCO_2 increase exceeds VO_2 as a result of muscle anaerobic metabolism). Identification of the anaerobic threshold can be made by a variety of methods including the V slope method and identification of the nadir for the ventilator equivalent for VO2 in relation to the rise in the ventilator equivalent for VCO2. If a patient achieves a respiratory exchange ratio (VCO_2/VO_2) ≥ 1.1 an adequate patient effort is generally considered to have been achieved. Irrespective of how the anaerobic threshold is identified its determination signals an adequate effort and at least a near maximal test.

In seminal studies, the peak VO_2 has been shown to provide significant prognostic information for heart failure severity, mortality, and transplant candidacy. The foundational study was performed in 1994 showing that heart failure patients with a peak $VO_2 \leq 14$ mL/kg/min had significantly lower survival [108]. This was in the era prior to current optimal therapy (beta blockers, ACE inhibitors, cardiac resynchronization, ICDs) though subsequent analyses have confirmed the importance of peak VO_2 [109–111]. A more useful peak VO2 threshold for heart transplant listing in the current era is less than 12 mL/kg/min [112].

A number of measurements other than peak VO_2 obtained during CPET provide valuable information. Ventilatory efficiency (VE/VCO_2) is the ratio of volume of expired air over a minute (in liters) to remove one liter of carbon dioxide. The slope of this line is useful even prior to reaching the VAT and has been studied in chronic heart failure patients, with values greater than 34–50 being an independent predictor of heart failure mortality [113–115]. An additional parameter is the oxygen uptake efficiency slope (OEUS), which is the slope of VO_2 and a logarithmically transformed VE. This parameter is not as well validated, with one study demonstrating an OEUS of less than 65% predicted being prognostic [116] and another showing a value of less than 1.47 being prognostic [117]. As peak VO2 is impacted by age, gender, and conditioning status use of percent predicted values may be advantageous in certain populations such as young patients (<age 40 yrs) or elderly women.

6.4.1.2 Six-Minute Walk Test

The six-minute walk test (6MWT) is an alternative to the full cardiopulmonary exercise test that can provide useful functional and prognostic information. This test is easier to perform as no sophisticated equipment is required other than a quiet corridor that is about 30 meters in length. Prior to beginning the walk test blood pressure, oxygen saturation, and heart rate are measured. The patient walks as far as they can for 6 min. An unencouraged test should be performed with the medical personnel observing or walking behind the patient i.e. not leading or setting the pace. At the termination of the test dyspnea is assessed using the Borg scale and heart rate, blood pressure, and oxygen saturation are recorded [118]. The total distance traveled is recorded and can be compared to age and gender specific reference ranges. The normal range, across all ages (up to 80 years) and genders, is 400–700 meters [119]. Generally a 6 min walk distance less than 300 m is associated with a worse prognosis [120–123], and together with changes in 6MWT has been used as a frequent clinical endpoint in clinical trials.

The 6MWT walk test has been shown to be mildly predictive of peak VO2 among patients with heart failure and in patients with severe heart failure as the test approaches maximal levels of exercise. A number of studies have shown that the 6MWT has a modest correlation with peak VO2 ($r = 0.59$ [124], $r = 0.64$ [120], $r = 0.65$ [122], $r = 0.76$ [125]), but these data do not support replacement of CPET with the 6MWT. Indeed, the CPET is the only test that gives reproducible hard data and with appropriate calibration, i.e. actual cut-off values useful in e.g. transplant selection.

6.4.1.3 Frailty Assessment

Many heart failure patients may be too ill to exercise and in those patients an assessment of frailty will help to assess prognosis. Frailty is a biologic syndrome characterized by a loss in overall function, reserve, and resistance to stressors leading to an increased susceptibility to adverse outcomes [126]. Heart failure patients are often elderly with multiple comorbid conditions, therefore, it is not surprising that prefrailty is present in 74–100% of HF patients and frailty is present among 19–65% [127–129]. Frailty is frequently diagnosed using the five component Fried Frailty Index [126].

Weight Loss: Unintentional weight loss of ≥10 pounds or ≥5% of body weight over the prior year
Weakness: Grip strength in the lowest 20%, adjusted for sex and BMI (averaged over three attempts)
Poor endurance and energy: Self-reported exhaustion, identified by two questions from the CES–D scale
Slowness: Time to walk 15 feet in the lowest 20%, adjusted or sex and height (>6–7 s)
Low physical activity: Lowest quintile of physical activity, as measured by kilocalorie expenditure (males <383 Kcals and females <270 Kcal)

Patients are classified as prefrail if they meet one or two criteria, frail if they meet three or more criteria, and not frail if they meet none of the criteria. Frailty has been shown to be an independent predictor of hospitalization [128, 129], mortality among patients with heart failure [127, 128, 130], and mortality following left ventricular assist device implantation [131].

6.4.2 Invasive Assessment

6.4.2.1 Endomyocardial Biopsy

The endomyocardial biopsy (EMB) may be useful in selected cases of heart failure and is recommended in patients with an unexplained cause of heart failure where the biopsy will provide diagnostic information that may change clinical care. The diagnostic yield varies due to sampling error and diagnostic limitations. A diagnosis may be determined using EMB half of the time [132, 133], though a treatable etiology is rarely identified. When viral myocarditis is suspected, the addition of viral polymerase chain reaction (PCR) may increase the sensitivity of the biopsy, as viral genomic sequences may be found in as many as two-thirds of patients with heart failure who do not meet the histopathological Dallas criteria [134, 135]. It has been suggested that these patients may have worse clinical outcomes [136], however the precise clinical impact of a virus present in the myocardium in the absence of myocardial inflammation is not presently known.

EMB is strongly recommended for patients with new-onset heart failure of fewer than 2 weeks duration with a normal sized or dilated ventricle, looking for giant cell, eosinophilic, or lymphocytic myocarditis. Similarly, among those with heart failure diagnosed within the last 3 months with a dilated ventricle without response to treatment or associated with arrhythmias EMB, is strongly recommended (Class I, LOE B) [137]. Performance of an EMB may be reasonable among patients with a suspicion of anthracycline induced cardiomyopathy, allergic/eosinophilic cardiomyopathy, restrictive cardiomyopathy from infiltration, and suspected arrhythmogenic right ventricular dysplasia/cardiomyopathy.

An EMB is performed through either femoral or internal jugular venous access and a small piece of tissue is taken from the septum of the right ventricle under fluoroscopic guidance. In total, five to seven biopsy specimens are recommended [137]. The most frequent complications of biopsy include access site issues (2–3%), conduction abnormalities (RBBB) and arrhythmia (2%), and perforation (0.5%) [138].

6.5 Hemodynamic Assessment

6.5.1 Invasive

Right heart catheterization (RHC) allows for direct measurements of hemodynamics. The use of invasive hemodynamic measurements in heart failure, once frequent, has become more selective after publication of the ESCAPE trial [139], which failed to show benefit of routine RHC in acute heart failure. Despite this, invasive hemodynamic monitoring remains an important part of the care of heart failure patients. Both major societies recommend RHC when physical exam is inadequate to determine filling pressures, patients with persistent hypoperfusion despite medical therapy, those with worsening renal function despite therapy, patients who require vasoactive medications, and those being considered

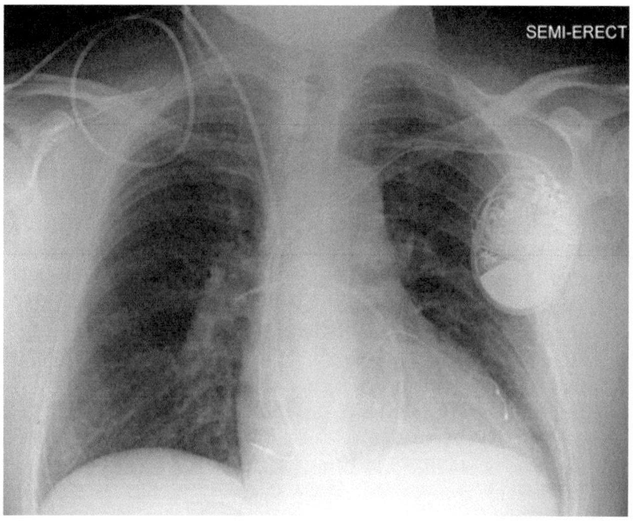

Fig. 6.6 Chest X-ray of Swan-Ganz catheter & CRT-D device

for mechanical circulatory support or heart transplantation [30, 31].

The pulmonary artery catheter is a balloon tipped pressure sensing catheter that requires venous access (internal jugular, brachial, or femoral) (Fig. 6.6). Following a careful zeroing and flushing of the catheter it is advanced with balloon inflated to the right atrium, typically 15–20 cm from the internal jugular vein, 40–50 cm from the femoral vein, or 45–50 cm from the brachial vein. The right atrial waveform has an "a" wave representing atrial contraction, a small "c" wave representing tricuspid valve closure, and a "v" wave representing atrial filling. Among all patients, a right atrial pressure less than 7 mm Hg is typically considered normal. The catheter is next advanced approximately 10 cm across the tricuspid valve to the right ventricle where the pressure waveform changes and the systolic pressure increases (normally less than 25/5 mm Hg). Advancement of the catheter another 10 cm results in positioning in the main pulmonary artery where the diastolic pressure increases (normally less than 25/10 mm Hg). In the absence of pre-capillary pulmonary hypertension, the PA diastolic pressure will approximate the pulmonary capillary wedge pressure (PCWP). The balloon tip catheter is then slowly advanced until the PCWP is obtained (normally less than 12 mm Hg) and the waveform appears similar to that in the right atrium, though with higher pressures and a smaller pulse pressure. The PCWP, which estimates the left atrial pressure, is identified by a decrease in pressure and characteristic waveform with both "a" and "v" waves. Prominent "v" waves may be present in mitral regurgitation, impair diastolic function, and ventricular septal defects.

Cardiac output may be calculated using either the Fick method or thermodilution. The Fick method is based on the principle that oxygen consumption of an organ can be measured by blood flow to the organ (cardiac output) and the arteriovenous difference of that substance. Oxygen consumption (mL/min) is either directly measured (metabolic cart) or estimated based on patient characteristics (age, gender, height, weight). Arteriovenous difference in oxygen concentration is determined using an arterial oxygen saturation and pulmonary artery or mixed venous oxygen saturation in the following equation: (1.36 mL O_2/g Hgb × Hgb [g/dL] × [S_AO_2−S_VO_2] × 10 [dL/L]). The Fick method is limited by accurate measurement of oxygen consumption, which is often estimated and not directly measured. Further the oxygen consumption of a patient at rest may be significantly different than during exercise, which may provide misleading information. However in the presence of severe tricuspid regurgitation use of Fick cardiac output is more accurate than thermodilution technique which is described below.

The thermodilution technique is based on the indicator thermodilution principle whereby the rate of blood flow is inversely proportional to the concentration of a substance downstream from its injection. In practice, a 10 mL bolus of saline is injected into the right ventricle and the thermistor at the tip of the PA catheter measures the temperature change over time. The resulting area under the temperature-time curve is inversely proportional to cardiac output. This technique is limited by tricuspid regurgitation (underestimates CO), intracardiac shunts (overestimates CO), and very low output states (overestimates CO). Cardiac output values may range from 4.8 to 7.3 L/min for the average adult but should be indexed to body surface area to produce a cardiac index (L/min/m^2). The normal range for cardiac index is 2.8–4.2 L/min/m^2.

Pulmonary artery catheters can provide useful hemodynamic data beyond simply cardiac output and filling pressures. Systemic vascular resistance can determined to aid in the differentiation of type of shock. Similarly pulmonary vascular resistance may be calculated. Lastly, right ventricular function can be interrogated through calculation of the right ventricular stroke work index or pulmonary artery pulsatility index.

6.5.2 Implantable Hemodynamic Monitors

Hemodynamic assessment through implanted devices is available through two main modalities: implantable hemodynamic monitoring and intrathoracic impedance monitoring. Implantable hemodynamic monitoring has been tried with a number of specific devices provide real-time monitoring of intracardiac filling pressures. One such device was the Medtronic Chronicle, a device that was similar to a permanent pacemaker with a subcutaneous generator and a transvenous pressure sensing lead implanted in the right ventricular apex. This device allowed for remote transmission of hemodynamic parameters including right ventricular systolic and diastolic pressure, estimated pulmonary artery diastolic pressure, heart rate, and right ventricular dP/dt. This device was studied in the single-blind COMPASS-HF trial [140], in which patients with New York Heart Association functional class III or IV were followed for 6 months with the device. The device was unable to demonstrate an ability to reduce heart failure hospitalizations and failed to achieve FDA approval.

A second implantable device, CardioMEMS, is an implanted pulmonary artery monitor that wirelessly transmits pulmonary artery pressures. This device is inserted through 11 Fr venous access and implanted in the pulmonary artery percutaneously. Following implantation, patients require 1 month of clopidogrel and lifelong aspirin. This device was studied in the single-blind CHAMPION trial, which demonstrated the device was able to decrease the risk of hospitalization for heart failure by 37% at 18 months. Device complication was experienced by 1.4% of patients. This device, which achieved Food and Drug Administration approval in 2014, currently costs almost $18,000 in the United States and cost-effectiveness has been debated [141].

Intrathoracic impedance monitoring is available with a number of existing cardiac resynchronization or implantable cardioverter defibrillators (Fig. 6.6). Intrathoracic impedance monitoring measures the resistance that an electrical signal experiences between the defibrillator can and the right ventricular lead, which will decrease with increased water content (better conduction). As such these devices note a decrease in impedance in the setting of increased pulmonary edema (lung water content). This monitoring has demonstrated the ability to identify patients at increased risk of hospitalization [142, 143], however it has not been shown to decrease heart failure related events [144, 145].

References

1. Wang CS, FitzGerald J, Schulzer M, Mak E, Ayas NT. Does this dyspneic patient in the emergency department have congestive heart failure? JAMA. 2005;294:1944–56.
2. Clark AL, Poole-Wilson PA, Coats AJ. Exercise limitation in chronic heart failure: central role of the periphery. J Am Coll Cardiol. 1996;28:1092–102.
3. Wilson JR, Martin JL, Ferraro N. Impaired skeletal muscle nutritive flow during exercise in patients with congestive heart failure: role of cardiac pump dysfunction as determined by the effect of dobutamine. Am J Cardiol. 1984;53:1308–15.
4. Wilson JR, Martin JL, Ferraro N, Weber KT. Effect of hydralazine on perfusion and metabolism in the leg during upright bicycle exercise in patients with heart failure. Circulation. 1983;68:425–32.
5. Anker SD, von Haehling S. Inflammatory mediators in chronic heart failure: an overview. Heart. 2004;90:464–70.
6. McPeak EM, Levine SA. The preponderance of right hydrothorax in congestive heart failure. Ann Intern Med. 1946;25:916–27.
7. Woodring JH. Distribution of pleural effusion in congestive heart failure: what is atypical? South Med J. 2005;98:518–23.
8. Leung RST, Bowman ME, Parker JD, Newton GE, Bradley TD. Avoidance of the left lateral decubitus position during sleep in patients with heart failure: relationship to cardiac size and function. J Am Coll Cardiol. 2003;41:227–30.
9. Lund LH, Williams JJ, Freda P, LaManca JJ, LeJemtel TH, Mancini DM. Ghrelin resistance occurs in severe heart failure and resolves after heart transplantation. Eur J Heart Fail. 2009;11:789–94.
10. Lund LH, Freda P, Williams JJ, LaManca JJ, LeJemtel TH, Mancini DM. Growth hormone resistance in severe heart failure resolves after cardiac transplantation. Eur J Heart Fail. 2009;11:525–8.
11. Anker SD, Chua TP, Ponikowski P, Harrington D, Swan JW, Kox WJ, Poole-Wilson PA, Coats AJ. Hormonal changes and catabolic/anabolic imbalance in chronic heart failure and their importance for cardiac cachexia. Circulation. 1997;96:526–34.
12. Javaheri S, Parker TJ, Liming JD, Corbett WS, Nishiyama H, Wexler L, Roselle GA. Sleep apnea in 81 ambulatory male patients with stable heart failure. Types and their prevalences, consequences, and presentations. Circulation. 1998;97:2154–9.
13. Padeletti M, Green P, Mooney AM, Basner RC, Mancini DM. Sleep disordered breathing in patients with acutely decompensated heart failure. Sleep Med. 2009;10:353–60.
14. Murugiah K, Wang Y, Desai NR, Spatz ES, Nuti SV, Dreyer RP, Krumholz HM. Trends in short- and long-term outcomes for Takotsubo cardiomyopathy among Medicare fee-for-service beneficiaries, 2007 to 2012. JACC Heart Fail. 2016;4:197–205.
15. Templin C, Ghadri JR, Diekmann J, Napp LC, Bataiosu DR, Jaguszewski M, Cammann VL, Sarcon A, Geyer V, Neumann CA, Seifert B, Hellermann J, Schwyzer M, Eisenhardt K, Jenewein J, Franke J, Katus HA, Burgdorf C, Schunkert H, Moeller C, Thiele H, Bauersachs J, Tschöpe C, Schultheiss H-P, Laney CA, Rajan L, Michels G, Pfister R, Ukena C, Böhm M, Erbel R, Cuneo A, Kuck K-H, Jacobshagen C, Hasenfuss G, Karakas M, Koenig W, Rottbauer W, Said SM, Braun-Dullaeus RC, Cuculi F, Banning A, Fischer TA, Vasankari T, Airaksinen KEJ, Fijalkowski M, Rynkiewicz A, Pawlak M, Opolski G, Dworakowski R, MacCarthy P, Kaiser C, Osswald S, Galiuto L, Crea F, Dichtl W, Franz WM, Empen K, Felix SB, Delmas C, Lairez O, Erne P, Bax JJ, Ford I, Ruschitzka F, Prasad A, Lüscher TF. Clinical features and outcomes of Takotsubo (stress) cardiomyopathy. N Eng J Med. 2015;373:929–38.
16. Sliwa K, Damasceno A, Mayosi BM. Epidemiology and etiology of cardiomyopathy in Africa. Circulation. 2005;112:3577–83.
17. Packer M. The neurohormonal hypothesis: a theory to explain the mechanism of disease progression in heart failure. J Am Coll Cardiol. 1992;20:248–54.
18. Stevenson L, Perloff JK. THe limited reliability of physical signs for estimating hemodynamics in chronic heart failure. JAMA. 1989;261:884–8.
19. Butman SM, Ewy GA, Standen JR, Kern KB, Hahn E. Bedside cardiovascular examination in patients with severe chronic heart failure: importance of rest or inducible jugular venous distension. J Am Coll Cardiol. 1993;22:968–74.
20. Drazner MH, Hamilton MA, Fonarow G, Creaser J, Flavell C, Warner SL. Relationship between right and left-sided filling pressures in 1000 patients with advanced heart failure. J Heart Lung Transplant. 1999;18:1126–32.
21. Drazner MH, Hellkamp AS, Leier CV, Shah MR, Miller LW, Russell SD, Young JB, Califf RM, Nohria A. Value of clinician assessment of hemodynamics in advanced heart failure: the ESCAPE trial. Circ Heart Fail. 2008;1:170–7.
22. Sochowski RA, Dubbin JD, Naqvi SZ. Clinical and hemodynamic assessment of the hepatojugular reflux. Am J Cardiol. 1990;66:1002–6.

23. Grayzel J. Gallop rhythm of the heart: II. Quadruple rhythm and its relation to summation and augmented gallops. Circulation. 1959;20:1053–62.
24. Drazner MH, Rame JE, Stevenson LW, Dries DL. Prognostic importance of elevated jugular venous pressure and a third heart sound in patients with heart failure. N Engl J Med. 2001;345:574–81.
25. Nohria A, Tsang SW, Fang JC, Lewis EF, Jarcho JA, Mudge GH, Stevenson LW. Clinical assessment identifies hemodynamic profiles that predict outcomes in patients admitted with heart failure. J Am Coll Cardiol. 2003;41:1797–804.
26. McKee PA, Castelli WP, McNamara PM, Kannel WB. The natural history of congestive heart failure: the Framingham study. N Engl J Med. 1971;285:1441–6.
27. Jorge S, Becquemin M-H, Delerme S, Bennaceur M, Isnard R, Achkar R, Riou B, Boddaert J, Ray P. Cardiac asthma in elderly patients: incidence, clinical presentation and outcome. BMC Cardiovasc Disord. 2007;7:16.
28. Nohria A, Lewis E, Stevenson L. Medical management of advanced heart failure. JAMA. 2002;287:628–40.
29. Maisel AS, Krishnaswamy P, Nowak RM, McCord J, Hollander JE, Duc P, Omland T, Storrow AB, Abraham WT, Wu AH, Clopton P, Steg PG, Westheim A, Knudsen CW, Perez A, Kazanegra R, Herrmann HC, McCullough PA. Rapid measurement of B-type natriuretic peptide in the emergency diagnosis of heart failure. N Engl J Med. 2002;347:161–7.
30. Ponikowski P, Voors AA, Anker SD, Bueno H, Cleland JGF, Coats AJS, Falk V, González-Juanatey JR, Harjola V-P, Jankowska EA, Jessup M, Linde C, Nihoyannopoulos P, Parissis JT, Pieske B, Riley JP, Rosano GMC, Ruilope LM, Ruschitzka F, Rutten FH, van der Meer P. 2016 ESC Guidelines for the diagnosis and treatment of acute and chronic heart failure. Eur Heart J. 2016; 37(27):2129–200.
31. Yancy CW, Jessup M, Bozkurt B, Butler J, Casey DE, Drazner MH, Fonarow GC, Geraci SA, Horwich T, Januzzi JL, Johnson MR, Kasper EK, Levy WC, Masoudi FA, McBride PE, McMurray JJV, Mitchell JE, Peterson PN, Riegel B, Sam F, Stevenson LW, Tang WHW, Tsai EJ, Wilkoff BL. 2013 ACCF/AHA guideline for the management of heart failure: a report of the American College of Cardiology Foundation/American Heart Association Task Force on Practice Guidelines. J Am Coll Cardiol. 2013;62:e147–239.
32. Rector TS, Kubo SH, Cohn JN. Patients' self-assessment of their congestive heart failure. Part 2: Content, reliability and validity of a new measure, the Minnesota Living with Heart Failure questionnaire. Heart Fail. 1987;3:198–209.
33. Rector TS, Cohn JN. Assessment of patient outcome with the Minnesota Living with Heart-Failure Questionnaire – reliability and validity during a randomized, double-blind, placebo-controlled trial of pimobendan. Am Heart J. 1992;124:1017–25.
34. Colucci WS, Packer M, Bristow MR, Gilbert EM, Cohn JN, Fowler MB, Krueger SK, Hershberger R, Uretsky BF, Bowers JA, SacknerBernstein JD, Young ST, Holcslaw TL, Lukas MA. Carvedilol inhibits clinical progression in patients with mild symptoms of heart failure. Circulation. 1996;94:2800–6.
35. Rector TS, Kubo SH, Cohn JN. Validity of the Minnesota Living with Heart-Failure questionnaire as a measure of therapeutic response to enalapril or placebo. Am J Cardiol. 1993;71:1106–7.
36. Sokos GG, Nikolaidis LA, Mankad S, Elahi D, Shannon RP. Glucagon-like peptide-1 infusion improves left ventricular ejection fraction and functional status in patients with chronic heart failure. J Card Fail. 2006;12:694–9.
37. Rector TS, Carson PE, Anand IS, McMurray JJ, Zile MR, McKelvie RS, Komajda M, Kuskowski M, Massie BM, Investigators ftI-PT. Assessment of long-term effects of irbesartan on heart failure with preserved ejection fraction as measured by the minnesota living with heart failure questionnaire in the irbesartan in heart failure with preserved systolic function (I-PRESERVE) trial. Circ Heart Fail. 2012;5:217–25.
38. Pagani FD, Miller LW, Russell SD, Aaronson KD, John R, Boyle AJ, Conte JV, Bogaev RC, MacGillivray TE, Naka Y, Mancini D, Massey HT, Chen L, Klodell CT, Aranda JM, Moazami N, Ewald GA, Farrar DJ, Frazier OH, HeartMate III. Extended mechanical circulatory support with a continuous-flow rotary left ventricular assist device. J Am Coll Cardiol. 2009;54:312–21.
39. Miller LW, Pagani FD, Russell SD, John R, Boyle AJ, Aaronson KD, Conte JV, Naka Y, Mancini D, Delgado RM, MacGillivray TE, Farrar DJ, Frazier OH, HeartMate IICI. Use of a continuous-flow device in patients awaiting heart transplantation. N Engl J Med. 2007;357:885–96.
40. Birks EJ, Tansley PD, Hardy J, George RS, Bowles CT, Burke M, Banner NR, Khaghani A, Yacoub MH. Left ventricular assist device and drug therapy for the reversal of heart failure. N Engl J Med. 2006;355:1873–84.
41. Rogers JG, Aaronson KD, Boyle AJ, Russell SD, Milano CA, Pagani FD, Edwards BS, Park S, John R, Conte JV, Farrar DJ, Slaughter MS, HeartMate III. Continuous flow left ventricular assist device improves functional capacity and quality of life of advanced heart failure patients. J Am Coll Cardiol. 2010;55:1826–34.
42. Leon AR, Greenberg JM, Kanuru N, Baker CM, Mera FV, Smith AL, Langberg JJ, DeLurgio DB. Cardiac resynchronization in patients with congestive heart failure and chronic atrial fibrillation – effect of upgrading to biventricular pacing after chronic right ventricular pacing. J Am Coll Cardiol. 2002;39:1258–63.
43. Gras D, Mabo P, Tang T, Luttikuis O, Chatoor R, Pedersen AK, Tscheliessnigg HH, Deharo JC, Puglisi A, Silvestre J, Kimber S, Ross H, Ravazzi A, Paul V, Skehan D. Multisite pacing as a supplemental treatment of congestive heart failure: preliminary results of the Medtronic Inc. InSync study. Pacing Clin Electrophysiol. 1998;21:2249–55.
44. Jessup M, Greenberg B, Mancini D, Cappola T, Pauly DF, Jaski B, Yaroshinsky A, Zsebo KM, Dittrich H, Hajjar RJ. Calcium upregulation by percutaneous administration of gene therapy in cardiac disease (CUPID): a phase 2 trial of intracoronary gene therapy of sarcoplasmic reticulum Ca2+-ATPase in patients with advanced heart failure. Circulation. 2011;124:304–U113.
45. Parajon T, Lupon J, Gonzalez B, Urrutia A, Altimir S, Coll R, Prats M, Valle V. Use of the Minnesota Living with Heart Failure quality of life questionnaire in Spain. Revista Espanola De Cardiologia. 2004;57:155–60.
46. Carvalho VO, Guimaraes GV, Carrara D, Bacal F, Bocchi EA. Validation of the Portuguese version of the Minnesota Living with Heart Failure Questionnaire. Arq Bras Cardiol. 2009;93:39–44.
47. Ho CC, Clochesy JM, Madigan E, Liu CC. Psychometric evaluation of the Chinese version of the Minnesota Living with Heart Failure Questionnaire. Nurs Res. 2007;56:441–8.
48. Quittan M, Wiesinger GF, Crevenna R, Nuhr MJ, Posch M, Hulsmann M, Muller D, Pacher R, Fialka-Moser V. Cross-cultural adaptation of the Minnesota living with heart failure questionnaire for German-speaking patients. J Rehabil Med. 2001;33:182–6.
49. Green CP, Porter CB, Bresnahan DR, Spertus JA. Development and evaluation of the Kansas City Cardiomyopathy Questionnaire: a new health status measure for heart failure. J Am Coll Cardiol. 2000;35:1245–55.
50. Nave-Leal E, Pais-Ribeiro J, Oliveira MM, da Silva N, Soares R, Fragata J, Ferreira R. Psychometric properties of the Portuguese version of the Kansas City Cardiomyopathy Questionnaire in dilated cardiomyopathy with congestive heart failure. Rev Port Cardiol. 2010;29:353–72.

51. Faller H, Steinbuchel T, Schowalter M, Spertus JA, Stork S, Angermann CE. The Kansas City Cardiomyopathy Questionnaire (KCCQ) – a new disease-specific quality of life measure for patients with chronic heart failure psychometric evaluation of the German version. Psychother Psychosom Med Psychol. 2005;55:200–8.
52. Miani D, Rozbowsky P, Gregori D, Pilotto L, Albanese MC, Fresco C, Fioretti PM. The Kansas City cardiomyopathy questionnaire: Italian translation and validation. Ital Heart J. 2003;4:620–6.
53. Comin-Colet J, Garin O, Lupon J, Manito N, Crespo-Leiro MG, Gomez-Bueno M, Ferrer M, Artigas R, Zapata A, Elosua R, Grp V-KS. Validation of the Spanish version of the Kansas city cardiomyopathy questionnaire. Revista Espanola De Cardiologia. 2011;64:51–8.
54. Davie AP, Francis CM, Love MP, Caruana L, Starkey IR, Shaw TR, Sutherland GR, McMurray JJ. Value of the electrocardiogram in identifying heart failure due to left ventricular systolic dysfunction. BMJ (Clinical Research Ed). 1996;312:222.
55. Devereux RB, Roman MJ, Palmieri V, Liu JE, Lee ET, Best LG, Fabsitz RR, Rodeheffer RJ, Howard BV. Prognostic implications of ejection fraction from linear echocardiographic dimensions: the Strong Heart Study. Am Heart J. 2003;146:527–34.
56. Nagueh SF, Bhatt R, Vivo RP, Krim SR, Sarvari SI, Russell K, Edvardsen T, Smiseth OA, Estep JD. Echocardiographic evaluation of hemodynamics in patients with decompensated systolic heart failure. Circ Cardiovasc Imaging. 2011;4:220–7.
57. Nagueh SF, Smiseth OA, Appleton CP, Byrd BF, III, Dokainish H, Edvardsen T, Flachskampf FA, Gillebert TC, Klein AL, Lancellotti P, Marino P, Oh JK, Popescu BA, Waggoner AD. Recommendations for the evaluation of left ventricular diastolic function by echocardiography: an update from the American Society of Echocardiography and the European Association of Cardiovascular Imaging. J Am Soc Echocardiogr. 2016;29:277–314.
58. Schinkel AFL, Bax JJ, Geleijnse ML, Boersma E, Elhendy A, Roelandt JRTC, Poldermans D. Noninvasive evaluation of ischaemic heart disease: myocardial perfusion imaging or stress echocardiography? Eur Heart J. 2003;24:789–800.
59. Pellikka PA, Nagueh SF, Elhendy AA, Kuehl CA and Sawada SG. American Society of Echocardiography recommendations for performance, interpretation, and application of stress echocardiography. J Am Soc Echocardiogr. 2007;20:1021–41.
60. Einstein AJ, Moser KW, Thompson RC, Cerqueira MD, Henzlova MJ. Radiation dose to patients from cardiac diagnostic imaging. Circulation. 2007;116:1290–305.
61. Parker MW, Iskandar A, Limone B, Perugini A, Kim H, Jones C, Calamari B, Coleman CI, Heller GV. Diagnostic accuracy of cardiac positron emission tomography versus single photon emission computed tomography for coronary artery disease: a bivariate meta-analysis. Circ Cardiovasc Imaging. 2012;5:700–7.
62. Bart BA, Shaw LK, McCants CB Jr, Fortin DF, Lee KL, Califf RM, O'Connor CM. Clinical determinants of mortality in patients with angiographically diagnosed ischemic or nonischemic cardiomyopathy. J Am Coll Cardiol. 1997;30:1002–8.
63. Meijboom WB, Meijs MF, Schuijf JD, Cramer MJ, Mollet NR, van Mieghem CA, Nieman K, van Werkhoven JM, Pundziute G, Weustink AC, de Vos AM, Pugliese F, Rensing B, Jukema JW, Bax JJ, Prokop M, Doevendans PA, Hunink MG, Krestin GP, de Feyter PJ. Diagnostic accuracy of 64-slice computed tomography coronary angiography: a prospective, multicenter, multivendor study. J Am Coll Cardiol. 2008;52:2135–44.
64. Miller JM, Rochitte CE, Dewey M, Arbab-Zadeh A, Niinuma H, Gottlieb I, Paul N, Clouse ME, Shapiro EP, Hoe J, Lardo AC, Bush DE, de Roos A, Cox C, Brinker J, Lima JA. Diagnostic performance of coronary angiography by 64-row CT. N Engl J Med. 2008;359:2324–36.
65. Budoff MJ, Dowe D, Jollis JG, Gitter M, Sutherland J, Halamert E, Scherer M, Bellinger R, Martin A, Benton R, Delago A, Min JK. Diagnostic performance of 64-multidetector row coronary computed tomographic angiography for evaluation of coronary artery stenosis in individuals without known coronary artery disease: results from the prospective multicenter ACCURACY (Assessment by Coronary Computed Tomographic Angiography of Individuals Undergoing Invasive Coronary Angiography) trial. J Am Coll Cardiol. 2008;52:1724–32.
66. Abdel-Aty H, Boye P, Zagrosek A, Wassmuth R, Kumar A, Messroghli D, Bock P, Dietz R, Friedrich MG, Schulz-Menger J. Diagnostic performance of cardiovascular magnetic resonance in patients with suspected acute myocarditis: comparison of different approaches. J Am Coll Cardiol. 2005;45:1815–22.
67. Smedema JP, Snoep G, van Kroonenburgh MP, van Geuns RJ, Dassen WR, Gorgels AP, Crijns HJ. Evaluation of the accuracy of gadolinium-enhanced cardiovascular magnetic resonance in the diagnosis of cardiac sarcoidosis. J Am Coll Cardiol. 2005;45:1683–90.
68. Vignaux O, Dhote R, Duboc D, Blanche P, Dusser D, Weber S, Legmann P. Clinical significance of myocardial magnetic resonance abnormalities in patients with sarcoidosis: a 1-year follow-up study. Chest. 2002;122:1895–901.
69. Sekiguchi M, Yazaki Y, Isobe M, Hiroe M. Cardiac sarcoidosis: diagnostic, prognostic, and therapeutic considerations. Cardiovasc Drugs Ther. 1996;10:495–510.
70. Greulich S, Deluigi CC, Gloekler S, Wahl A, Zurn C, Kramer U, Nothnagel D, Bultel H, Schumm J, Grun S, Ong P, Wagner A, Schneider S, Nassenstein K, Gawaz M, Sechtem U, Bruder O, Mahrholdt H. CMR imaging predicts death and other adverse events in suspected cardiac sarcoidosis. JACC Cardiovasc Imaging. 2013;6:501–11.
71. Januzzi JL, van Kimmenade R, Lainchbury J, Bayes-Genis A, Ordonez-Llanos J, Santalo-Bel M, Pinto YM, Richards M. NT-proBNP testing for diagnosis and short-term prognosis in acute destabilized heart failure: an international pooled analysis of 1256 patients: the International Collaborative of NT-proBNP Study. Eur Heart J. 2006;27:330–7.
72. Hartmann F, Packer M, Coats AJ, Fowler MB, Krum H, Mohacsi P, Rouleau JL, Tendera M, Castaigne A, Anker SD, Amann-Zalan I, Hoersch S, Katus HA. Prognostic impact of plasma N-terminal pro-brain natriuretic peptide in severe chronic congestive heart failure: a substudy of the Carvedilol Prospective Randomized Cumulative Survival (COPERNICUS) trial. Circulation. 2004;110:1780–6.
73. Fonarow GC, Peacock WF, Phillips CO, Givertz MM, Lopatin M. Admission B-type natriuretic peptide levels and in-hospital mortality in acute decompensated heart failure. J Am Coll Cardiol. 2007;49:1943–50.
74. Horwich TB, Patel J, MacLellan WR, Fonarow GC. Cardiac troponin I is associated with impaired hemodynamics, progressive left ventricular dysfunction, and increased mortality rates in advanced heart failure. Circulation. 2003;108:833–8.
75. Hershberger RE, Lindenfeld J, Mestroni L, Seidman CE, Taylor MRG, Towbin JA. Genetic evaluation of cardiomyopathy—a Heart Failure Society of America Practice Guideline. J Card Fail. 2009;15:83–97.
76. Richard P, Charron P, Carrier L, Ledeuil C, Cheav T, Pichereau C, Benaiche A, Isnard R, Dubourg O, Burban M, Gueffet JP, Millaire A, Desnos M, Schwartz K, Hainque B, Komajda M. Hypertrophic cardiomyopathy: distribution of disease genes, spectrum of mutations, and implications for a molecular diagnosis strategy. Circulation. 2003;107:2227–32.
77. Maron BJ, Maron MS, Semsarian C. Genetics of hypertrophic cardiomyopathy after 20 years: clinical perspectives. J Am Coll Cardiol. 2012;60:705–15.

78. Landstrom AP, Ho CY, Ackerman MJ. Mutation type is not clinically useful in predicting prognosis in hypertrophic cardiomyopathy response to Landstrom and Ackerman. Circulation. 2010;122:2441–50.
79. Arbustini E, Narula N, Tavazzi L, Serio A, Grasso M, Favalli V, Bellazzi R, Tajik JA, Bonow RO, Fuster V, Narula J. The MOGE(S) classification of cardiomyopathy for clinicians. J Am Coll Cardiol. 2014;64:304–18.
80. Arbustini E, Narula N, Dec GW, Reddy KS, Greenberg B, Kushwaha S, Marwick T, Pinney S, Bellazzi R, Favalli V, Kramer C, Roberts R, Zoghbi WA, Bonow R, Tavazzi L, Fuster V, Narula J. The MOGE(S) classification for a phenotype-genotype nomenclature of cardiomyopathy: endorsed by the world heart federation. J Am Coll Cardiol. 2013;62:2046–72.
81. Benedict CR, Johnstone DE, Weiner DH, Bourassa MG, Bittner V, Kay R, Kirlin P, Greenberg B, Kohn RM, Nicklas JM, et al. Relation of neurohumoral activation to clinical variables and degree of ventricular dysfunction: a report from the Registry of Studies of Left Ventricular Dysfunction. SOLVD Investigators. J Am Coll Cardiol. 1994;23:1410–20.
82. Gheorghiade M, Abraham WT, Albert NM, Gattis Stough W, Greenberg BH, O'Connor CM, She L, Yancy CW, Young J, Fonarow GC. Relationship between admission serum sodium concentration and clinical outcomes in patients hospitalized for heart failure: an analysis from the OPTIMIZE-HF registry. Eur Heart J. 2007;28:980–8.
83. Lee WH, Packer M. Prognostic importance of serum sodium concentration and its modification by converting-enzyme inhibition in patients with severe chronic heart failure. Circulation. 1986;73:257–67.
84. Adams KF Jr, Fonarow GC, Emerman CL, LeJemtel TH, Costanzo MR, Abraham WT, Berkowitz RL, Galvao M, Horton DP. Characteristics and outcomes of patients hospitalized for heart failure in the United States: rationale, design, and preliminary observations from the first 100,000 cases in the Acute Decompensated Heart Failure National Registry (ADHERE). Am Heart J. 2005;149:209–16.
85. Heywood JT, Fonarow GC, Costanzo MR, Mathur VS, Wigneswaran JR, Wynne J. High prevalence of renal dysfunction and its impact on outcome in 118,465 patients hospitalized with acute decompensated heart failure: a report from the ADHERE database. J Card Fail. 2007;13:422–30.
86. Ezekowitz J, McAlister FA, Humphries KH, Norris CM, Tonelli M, Ghali WA, Knudtson ML. The association among renal insufficiency, pharmacotherapy, and outcomes in 6,427 patients with heart failure and coronary artery disease. J Am Coll Cardiol. 2004;44:1587–92.
87. Smith GL, Lichtman JH, Bracken MB, Shlipak MG, Phillips CO, DiCapua P, Krumholz HM. Renal impairment and outcomes in heart failure: systematic review and meta-analysis. J Am Coll Cardiol. 2006;47:1987–96.
88. Al-Ahmad A, Rand WM, Manjunath G, Konstam MA, Salem DN, Levey AS, Sarnak MJ. Reduced kidney function and anemia as risk factors for mortality in patients with left ventricular dysfunction. J Am Coll Cardiol. 2001;38:955–62.
89. Nanas JN, Matsouka C, Karageorgopoulos D, Leonti A, Tsolakis E, Drakos SG, Tsagalou EP, Maroulidis GD, Alexopoulos GP, Kanakakis JE, Anastasiou-Nana MI. Etiology of anemia in patients with advanced heart failure. J Am Coll Cardiol. 2006;48:2485–9.
90. Androne AS, Katz SD, Lund L, LaManca J, Hudaihed A, Hryniewicz K, Mancini DM. Hemodilution is common in patients with advanced heart failure. Circulation. 2003;107:226–9.
91. Horwich TB, Fonarow GC, Hamilton MA, MacLellan WR, Borenstein J. Anemia is associated with worse symptoms, greater impairment in functional capacity and a significant increase in mortality in patients with advanced heart failure. J Am Coll Cardiol. 2002;39:1780–6.
92. Ezekowitz JA, McAlister FA, Armstrong PW. Anemia is common in heart failure and is associated with poor outcomes: insights from a cohort of 12 065 patients with new-onset heart failure. Circulation. 2003;107:223–5.
93. Bacon BR, Adams PC, Kowdley KV, Powell LW, Tavill AS. Diagnosis and management of hemochromatosis: 2011 practice guideline by the American Association for the Study of Liver Diseases. Hepatology (Baltimore, Md). 2011;54:328–43.
94. Klein I, Ojamaa K. Thyroid hormone and the cardiovascular system. N Engl J Med. 2001;344:501–9.
95. Sandler G, Wilson GM. The nature and prognosis of heart disease in thyrotoxicosis. A review of 150 patients treated with 131I. Q J Med. 1959;28:347–69.
96. Witte KK, Clark AL, Cleland JG. Chronic heart failure and micronutrients. J Am Coll Cardiol. 2001;37:1765–74.
97. Aquilani R, Opasich C, Verri M, Boschi F, Febo O, Pasini E, Pastoris O. Is nutritional intake adequate in chronic heart failure patients? J Am Coll Cardiol. 2003;42:1218–23.
98. Horwich TB, Kalantar-Zadeh K, MacLellan RW, Fonarow GC. Albumin levels predict survival in patients with systolic heart failure. Am Heart J. 2008;155:883–9.
99. Barbaro G, Di Lorenzo G, Grisorio B, Barbarini G. Incidence of dilated cardiomyopathy and detection of HIV in myocardial cells of HIV-positive patients. N Engl J Med. 1998;339:1093–9.
100. Cerrato E, D'Ascenzo F, Biondi-Zoccai G, Calcagno A, Frea S, Grosso Marra W, Castagno D, Omede P, Quadri G, Sciuto F, Presutti D, Frati G, Bonora S, Moretti C, Gaita F. Cardiac dysfunction in pauci symptomatic human immunodeficiency virus patients: a meta-analysis in the highly active antiretroviral therapy era. Eur Heart J. 2013;34:1432–6.
101. Quarta CC, Kruger JL, Falk RH. Cardiac amyloidosis. Circulation. 2012;126:e178–82.
102. The Criteria Committee of the New York Heart Association. Nomenclature and criteria for diagnosis of diseases of the heart and great vessels. 9th ed. Boston: Little, Brown & Co; 1994.
103. Packer M, O'Connor CM, Ghali JK, Pressler ML, Carson PE, Belkin RN, Miller AB, Neuberg GW, Frid D, Wertheimer JH, Cropp AB, DeMets DL. Effect of amlodipine on morbidity and mortality in severe chronic heart failure. N Engl J Med. 1996;335:1107–14.
104. Thibodeau JT, Mishkin JD, Patel PC, Mammen PPA, Markham DW, Drazner MH. IIIB or not IIIB: a previously unanswered question. J Card Fail. 2012;18:367–72.
105. Raphael C, Briscoe C, Davies J, Whinnett ZI, Manisty C, Sutton R, Mayet J, Francis DP. Limitations of the New York Heart Association functional classification system and self-reported walking distances in chronic heart failure. Heart. 2007;93:476–82.
106. Goda A, Williams P, Mancini D, Lund LH. Selecting patients for heart transplantation: comparison of the Heart Failure Survival Score (HFSS) and the Seattle heart failure model (SHFM). J Heart Lung Transplant. 2011;30:1236–43.
107. Harrington D, Anker SD, Chua TP, Webb-Peploe KM, Ponikowski PP, Poole-Wilson PA, Coats AJ. Skeletal muscle function and its relation to exercise tolerance in chronic heart failure. J Am Coll Cardiol. 1997;30:1758–64.
108. Mancini DM, Eisen H, Kussmaul W, Mull R, Edmunds LH Jr, Wilson JR. Value of peak exercise oxygen consumption for optimal timing of cardiac transplantation in ambulatory patients with heart failure. Circulation. 1991;83:778–86.
109. O'Neill JO, Young JB, Pothier CE, Lauer MS. Peak oxygen consumption as a predictor of death in patients with heart failure receiving beta-blockers. Circulation. 2005;111:2313–8.
110. Butler J, Khadim G, Paul KM, Davis SF, Kronenberg MW, Chomsky DB, Pierson RN 3rd, Wilson JR. Selection of patients

for heart transplantation in the current era of heart failure therapy. J Am Coll Cardiol. 2004;43:787–93.
111. Goda A, Lund LH, Mancini D. The Heart Failure Survival Score outperforms the peak oxygen consumption for heart transplantation selection in the era of device therapy. J Heart Lung Transplant. 2011;30:315–25.
112. Mehra MR, Canter CE, Hannan MM, Semigran MJ, Uber PA, Baran DA, Danziger-Isakov L, Kirklin JK, Kirk R, Kushwaha SS, Lund LH, Potena L, Ross HJ, Taylor DO, Verschuuren EA, Zuckermann A. The 2016 International Society for Heart Lung Transplantation listing criteria for heart transplantation: a 10-year update. J Heart Lung Transplant. 2016;35:1–23.
113. MacGowan GA, Janosko K, Cecchetti A, Murali S. Exercise-related ventilatory abnormalities and survival in congestive heart failure. Am J Cardiol. 1997;79:1264–6.
114. Robbins M, Francis G, Pashkow FJ, Snader CE, Hoercher K, Young JB, Lauer MS. Ventilatory and heart rate responses to exercise: better predictors of heart failure mortality than peak oxygen consumption. Circulation. 1999;100:2411–7.
115. Chua TP, Ponikowski P, Harrington D, Anker SD, Webb-Peploe K, Clark AL, Poole-Wilson PA, Coats AJ. Clinical correlates and prognostic significance of the ventilatory response to exercise in chronic heart failure. J Am Coll Cardiol. 1997;29:1585–90.
116. Sun XG, Hansen JE, Stringer WW. Oxygen uptake efficiency plateau best predicts early death in heart failure. Chest. 2012;141:1284–94.
117. Davies LC, Wensel R, Georgiadou P, Cicoira M, Coats AJ, Piepoli MF, Francis DP. Enhanced prognostic value from cardiopulmonary exercise testing in chronic heart failure by non-linear analysis: oxygen uptake efficiency slope. Eur Heart J. 2006;27:684–90.
118. ATS statement: guidelines for the six-minute walk test. Am J Respir Crit Care Med. 2002;166:111–7.
119. Casanova C, Celli BR, Barria P, Casas A, Cote C, de Torres JP, Jardim J, Lopez MV, Marin JM, Montes de Oca M, Pinto-Plata V, Aguirre-Jaime A. The 6-min walk distance in healthy subjects: reference standards from seven countries. Eur Respir J. 2011;37:150–6.
120. Cahalin LP, Mathier MA, Semigran MJ, Dec GW, DiSalvo TG. The six-minute walk test predicts peak oxygen uptake and survival in patients with advanced heart failure. Chest. 1996;110:325–32.
121. Passantino A, Lagioia R, Mastropasqua F, Scrutinio D. Short-term change in distance walked in 6 min is an indicator of outcome in patients with chronic heart failure in clinical practice. J Am Coll Cardiol. 2006;48:99–105.
122. Roul G, Germain P, Bareiss P. Does the 6-minute walk test predict the prognosis in patients with NYHA class II or III chronic heart failure? Am Heart J. 1998;136:449–57.
123. Shah MR, Hasselblad V, Gheorghiade M, Adams KF Jr, Swedberg K, Califf RM, O'Connor CM. Prognostic usefulness of the six-minute walk in patients with advanced congestive heart failure secondary to ischemic or nonischemic cardiomyopathy. Am J Cardiol. 2001;88:987–93.
124. Opasich C, Pinna GD, Mazza A, Febo O, Riccardi R, Riccardi PG, Capomolla S, Forni G, Cobelli F, Tavazzi L. Six-minute walking performance in patients with moderate-to-severe heart failure – is it a useful indicator in clinical practice? Eur Heart J. 2001;22:488–96.
125. Zugck C, Kruger C, Durr S, Gerber SH, Haunstetter A, Hornig K, Kubler W, Haass M. Is the 6-minute walk test a reliable substitute for peak oxygen uptake in patients with dilated cardiomyopathy? Eur Heart J. 2000;21:540–9.
126. Fried LP, Tangen CM, Walston J, Newman AB, Hirsch C, Gottdiener J, Seeman T, Tracy R, Kop WJ, Burke G, McBurnie MA. Frailty in older adults: evidence for a phenotype. J Gerontol Ser A Biol Med Sci. 2001;56:M146–57.
127. Jha SR, Hannu MK, Chang S, Montgomery E, Harkess M, Wilhelm K, Hayward CS, Jabbour A, Spratt PM, Newton P, Davidson PM, Macdonald PS. The prevalence and prognostic significance of frailty in patients with advanced heart failure referred for heart transplantation. Transplantation. 2016;100:429–36.
128. Madan SA, Fida N, Barman P, Sims D, Shin J, Verghese J, Pina I, Jorde U, Patel SR. Frailty assessment in advanced heart failure. J Card Fail. 2016;22:840–4.
129. McNallan SM, Singh M, Chamberlain AM, Kane RL, Dunlay SM, Redfield MM, Weston SA, Roger VL. Frailty and healthcare utilization among patients with heart failure in the community. JACC Heart Fail. 2013;1:135–41.
130. Lupón J, González B, Santaeugenia S, Altimir S, Urrutia A, Más D, Díez C, Pascual T, Cano L, Valle V. Prognostic implication of frailty and depressive symptoms in an outpatient population with heart failure. Revista Española de Cardiología (English Edition). 2008;61:835–42.
131. Dunlay SM, Park SJ, Joyce LD, Daly RC, Stulak JM, McNallan SM, Roger VL, Kushwaha SS. Frailty and outcomes after implantation of left ventricular assist device as destination therapy. J Heart Lung Transplant. 2014;33:359–65.
132. Felker GM, Thompson RE, Hare JM, Hruban RH, Clemetson DE, Howard DL, Baughman KL, Kasper EK. Underlying causes and long-term survival in patients with initially unexplained cardiomyopathy. N Engl J Med. 2000;342:1077–84.
133. Kindermann I, Kindermann M, Kandolf R, Klingel K, Bultmann B, Muller T, Lindinger A, Bohm M. Predictors of outcome in patients with suspected myocarditis. Circulation. 2008;118:639–48.
134. Kuhl U, Pauschinger M, Noutsias M, Seeberg B, Bock T, Lassner D, Poller W, Kandolf R, Schultheiss HP. High prevalence of viral genomes and multiple viral infections in the myocardium of adults with "idiopathic" left ventricular dysfunction. Circulation. 2005;111:887–93.
135. Pauschinger M, Bowles NE, Fuentes-Garcia FJ, Pham V, Kühl U, Schwimmbeck PL, Schultheiss H-P, Towbin JA. Detection of adenoviral genome in the myocardium of adult patients with idiopathic left ventricular dysfunction. Circulation. 1999;99:1348–54.
136. Why HJ, Meany BT, Richardson PJ, Olsen EG, Bowles NE, Cunningham L, Freeke CA, Archard LC. Clinical and prognostic significance of detection of enteroviral RNA in the myocardium of patients with myocarditis or dilated cardiomyopathy. Circulation. 1994;89:2582–9.
137. Cooper LT, Baughman KL, Feldman AM, Frustaci A, Jessup M, Kuhl U, Levine GN, Narula J, Starling RC, Towbin J, Virmani R. the role of endomyocardial biopsy in the management of cardiovascular diseasea scientific statement From the American Heart Association, the American College of Cardiology, and the European Society of Cardiology Endorsed by the Heart Failure Society of America and the Heart Failure Association of the European Society of Cardiology. J Am Coll Cardiol. 2007;50:1914–31.
138. Deckers JW, Hare JM, Baughman KL. Complications of transvenous right ventricular endomyocardial biopsy in adult patients with cardiomyopathy: a seven-year survey of 546 consecutive diagnostic procedures in a tertiary referral center. J Am Coll Cardiol. 1992;19:43–7.
139. The EI and Coordinators ES. Evaluation study of congestive heart failure and pulmonary artery catheterization effectiveness: the escape trial. JAMA. 2005;294:1625–33.
140. Bourge RC, Abraham WT, Adamson PB, Aaron MF, Aranda JJM, Magalski A, Zile MR, Smith AL, Smart FW, O'Shaughnessy MA, Jessup ML, Sparks B, Naftel DL, Stevenson LW. Randomized controlled trial of an implantable continuous hemodynamic monitor in patients with advanced heart failure. The COMPASS-HF study. J Am Coll Cardiol. 2008;51:1073–9.

141. Sandhu AT, Goldhaber-Fiebert JD, Owens DK, Turakhia MP, Kaiser DW, Heidenreich PA. Cost-effectiveness of implantable pulmonary artery pressure monitoring in chronic heart failure. JACC Heart Fail. 2016;4:368–75.
142. Packer M, Abraham WT, Mehra MR, Yancy CW, Lawless CE, Mitchell JE, Smart FW, Bijou R, O'Connor CM, Massie BM, Pina IL, Greenberg BH, Young JB, Fishbein DP, Hauptman PJ, Bourge RC, Strobeck JE, Murali S, Schocken D, Teerlink JR, Levy WC, Trupp RJ, Silver MA. Utility of impedance cardiography for the identification of short-term risk of clinical decompensation in stable patients with chronic heart failure. J Am Coll Cardiol. 2006;47:2245–52.
143. Whellan DJ, Ousdigian KT, Al-Khatib SM, Pu W, Sarkar S, Porter CB, Pavri BB, O'Connor CM. Combined heart failure device diagnostics identify patients at higher risk of subsequent heart failure hospitalizations: results from PARTNERS HF (Program to access and review trending information and evaluate correlation to symptoms in patients with heart failure) study. J Am Coll Cardiol. 2010;55:1803–10.
144. Boriani G, Da Costa A, Ricci RP, Quesada A, Favale S, Iacopino S, Romeo F, Risi A, di SSL M, Navarro X, Biffi M, Santini M, Burri H. The MOnitoring Resynchronization dEvices and CARdiac patiEnts (MORE-CARE) randomized controlled trial: phase 1 results on dynamics of early intervention with remote monitoring. J Med Internet Res. 2013;15:e167.
145. van Veldhuisen DJ, Braunschweig F, Conraads V, Ford I, Cowie MR, Jondeau G, Kautzner J, Aguilera RM, Lunati M, Yu CM, Gerritse B, Borggrefe M. Intrathoracic impedance monitoring, audible patient alerts, and outcome in patients with heart failure. Circulation. 2011;124:1719–26.

Part V

Therapeutics

Pharmacotherapy in Heart Failure (I): Renin-Angiotensin-Aldosterone System (incl. ARNI), Diuretics, Digoxin and Statins

7

Hans-Peter Brunner-La Rocca

Different medication has proven efficacy to reduce both morbidity and mortality in patients with heart failure. However, this is only true in patients with reduced left-ventricular ejection fraction (LVEF). Most studies used an LVEF of 35% and some 40% as cut-off. In patients with normal ejection fraction (i.e. 50% or more), however, no effective medical treatment is known. In the group in between, evidence is also limited. This resulted in the definition of three groups of heart failure based on LVEF in the new European guidelines on heart failure [1]: HFrEF = heart failure with reduced ejection fraction (i.e. LVEF<40%), HFpEF = heart failure with preserved ejection fraction (i.e. LVEF≥50%), and HFmrEF = heart failure with mid-range ejection fraction (i.e. LVEF 40–49%). The main reason for newly defining this additional group is to stimulate research in this so far under-represented group. However in clinical practice, LVEF is usually determined by the use of echocardiography and inaccuracy of measurements is larger than the range of HFmrEF [2]. Moreover, some of the larger treatment trials included patients with relatively preserved LVEF with little evidence that treatment is not effective in this group [3]. This is also in line with the recent post-hoc analysis of TOP CAT where the effect of spironolactone in HFpEF patients was studied [4]. Patients with LVEF with 45% and higher were included. The post-hoc analysis showed a potential benefit in those with mildly reduced LVEF, but not in those with fully preserved LVEF. In addition, a recent meta-analysis of large trial investigating blockers of the renin-angiotensin-aldosterone system found significant interactions of effect and LVEF, with only patients with fully preserved LVEF not showing any benefit [5]. Therefore until additional research is being done, it seems advisable in clinical practice to separate patients in those with normal LVEF (i.e. LVEF≥50%) and reduced LVEF. It may be expected that evidence will remain poor in HFmrEF patients in the up-coming years and as a consequence, this pragmatic approach will remain valid for quite some time.

Several classes of drugs have been studied extensively in patients with HFrEF and / or are being used in patients with heart failure in general. This chapter discusses the use of several of these classes of drugs; the use of beta-blockers, ivabradine and hydralazine/nitrates is discussed in a separate chapter of this book.

7.1 Treatment of HFpEF

It is important to note that the positive effects discussed apply to patients with reduced LVEF only. Both ACE-inhibitors and ARBs have failed to show any benefit in patients with preserved LVEF (HFpEF) [6–8]. The same is also true for MRA's as spironolactone treatment in HF patients with LVEF of 45% (TOPCAT study) failed to show a significant improvement [9]. Although it has been claimed that different selection of patients in Russia and Georgia, where no effect of spironolactone was seen, may explain this failure [10], an at least as likely reason is that spironolactone may not improve outcome if LVEF fully preserved, i.e. really normal [4]. Also, the use of β-blockers have not been studied in sufficiently large prospective randomised controlled trials. There is some indirect evidence that treatment effects of standard heart failure medication in HFpEF is significantly different as compared to HFrEF. Thus, intensifying heart failure medication in HFpEF did not improve outcome whereas it did in HFrEF [11]. Co-morbidities play an important role in patients with HFpEF, as a cause of HFpEF but also as a cause of symptoms not necessarily directly related cardiac dysfunction [12]. Inflammation has been suggested as important common underlying mechanism in HFpEF, as most of the co-morbidities often seen in HFpEF may cause inflammation, supported by experimental evidence [13]. There are also some early studies suggesting that treating heart failure might prevent HFpEF, but evidence that inflammation is the key factor in HFpEF is far from being

H.-P. Brunner-La Rocca (✉)
Department of Cardiology, Maastricht University Medical Center, Maastricht, The Netherlands
e-mail: hp.brunnerlarocca@mumc.nl

D. S. Feldman, P. Mohacsi (eds.), *Heart Failure*, Cardiovascular Medicine, https://doi.org/10.1007/978-3-319-98184-0_7

sufficiently solid [14]. Also, data from a phase II study using sacubitril/valsartan (see below) are promising [15], but the real proof of a sufficiently large outcome trial is still missing. Therefore, it still remains unclear how patients with HFpEF should be treated apart from treating underlying disease and co-morbidities as well as decongestion by diuretics.

7.2 Inhibition of the Renin-Angiotensin-Aldosterone System (RAAS)

Several classes of drugs inhibit parts of the RAAS. Figure 7.1 provides an overview of the RAAS, the interaction and links with other (neurohumoral) systems as well as the mode of action of the different classes of drugs. Although widely studied, not all aspects of the RAAS are fully elucidated. Thus, angiotensin-II 1–7 and other fragments of angiotensin are less well studied, but may play an important role. In addition, whereas the effects of the stimulation and blockade of the type-1 angiotensin-II receptor is well studied, the effects of stimulation of the type-2 receptor is less well known. Thus, the inhibition of the effects of angiotensin-II either by receptor blockade of the type 1 receptor or inhibition of the formation of angiotensin-II by angiotensin-converting-enzyme (ACE)-inhibition may only be part of the effects of these drugs. Still, it is generally believed that the main effects of these two classes of drugs are mediated via this pathway. Moreover, inhibition of the effects of aldosterone is important.

The important medication inhibiting the effects of the RAAS are the following groups: inhibition of the angiotensin-converting enzyme (ACE-inhibitor), type-1 angiotensin-II receptor blockade (ARB), antagonism of the mineralocorticoid receptor (MRA), renin-inhibition (aliskiren) and the new combination of ARB and neprilysin-inhibition (ARNI). Newer compounds may affect other parts of the RAAS, but they are not being used in clinical practice yet. A brief outlook will be given at the end of this chapter.

7.3 Combining Drugs Affecting the RAAS

Though working on the same system, i.e. RAAS, some combinations are clinically important. This refers to combining MRA with any other class mentioned. The rational for this was the fact that aldosterone escape was found to occur after some months of starting ACE-inhibition [16]. Therefore, the addition of MRA to ACE-inhibition was studied. The first large trial to study this was the RALES trials, showing significant improvement of outcome by adding spironolactone to ACE-inhibition in patients with advanced heart failure (NYHA III and IV) and reduced LVEF [17]. Later, the MRA eplerenone was studied after myocardial infarction complicated by heart failure (EPHESUS) or in less advanced heart failure (NYHA II) with reduced LVEF (EMPHASIS-HF), both studies showing significant improvement in outcome [18, 19]. Based on these results, the combination of MRA with one of the other drugs of the RAAS is considered as standard in all symptomatic patients with LVEF of 35% or less [1, 20].

It is important to note that other combinations are less meaningful or even contraindicated. Thus, the combined use of ACE-inhibition and ARB may only be used if patients are intolerant to MRA's and the introduction of ARNI will further reduce the clinical use of this combination. It is even contraindicated if MRAs are used [1, 20]. ARNI must not be combined with ACE-inhibitors as this combination has not been studied and is expected to result in significant increased frequency of life-threatening angioedema, as found for the combination of ACE-inhibition and neprilysin-inhibition [21]. This is related to the fact that both neprilysin- and ACE-inhibition inhibit the breakdown of bradykinin. Although

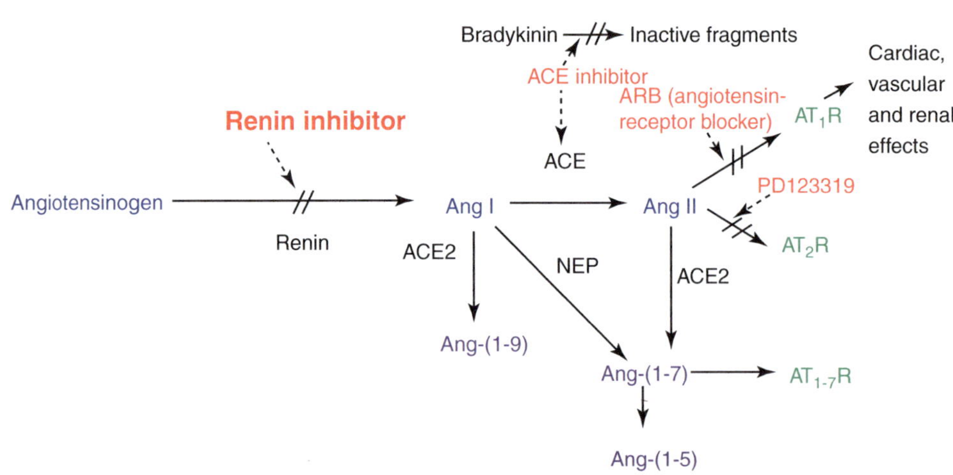

Fig. 7.1 Overview of the renin-angiotensin-system

bradykinin may contribute to the cardioprotective effects of ACE-inhibition [22], substantial rise in bradykinin-levels are responsible for angioedema in susceptible patients [23].

Renin-inhibition (currently the only available oral renin-inhibitor is aliskiren) in combination with ACE-inhibition and ARB does not add any benefit and may result in more significant side effects [24, 25]. Combining renin-inhibition with ARNI has not been studied, but given the possibly harmful effects when combining with ARB, it is highly unlikely that this combination is of any benefit.

7.4 ACE-inhibition

The classical RAAS inhibitors recommended in the treatment of chronic HF are the ACE-inhibitors, which inhibit the conversion of angiotensin-I in angiotensin-II. This effect leads to a reduction of AII-mediated response, such as vasoconstriction, the release of aldosterone and the sympathetic nervous system (SNS) activation [26]. The vasodilator effect of ACE-inhibition is not associated with reflex tachycardia [27], as the SNS is inhibited and possibly the parasympathetic system activated. In addition, the use of ACE-inhibitors has also been shown to increase the levels of a tetrapeptide (N-acetyl-seryl-aspartyl-lysyl proline), probably responsible for the antifibrotic effects [28]. Due to reflex increase, ACE-inhibition increase the Angiotensin-I levels and its conversion to angiotensin 1–7 that entails a further improvement of cardiovascular effects [29].

ACE-inhibitors have been introduced in the 1980's. In 1987, the CONSENSUS study was published showing that ACE-inhibition reduces mortality in patients with advance heart failure [30]. Interestingly, LVEF was not measured in this study and was obviously also no inclusion criterion, in contrast to all consecutive trials. Given the fact that HFpEF was less common in the 80's than it is nowadays, the majority of patients in CONSENSUS probably had HFrEF. In the early 1990's, several large randomised controlled trials investigated the effects of ACE-inhibitors on prognosis in patients with HFrEF, either in chronic stage or after acute myocardial infarction [31–36]. As cut-off value, LVEF of 35% and in some of 40% was used, apart from the AIRE trial that included post-infarct patients based on clinical signs of heart failure only [34]. The studies consistently showed an improvement in morbidity and mortality of approximately 20% [37]. It became clear that the underlying cause of heart failure is not important to see the beneficial effects of ACE-inhibition. Importantly, this is also true early after myocardial infarction. This may just not be the case for the very first day after infarction as found in the CONSENSUS II trial [38].

Specific target doses were used in all of these trials. In general, these target doses were relatively high, which may not always be achieved in clinical practice. As often this is related to some preferences by patients or treating physicians or fear of side effects rather than real intolerability, the question arises as to whether dose of ACE-inhibition is of importance. There were some small studies in the 90's suggesting some benefit [39], but there is only one larger trial that investigated this question [40]. Thus, the ATLAS trial compared the effects of low (i.e. 2.5 to 5 mg) versus high (i.e. 32.5 to 35 mg) of lisinopril (mean difference between the two groups 19 mg) in patients with LVEF of 30% or lower on morbidity and mortality. Whereas mortality was not significantly reduced (8% lower risk of death, $p = 0.13$), the primary combined endpoint of death or all-cause hospitalisation (12% reduction, $p = 0.002$) and heart failure hospitalisations (24% reduction, $p = 0.002$) were significantly reduced. Therefore, there seem to be a dose effect of ACE-inhibition in heart failure, but this effect may be slightly less than the use of any ACE-inhibitor as compared not using ACE-inhibition at all. In addition, high doses seem to be related to more side effects [40], which may be related to plasma levels of ACE-inhibitors [41]. Therefore, if side effect limit the use of medication in HFrEF, it seems to be preferable to use all recommended drugs in low doses instead of just one or two at higher doses. Nevertheless, any attempt should be made to uptitrate medication to achieve recommended disease as far as possible [1].

7.4.1 Are All ACE-inhibitors Similar?

ACE-inhibitors have different pharmacokinetics, which obviously need to be considered when prescribing them (see Table 7.1). In clinical practice, the most important problem is the fact that most of the ACE-inhibitors do not have a sufficiently long half-life to allow once daily dose regimens without significant variation in plasma levels [42]. Still, they are often used once daily which may, at least in theory, affect efficacy and tolerability of them. If this really results in clinically meaningful effects is not entirely clear as there are no sufficiently large studies addressing this point sufficiently. A small study (total of 115 patients) using the ARB valsartan concluded that once daily dosing of valsartan has similar effects and tolerability as twice daily dosing [43]. However, personal experience suggests that dividing ACE-inhibition during the day without changing the total daily dose may help to reduce symptoms of hypotension in some patients (unpublished data).

Possibly, such differences might explain some differences in the effects on outcome of different ACE-inhibitors. Moreover, penetration of ACE-inhibitors to tissue has been claimed to explain different effects of them. However, it has not been investigated as to whether different ACE-inhibitors result in differences in clinically meaningful outcome. Thus, head-to-head comparisons of difference ACE-inhibitors in

Table 7.1 Different drugs, start and target dose, and basic pharmacokinetics of RAAS used in patients with HFrEF

Drug	Prodrug	Start dose	Target dose	T ½ (h)[a]	Main elimination
ACE-inhibitors					
Captopril	No	6.25 mg t.i.d.	50 mg t.i.d	2	Renal
Enalapril	Yes	2.5 mg b.i.d.	10–20 mg b.i.d.	11	Renal
Lisinopril	No	2.5–5 mg o.d.	30–35 mg o.d.	12	Renal
Ramipril	Yes	1.25–2.5 mg o.d.	5 mg b.i.d.	13–17	Renal
Trandolapril	Yes	0.5 mg o.d.	4 mg o.d.	16–24	Feces/renal
Perindopril	Yes	1–2 mg o.d.	8–10 mg o.d.	17–25	Renal
Fosinopril	Yes	5 mg o.d.	20 mg b.i.d.	12	Hepatic/renal
Quinapril	Yes	2.5 mg o.d.	40 mg o.d.	25	Renal
Angiotensin-II type 1 receptor antagonist (ARB)					
Candesartan	No	4 mg o.d.	16 mg b.i.d.	9	Hepatic/renal
Valsartan	No	40 mg b.i.d.	160 mg b.i.d.	6	Faeces
Losartan	No	12.5 mg b.i.d.	50 mg t.i.d.	2 (active metab. 6–9)	Faeces (renal)
Renin-inhibitor					
Aliskiren	No	75 mg o.d.	300 mg o.d.	40 (+)	Faeces
Mineralocorticoid receptor antagonists (MRA)					
Spironolactone	No	12.5–25 mg o.d.	50 mg o.d.	10–35 (active metabolite)	Hepatic
Eplerenone	No	25 mg o.d.	50 mg o.d.	3–5	Hepatic
Angiotensin-II type 1 receptor antagonist / neprilysin-inhibitor					
Sacubitril/valsartan	No	24/26 mg b.i.d.	97/103 mg b.i.d.	12/10	Hepatic/renal hepatic

[a]Active substance or active metabolite determining duration of action

sufficiently large trials are lacking and a large meta-analysis of ACE-inhibitor trials came to the conclusion that it is likely that ACE-inhibitors depict a class effect [37], which is supported by some cohort studies [44]. There are, however, cohort studies, suggesting that some ACE-inhibitors are more effective than others [45, 46]. If such potential differences are clinically meaningful is not clear. The guidelines recommend several ACE-inhibitors that have been sufficiently investigated in clinical trials at reasonable dose without any preference for a specific drug (Table 7.1) [1, 20].

7.5 Angiotensin Type 1 Receptor Blockers (ARB)

Theoretically, there may be a large difference in the effects of ARBs and ACE-inhibitors. Thus, ARBs only block the angiotensin-II effects via the type 1 receptor, leaving the type 2 receptor unopposed. Moreover, ARBs cause significant increase in angiotensin-II levels, which may result in increased levels of other angiotensins such as angiotensin-III and angiotensin 1–7 [47], although the latter may also be elevated when using ACE-inhibition due to decreased metabolism [48]. As shown in Fig. 7.1, the renin-angiotensin-system is much more complex than simply the effects of angiotensin-II acting on the type 1 receptor. There is significant literature on this topic since more than 20 years [47, 49], but the clinical consequences of all the different parts of the renin-angiotensin-system is still poorly understood. Surprisingly enough, there is little evidence that the effects comparing ACE-inhibition and ARBs differ regarding clinical efficacy, whereas side effects are less prevalent with ARB than with ACE-inhibitors. The latter is related to the additional effects of ACE-inhibition on kinin metabolism resulting in increased cough and angioedema. Despite that, effects on morbidity and mortality seem to be more or less identical, in heart failure, but also in other cardiovascular diseases. There has been a debate as to whether patients treated with ARB are more prone to develop atherosclerosis and myocardial infarction as compare to those treated with ACE-inhibitors. However, this debate is still far from being resolved and ARBs are considered as good alternative in patients not tolerating ACE-inhibitors [1].

Given the different mode of action, ARBs were first considered as add-on to standard therapy including ACE-inhibition in heart failure (and other diseases, the latter not being covered in this chapter). Thus, the majority of patients included in the large Val-HeFT trial were on ACE-inhibition, but the added effects on top of ACE-inhibition seemed rather limited [50], in contrast to those that were ACE-inhibitor intolerant [51]. This difference was also found in the CHARM program [52, 53] although the interpretation by the investigators was rather different [54]. In addition, the VALIANT study in patients after myocardial infarction and symptoms of heart failure and/or LVEF of <40% showed equal effects when comparing the ACE-inhibitor captopril with valsartan, whereas the combined treatment did not result in an additional benefit and increased the risk of adverse events [55]. The findings resulted in a general recommendation to use ARBs in patients that are intolerant to ACE-inhibition [1, 20]. However, the combined use is of limited value and in combination with MRA potentially even harmful. Given the positive effects of MRA in these patients (see below), adding MRA to ACE-inhibition (or ARB if ACE-inhibition intolerant) is therefore the primary recommendation.

The potential effect of low versus high dose of ARB has been studied in the HEAAL trial [56], showing very similar results as found in the ATLAS trial for ACE-inhibition [40]. Thus, high dose of the ARB losartan (i.e. 150 mg) as compared to low-dose losartan (i.e. 50 mg) resulted in a 10% reduction of the combined endpoint death or hospital admission due to heart failure, at the cost of an increase in side effects such as hypotension and renal failure [56]. This benefit was mainly driven by reduction in heart failure related hospitalisations. This beneficial effect of high dose losartan might explain the trend in more events of losartan 50 mg daily as compared to captopril 50 mg three times daily in the ELITE-II trial [57], suggesting equal effects of ARB and ACE-inhibition in HFrEF if adequately doses are used. This is in line with the results of the CHARM program and the Val-HeFT trial as discussed above [51, 52].

Despite little evidence of differences between drugs apart from pharmacokinetics, it is generally recommended to only use those ARBs studied in the large heart failure trials (Table 7.1).

7.6 Renin Inhibition

Stopping the detrimental effects of the renin-angiotensin system at the most upstream and rate-limiting step of the cascade may offer theoretical advantages for cardiovascular protection [58]. Renin has a high specificity to its substrate, angiotensinogen, whereas ACE is not the only pathway for conversion of angiotensin-I to angiotensin-II. Renin inhibition does not affect kinin metabolism, which is responsible for some side effects of ACE-inhibition. However for a long time, there was no oral compound available to directly inhibit renin with sufficient potency, bioavailability and duration of action. Aliskiren is the first and so far only clinically available oral renin-inhibitor that fulfils these three prerequisite for use in clinical practice. It is registered for the treatment of hypertension. There have been some studies investigating the effects of aliskiren in patients with heart failure [24, 25, 59]. None of these studies convincingly showed a clinical benefit of aliskiren in heart failure. Therefore, the question arises as to whether aliskiren should have any role in treating heart failure. The most recent guidelines of the ESC state that "aliskiren (direct renin inhibitor) failed to improve outcomes for patients hospitalized for HF at 6 months or 12 months in one study and is not presently recommended as an alternative to an ACE-inhibitor or ARB" [1]. This statement is based on the ASTRONAUT study that investigated effects up to 1 year of aliskiren on top of standard therapy [24]. Thus, the study did not investigate aliskiren as alternative to ACE-inhibitor or ARB.

In April 2016, the ATMOSPHERE trial was published that investigated the effects of aliskiren, both as add-on to ACE-inhibition and as alternative in 7784 symptomatic patients with heart failure and reduced LVEF (≤35%) [25]. The trial did not find superiority of the combination but more side effects as compared to the ACE-inhibitor enalapril alone (primary endpoint: hazard ratio [HR] 0.93 [95%-CI 0.85–1.03], $p = 0.17$). In addition, the formal non-inferiority criteria was not met for aliskiren alone versus enalapril despite similar numbers of endpoints in the two groups (primary endpoint: HR = 0.99 [95%-CI 0.90–1.10], $p = 0.91$ for superiority). Thus, although the non-inferiority margin of 1.104 was met with the use of the 95% confidence interval, the one-sided p-value of 0.0184 did not fulfil the prespecified requirement of a p-value of ≤0.0123 [25]. An important reason for this is the fact that patients with diabetes had to be withdrawn from the study during the trial because ALTITUDE [60] and ASTRONAUT [24] raised some safety concerns in these patients, despite the advice by the steering committee to continue with the original protocol [61, 62]. The concerns were not confirmed in ATMOSPHERE and no relevant subgroup interactions were noted. Importantly, this action by the authorities supported by the sponsor of the trial caused an important discussion about the importance of trust in data safety monitoring boards of large trials and the independence of such trials to guarantee integrity of trials [63–65].

7.6.1 How to Use Aliskiren in Heart Failure?

Aliskiren is advisable to be used if patients are intolerant to both ACE-inhibitors and ARBs. This might also refer to patients experiencing angioedema, as angioedema occurs less, but still sometimes when using ARBs. As it is a life-threating side effect, ARBs should not be used in patient with history of angioedema. For aliskiren, theoretically angioedema may not occur as it does not interfere with bradykinin [66], but it has been reported as well in patients taking aliskiren [67, 68]. Therefore, extreme caution should be applied in such patients.

Although the non-inferiority criteria of aliskiren compared to enalapril was not met in ATMOSPHERE, the results suggest equal effects, but less side-effects of aliskiren as compared to the ACE-inhibitor enalapril [25]. Importantly, formal non-inferiority was not tested for ARBs as compared to ACE-inhibition. Despite this, ARBs are recommended as alternative to ACE-inhibition [1, 20], based on the results of CHARM-Alternative [52] and the post-hoc analysis of the Val-HeFT trial in those not on ACE-inhibition [51]. Although such study comparing placebo with a direct renin-inhibitor in patients not receiving any ACE-inhibition or ARB is not available and will most likely never be, it is almost certain that aliskiren improves outcome in patients with HFrEF as compared to placebo, i.e. in patients not receiving ACE-inhibition or ARB. In the ATMOSPHERE trial, there was no clinically relevant suggestion based on sub-group analyses that the effects may be dependent on baseline characteristics including age, gender and the presence of diabetes mellitus. Still, the average age (63 years) was app. 10 years less than in cohort studies and the proportion of women included was low (i.e. 22%) [25]. Still, this is true for most studies investigating drug effects in HFrEF patients.

7.6.2 ACE-inhibition, ARB or Aliskiren?

Given the available evidence, ACE-inhibition should be first choice in patients with HFrEF (LVEF≤40%) as recommended by the guidelines [1, 20]. If patients are intolerant to ACE-inhibition, ARB is the recommended alternative unless patients experience angioedema. If patients are intolerant to ARB as well, aliskiren should be given, starting with 75 mg per day with 2 step uptitration to 300 mg once daily. Higher starting dose may be used if patient are already on ACE-inhibition or ARB and medication is switched to aliskiren. As ARNI also contain an ARB (i.e. valsartan), ARNI are no alternative for patients intolerant to both ACE-inhibition and ARB.

7.7 Mineralocorticoid Receptor Antagonists (MRA)

Due to the aldosterone escape despite using ACE-inhibition, the hypothesis was raised that the addition of MRA may further improve prognosis in patients with HFrEF [16]. This hypothesis was confirmed in 1999, when the RALES trial was published [17]. Thus, spironolactone resulted in a substantial, approximately 30% relative risk reduction, irrespective of the endpoint being used. The RALES study, however, had some shortcomings that limited its use in patients with HFrEF, resulting in limited use up to now [69]. Thus, only patients with advanced HFrEF were investigated, i.e. patients in NYHA-class III and IV. Moreover, only very few patients were on β-blockers since large RCT showing the positive effects of β-blockers in HFrEF were running at the same time as RALES. Side-effects also limited its use. On the one hand, hyperkalaemia may occur when using MRA. In fact, a report in 2004 showed the increased incidence of hyperkalaemia resulting in hospital admission after the publication of RALES [70] although severe hyperkalaemia was not more common with spironolactone than with placebo in RALES [17]. Patients with renal dysfunction and high levels of potassium prior to start are of particular risk. Because of this risk, guidelines recommend early and repeated controls of serum potassium (in addition to renal function) with use of MRA. Unfortunately, this advice is often not followed in clinical practice even more than 15 years after the introduction of MRA as standard for HFrEF treatment [71]. On the other hand, gynaecomastia is an important side effect of spironolactone that is particularly disturbing in men. In RALES, as many as 10% of men had either gynaecomastia, breast pain or both [17]. However, it may occur even more often with the use of spironolactone and mastodynia may occur in women [72].

Therefore, the use of more selective MRA and the use of MRA in less symptomatic patients with HFrEF was eagerly awaited. It took, however, 4 years until results regarding the more selective MRA eplerenone were reported in patients with heart failure after myocardial infarction (EPHESUS) [73] and 12 years in HFrEF patients with NYHA II symptoms (EMPHASIS-HF) [19]. In EPHESUS, patient 3 to 14 days after acute myocardial infarction with LVEF of ≤40% and either clinical signs of heart failure or the presence of diabetes mellitus were included. They received 25 to 50 mg of eplerenone versus placebo. There was a significant reduction of all endpoints, including all cause death ($HR = 0.85$, $p = 0.008$), but the effects were smaller than seen in RALES. The reduction in cardiovascular death was in large parts due to reduction in sudden cardiac death, which might be explained by the reduced rate of significant hypokalaemia in the eplerenone group. This could be in line with the findings that positive effects were larger in patients having hypokalemia at baseline [73]. Moreover, heart failure hospitalisations were significantly reduced. The potential reasons for the observed reduction in events is obviously speculative, but based on animal studies, different mechanisms might play a role.

For a long time, it was unclear if MRA's are also beneficial in stabile heart failure patients with little symptoms (i.e. NYHA II). Still, MRA's were used in such patients [74], particularly in those with low serum potassium levels. Moreover, spironolactone has been shown to be of added value in patients with ascites, which is why it was and still is used in higher doses in patients with refractory oedema related right heart failure. Still, it must be noted that this approach has not been properly tested in sufficiently large treatment trials. The uncertainty regarding the use of MRA's in heart failure patients was reduced by the publication of the EMPHASIS-HF trial [19]. This trial finally resolved the debate as to whether MRA's are also helpful in less symptomatic HFrEF patients. The effect on relative reduction of all endpoints including mortality was almost as large as found in RALES. E.g. all-cause mortality was reduced by 24% and the combined primary endpoint by 37% [19]. Interestingly, average age was higher in this trial than in most other heart failure treatment trials (i.e. mean age 69 years), patients were well treated (i.e. most were on either ACE-inhibitor or ARB and on β–blocker), and effects were similar in all subgroups and independent of underlying treatment.

Taken together, MRA's are standard therapy in patients with heart failure and LVEF of 35% or less if they remain symptomatic despite treatment with ACE-I/ARB and β-blockade. In clinical practice, however, they are often used before ACE-I/ARB and β-blockade are fully uptitrated, particularly if serum potassium is low. Such practice may speed up establishment of standard therapy, but has not been tested to be superior as compared to the approach suggested by the guidelines; i.e. establishment of ACE-I/ARB and β-blockade first and only then start with MRA if still symptomatic [1]. On the other hand, MRA's are still not used in a significant number of patients that fulfil the criteria for their use [74, 75].

7.8 Angiotensin-II Receptor / neprilysin Inhibition (ARNI)

Effects of angiotensin-II 1–7 and other fragments of angiotensin as well as the stimulation of the angiotensin type-2 receptor might be particularly important if metabolism of angiotensin-II is inhibited by the use of neprilysin-inhibitors (e.g. sacubitril), but the type-1 receptor is blocked (e.g. by valsartan). This new concept in the treatment of heart failure is called ARNI. Currently, there is only one drug commercially available that has these two effects, i.e. Entresto.

Entresto is a single molecule comprising molecular moieties of valsartan and the NEP inhibitor prodrug sacubitril (1:1 ratio) [76]. In healthy participants (n = 80), oral administration of Entresto of single-dose (200–1200 mg) and multiple-dose (50–900 mg once daily for 14 days) resulted in peak plasma concentrations that were reached rapidly for valsartan (1.6–4.9 h), sacubitril (0.5–1.1 h) and its active metabolite LBQ657 (1.8–3.5 h) [76]. Entresto treatment was associated with increases in plasma cGMP, renin concentration and activity, and angiotensin II, providing evidence for NEP inhibition and angiotensin receptor blockade. In a randomized, open-label crossover study in healthy participants (n = 56), oral Entresto 194/206 mg and valsartan 320 mg were shown to provide similar exposure to valsartan (geometric mean ratio [90% confidence interval]: AUC (0-infinity) 0.90 [0.82–0.99]) [76]. Thus, the available doses of 24/26 mg, 49/51 mg and 97/103 mg correspond to 40, 80 and 160 mg valsartan.

Entresto was studied in more than 8000 patients with HFrEF, clearly showing superiority above treatment with ACE-inhibitor enalapril in appropriate doses [77]. Importantly, not only the combined morbidity/mortality endpoint was reduced by 20% (NNT 21), but also death from any cause alone was significantly reduced by 16% (NNT 45). This reduction was similar in all predefined subgroups [77], was independent of the individual risk of the participating patients [78], and prevented progression of disease in surviving patients [79]. Obviously, Entresto was not compared to placebo as this was ethically not possible. However, effects of Entresto as compared to placebo were theoretically calculated considering the effects of enalapril in SOLVD-T [31] and candesartan in CHARM-Alternative [52], resulting in an estimated risk reduction as compared to placebo of the primary endpoint of app. 40% and cardiovascular death of app. 1/3 [80]. Entresto was generally well tolerated and even improved renal function as compared to enalapril [77]. There are, however, some safety concerns, which are addressed below.

Entresto is also promising in patients with HFpEF. Thus, a phase 2 study showed larger reduction in NT-proBNP and NYHA-class after 36 weeks of treatment with Entresto as compared to valsartan alone [15]. These effects were independent of reduction in systolic blood pressure [81]. This is important as the blood pressure lowering effect exceeds that of valsartan alone [82]. As hypertension is an important, but certainly not the only factor in the pathophysiology of HFpEF [14] and all previous attempts to improve prognosis in HFpEF by inhibition of RAAS failed [6, 7, 9], effects of new compounds for potential treatment in HFpEF to improve outcome should have effects in addition to pure blood pressure reduction. Still, it is obvious that the ongoing phase 3 study must be awaited and this trial needs to show improvement in prognosis until Entresto can be recommended for treatment of HFpEF.

7.8.1 Potential Safety Concerns

There are some safety concerns about the use of Entresto. Thus, hypotension may limit the use of Entresto in patients with heart failure. In the PARADIGM-HF trial, symptomatic hypotension occurred app. 5% more often with Entresto 97/103 mg twice daily (average daily dose 182/193 mg) as compared to enalapril 10 mg twice daily (average daily dose 18.9 mg), but severe hypotension relatively rare [77]. However, it needs to be noted that only patients that tolerated at least 10 mg daily equivalent of enalapril were included in the trial and that there was an active run-in period prior to randomisation. Thus, those really intolerant to either Entresto or high dose of ACE-inhibition were not included. Given the fact that the average age of patients included in the

PARADIGM-HF trial was app. 10 years younger than in patients seen in daily care and that area under plasma concentration time curves of both valsartan and the active metabolite LBQ657 were slightly increased with age [83], hypotension might be more often seen in clinical practice than reported in the trials.

Another potential safety concern is the development of angioedema in patients taking Entresto. Angioedema was one of the major reasons why the combination of ACE-inibition and neprilysin-inhibition finally failed [84]. However, the combination with an ARB instead of an ACE-inhibitor may reduce the risk of angioedema although ARB may also increase bradykinin levels [85]. Angioedema has not been a problem so far in treatment trials of Entresto [77, 86]. However, patients were preselected and previous angioedema was an exclusion criterion in these trials. Therefore, the real incidence of angioedema with the use of Entresto is not yet known. Therefore, similar caution as with ACE-inhibitors is required and patients with a history of angioedema must not be treated with Entresto.

Finally, neprilysin may be one of multiple enzymes involved in the proteolytic degradation of amyloid-β (Aβ) [87]. There are many other proteases with Aβ-degrading properties including angiotensin converting enzyme [88]. The relative contribution of individual enzymes to the proteolytic degradation of Aβ remains unknown. The potential exists that treatment with Entresto through inhibition of neprilysin by LBQ657, may result in accumulation of aggregation-prone Aβ subtypes (e.g. Aβ 1–42 and Aβ 1–40) that are found in senile plaques in the brain of patients with Alzheimer's disease [89]. Although the role of Aβ in the pathophysiology of AD is not conclusively defined [90], the fact that LBQ657 crosses the blood-brain-barrier in low, but biologically active concentrations [91] is of potential concern. Still, no changes in the cerebrospinal fluid concentrations of the aggregable Aβ were found [91]. Thus, it is still unclear if this is potentially of clinical relevance, which only long-term results will reveal. So far, there is no evidence that this is the case. Given the poor prognosis of HFrEF and the convincing results regarding outcome, however, the benefit outweighs these potential concerns.

7.9 Safety Concerns When Using RAAS Blockers

Profiles of side effects are relatively similar in all drug addressing the RAAS (Table 7.2), as also discussed in the different paragraphs of the different agents. Thus, all may result in worsening renal function and may cause hyperkalaemia [1]. Therefore, particular attention is required regarding renal function and potassium levels, not only if these drugs are started and uptitrated, but also on a regular basis during chronic treatment. In general, blood chemistry (creatinine, urea/BUN, K+) is recommended 1–2 weeks after start and after uptitration and in 4 months intervals thereafter (see Web table of [1]). In clinical practice, controls are often less. Importantly, it has not been tested which intervals are required to be safe and to achieve best outcome at lowest costs. Therefore, such recommendations are expert opinion only. It is important to note that risk for significant worsening renal function and hyperkalaemia is not equal in all patients and highly depend on underlying risk. It is particularly high in patients with renal dysfunction and in patients with high potassium levels. Also, potential drug interactions must be considered. This includes NSAID's, K + −sparing agents, K + −supplements, and trimethoprim. Potassium levels up to 5.5 mmol/l are acceptable; higher levels may require dose reduction or even discontinuation and very close monitoring. Patients need to be advised to avoid drugs mentioned above and to report side effects and deterioration immediately.

Another important side effect is hypotension, which is dose-dependent (e.g. [56]). However, the probably most common unjustified cause of withdrawing RAAS-blockers is asymptomatic hypotension. Slight orthostatic reaction is common in heart failure and not necessarily related to drug treatment. It is usually acceptable. With improvement of heart failure, such symptoms often disappear. If unacceptable symptomatic hypotension occurs, concomitant medication should be reconsidered. Thus, drugs such nitrates and ca-antagonists may be given for improving symptoms, but do not improve prognosis in HFrEF. Possibly, diuretics may be given in lower doses or even withdrawn if fluid overload is absent.

Table 7.2 Common side effects of drug affecting the RAAS

	ACE-inhibitors	ARBs	Aliskiren	MRAs	Entresto
Hypotension	++	++	++	+	+++
Hyperkalaemia	+	+	+	++	(+)
WRF	++	++	++	++	++
Cough	++	–	–	–	+
Gynaecomastia	–	–	–	++[a]	–
Angioedema	+	(+)	(+)?	–	+?

[a]spironolactone only. *WRF* worsening renal function

Cough is a common side effect of ACE-inhibitors, but is also a very common sign of heart failure. In fact, dose of ACE-inhibitor may not be related to cough as higher doses are more efficacious treatment of heart failure [39]. Thus, patients should be evaluated carefully if cough is caused by heart failure. Moreover, often heart failure patients have concomitant pulmonary disease.

General recommendations on how to use these drugs are nicely summarised in the Web table of [1].

7.10 Are Effects Similar in All Patients?

Generally spoken, there are very little differences in various subgroup analyses of the large treatment trials. There is no evidence of important differences regarding effects between drugs of the same class as mentioned above. If some studies found some trends in different effects in subgroups, such differences were not confirmed in other studies. Therefore, there is no evidence that use of RAAS-blockers should not be given in particular subgroups of patients. This statement obviously does not apply to absolute contraindications of these drugs such as allergic reactions, bilateral renal stenosis (all but MRA's), angioedema (particularly ACE-inhibitors and ARNI), and pregnancy (all but MRA's).

However, it must be noted that evidence is less or not present in some subgroups of patients, which is true not only for RAAS-blockers, but also other treatment. This is particularly true in very elderly patients that have been largely excluded from the large trials. This also applies to patients with significant co-morbidities. It may be that effects in such patients are less [11]. In clinical practice, it is important to consider side effects, changes in metabolism (e.g. most ACE inhibitors are renally excreted and dose needs to be adjusted to renal function), interaction with other treatment, but also individual preferences of patients. It might be that patients with significant co-morbidities might have specific preferences. Importantly, such preferences regarding priority of treatment are not predicable and should be discussed individually with patients [92].

7.11 New Agents Addressing the RAAS

There are several new drugs under investigation that act via the RAAS [26]. An important group of drugs refers to new blockers of the mineralocorticoid receptor. Several new non-steroidal MRA's have been developed to maintain the protective cardio-vascular effect, while reducing the occurrence of side effects. They encompass finerenone (BAY 94-8862), SM-0368229, PF-3882845 and BR-4628 [26]. The agent best studied in heart failure is finerenone. It has been investigated in two phase 2 trial in patients with reduced LVEF [93, 94]. Patients also had to have chronic kidney disease [93] or diabetes and/or chronic kidney disease (but eGFR of >30 ml/min/1.73m^2) [94]. The first study showed that finerenone decreased levels of BNP, N-terminal proBNP and albuminuria at least as much as spironolactone whereas worsening renal failure and hyperkalaemia were less common [93]. Very recently, different doses of finerenone was compared with eplerenone, showing comparable effects on NT-proBNP levels, equal safety and numerically less combined endpoints of morbidity and mortality in higher doses [94]. The second highest dose even resulted in a significant reduction of this combined clinical endpoint, but obviously, the study was not powered to show such differences. Thus, the studies are very promising and a large phase 3 trial has to show if newer MRA's are superior and/or safer than currently available MRA's including eplerenone. Importantly, other new MRA's have additional properties (i.e. SM-368229 partial agonist activity; BR-4628 also blocks the L-type calcium-channels [26], but further studies must show to what extent these additional effects are of relevance. Aldosterone synthesis inhibition (FAD286A, LCI699, CYP11B2) is an alternative to receptor blockade. The reduction in aldosterone levels translated into improvement in organ damage [95], but possibly only a modest blood pressure reduction [96]. Studies have to show to what extent this is relevant. Theoretically, little effects on blood pressure with sufficient organ protection might be interesting for treating HFrEF patients, which often are hypotensive.

Human recombinant ACE2 (hrACE2) may be beneficial as it degrades among other angiotensin-II to angiotensin 1-7 (Ang 1-7), which acts through the MAS1 receptor and has vasodilatory and anti-fibrotic properties that counterbalance the action of angiotensin-II and aldosterone [97, 98]. ACE2 and Ang 1-7 have emerged as a key protective pathway against HF with both reduced and preserved ejection fraction. Recombinant human ACE2 has been tested in phase I and II clinical trials without adverse effects while lowering plasma angiotensin II and increasing Ang 1-7 levels and has important clinical potential as nicely summarised in a comprehensive review article [98]. Another option to increase Ang 1-7 levels involves the inhibition of its degradation. The simultaneous administration of Ang 1-7 and hydroxipropyl-β-cyclodextrin seems to protect Ang 1-7 from degradation and act as a system to slow drug release. This formulation in animal models has demonstrated a reduction in blood pressure [99]. This innovative particle engineering approach which synergistically coalesce two principally different solubility enhancement strategies namely ternary β-cyclodextrin complexation and top-down nanonization in a unit process may also improve solubility and reduce in vivo variability in pharmacokinetic parameters irrespective to physiological pH conditions and thereby bioavailability of other drugs [100]. Finally, a therapeutic strategy to enhance Ang 1-7 effects involves the development of MAS1 receptor agonists. The non-peptide compound AVE 0991 has shown similar protective effects of Ang 1-7 [101].

In view of the beneficial effects of the angiotensin-II type 2 (AT2) receptor activation, non-peptide agonists were developed. Compound 21 is a selective non-peptide AT2 agonist that has shown to reduce the collagen in the extracellular matrix and vascular tissue, oxidative stress, and inflammatory cell infiltration. Moreover, it may induce in animal models of myocardial infarction an improvement of cardiac function [102]. However, it has not yet been tested in human. Finally, a new therapeutic strategy is the formation of vaccines against renin, angiotensin-I, angiotensin-II and angiotensin-II type 1 receptors. However, only relatively small trials are available, not yet showing uniform results and some safety concerns have been raised. Moreover, it has not yet been clear, which is the best target for this approach. Thus, both efficacy and safety needs to be shown in large outcome trials [103].

7.12 Diuretics

Diuretics were introduced in the treatment of heart failure more than 50 years ago. Diuretics are a mainstay in the treatment of both HFrEF and HFpEF (and HFmrEF) [1]. If patients are fluid overloaded, diuretics are recommended. Moreover, they are first line treatment in acute decompensated heart failure (ADHF), irrespectively as to whether heart failure is present for the first time or previous episodes have occurred [1]. During acute episodes, intravenous treatment with loop diuretics is often required, because oral treatment may be less effective [104]. In fact, oral bioavailability may decrease in volume overloaded patients, particularly if right-sided decompensation is present. Higher doses (app. 2.5 times the dose previous oral dose) are slightly more effective than lower doses (equivalent to patient's oral dose), but it does not matter if loop diuretics are given as a continuous infusion or as bolus every 12 h [105].

Despite the importance of diuretics in the treatment of heart failure, they have never been tested in appropriate randomised trials to show their prognostic effect. Moreover, diuretics may significantly hamper renal function, particularly if given in (too) high doses. Obviously, the problem with a prospective trial comparing (loop) diuretics with placebo in heart failure is the fact that diuretics are used to (acutely) treat congestion and it may be an ethical problem to withhold diuretics in such patients. After the introduction of ACE-inhibitors in the treatment of HFrEF, there have been some small studies to test if diuretics may be reduced / stopped if ACE-inhibition is used. However, the need for reinstalling diuretic therapy was not different in patients treated with ACE-inhibitors from those receiving placebo [106]. Thus, one may argue that withholding diuretics is simply not possible in a significant number of heart failure patients (both HFrEF and HFpEF) due to symptoms. However, it may also be argued that withholding diuretics is possible in a significant proportion of stable heart failure patients and should therefore be attempted. It is unlikely that such a trial will be done in the future. A Cochrane review suggested some beneficial effects of diuretics on morbidity and even mortality [107], but this metanalysis was recently withdrawn because several studies included did not meet the diagnostic criteria for inclusion [108]. Still, there has been an RCT on the comparison of two loop diuretics, showing significant better outcome when using torasemide than furosemide [109]. Unfortunately, this trial has not been double-blinded and relatively low risk patients have been included, raising the question as to whether a substantial number of included patients were in real need of loop diuretic therapy.

As a consequence, diuretic therapy are given based on clinical signs and symptoms of volume overload and effects on renal function (and electrolytes). Although not based on adequate studies, it is generally recommended to use (loop) diuretics in the lowest achievable dose to keep the patients euvolaemic and to even stop them if possible. Patients can be trained to self-adjust their diuretic dose based on monitoring of symptoms/signs of congestion and daily weight measurements [1]. Figure 7.2 provides a scheme to show that both volume depletion and volume overload can result in worsening renal function [110], highlighting the need for individualised balance in euvolaemia. Unfortunately, response to diuretic therapy in individual patients can hardly be predicted, indicating that close monitoring of volume state and renal function is crucial. Still, if patients are significantly volume overloaded, chances that diuretic therapy results in increase in eGFR is obviously larger.

Loop diuretics produce a more intense and shorter diuresis than thiazides, although they act synergistically and the combination may be used to treat resistant oedema. However, adverse effects are more likely and these combinations should only be used with care and appropriate monitoring, including measurement of renal function and electrolytes. Importantly, the risk of hypokamaemia is significant when using this combination.

Important side effects of loop diuretic therapy include hypotension, worsening of renal function, hypokalaemia, dehydration, and gout. Hyponatraemia may be a side effect, but also a sign of worsening heart failure. Therefore, monitoring is important and similar to the use of RAAS-blockers.

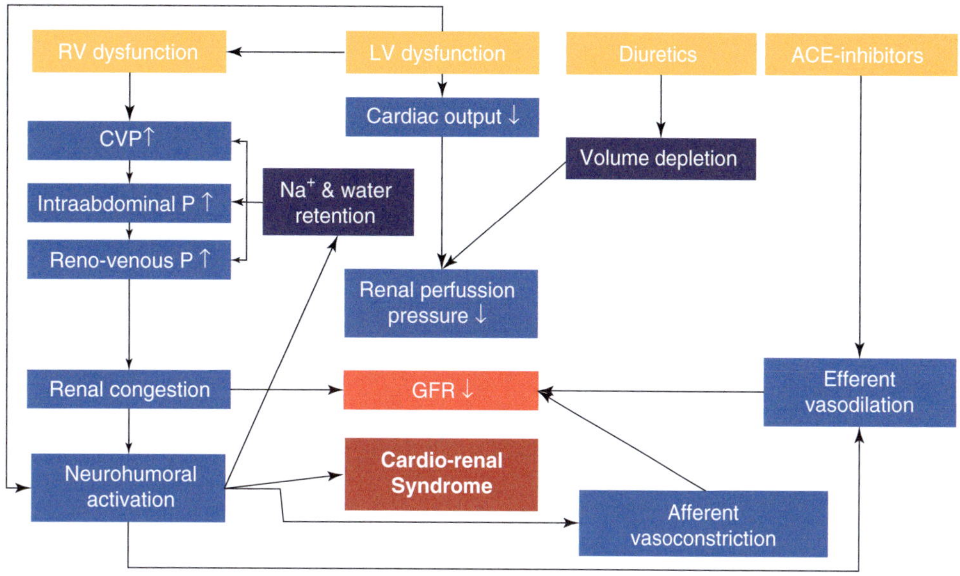

Fig. 7.2 Cardiorenal interaction resulting cardio-renal syndrome. (Adapted from [110])

7.13 Digoxin

Digitalis (foxglove) has been being used for the treatment of heart failure for already more than 200 years. For a long time, it was the only effective treatment available, before diuretics were discovered. Before the introduction of ACE-inhibitors into the treatment of heart failure, the combination of digoxin and diuretics was the standard therapy in heart failure patients, often with dismal outcome. After the introduction of ACE-inhibitors, there were some studies investigating the effects of withdrawal of digoxin. These studies showed an increased risk of hospitalisation due to heart failure after withdrawal of digoxin [111, 112], but were not sufficiently large to investigate effects on mortality. In addition, a recent metanalysis did not found any effects on mortality and all-cause hospitalisation after withdrawal [113]. In 1997, the large DIG-trial was published, which still is the only sufficiently large morbidity and mortality trial investigating digoxin in heart failure [114]. Again, no effects on mortality was found, but a significant reduction in heart failure related hospitalisations (absolute risk reduction of 7.9%). As a consequence, digoxin was primarily considered for symptomatic treatment for heart failure [115] and over the years, its use has been downgraded as second line treatment only [1].

Several aspects of the use of digoxin in heart failure needs to be considered. (1) digoxin has only been prospectively investigated in a significant number of patients in sinus rhythm, but not in atrial fibrillation [114]. Although digoxin is often mentioned as important part of treatment in patients with heart failure and atrial fibrillation [1], this has not been properly tested. A metanalysis of observational data even suggested an increased mortality with the use of digoxin in such patients [116], whereas other metanalyses concluded that digoxin has a neural effect [117, 118]. None, however, concluded that digoxin may improve outcome in HF patients with atrial fibrillation. (2) A post-hoc analysis of the DIG trial suggested that plasma levels may be important for predicting the response to digoxin in heart failure patients with sinus rhythm. Thus, whereas in patients with low digoxin plasma levels (i.e. 0.6–0.9 ng/L) prognosis was improved, the opposite was the case with higher digoxin levels [119], which were still in the therapeutic range. Plasma levels were dependent several factors, i.e. dose of digoxin, renal dysfunction, female sex, age, use of diuretics and pulmonary congestions, and lower body mass index [119]. In addition to measuring digoxin levels when used, optimal dose may be assessed by considering renal function [120]. (3) The DIG-trial was performed when only ACE-inhibitors were part of the standard therapy in HFrEF, but not β-blockers and MRAs. Thus, it remains speculative if the effects found in the DIG-trial are directly applicable to the current situation, where standard therapy is much broader. (4) In order to resolve this problem, there is an ongoing trial to test the use of digitalis in heart failure in modern times by testing digitoxin versus placebo in 2200 HFrEF patients (DIGIT-HF trial; digit-hf.de). (5) Digoxin is also not properly tested in HFpEF patients, irrespectively of the underlying rhythm. Still, almost 1000 patients of the DIG-trial had a preserved LVEF with a non-significant positive effect of digoxin, comparable to the effects found in CHARM-preserved [121]. Obviously, this is not sufficient to recommend standard digoxin use in HFpEF patients.

Thus, when should digoxin been used in heart failure? Following the current guidelines, digoxin may be considered in patients with HFrEF and sinus rhythm if they remain significantly symptomatic despite standard therapy including all drugs improving prognosis and devices [1]. It is obvious that standard therapy must be given as far as possible before considering digoxin. However, if patients remain symptomatic and/or are difficult to treat with standard therapy (e.g. hypotension) digoxin may be considered. Based on personal experience of the author, some patients respond with significant and obvious improvement to digoxin whereas other do not respond at all. It is, however, impossible to predict this response. Thus, digoxin may be tried in the patients mentioned above to optimise heart failure treatment, particularly in those that are difficult to treat with standard therapy.

If treated with digoxin, it is recommended to use low doses only, adjusted for renal function [120], and to measure plasma levels when established (target 0.6–0.9 ng/L). Potential interactions need to be considered. In particular, it is important to know that the use of amiodarone may double plasma levels of digoxin.

7.14 Statins

Inflammation, oxidative stress and endothelial and platelet dysfunction predispose to HF development and progression and statins have shown to reduce these effects. In fact, statins have been shown to reduce HF incidence possibly via their pleiotropic actions on these mechanisms [122]. However, once heart failure is established, the effects of statins are less certain. In fact in patients with HFrEF, two large randomised controlled trials did not find any beneficial effects of statin therapy, even in patients with coronary artery disease as underlying cause of HF [123, 124]. In both of these trials, rosuvastatin was investigated. Although the primary endpoint was not reduced, rosuvastatin did not increase risk, there were no serious safety concerns and it may reduce cardiovascular hospitalisation [123, 124]. Given the neutral findings on the primary endpoints and the fact that most of the statins are out of patent, it is unlikely that an additional large RCT will be carried out to investigate the potential use of statins in (subgroups of) patients with HFrEF.

This may be different for HFpEF, but data are not yet sufficient to recommend statin use as standard therapy. Still, initial findings and post-hoc analyses look promising [125, 126]. It must be mentioned, however, that many substances looked promising in HFpEF patients when analysed in registries or post-hoc analyses, but were finally not successful in RCT's. Therefore, such trials must be awaited until statin therapy may be recommended.

References

1. Ponikowski P, Voors AA, Anker SD, Bueno H, Cleland JG, Coats AJ, Falk V, Gonzalez-Juanatey JR, Harjola VP, Jankowska EA, Jessup M, Linde C, Nihoyannopoulos P, Parissis JT, Pieske B, Riley JP, Rosano GM, Ruilope LM, Ruschitzka F, Rutten FH, van der Meer P. 2016 ESC guidelines for the diagnosis and treatment of acute and chronic heart failure: the task force for the diagnosis and treatment of acute and chronic heart failure of the European Society of Cardiology (ESC)developed with the special contribution of the heart failure association (HFA) of the ESC. Eur Heart J. 2016;18(8):891–975.
2. Kaufmann BA, Min SY, Goetschalckx K, Bernheim AM, Buser PT, Pfisterer ME, Brunner-La Rocca HP. How reliable are left ventricular ejection fraction cut offs assessed by echocardiography for clinical decision making in patients with heart failure? Int J Cardiovasc Imaging. 2013;29(3):581–8.
3. Flather MD, Shibata MC, Coats AJ, van Veldhuisen DJ, Parkhomenko A, Borbola J, Cohen-Solal A, Dumitrascu D, Ferrari R, Lechat P, Soler-Soler J, Tavazzi L, Spinarova L, Toman J, Bohm M, Anker SD, Thompson SG, Poole-Wilson PA. Randomized trial to determine the effect of nebivolol on mortality and cardiovascular hospital admission in elderly patients with heart failure (SENIORS). Eur Heart J. 2005;26(3):215–25.
4. Solomon SD, Claggett B, Lewis EF, Desai A, Anand I, Sweitzer NK, O'Meara E, Shah SJ, McKinlay S, Fleg JL, Sopko G, Pitt B, Pfeffer MA. Influence of ejection fraction on outcomes and efficacy of spironolactone in patients with heart failure with preserved ejection fraction. Eur Heart J. 2016;37(5):455–62.
5. Emdin CA, Callender T, Cao J, McMurray JJ, Rahimi K. Meta-analysis of large-scale randomized trials to determine the effectiveness of inhibition of the renin-angiotensin aldosterone system in heart failure. Am J Cardiol. 2015;116(1):155–61.
6. Massie BM, Carson PE, McMurray JJ, Komajda M, McKelvie R, Zile MR, Anderson S, Donovan M, Iverson E, Staiger C, Ptaszynska A. Irbesartan in patients with heart failure and preserved ejection fraction. N Engl J Med. 2008;359(23):2456–67.
7. Cleland JG, Tendera M, Adamus J, Freemantle N, Polonski L, Taylor J. The perindopril in elderly people with chronic heart failure (PEP-CHF) study. Eur Heart J. 2006;27(19):2338–45.
8. Yusuf S, Pfeffer MA, Swedberg K, Granger CB, Held P, McMurray JJ, Michelson EL, Olofsson B, Ostergren J. Effects of candesartan in patients with chronic heart failure and preserved left-ventricular ejection fraction: the CHARM-preserved trial. Lancet. 2003;362(9386):777–81.
9. Pitt B, Pfeffer MA, Assmann SF, Boineau R, Anand IS, Claggett B, Clausell N, Desai AS, Diaz R, Fleg JL, Gordeev I, Harty B, Heitner JF, Kenwood CT, Lewis EF, O'Meara E, Probstfield JL, Shaburishvili T, Shah SJ, Solomon SD, Sweitzer NK, Yang S, McKinlay SM. Spironolactone for heart failure with preserved ejection fraction. N Engl J Med. 2014;370(15):1383–92.
10. Pfeffer MA, Claggett B, Assmann SF, Boineau R, Anand IS, Clausell N, Desai AS, Diaz R, Fleg JL, Gordeev I, Heitner JF, Lewis EF, O'Meara E, Rouleau JL, Probstfield JL, Shaburishvili T, Shah SJ, Solomon SD, Sweitzer NK, McKinlay SM, Pitt B. Regional variation in patients and outcomes in the treatment of preserved cardiac function heart failure with an aldosterone antagonist (TOPCAT) trial. Circulation. 2015;131(1):34–42.
11. Brunner-La Rocca HP, Eurlings L, Richards AM, Januzzi JL, Pfisterer ME, Dahlstrom U, Pinto YM, Karlstrom P, Erntell H, Berger R, Persson H, O'Connor CM, Moertl D, Gaggin HK, Frampton CM, Nicholls MG, Troughton RW. Which heart failure patients profit from natriuretic peptide guided therapy? A meta-analysis from individual patient data of randomized trials. Eur J Heart Fail. 2015;17(12):1252–61.

12. Senni M, Paulus WJ, Gavazzi A, Fraser AG, Diez J, Solomon SD, Smiseth OA, Guazzi M, Lam CS, Maggioni AP, Tschope C, Metra M, Hummel SL, Edelmann F, Ambrosio G, Stewart Coats AJ, Filippatos GS, Gheorghiade M, Anker SD, Levy D, Pfeffer MA, Stough WG, Pieske BM. New strategies for heart failure with preserved ejection fraction: the importance of targeted therapies for heart failure phenotypes. Eur Heart J. 2014;35(40):2797–815.
13. Paulus WJ, Tschope C. A novel paradigm for heart failure with preserved ejection fraction: comorbidities drive myocardial dysfunction and remodeling through coronary microvascular endothelial inflammation. J Am Coll Cardiol. 2013;62(4):263–71.
14. van Empel V, Brunner-La Rocca HP. Inflammation in HFpEF: key or circumstantial? Int J Cardiol. 2015;189:259–63.
15. Solomon SD, Zile M, Pieske B, Voors A, Shah A, Kraigher-Krainer E, Shi V, Bransford T, Takeuchi M, Gong J, Lefkowitz M, Packer M, McMurray JJ. The angiotensin receptor neprilysin inhibitor LCZ696 in heart failure with preserved ejection fraction: a phase 2 double-blind randomised controlled trial. Lancet. 2012;380(9851):1387–95.
16. Pitt B. "Escape" of aldosterone production in patients with left ventricular dysfunction treated with an angiotensin converting enzyme inhibitor: implications for therapy. Cardiovasc Drugs Ther. 1995;9(1):145–9.
17. Pitt B, Zannad F, Remme WJ, Cody R, Castaigne A, Perez A, Palensky J, Wittes J. The effect of spironolactone on morbidity and mortality in patients with severe heart failure. Randomized Aldactone evaluation study investigators. N Engl J Med. 1999;341(10):709–17.
18. Pitt B, Williams G, Remme W, Martinez F, Lopez-Sendon J, Zannad F, Neaton J, Roniker B, Hurley S, Burns D, Bittman R, Kleiman J. The EPHESUS trial: eplerenone in patients with heart failure due to systolic dysfunction complicating acute myocardial infarction. Eplerenone post-AMI heart failure efficacy and survival study. Cardiovasc Drugs Ther. 2001;15(1):79–87.
19. Zannad F, McMurray JJ, Krum H, van Veldhuisen DJ, Swedberg K, Shi H, Vincent J, Pocock SJ, Pitt B. Eplerenone in patients with systolic heart failure and mild symptoms. N Engl J Med. 2011;364(1):11–21.
20. Yancy CW, Jessup M, Bozkurt B, Masoudi FA, Butler J, McBride PE, Casey DE Jr, McMurray JJ, Drazner MH, Mitchell JE, Fonarow GC, Peterson PN, Geraci SA, Horwich T, Januzzi JL, Johnson MR, Kasper EK, Levy WC, Riegel B, Sam F, Stevenson LW, Tang WH, Tsai EJ, Wilkoff BL. 2013 ACCF/AHA guideline for the management of heart failure: a report of the American College of Cardiology Foundation/American Heart Association task force on practice guidelines. J Am Coll Cardiol. 2013;62:e147–239.
21. Coats AJ. Omapatrilat – the story of overture and octave. Int J Cardiol. 2002;86(1):1–4.
22. Xu J, Carretero OA, Shesely EG, Rhaleb NE, Yang JJ, Bader M, Yang XP. The kinin B1 receptor contributes to the cardioprotective effect of angiotensin-converting enzyme inhibitors and angiotensin receptor blockers in mice. Exp Physiol. 2009;94(3):322–9.
23. Nussberger J, Cugno M, Amstutz C, Cicardi M, Pellacani A, Agostoni A. Plasma bradykinin in angio-oedema. Lancet. 1998;351:1693–7.
24. Gheorghiade M, Bohm M, Greene SJ, Fonarow GC, Lewis EF, Zannad F, Solomon SD, Baschiera F, Botha J, Hua TA, Gimpelewicz CR, Jaumont X, Lesogor A, Maggioni AP. Effect of aliskiren on postdischarge mortality and heart failure readmissions among patients hospitalized for heart failure: the ASTRONAUT randomized trial. JAMA. 2013;309(11):1125–35.
25. McMurray JJ, Krum H, Abraham WT, Dickstein K, Kober LV, Desai AS, Solomon SD, Greenlaw N, Ali MA, Chiang Y, Shao Q, Tarnesby G, Massie BM. Aliskiren, Enalapril, or Aliskiren and Enalapril in heart failure. N Engl J Med. 2016;374(16):1521–32.
26. Mollace V, Gliozzi M, Capuano A, Rossi F. Modulation of RAAS-natriuretic peptides in the treatment of HF: old guys and newcomers. Int J Cardiol. 2017;226:126–31.
27. Reid IA. Interactions between ANG II, sympathetic nervous system, and baroreceptor reflexes in regulation of blood pressure. Am J Phys. 1992;262(6 Pt 1):E763–78.
28. Gonzalez GE, Rhaleb NE, Nakagawa P, Liao TD, Liu Y, Leung P, Dai X, Yang XP, Carretero OA. N-acetyl-seryl-aspartyl-lysyl-proline reduces cardiac collagen cross-linking and inflammation in angiotensin II-induced hypertensive rats. Clin Sci (Lond). 2014;126(1):85–94.
29. Luque M, Martin P, Martell N, Fernandez C, Brosnihan KB, Ferrario CM. Effects of captopril related to increased levels of prostacyclin and angiotensin-(1-7) in essential hypertension. J Hypertens. 1996;14(6):799–805.
30. The CONSENSUS Trial Study Group. Effects of enalapril on mortality in severe congestive heart failure. Results of the cooperative north Scandinavian Enalapril survival study (CONSENSUS). N Engl J Med. 1987;316(23):1429–35.
31. The SOLVD Investigators. Effect of enalapril on survival in patients with reduced left ventricular ejection fractions and congestive heart failure. N Engl J Med. 1991;325(5):293–302.
32. The SOLVD Investigators. Effect of enalapril on mortality and the development of heart failure in asymptomatic patients with reduced left ventricular ejection fractions. N Engl J Med. 1992;327(10):685–91.
33. Pfeffer MA, Braunwald E, Moye LA, Basta L, Brown EJ Jr, Cuddy TE, Davis BR, Geltman EM, Goldman S, Flaker GC. Effect of captopril on mortality and morbidity in patients with left ventricular dysfunction after myocardial infarction. Results of the survival and ventricular enlargement trial. The SAVE investigators. N Engl J Med. 1992;327(10):669–77.
34. Hall AS, Murray GD, Ball SG. Follow-up study of patients randomly allocated ramipril or placebo for heart failure after acute myocardial infarction: AIRE extension (AIREX) study. Acute infarction ramipril efficacy. Lancet. 1997;349(9064):1493–7.
35. ISIS-4: a randomised factorial trial assessing early oral captopril, oral mononitrate, and intravenous magnesium sulphate in 58,050 patients with suspected acute myocardial infarction. ISIS-4 (fourth international study of infarct survival) collaborative group. Lancet. 1995;345(8951):669–85.
36. Kober L, Torp P, Carlsen JE, Bagger H, Eliasen P, Lyngborg K, Videbaek J, Cole DS, Auclert L, Pauly NC, Aliot E. A clinical trial of the angiotensin-converting-enzyme inhibitor trandolapril in patients with left ventricular dysfunction after myocardial infarction. Trandolapril Cardiac Evaluation (TRACE) study group. N Engl J Med. 1995;333(25):1670–6.
37. Garg R, Yusuf S. Overview of randomized trials of angiotensin-converting enzyme inhibitors on mortality and morbidity in patients with heart failure. Collaborative group on ACE inhibitor trials. JAMA. 1995;273(18):1450–6.
38. Swedberg K, Held P, Kjekshus J, Rasmussen K, Ryden L, Wedel H. Effects of the early administration of enalapril on mortality in patients with acute myocardial infarction. Results of the Cooperative New Scandinavian Enalapril Survival Study II (CONSENSUS II). N Engl J Med. 1992;327(10):678–84.
39. Brunner-La Rocca HP, Weilenmann D, Kiowski W, Maly FE, Candinas R, Follath F. Within-patient comparison of effects of different dosages of enalapril on functional capacity and neurohormone levels in patients with chronic heart failure. Am Heart J. 1999;138(4 Pt 1):654–62.
40. Packer M, Poole-Wilson PA, Armstrong PW, Cleland JG, Horowitz JD, Massie BM, Ryden L, Thygesen K, Uretsky BF. Comparative effects of low and high doses of the angiotensin-converting enzyme inhibitor, lisinopril, on morbidity

and mortality in chronic heart failure. ATLAS Study Group Circulation. 1999;100(23):2312–8.
41. Brunner-La Rocca HP, Weilenmann D, Kiowski W, Maly FE, Follath F. Plasma levels of enalaprilat in chronic therapy of heart failure: relationship to adverse events. J Pharmacol Exp Ther. 1999;289(1):565–71.
42. Song JC, White CM. Clinical pharmacokinetics and selective pharmacodynamics of new angiotensin converting enzyme inhibitors: an update. Clin Pharmacokinet. 2002;41(3):207–24.
43. Anand IS, Deswal A, Kereiakes DJ, Purkayastha D, Zappe DH. Comparison of once-daily versus twice-daily dosing of valsartan in patients with chronic stable heart failure. Vasc Health Risk Manag. 2010;6:449–55.
44. Tu K, Mamdani M, Kopp A, Lee D. Comparison of angiotensin-converting enzyme inhibitors in the treatment of congestive heart failure. Am J Cardiol. 2005;95(2):283–6.
45. Pilote L, Abrahamowicz M, Rodrigues E, Eisenberg MJ, Rahme E. Mortality rates in elderly patients who take different angiotensin-converting enzyme inhibitors after acute myocardial infarction: a class effect? Ann Intern Med. 2004;141(2):102–12.
46. Pilote L, Abrahamowicz M, Eisenberg M, Humphries K, Behlouli H, Tu JV. Effect of different angiotensin-converting-enzyme inhibitors on mortality among elderly patients with congestive heart failure. CMAJ. 2008;178(10):1303–11.
47. Yugandhar VG, Clark MA. Angiotensin III: a physiological relevant peptide of the renin angiotensin system. Peptides. 2013;46:26–32.
48. Chappell MC, Pirro NT, Sykes A, Ferrario CM. Metabolism of angiotensin-(1-7) by angiotensin-converting enzyme. Hypertension. 1998;31(1 Pt 2):362–7.
49. Brunner-La Rocca HP, Vaddadi G, Esler MD. Recent insight into therapy of congestive heart failure: focus on ACE inhibition and angiotensin-II antagonism. J Am Coll Cardiol. 1999;33(5):1163–73.
50. Cohn JN, Tognoni G. A randomized trial of the angiotensin-receptor blocker valsartan in chronic heart failure. N Engl J Med. 2001;345(23):1667–75.
51. Maggioni AP, Anand I, Gottlieb SO, Latini R, Tognoni G, Cohn JN. Effects of valsartan on morbidity and mortality in patients with heart failure not receiving angiotensin-converting enzyme inhibitors. J Am Coll Cardiol. 2002;40(8):1414–21.
52. Granger CB, McMurray JJ, Yusuf S, Held P, Michelson EL, Olofsson B, Ostergren J, Pfeffer MA, Swedberg K. Effects of candesartan in patients with chronic heart failure and reduced left-ventricular systolic function intolerant to angiotensin-converting-enzyme inhibitors: the CHARM-alternative trial. Lancet. 2003;362(9386):772–6.
53. McMurray JJ, Ostergren J, Swedberg K, Granger CB, Held P, Michelson EL, Olofsson B, Yusuf S, Pfeffer MA. Effects of candesartan in patients with chronic heart failure and reduced left-ventricular systolic function taking angiotensin-converting-enzyme inhibitors: the CHARM-added trial. Lancet. 2003;362(9386):767–71.
54. Pfeffer MA, Swedberg K, Granger CB, Held P, McMurray JJ, Michelson EL, Olofsson B, Ostergren J, Yusuf S, Pocock S. Effects of candesartan on mortality and morbidity in patients with chronic heart failure: the CHARM-overall programme. Lancet. 2003;362(9386):759–66.
55. Pfeffer MA, McMurray JJ, Velazquez EJ, Rouleau JL, Kober L, Maggioni AP, Solomon SD, Swedberg K, Van De Werf F, White H, Leimberger JD, Henis M, Edwards S, Zelenkofske S, Sellers MA, Califf RM. Valsartan, captopril, or both in myocardial infarction complicated by heart failure, left ventricular dysfunction, or both. N Engl J Med. 2003;349(20):1893–906.
56. Konstam MA, Neaton JD, Dickstein K, Drexler H, Komajda M, Martinez FA, Riegger GA, Malbecq W, Smith RD, Guptha S, Poole-Wilson PA. Effects of high-dose versus low-dose losartan on clinical outcomes in patients with heart failure (HEAAL study): a randomised, double-blind trial. Lancet. 2009;374(9704):1840–8.
57. Pitt B, Poole-Wilson PA, Segal R, Martinez FA, Dickstein K, Camm AJ, Konstam MA, Riegger G, Klinger GH, Neaton J, Sharma D, Thiyagarajan B. Effect of losartan compared with captopril on mortality in patients with symptomatic heart failure: randomised trial--the losartan heart failure survival study ELITE II. Lancet. 2000;355(9215):1582–7.
58. Gradman AH, Schmieder RE, Lins RL, Nussberger J, Chiang Y, Bedigian MP. Aliskiren, a novel orally effective renin inhibitor, provides dose-dependent antihypertensive efficacy and placebo-like tolerability in hypertensive patients. Circulation. 2005;111(8):1012–8.
59. McMurray JJ, Pitt B, Latini R, Maggioni AP, Solomon SD, Keefe DL, Ford J, Verma A, Lewsey J. Effects of the oral direct renin inhibitor aliskiren in patients with symptomatic heart failure. Circ Heart Fail. 2008;1(1):17–24.
60. Parving HH, Brenner BM, McMurray JJ, de Zeeuw D, Haffner SM, Solomon SD, Chaturvedi N, Persson F, Desai AS, Nicolaides M, Richard A, Xiang Z, Brunel P, Pfeffer MA. Cardiorenal end points in a trial of aliskiren for type 2 diabetes. N Engl J Med. 2012;367(23):2204–13.
61. McMurray JJ, Abraham WT, Dickstein K, Kober L, Massie BM, Krum H. Aliskiren, ALTITUDE, and the implications for ATMOSPHERE. Eur J Heart Fail. 2012;14(4):341–3.
62. Krum H, Massie B, Abraham WT, Dickstein K, Kober L, McMurray JJ. Losing ALTITUDE? How should ASTRONAUT launch into ATMOSPHERE. Eur J Heart Fail. 2013;15(11):1205–7.
63. Swedberg K, Borer JS, Pitt B, Pocock S, Rouleau J. Challenges to data monitoring committees when regulatory authorities intervene. N Engl J Med. 2016;374(16):1580–4.
64. Tougas G, Aftring RP. Novartis reply to the ATMOSPHERE data monitoring committee. N Engl J Med. 2016;374(16):1586–7.
65. Salmonson T, Janssen H, Sudhop T, Stahl E. Regulatory reply to the ATMOSPHERE data monitoring committee. N Engl J Med. 2016;374(16):1585–6.
66. Joseph K, Tholanikunnel TE, Kaplan AP. In vitro comparison of bradykinin degradation by aliskiren, a renin inhibitor, and an inhibitor of angiotensin-converting enzyme. J Renin-Angiotensin-Aldosterone Syst. 2015;16(2):321–7.
67. Ali AK. Pharmacovigilance analysis of adverse event reports for aliskiren hemifumarate, a first-in-class direct renin inhibitor. Ther Clin Risk Manag. 2011;7:337–44.
68. White WB, Bresalier R, Kaplan AP, Palmer BF, Riddell RH, Lesogor A, Chang W, Keefe DL. Safety and tolerability of the direct renin inhibitor aliskiren in combination with angiotensin receptor blockers and thiazide diuretics: a pooled analysis of clinical experience of 12,942 patients. J Clin Hypertens (Greenwich). 2011;13(7):506–16.
69. Lachaine J, Beauchemin C, Ramos E. Use, tolerability and compliance of spironolactone in the treatment of heart failure. BMC Clin Pharmacol. 2011;20:4–11.
70. Juurlink DN, Mamdani MM, Lee DS, Kopp A, Austin PC, Laupacis A, Redelmeier DA. Rates of hyperkalemia after publication of the randomized Aldactone evaluation study. N Engl J Med. 2004;351(6):543–51.
71. Allen LA, Shetterly SM, Peterson PN, Gurwitz JH, Smith DH, Brand DW, Fairclough DL, Rumsfeld JS, Masoudi FA, Magid DJ. Guideline concordance of testing for hyperkalemia and kidney dysfunction during initiation of mineralocorticoid receptor antagonist therapy in patients with heart failure. Circ Heart Fail. 2014;7(1):43–50.
72. Parthasarathy HK, Menard J, White WB, Young WF Jr, Williams GH, Williams B, Ruilope LM, McInnes GT, Connell JM, MacDonald TM. A double-blind, randomized study comparing

the antihypertensive effect of eplerenone and spironolactone in patients with hypertension and evidence of primary aldosteronism. J Hypertens. 2011;29(5):980–90.
73. Pitt B, Remme W, Zannad F, Neaton J, Martinez F, Roniker B, Bittman R, Hurley S, Kleiman J, Gatlin M. Eplerenone, a selective aldosterone blocker, in patients with left ventricular dysfunction after myocardial infarction. N Engl J Med. 2003;348(14):1309–21.
74. Thorvaldsen T, Benson L, Dahlstrom U, Edner M, Lund LH. Use of evidence-based therapy and survival in heart failure in Sweden 2003-2012. Eur J Heart Fail. 2016;18(5):503–11.
75. Maggioni AP, Anker SD, Dahlstrom U, Filippatos G, Ponikowski P, Zannad F, Amir O, Chioncel O, Leiro MC, Drozdz J, Erglis A, Fazlibegovic E, Fonseca C, Fruhwald F, Gatzov P, Goncalvesova E, Hassanein M, Hradec J, Kavoliuniene A, Lainscak M, Logeart D, Merkely B, Metra M, Persson H, Seferovic P, Temizhan A, Tousoulis D, Tavazzi L. Are hospitalized or ambulatory patients with heart failure treated in accordance with European society of cardiology guidelines? Evidence from 12,440 patients of the ESC heart failure long-term registry. Eur J Heart Fail. 2013;15(10):1173–84.
76. Gu J, Noe A, Chandra P, Al-Fayoumi S, Ligueros-Saylan M, Sarangapani R, Maahs S, Ksander G, Rigel DF, Jeng AY, Lin TH, Zheng W, Dole WP. Pharmacokinetics and pharmacodynamics of LCZ696, a novel dual-acting angiotensin receptor-neprilysin inhibitor (ARNi). J Clin Pharmacol. 2010;50(4):401–14.
77. McMurray JJ, Packer M, Desai AS, Gong J, Lefkowitz MP, Rizkala AR, Rouleau JL, Shi VC, Solomon SD, Swedberg K, Zile MR. Angiotensin-neprilysin inhibition versus enalapril in heart failure. N Engl J Med. 2014;371(11):993–1004.
78. Simpson J, Jhund PS, Silva Cardoso J, Martinez F, Mosterd A, Ramires F, Rizkala AR, Senni M, Squire I, Gong J, Lefkowitz MP, Shi VC, Desai AS, Rouleau JL, Swedberg K, Zile MR, McMurray JJ, Packer M, Solomon SD. Comparing LCZ696 with enalapril according to baseline risk using the MAGGIC and EMPHASIS-HF risk scores: an analysis of mortality and morbidity in PARADIGM-HF. J Am Coll Cardiol. 2015,66(19):2059–71.
79. Packer M, Jj MM, Desai AS, Gong J, Lefkowitz MP, Rizkala AR, Rouleau JL, Shi VC, Solomon SD, Swedberg K, Zile M, Andersen K, Arango JL, Arnold JM, Belohlavek J, Bohm M, Boytsov S, Burgess LJ, Cabrera W, Calvo C, Chen CH, Dukat A, Duarte YC, Erglis A, Fu M, Gomez E, Gonzalez-Medina A, Hagege AA, Huang J, Katova T, Kiatchoosakun S, Kim KS, Kozan O, Llamas EB, Martinez F, Merkely B, Mendoza I, Mosterd A, Negrusz-Kawecka M, Peuhkurinen K, Ramires FJ, Refsgaard J, Rosenthal A, Senni M, Sibulo AS Jr, Silva-Cardoso J, Squire IB, Starling RC, Teerlink JR, Vanhaecke J, Vinereanu D, Wong RC. Angiotensin receptor neprilysin inhibition compared with enalapril on the risk of clinical progression in surviving patients with heart failure. Circulation. 2015;131(1):54–61.
80. McMurray J, Packer M, Desai A, Gong J, Greenlaw N, Lefkowitz M, Rizkala A, Shi V, Rouleau J, Solomon S, Swedberg K, Zile MR, Andersen K, Arango JL, Arnold M, Belohlavek J, Bohm M, Boytsov S, Burgess L, Cabrera W, Chen CH, Erglis A, Fu M, Gomez E, Gonzalez A, Hagege AA, Katova T, Kiatchoosakun S, Kim KS, Bayram E, Martinez F, Merkely B, Mendoza I, Mosterd A, Negrusz-Kawecka M, Peuhkurinen K, Ramires F, Refsgaard J, Senni M, Sibulo AS Jr, Silva-Cardoso J, Squire I, Starling RC, Vinereanu D, Teerlink JR, Wong R. A putative placebo analysis of the effects of LCZ696 on clinical outcomes in heart failure. Eur Heart J. 2015;36(7):434–9.
81. Jhund PS, Claggett B, Packer M, Zile MR, Voors AA, Pieske B, Lefkowitz M, Shi V, Bransford T, McMurray JJ, Solomon SD. Independence of the blood pressure lowering effect and efficacy of the angiotensin receptor neprilysin inhibitor, LCZ696, in patients with heart failure with preserved ejection fraction: an analysis of the PARAMOUNT trial. Eur J Heart Fail. 2014;16(6):671–7.
82. Ruilope LM, Dukat A, Bohm M, Lacourciere Y, Gong J, Lefkowitz MP. Blood-pressure reduction with LCZ696, a novel dual-acting inhibitor of the angiotensin II receptor and neprilysin: a randomised, double-blind, placebo-controlled, active comparator study. Lancet. 2010;375(9722):1255–66.
83. Gan L, Langenickel T, Petruck J, Kode K, Rajman I, Chandra P, Zhou W, Rebello S, Sunkara G. Effects of age and sex on the pharmacokinetics of LCZ696, an angiotensin receptor neprilysin inhibitor. J Clin Pharmacol. 2016;56(1):78–86.
84. Coats A. Omapatrilat- the story of overture and octave. Int J Cardiol. 2002;86(1):1.
85. Campbell DJ, Krum H, Esler MD. Losartan increases bradykinin levels in hypertensive humans. Circulation. 2005;111(3):315–20.
86. Kario K, Sun N, Chiang FT, Supasyndh O, Baek SH, Inubushi-Molessa A, Zhang Y, Gotou H, Lefkowitz M, Zhang J. Efficacy and safety of LCZ696, a first-in-class angiotensin receptor neprilysin inhibitor, in Asian patients with hypertension: a randomized, double-blind, placebo-controlled study. Hypertension. 2014;63(4):698–705.
87. Takaki Y, Iwata N, Tsubuki S, Taniguchi S, Toyoshima S, Lu B, Gerard NP, Gerard C, Lee HJ, Shirotani K, Saido TC. Biochemical identification of the neutral endopeptidase family member responsible for the catabolism of amyloid beta peptide in the brain. J Biochem. 2000;128(6):897–902.
88. Baranello RJ, Bharani KL, Padmaraju V, Chopra N, Lahiri DK, Greig NH, Pappolla MA, Sambamurti K. Amyloid-beta protein clearance and degradation (ABCD) pathways and their role in Alzheimer's disease. Curr Alzheimer Res. 2015;12(1):32–46.
89. Iwatsubo T, Odaka A, Suzuki N, Mizusawa H, Nukina N, Ihara Y. Visualization of a beta 42(43) and a beta 40 in senile plaques with end-specific a beta monoclonals: evidence that an initially deposited species is a beta 42(43). Neuron. 1994;13(1):45–53.
90. Sorrentino P, Iuliano A, Polverino A, Jacini F, Sorrentino G. The dark sides of amyloid in Alzheimer's disease pathogenesis. FEBS Lett. 2014;588(5):641–52.
91. Langenickel TH, Tsubouchi C, Ayalasomayajula S, Pal P, Valentin MA, Hinder M, Jhee S, Gevorkyan H, Rajman I. The effect of LCZ696 on amyloid-beta concentrations in cerebrospinal fluid in healthy subjects. Br J Clin Pharmacol. 2016;81(5):878–90.
92. Brunner La Rocca HP, Rickenbacher P, Muzzarelli S, Schindler R, Maeder MT, Jeker U, Kiowski W, Leventhal ME, Pfister O, Osswald S, Pfisterer ME, Rickli H. End-of-life preferences of elderly patients with chronic heart failure. Eur Heart J. 2012;33(6):752–9.
93. Pitt B, Kober L, Ponikowski P, Gheorghiade M, Filippatos G, Krum H, Nowack C, Kolkhof P, Kim SY, Zannad F. Safety and tolerability of the novel non-steroidal mineralocorticoid receptor antagonist BAY 94-8862 in patients with chronic heart failure and mild or moderate chronic kidney disease: a randomized, double-blind trial. Eur Heart J. 2013;34(31):2453–63.
94. Filippatos G, Anker SD, Bohm M, Gheorghiade M, Kober L, Krum H, Maggioni AP, Ponikowski P, Voors AA, Zannad F, Kim SY, Nowack C, Palombo G, Kolkhof P, Kimmeskamp-Kirschbaum N, Pieper A, Pitt B. A randomized controlled study of finerenone vs. eplerenone in patients with worsening chronic heart failure and diabetes mellitus and/or chronic kidney disease. Eur Heart J. 2016;37(27):2105–14.
95. Lea WB, Kwak ES, Luther JM, Fowler SM, Wang Z, Ma J, Fogo AB, Brown NJ. Aldosterone antagonism or synthase inhibition reduces end-organ damage induced by treatment with angiotensin and high salt. Kidney Int. 2009;75(9):936–44.
96. Romero CA, Orias M, Weir MR. Novel RAAS agonists and antagonists: clinical applications and controversies. Nat Rev Endocrinol. 2015;11(4):242–52.

97. Parajuli N, Ramprasath T, Patel VB, Wang W, Putko B, Mori J, Oudit GY. Targeting angiotensin-converting enzyme 2 as a new therapeutic target for cardiovascular diseases. Can J Physiol Pharmacol. 2014;92(7):558–65.
98. Patel VB, Zhong JC, Grant MB, Oudit GY. Role of the ACE2/angiotensin 1-7 Axis of the renin-angiotensin system in heart failure. Circ Res. 2016;118(8):1313–26.
99. Bertagnolli M, Casali KR, De Sousa FB, Rigatto K, Becker L, Santos SH, Dias LD, Pinto G, Dartora DR, Schaan BD, Milan RD, Irigoyen MC, Santos RA. An orally active angiotensin-(1-7) inclusion compound and exercise training produce similar cardiovascular effects in spontaneously hypertensive rats. Peptides. 2014;51:65–73.
100. Sangwai M, Vavia P. Amorphous ternary cyclodextrin nanocomposites of telmisartan for oral drug delivery: improved solubility and reduced pharmacokinetic variability. Int J Pharm. 2013;453(2):423–32.
101. Ferreira AJ, Jacoby BA, Araujo CA, Macedo FA, Silva GA, Almeida AP, Caliari MV, Santos RA. The nonpeptide angiotensin-(1–7) receptor mas agonist AVE-0991 attenuates heart failure induced by myocardial infarction. Am J Physiol Heart Circ Physiol. 2007;292(2):H1113–9.
102. Unger T, Dahlof B. Compound 21, the first orally active, selective agonist of the angiotensin type 2 receptor (AT2): implications for AT2 receptor research and therapeutic potential. J Renin-Angiotensin-Aldosterone Syst. 2010;11(1):75–7.
103. Campbell DJ. Vaccination against high blood pressure. Curr Pharm Des. 2012;18(7):1005–10.
104. Sica DA. Pharmacotherapy in congestive heart failure: drug absorption in the management of congestive heart failure: loop diuretics. Congest Heart Fail. 2003;9(5):287–92.
105. Felker GM, Lee KL, Bull DA, Redfield MM, Stevenson LW, Goldsmith SR, Lewinter MM, Deswal A, Rouleau JL, Ofili EO, Anstrom KJ, Hernandez AF, McNulty SE, Velazquez EJ, Kfoury AG, Chen HH, Givertz MM, Semigran MJ, Bart BA, Mascette AM, Braunwald E, O'Connor CM. Diuretic strategies in patients with acute decompensated heart failure. N Engl J Med. 2011;364(9):797–805.
106. Grinstead WC, Francis MJ, Marks GF, Tawa CB, Zoghbi WA, Young JB. Discontinuation of chronic diuretic therapy in stable congestive heart failure secondary to coronary artery disease or to idiopathic dilated cardiomyopathy. Am J Cardiol. 1994;73(12):881–6.
107. Faris RF, Flather M, Purcell H, Poole-Wilson PA, Coats AJ. Diuretics for heart failure. Cochrane Database Syst Rev. 2012;15(2):Cd003838.
108. Faris RF, Flather M, Purcell H, Poole-Wilson PA, Coats AJ. WITHDRAWN: diuretics for heart failure. Cochrane Database Syst Rev. 2016;4:Cd003838.
109. Cosin J, Diez J. Torasemide in chronic heart failure: results of the TORIC study. Eur J Heart Fail. 2002;4(4):507–13.
110. Gnanaraj F, von Haehling S, Anker SD, Raj DS, Radhakrishnan J. The relevance of congestion in the cardio-renal syndrome. Kidney Int. 2013;83(3):384–91.
111. Packer M, Gheorghiade M, Young JB, Costantini PJ, Adams KF, Cody RJ, Smith LK, Van Voorhees L, Gourley LA, Jolly MK. Withdrawal of digoxin from patients with chronic heart failure treated with angiotensin-converting-enzyme inhibitors. RADIANCE study. N Engl J Med. 1993;329(1):1–7.
112. Uretsky BF, Young JB, Shahidi FE, Yellen LG, Harrison MC, Jolly MK. Randomized study assessing the effect of digoxin withdrawal in patients with mild to moderate chronic congestive heart failure: results of the PROVED trial. PROVED investigative group. J Am Coll Cardiol. 1993;22(4):955–62.
113. Hopper I, Samuel R, Hayward C, Tonkin A, Krum H. Can medications be safely withdrawn in patients with stable chronic heart failure? Systematic review and meta-analysis. J Card Fail. 2014;20(7):522–32.
114. The effect of digoxin on mortality and morbidity in patients with heart failure. The Digitalis investigation group. N Engl J Med. 1997;336(8):525–33.
115. Remme WJ, Swedberg K. Guidelines for the diagnosis and treatment of chronic heart failure. Eur Heart J. 2001;22(17):1527–60.
116. Turakhia MP, Santangeli P, Winkelmayer WC, Xu X, Ullal AJ, Than CT, Schmitt S, Holmes TH, Frayne SM, Phibbs CS, Yang F, Hoang DD, Ho PM, Heidenreich PA. Increased mortality associated with digoxin in contemporary patients with atrial fibrillation: findings from the TREAT-AF study. J Am Coll Cardiol. 2014;64(7):660–8.
117. Ziff OJ, Lane DA, Samra M, Griffith M, Kirchhof P, Lip GY, Steeds RP, Townend J, Kotecha D. Safety and efficacy of digoxin: systematic review and meta-analysis of observational and controlled trial data. BMJ. 2015;351:h4451.
118. Chamaria S, Desai AM, Reddy PC, Olshansky B, Dominic P. Digoxin use to control ventricular rate in patients with atrial fibrillation and heart failure is not associated with increased mortality. Cardiol Res Pract. 2015;2015:314041.
119. Ahmed A, Rich MW, Love TE, Lloyd-Jones DM, Aban IB, Colucci WS, Adams KF, Gheorghiade M. Digoxin and reduction in mortality and hospitalization in heart failure: a comprehensive post hoc analysis of the DIG trial. Eur Heart J. 2006;27(2):178–86.
120. Muzzarelli S, Stricker H, Pfister O, Foglia P, Moschovitis G, Mombelli G, Brunner-La RH. Individual dosage of digoxin in patients with heart failure. QJM. 2011;104(4):309–17.
121. Ahmed A, Young JB, Gheorghiade M. The underuse of digoxin in heart failure, and approaches to appropriate use. CMAJ. 2007;176(5):641–3.
122. Katsiki N, Doumas M, Mikhailidis DP. Lipids, statins and heart failure: an update. Curr Pharm Des. 2016;22(31):4796–806.
123. Kjekshus J, Apetrei E, Barrios V, Bohm M, Cleland JG, Cornel JH, Dunselman P, Fonseca C, Goudev A, Grande P, Gullestad L, Hjalmarson A, Hradec J, Janosi A, Kamensky G, Komajda M, Korewicki J, Kuusi T, Mach F, Mareev V, McMurray JJ, Ranjith N, Schaufelberger M, Vanhaecke J, van Veldhuisen DJ, Waagstein F, Wedel H, Wikstrand J. Rosuvastatin in older patients with systolic heart failure. N Engl J Med. 2007;357(22):2248–61.
124. Tavazzi L, Maggioni AP, Marchioli R, Barlera S, Franzosi MG, Latini R, Lucci D, Nicolosi GL, Porcu M, Tognoni G. Effect of rosuvastatin in patients with chronic heart failure (the GISSI-HF trial): a randomised, double-blind, placebo-controlled trial. Lancet. 2008;372(9645):1231–9.
125. Nochioka K, Sakata Y, Miyata S, Miura M, Takada T, Tadaki S, Ushigome R, Yamauchi T, Takahashi J, Shimokawa H. Prognostic impact of statin use in patients with heart failure and preserved ejection fraction. Circ J. 2015;79(3):574–82.
126. Fukuta H, Goto T, Wakami K, Ohte N. The effect of statins on mortality in heart failure with preserved ejection fraction: a meta-analysis of propensity score analyses. Int J Cardiol. 2016;214:301–6.

8 Pharmacotherapy in Heart Failure (II): Beta Adrenergic Blocking Drugs, Ivabradine, Hydralazine and Nitrates

Shirin Zarafshar and Michael B Fowler

8.1 Beta Adrenergic Blocking Drugs

Sympathetic nervous system activation is a cardinal feature of heart failure. Cannon [1] first described this component of the autonomic nervous system as the "fight or flight response" which became activated to react to short bursts of activity associated with "pain, hunger, fear or rage." The principal responses seen in the cardiovascular system are an increase in heart rate and myocardial contractility, an increase in peripheral vasoconstriction, and other alterations in vascular tone causing redirection of blood flow to vital organs. Chidsey [2] was one of the earliest investigators to demonstrate that heart failure was accompanied by chronic activation of the sympathetic nervous system. This was at one time felt to be a beneficial response, helping to restore cardiac output through inotropic and chronotropic actions which were held to be beneficial to the failing heart. Beta adrenergic blocking drugs were believed to be contraindicated in heart failure and labeled as such. An improved understanding of the potential detrimental effects of chronic sympathetic activation emerged with new insights into the pathophysiology of heart failure, and from small clinical studies which suggested patients with heart failure could benefit from treatment with beta adrenergic blockade.

Cohn, who was at the forefront of recognizing the adverse hemodynamic consequences of the increase in peripheral resistance that occurs in heart failure, demonstrated an inverse relationship between circulating levels of norepinephrine and survival in patients with chronic congestive heart failure [3]. Studies on failing human myocardium obtained at the time of cardiac transplantation, led by Michael Bristow, revealed profound alterations in the sensitivity to chronic sympathetic activation. He demonstrated that failing myocardium had selective down regulation of beta-1 adrenergic receptors leading to catecholamine subsensitivity [4].

Chronic heart failure was being increasingly recognized as a condition characterized by an exuberant response of the neuronal hormonal system that normally regulates contractility, the response to injury, and regulation of salt and water balance [5]. Although natriuretic peptides and other vasodilator hormones become activated, the dominant influence of the complex series of responses to the heart failure state is one of vasoconstriction, salt and water retention, and a progressive myocardial remodeling process that contributes to disease progression. This pathophysiology is relatively well understood and accepted in patients where the response to injury is heart failure with reduced ejection fraction. It is this group of patients that have been shown to respond to anti-adrenergic therapy with beta adrenergic blocking drugs. These patients also require therapy directed against the renin-angiotensin-aldosterone system and will also respond to vasodilator therapy, specifically combination therapy with hydralazine and nitrates. Recently patients who have been shown to have a persistent relative tachycardia in sinus rhythm despite optimal tolerated doses of beta adrenergic blocking drugs have been demonstrated to have modest clinical benefit when ivabradine, a drug that slows heart rate in sinus rhythm, is given.

8.2 Beta Adrenergic Blocking Drugs: Early Studies

In 1975 Waagstein [6] reported for the first time that patients with idiopathic dilated cardiomyopathy had improvements in parameters of systolic and diastolic function and appeared to tolerate and improve clinically when treated with beta-1 selective beta blocking drugs. The same group from Gothenburg, Sweden subsequently reported in small single center studies that patients appeared to derive long-term benefit from this therapy. Studies from Stanford showed an improvement in left ventricular ejection fraction, restoration

S. Zarafshar (✉) · M. B. Fowler
Department of Cardiovascular Medicine, Stanford University, Stanford, CA, USA
e-mail: shirin@stanford.edu

D. S. Feldman, P. Mohacsi (eds.), *Heart Failure*, Cardiovascular Medicine, https://doi.org/10.1007/978-3-319-98184-0_8

of myocardial beta −1 adrenergic receptor density, and an apparent recovery of contractile responses to dobutamine following therapy with metoprolol tartrate [7]. The first randomized trial to evaluate the effect of beta blockade in patients with heart failure was a single center study by Engelmeier [8] which appeared to confirm a clinical benefit. The MDC study was the first multi-center study of metoprolol tartrate in patients with dilated cardiomyopathy [9]. The study found that patients randomized to metoprolol were less likely to die or be listed for cardiac transplantation. These early studies and a greater appreciation of the potential detriment from chronic sympathetic over-activity resulted in a series of pivotal studies which clearly established that patients with chronic heart failure, irrespective of etiology, and a reduced ejection fraction, had an important reduction in the risk of death and reduced risk of hospitalization for any reason, and specifically for heart failure exacerbation, when treated with certain beta blocking drugs.

8.3 Beta Adrenergic Blocking Drugs: Randomized Trials

Evidence supporting the routine use of certain beta adrenergic blocking drugs in patients with heart failure and a reduced ejection fraction is provided by four randomized trials order which demonstrated an important statistically significant benefit. The original study was a four-component trial designed to establish the safety and efficacy of carvedilol in heart failure. On the basis of the six-minute walk test, patients were separately randomized into trials designed to evaluate the drug in mild, moderate, and severe heart failure. Two moderate heart failure severity trial designs were completed; one, although recruiting a relatively small number of patients, remains the only study which specifically explored the dose response to beta adrenergic blocking drugs [10]. An independent data safety board recommended early discontinuation of the US carvedilol trials program when the mortality was observed to be 65% lower in the patients randomized to carvedilol compared to the placebo group [11]. Patients recruited into this trial needed a systolic blood pressure greater than 85 mmHg and deemed stable outpatients. They had to be on optimal doses of diuretics and receiving treatment, if tolerated with an ACE inhibitor. Patients were required have a reduced left ventricle ejection fraction to enter the trial (HFrEF). Patients with major impairment of renal or hepatic function were excluded. The placebo annualized mortality of approximately 10% is consistent with other trials in NYHA functional class II heart failure. MERIT HF [12] and CIBIS 2 [13] were multi-center randomized trials designed as survival trials. Entry criteria were similar to those of the US carvedilol trials program. None of these trials were designed with a run-in period. All these studies recruited patients with HFrEF of ischemic or non-ischemic etiology. The results from these studies show an important, approximately 35% reduction in mortality with carvedilol, metoprolol succinate, or bisoprolol. All-cause and heart failure re-hospitalization was reduced. Patients with ischemic or non-ischemic etiology of heart failure appeared to derive a similar benefit. Although the CIBS study purported to enroll patients with class II and III heart failure, the approximately 10% per year mortality in the placebo arm was more characteristic of a patient population with class II heart failure. In order to address the concern that patients with advanced heart failure may not benefit, the COPERNICUS study was designed to evaluate the role of carvedilol in patients with severe heart failure. Patients had to have an LVEF of less than 25% to be eligible for this study. This study achieved its primary endpoint and survival in the carvedilol group was improved by a remarkable 34% [14]. Again the risk of hospitalization was reduced. In this study the initial dose of carvedilol was 3.125 mg twice daily, gradually up titrated to a target dose of 25 mg twice daily. In this patient population, the placebo annualized mortality was 18.5%. Although this is by far the most severe heart failure patient population ever evaluated in a large, multicenter, randomized trial of beta adrenergic blocking therapy, this mortality rate is still considerably lower than that described in refractory heart failure patients who are experiencing frequent readmission where the six-month mortality may be as high as 50%.

8.4 Beta Adrenergic Blocking Drugs: Specific Properties

More than perhaps most classes of drugs, beta adrenergic blocking drugs exhibit multiple differences in their pharmacology. All the drugs shown in randomized trials to be beneficial are lipophilic. This confers a lidocaine-like membrane stabilizing effect, and means that these drugs cross the blood brain barrier. They cross the placental barrier and will present in breast milk. Beta-one selective agents, such as metoprolol and bisoprolol, will not tend to increase peripheral resistance. This vasoconstriction is a detrimental effect of beta-2 adrenergic receptor blockade, particularly in patients with heart failure seen with non-selective agents due to blocking of peripheral beta-2 adrenergic receptors, which are vasodilatory. Carvedilol, which is a nonselective agent, is free from this disadvantage due to the peripheral vasodilatation caused by the blocking alpha-1 adrenergic receptors. Other differences between agents including possible different actions on beta receptor density, and other ancillary properties such as an anti-oxidant effect, lend caution to regarding all beta adrenergic blocking drugs as being necessarily equally effective or having exactly similar impact in patients. In a hypertensive patient population with type II diabetes the vasodilatation from carvedilol compared to metoprolol was the probable explanation all improvements in insulin sensitivity and differences in hemoglobin A-1 C reported when comparing the two agents (GEMINI trial [15]). In the longest trial of beta-adrenergic blocking drugs in heart failure, the COMET study compared metoprolol with carvedilol [16]. The study has been criticized because the short acting salt (tartrate) of metoprolol was used although this does not have an impact on the beta receptor blocking properties of metoprolol, but does influence the pharmacokinetics. One major limitation of this comparison study between two agents in the same class is that metoprolol tartrate had only been used in one randomized multicenter trial in heart failure (MDC trial) and that an effective dose of the tartrate salt had never been established. This study demonstrated that the majority of patients on a comprehensive medical regime, which included carvedilol or metoprolol, will die from heart failure. Out of a total of 3209 patients, 1112 patients (600 of the patients randomized to metoprolol and 512 of the patients randomized to carvedilol) died during a mean follow-up of 5 years [16]. It was possible to achieve a mean heart rate in this study in the 70s, which demonstrated that the majority of patients treated with the blocking drugs under the circumstances of a clinical trial could be titrated to the dose of either drug which achieved goal target heart rate without resorting to the additional use of ivabradine (*vide infra*).

8.5 Beta Adrenergic Blocking Drugs: Limitations in the Clinical Trials Evidence.

The US heart failure guidelines have divided patients with symptomatic heart failure into stage C and stage D categories. The stage D patients are the group with refractory heart failure. The recommendation from the AHA/ACC guidelines is for these end-stage patients to remain on the drugs that have been shown to be beneficial in randomized trials of stable patients with class C heart failure. There is no good direct evidence supporting this recommendation. Various lines of evidence support the contention that even patients much sicker than those recruited into the COPERNICUS trial are likely benefiting from beta blocking drugs. The observation by Fonarow that patients who are admitted to hospital with an acute exacerbation of heart failure have better outcomes if they were kept on beta adrenergic blocking drugs is important, but propensity analysis may not have able to separate the clinical features associated with a poor prognosis that contributed to what was likely an appropriate decision to discontinue therapy with beta blocking drugs during the hospitalization [17]. Similarly, the incorporation of the absence of therapy with a beta blocking drug to an adverse outcome in the Seattle heart failure score does not necessarily imply that patients who have become intolerant to beta blocking drugs would be better served if they were continued on therapy they appeared not to tolerate. Although there is no clinical trials evidence supporting the use of sympathetically-mediated inotropic agents, dobutamine or milrinone are frequently found to be useful in treating patients with acute decompensated heart failure, especially those with evidence of a low cardiac output state. Some investigators have claimed benefit from a combined use of beta adrenergic blocking drugs with enoximone, a phosphodiesterase inhibitor [18], although this benefit has not been shown in any multicenter clinical trials. Not all trials of beta adrenergic blocking drugs or of studies that modulate and reduce sympathetic exposure to the failing heart have been beneficial. Bucindolol was explored in a dose ranging study where the greatest improvement left ventricular ejection fraction appeared to be greatest at the highest dose. This was the target dose selected in the BEST study [19]. The study did not reach its primary endpoint of survival. Subsequent analysis appeared to show that the response was determined by specific beta adrenergic pathway polymorphisms [20]. It is consistent with the trial data that the dose selected in the BEST trial may have been too high and that modulation of excess catecholamine exposure is needed to strike the balance between harm and benefit. This hypothesis is to some extent supported in clinical practice where patients who have previously tolerated and appeared to benefit from high doses adrenergic blocking drugs require and seem to initially benefit when dose reductions are forced by disease progression. Many of these patients will initially improve with a dose reduction with recovery from severe symptomatic hypotension and clinical and laboratory evidence of a low output state. In many patients a forced reduction in the dose of a previously well-tolerated beta adrenergic blocking drug is often an indicator of a slide into terminal refractory stage D heart failure. This can be used as a relatively reliable indicator of a poor prognosis and used to initiate the process of evaluating selected patients for mechanical support and cardiac transplantation. Further evidence that some level of adrenergic activity may be beneficial can be derived from the results of the MOXCON trial in which moxonidine, a central inhibitor of norepinephrine, reduced circulating norepinephrine levels but increased mortality [21].

8.6 Beta Adrenergic Blocking Drugs: Special Populations

Beta adrenergic blocking drugs benefit in patients with heart failure and a reduced ejection fraction appears to be consistent across various patient groups. Specific trials designed to compare the benefit in patients in specific patient populations have not been performed but subgroup analysis in general has confirmed that the benefit is preserved between the sexes, in patients of different ethnicity, and in subgroups with diabetes. Not all of these analyses have necessarily shown an equal benefit but interpretation of data from subgroup analysis, even if this subgroup analysis was prespecified, is fraught with the potential to provide misleading information. For instance, although the Merit-HF failure study did not appear to show benefit in the patients recruited in the United States or in women, studies with carvedilol have established that women and men drive equal benefit [22]. African-American populations have been shown to benefit in subgroup analysis of carvedilol studies [23]. Small studies have suggested that an Asian population may not tolerate the full target dosages are beta adrenergic blocking drugs shown to be effective in United States and European populations [24]. Interpretation of this data is difficult, and in general it would seem appropriate to treat all patient population with heart failure at a reduced ejection fraction with one of the approved agents and up tirate to maximum tolerated dose if the target dose cannot be reached.

Various studies and registry data have suggested that patients who remain on low doses of beta adrenergic blocking drugs fare less well than patient up titrated to the target dosages used in the trials, and that adrenergic blocker benefits are dose-related [25]. Two factors probably contribute to this observation. First, patients not up titrated likely are not receiving the maximum potential benefit. Second, the patients who really do not tolerate up titration are likely to have more advanced disease with hypotension and possibly symptoms of fatigue with evidence of a low output state preventing successful dose escalation. These patients will have a worse prognosis than individuals with less advanced disease. It remains far from certain that forcing patients to a high dose of a adrenergic blocking drug for which there appears to be true evidence of intolerance would be beneficial to that patient. It is worth noting that in the randomized trials not all patients in the study reached target dose and that the positive results seen in these studies included patients who were maintained below target dose due to intolerance. It is necessary for the treating physician to work closely with each individual patient to titrate to the highest possible tolerate dose while at the same time accepting that some patients may be optimally managed a doses below target.

Elderly patients with heart failure have specifically been evaluated. The SENIORS trial compared nevibolol with placebo in patients who were 70 years old or greater [26]. Although the study was relatively small (2128 patients), it did demonstrate improvement in the combined endpoint of mortality and cardiovascular admission. Uniquely this study did recruit patients with clinical heart failure regardless of ejection fraction. In a pre-specified subgroup analysis, the preserved ejection fraction patient population apparently showed equal benefit to the patient group with reduced left ventricle ejection fraction. This finding has not been replicated. A relatively small study of carvedilol in patients with preserved ejection fraction, the Japanese diastolic heart failure study (J-DHF) showed no difference between carvedilol and a control group for a combined primary outcome of cardiovascular death or unplanned hospitalization for heart failure [27]. During a mean follow-up of 3.2 years, 29 patients in the carvedilol group and 34 patients in the control group met this primary endpoint. Chronotropic incompetence may contribute to the pathophysiology of heart failure with a preserved ejection fraction. Patients in this group category would likely not benefit from the heart rate lowering effects of beta adrenergic blocking drugs. Similarly, patients who have heart failure and a preserved left ventricular ejection fraction with radiation-induced heart disease often have striking tachycardia but appear to be harmed when beta adrenergic blocking drugs are prescribed (personal observation). Presumably in this patient population, stroke volume is low and fixed and cardiac output is dependent on heart rate. Conversely some patients with heart failure and a preserved ejection fraction, classically those with mitral stenosis dependent on heart rate lowering to adequately fill the ventricle. Perhaps the first use of beta adrenergic blocking drugs in heart failure was in patients with rheumatic mitral stenosis. It is likely that some patients with heart failure and a preserved left ventricle ejection fraction will benefit from beta adrenergic blocking drugs but the precise patient population and the patient-specific characteristics which support their use has yet to be determined.

8.7 Beta Adrenergic Blocking Drugs: Practical Considerations

Treatment guidelines, evidence from randomized trials, and even practice performance measures strongly advocate the routine use of beta adrenergic blocking drugs in all patients with heart failure with reduced ejection fraction. It is appropriate to initiate therapy as soon as the patient is approaching optimal volume status. In patients with hypertension and who are clearly well perfused, beta adrenergic blocking drugs should be initiated at the recommended initial starting dose. In patients who remain hypertensive after initiation of therapy, a higher starting dose could be considered and up titration should be rapid. Conversely, those patients with low blood pressure and tenuous clinical status may require lower-than-recommended initial doses and slower up titration of therapy. Although very few hospitalized patients were entered into randomized trials and the majority of trials specifically recruited patients who are felt to be stable, patients do seem to tolerate the initiation of therapy in hospital with little adverse impact on the duration of hospital stay [28].

Most patients with chronic congestive heart failure will tolerate up titration to the target dose of the specific heart failure trials. Patients will need to be seen frequently during this up titration phase to adjust concomitant medications and especially to prevent over-diuresis so that a relative degree of hypovolemia with hypotension is not wrongly attributed to beta adrenergic therapy up titration. Strategies to improve the proportion of patients who can be up titrated to target dosages include changing the timing of other drugs that might lower blood pressure. Once daily angiotensin-converting enzyme inhibitors or angiotensin receptor blockers could be given in the evening before bed while carvedilol could be given twice daily with food or metoprolol succinate in the morning. Once patients become tolerant to the titrated dose, some of these complex timing strategies can often be abandoned in favor of a more convenient and more easily adherent medication schedule.

Patients with left bundle branch block and a QRS duration of great than 150 milliseconds with hypotension and evidence of a low output state may not initially tolerate anti-adrenergic therapy. In this particular patient population, a relatively early implantation of a biventricular pacing device to provide cardiac resynchronization therapy (CRT) will sometimes improve the clinical stability and hemodynamics of a patient to the extent where beta adrenergic blocking drugs can be initiated and successfully up titrated.

In general, the group of patients who have responded well to beta adrenergic blocking drug, should remain on therapy indefinitely. Patients who discontinue beta adrenergic blocking drugs and the other neurohormonal antagonists that have been associated with recovery of left ventricular ejection fraction are at risk of re-development of LV dysfunction and recurrent overt heart failure symptoms. Exceptions might be a patient who recovered from a proven episode of acute myocarditis or heart failure associated with preeclampsia where there are credible reasons for a patient to want to discontinue therapy that is usually well-tolerated and which has been associated with recovery from a serious condition.

In general patients need to be encouraged to take beta adrenergic blocking drugs for the rest of their life when they have been prescribed for heart failure. The majority of patients with heart failure will die from heart failure despite the successful new therapies introduced over the last 30 years. The benefits of beta adrenergic blocking drugs specifically have to be explained to patients and some need to be coached to tolerate the relatively minor symptoms of postural hypotension that so often accompanies their use, particularly in patients who do not have background hypertension.

8.8 Ivabradine

Ivabradine has been developed to treat those patients who are unable to achieve a heart rate less than 70 beats per minute at rest. This new class of medication inhibits the "funny" channel (I_f) in the sinoatrial node, thereby reducing heart rate by a mechanism other than beta 1 inhibition. However, conduction outside the sinoatrial node is not affected, and there is no effect on contractility or repolarization. The SHIFT trial demonstrated improvement for all-cause hospitalization or heart failure hospitalization [29]. However, there was no significant difference in all-cause or cardiovascular mortality between those patients treated with standard medical therapy vs standard medical therapy and ivabradine. Furthermore, the reported benefit of ivabradine was considerably stronger in non-ischemic heart failure patients as compared to ischemic heart failure patients (hazard ratio 0.72 for non ischemics vs hazard ratio 0.87 for ischemics). This raises concern that ivabradine may not be as effective for those patients with ischemic cardiomyopathy [30]. Of note, the SHIFT trial excluded patients who had suffered myocardial infarction in the 60 days prior to enrollment. Nevertheless, the current ACC/AHA recommendations give ivabradine a Class IIa indication for heart failure patients of any etiology on maximally tolerated beta adrenergic blocking drugs with resting heart rate in sinus rhythm greater than 70 beats per minute [31].

8.9 Hydralazine and Nitrates

Early hemodynamic studies of heart failure patients demonstrated increased peripheral vascular resistance [32]. Patients with acute myocardial infarction were one of the first groups studied for acute afterload reduction [33]. A small study of 15 patients demonstrated that nitroprusside infusion helped reduce chest pain, dyspnea, and clinical signs of left ventricular failure in those patients with reduced cardiac index. Efforts to identify oral agents that could help patients with chronically reduced cardiac index included studies of minoxidil, prazosin, and phentolamine [34–36]. These oral agents were not as effective as nitroprusside infusions, however, and eventually combination therapy with hydralazine (a direct arterial vasodilator) and isosorbide dinitrate (ISDN, a relatively long- acting nitrate) were explored after initial exploratory studies of each medication as solitary treatment seemed promising [37, 38]. Two larger studies, V-HeFT I and V-HeFT II were designed to study possible mortality benefits of hydralazine/nitrate therapy. V-HeFT I randomized 642 men with systolic dysfunction to hydralazine (37.5 mg)/ISDN (20 mg), prazosin, or placebo while receiving digoxin and diuretics as standard medical therapy. This study showed decreased mortality at 2 years among those patients treated with hydralazine/ISDN whereas those patients treated with prazosin did not show mortality benefit or improvement in left ventricular ejection fraction [39]. Six years later, the V-HeFT II trial reported that 804 men randomized to enalapril (20 mg) vs. hydralazine (37.5 mg)/ISDN (40 mg) showed significant mortality reduction as compared to placebo. However, those patients treated with enalapril had lower mortality rates as compared to hydralazine/ISDN. On the other hand, peak VO2 and ejection fraction changes were more favorable among those patients treated with hydralazine/ISDN rather than enalapril. The authors concluded that the differential benefits of each regimen might make treatment with all three agents the most efficacious [40].

Retrospective analyses of the V-HeFTI and V-HeFT II studies suggested that African-American patients derived more benefit from hydralazine/ISDN than white patients. The A-HeFT trial was designed to examine if African-American patients with class III-class IV heart failure would benefit more from hydralazine (37.5 mg)/ISDN (20 mg) therapy rather than placebo, in addition to standard medical therapy (ACE inhibitors, aldosterone antagonists, diuretics, and digoxin, [41]). The study of 1050 patients was ended early after the mortality rate in the placebo group was found to be significantly higher than the hydralazine/ISDN group (10% vs 6%, $p = 0.02$). This lead to the first race-based guideline recommendation for heart failure therapy, and the first race-based Federal Drug Administration drug approval. However, the A-HeFT trial was not designed to test whether hydralazine/ISDN was more efficacious than ACE inhibitors or angiotensin receptor blockers. On the other hand, for those patients who are unable to take ACE inhibitors or angiotension receptor blockers, hydralazine/nitrates remain an important heart failure therapy for patients of all ethnicities.

References

1. Cannon W. Bodily changes in pain, hunger, fear, and rage. Philadelphia: Saunders; 1929.
2. Chidsey CA, Braunwald E, Morrow AG. Catecholamine excretion and cardiac stores of norepinephrine in congestive heart failure. Am J Med. 1965;39:442–51.
3. Cohn JN, Levine TB, Olivari MT, Garberg V, Lura D, Francis GS, et al. Plasma norepinephrine as a guide to prognosis in patients with chronic congestive heart failure. N Engl J Med. 1984;311(13):819–23.
4. Bristow MR, Ginsburg R, Minobe W, Cubicciotti RS, Sageman WS, Lurie K, et al. Decreased catecholamine sensitivity and beta-adrenergic-receptor density in failing human hearts. N Engl J Med. 1982;307(4):205–11.
5. Cohn JN, Levine TB, Francis GS, Goldsmith S. Neurohumoral control mechanisms in congestive heart failure. Am Heart J. 1981;102(3 Pt 2):509–14.
6. Waagstein F, Hjalmarson A, Varnauskas E, Wallentin I. Effect of chronic beta-adrenergic receptor blockade in congestive cardiomyopathy. Br Heart J. 1975;37(10):1022–36.
7. Heilbrunn SM, Shah P, Bristow MR, Valantine HA, Ginsburg R, Fowler MB. Increased beta-receptor density and improved hemodynamic response to catecholamine stimulation during long-term metoprolol therapy in heart failure from dilated cardiomyopathy. Circulation. 1989;79(3):483–90.
8. Engelmeier RS, O'Connell JB, Walsh R, Rad N, Scanlon PJ, Gunnar RM. Improvement in symptoms and exercise tolerance by metoprolol in patients with dilated cardiomyopathy: a double-blind, randomized, placebo-controlled trial. Circulation. 1985;72(3):536–46.
9. Waagstein F, Bristow MR, Swedberg K, Camerini F, Fowler MB, Silver MA, et al. Beneficial effects of metoprolol in idiopathic dilated cardiomyopathy. Metoprolol in Dilated Cardiomyopathy (MDC) Trial Study Group. Lancet. 1993;342(8885):1441–6.
10. Bristow MR, O'Connell JB, Gilbert EM, French WJ, Leatherman G, Kantrowitz NE, et al. Dose-response of chronic beta-blocker treatment in heart failure from either idiopathic dilated or ischemic cardiomyopathy. Bucindolol Investigators. Circulation. 1994;89(4):1632–42.
11. Packer M, Bristow MR, Cohn JN, Colucci WS, Fowler MB, Gilbert EM, et al. The effect of carvedilol on morbidity and mortality in patients with chronic heart failure. U.S. Carvedilol Heart Failure Study Group.[see comment]. N Engl J Med. 1996;334(21):1349–55.
12. MERIT-HF group. Effect of metoprolol CR/XL in chronic heart failure: Metoprolol CR/XL Randomised Intervention Trial in Congestive Heart Failure (MERIT-HF). Lancet. 1999;353(9169):2001–2007.
13. CIBIS-II Investigators and Committees. The Cardiac Insufficiency Bisoprolol Study II (CIBIS-II): a randomised trial. Lancet. 1999;353(9146):9–13.
14. Packer M, Coats AJ, Fowler MB, Katus HA, Krum H, Mohacsi P, et al. Effect of carvedilol on survival in severe chronic heart failure. [see comment]. N Engl J Med. 2001;344(22):1651–8.
15. Bakris GL, Fonseca V, Katholi RE, McGill JB, Messerli FH, Phillips RA, et al. Metabolic effects of carvedilol vs metoprolol in patients with type 2 diabetes mellitus and hypertension: a randomized controlled trial. JAMA. 2004;292(18):2227–36.
16. Poole-Wilson PA, Swedberg K, Cleland JG, Di Lenarda A, Hanrath P, Komajda M, et al. Comparison of carvedilol and metoprolol on clinical outcomes in patients with chronic heart failure in the Carvedilol Or Metoprolol European Trial (COMET): randomised controlled trial. Lancet. 2003;362(9377):7–13.
17. Fonarow GC, Abraham WT, Albert NM, Gattis WA, Gheorghiade M, Greenberg B, et al. Organized program to initiate lifesaving treatment in hospitalized patients with heart failure (OPTIMIZE-HF): rationale and design. Am Heart J. 2004;148(1):43–51.
18. Gilbert EM, Hershberger RE, Wiechmann RJ, Movsesian MA, Bristow MR. Pharmacologic and hemodynamic effects of combined beta-agonist stimulation and phosphodiesterase inhibition in the failing human heart. Chest. 1995;108(6):1524–32.
19. Beta-Blocker Evaluation of Survival Trial I. A trial of the beta-blocker bucindolol in patients with advanced chronic heart failure. N Engl J Med. 2001;344(22):1659–67.
20. Port JD, Bristow MR. Altered beta-adrenergic receptor gene regulation and signaling in chronic heart failure. J Mol Cell Cardiol. 2001;33(5):887–905.
21. Cohn JN, Pfeffer MA, Rouleau J, Sharpe N, Swedberg K, Straub M, et al. Adverse mortality effect of central sympathetic inhibition with sustained-release moxonidine in patients with heart failure (MOXCON). Eur J Heart Fail. 2003;5(5):659–67.
22. Ghali JK, Pina IL, Gottlieb SS, Deedwania PC, Wikstrand JC. Metoprolol CR/XL in female patients with heart failure: analysis of the experience in metoprolol extended-release random-

ized intervention trial in heart failure (MERIT-HF). Circulation. 2002;105(13):1585–91.
23. Shekelle PG, Rich MW, Morton SC, Atkinson CS, Tu W, Maglione M, et al. Efficacy of angiotensin-converting enzyme inhibitors and beta-blockers in the management of left ventricular systolic dysfunction according to race, gender, and diabetic status: a meta-analysis of major clinical trials. J Am Coll Cardiol. 2003;41(9):1529–38.
24. Hori M, Sasayama S, Kitabatake A, Toyo-Oka T, Handa S, Yokoyama M, et al. Low-dose carvedilol improves left ventricular function and reduces cardiovascular hospitalization in Japanese patients with chronic heart failure: the multicenter carvedilol heart failure dose assessment (MUCHA) trial. Am Heart J. 2004;147(2):324–30.
25. Bristow MR, Gilbert EM, Abraham WT, Adams KF, Fowler MB, Hershberger RE, et al. Carvedilol produces dose-related improvements in left ventricular function and survival in subjects with chronic heart failure. MOCHA Investigators Circulation. 1996;94(11):2807–16.
26. Flather MD, Shibata MC, Coats AJ, Van Veldhuisen DJ, Parkhomenko A, Borbola J, et al. Randomized trial to determine the effect of nebivolol on mortality and cardiovascular hospital admission in elderly patients with heart failure (SENIORS). Eur Heart J. 2005;26(3):215–25.
27. Yamamoto K, Origasa H, Hori M, Investigators JD. Effects of carvedilol on heart failure with preserved ejection fraction: the Japanese diastolic heart failure study (J-DHF). Eur J Heart Fail. 2013;15(1):110–8.
28. Fonarow GC. The role of in-hospital initiation of cardioprotective therapies to improve treatment rates and clinical outcomes. Rev Cardiovasc Med. 2002;3(Suppl 3):S2–S10.
29. Swedberg K, Komajda M, Bohm M, Borer JS, Ford I, Dubost-Brama A, et al. Ivabradine and outcomes in chronic heart failure (SHIFT): a randomised placebo-controlled study. Lancet. 2010;376(9744):875–85.
30. McMurray JJ. It is BEAUTIFUL we should be concerned about, not SIGNIFY: is ivabradine less effective in ischaemic compared with non-ischaemic LVSD? Eur Heart J. 2015;36(31):2047–9.
31. Yancy CW, Jessup M, Bozkurt B, Butler J, Casey DE Jr, Colvin MM, et al. 2016 ACC/AHA/HFSA focused update on new pharmacological therapy for heart failure: an update of the 2013 ACCF/AHA guideline for the management of heart failure: a report of the American College of Cardiology/American Heart Association task force on clinical practice guidelines and the Heart Failure Society of America. J Am Coll Cardiol. 2016;68(13):1476–88.
32. Cohn JN. Blood pressure and cardiac performance. Am J Med. 1973;55(3):351–61.
33. Franciosa JA, Limas CJ, Guiha NH, Rodriguera E, Cohn JN. Improved left ventricular function during nitroprusside infusion in acute myocardial infarction. Lancet. 1972;1(7752):650–4.
34. Franciosa JA, Cohn JN. Effects of minoxidil on hemodynamics in patients with congestive heart failure. Circulation. 1981;63(3):652–7.
35. Miller RR, Awan NA, Maxwell KS, Mason DT. Sustained reduction of cardiac impedance and preload in congestive heart failure with the antihypertensive vasodilator prazosin. N Engl J Med. 1977;297(6):303–7.
36. Schreiber R, Maier PT, Gunnar RM, Loeb HS. Hemodynamic improvement following a single dose of oral phentolamine. Administration in patients with chronic low output cardiac failure. Chest. 1979;76(5):571–5.
37. Massie B, Chatterjee K, Werner J, Greenberg B, Hart R, Parmley WW. Hemodynamic advantage of combined administration of hydralazine orally and nitrates nonparenterally in the vasodilator therapy of chronic heart failure. Am J Cardiol. 1977;40(5):794–801.
38. Pierpont GL, Cohn JN, Franciosa JA. Combined oral hydralazine-nitrate therapy in left ventricular failure. Hemodynamic equivalency to sodium nitroprusside. Chest. 1978;73(1):8–13.
39. Cohn JN, Archibald DG, Ziesche S, Franciosa JA, Harston WE, Tristani FE, et al. Effect of vasodilator therapy on mortality in chronic congestive heart failure. Results of a veterans administration cooperative study. N Engl J Med. 1986;314(24):1547–52.
40. Cohn JN, Johnson G, Ziesche S, Cobb F, Francis G, Tristani F, et al. A comparison of enalapril with hydralazine-isosorbide dinitrate in the treatment of chronic congestive heart failure. N Engl J Med. 1991;325(5):303–10.
41. Taylor AL, Ziesche S, Yancy C, Carson P, D'Agostino R Jr, Ferdinand K, et al. Combination of isosorbide dinitrate and hydralazine in blacks with heart failure. N Engl J Med. 2004;351(20):2049–57.

Device Therapy in the Heart Failure

9

Troy Rhodes and Raul Weiss

9.1 Introduction

In patients with heart failure (HF), the two main causes of death are sudden cardiac death (SCD) and progressive pump failure. In the Framingham Heart Study, HF increased overall and SCD mortality fivefold [1]. In patients with Class II or III HF, the mode of death is more likely be to "sudden" while in patients with Class IV HF, it is more likely to be due to pump failure [2]. The most common cause of SCD is the degeneration of ventricular tachycardia (VT) to ventricular fibrillation (VF), although pulseless electrical activity (PEA) and bradyarrhythmias account for up to one-third of cases [3]. Electrical defibrillation is the only effective approach for terminating VF. Following success with external defibrillation, an implantable defibrillator was developed in the mid-1960s and the first automatic internal defibrillator was implanted in humans in 1980 [4, 5].

Primary prevention of SCD refers to a therapy intended to prevent SCD who have not yet experienced symptomatic sustained VT or VF or sudden cardiac arrest (SCA) but are at increased risk for such events due to their heart failure since SCD may be the first presentation of a ventricular arrhythmia. The role of a primary prevention implantable cardioverter-defibrillator (ICD) depends upon the severity and etiology of the left ventricular (LV) dysfunction and the severity of clinical heart failure. Patients with heart failure who experience sustained ventricular tachycardia or SCA are at high risk for recurrence and will typically have an ICD implanted for secondary prevention of SCD. This chapter will discuss device therapy in HF, clinical trials and guidelines for implantation of ICDs and cardiac resynchronization therapy (CRT), ambulatory device monitoring, and the management of patients with VT and ICD therapies.

T. Rhodes
Division of Cardiovascular Medicine, University of Iowa Hospitals and Clinics, Iowa City, IA, USA

R. Weiss (✉)
David Heart and Lung Research Institute, Ohio State University Medical Center, Columbus, OH, USA
e-mail: raul.weiss@osumc.edu

9.2 Implantable Cardioverter Defibrillators (ICDs)

9.2.1 Ischemic Cardiomyopathy

Patients who have had a myocardial infarction (MI) leading to a reduced systolic function are at increased risk of SCD, most commonly due to ventricular tachyarrhythmias, and prophylactic ICD implantation in selected patients with ischemic cardiomyopathy reduces mortality. ICD therapy for primary prevention of SCD in patients with ischemic cardiomyopathy due is recommended for those with LV ejection fraction (LVEF) $\leq$ 35% with New York Association (NYHA) functional Class II or III and those with LVEF $\leq$ 30% with NYHA I symptoms. Patients should be at least 40 days post MI and more than 3 months following revascularization and on guideline-directed medical therapy (GDMT) since these interventions may lead to significant improvement in systolic function and heart failure class and potentially eliminate the need for a primary prevention device. The indications for ICD implantation were derived from the inclusion criteria of several major randomized trials enrolling patients with ischemic cardiomyopathy in the first weeks (early) and more than 4–6 weeks following MI (late) [6].

The Multicenter Automatic Defibrillator Implantation Trial (MADIT-I) was the first randomized clinical trial (RCT) to show the role of ICDs in primary prevention of SCD in asymptomatic patients with prior MI, nonsustained VT (NSVT) on ambulatory monitoring, LVEF $\leq$ 35%, and inducible sustained monomorphic VT (SMVT) during electrophysiology study (EPS) that remained inducible following the administration of procainamide. Patients were randomly assigned to pharmacologic therapy including an anti-arrhythmic medication at the discretion of the clinician

D. S. Feldman, P. Mohacsi (eds.), *Heart Failure*, Cardiovascular Medicine, https://doi.org/10.1007/978-3-319-98184-0_9

(most commonly amiodarone) or to ICD therapy were followed an average of 27 months. There was a significant reduction in overall mortality, cardiac mortality, and arrhythmic deaths in the ICD group with an average survival of 3.7 years compared to 2.8 years in those receiving medical therapy. Subset analysis showed a survival benefit for ICD for patients with LVEF < 26%, more severe CHF or QRS duration of ≥120 ms. MADIT-I was limited by a small number of patients (<200) and events, a low incidence of subsequent NSVT on ambulatory monitoring, only enrolling patients with inducible VT not suppressed or slowed by procainamide, and higher beta-blocker use in the ICD group. While a landmark study for the use of ICDs in primary prevention of SCD, MADIT-I has been supplanted by subsequent trials [7].

The Multicenter Automatic Defibrillator Implantation Trial II (MADIT-II) randomized 1232 patients with prior MI (>30 days and more than 3 months if bypass surgery had been performed) and LVEF ≤ 30% to prophylactic ICD or conventional therapy. MADIT-II addressed some of the limitations of MADIT-I by eliminating the requirement of EP study and the presence of NSVT. After an average follow-up of 20 months, the study was stopped early due to the survival benefit of ICD therapy. Those receiving an ICD had a significantly reduced all-cause mortality of over 5% compared to conventional therapy (14.2% vs 19.8%); the survival benefit was seen in all patient groups and was entirely due to a reduction in sudden cardiac death. There was a nonsignificant trend toward greater benefit in patients with a QRS > 150 ms. An unexpected finding was a higher rate of HF hospitalizations in the ICD group (20% vs 15%), possibly due to a higher incidence of HF progression with the prevention of SCD, myocardial injury as a result of ICD shocks, and the negative impact of unintentional right ventricular pacing [8].

The Coronary Artery Bypass Graft (CABG) Patch trial randomized 900 patients to an epicardial ICD implanted at the time of bypass surgery or medical therapy. Patients had a LVEF <36% with severe CAD requiring surgical revascularization, abnormal signal-averaged ECG, but no history of sustained ventricular tachyarrhythmia or syncope. There was no significant difference in overall or cardiovascular mortality with an average follow-up of 32 months. It is likely that ICD therapy did not improve mortality due to the beneficial effect of coronary revascularization itself in the prevention of sudden cardiac death. It is worth noting the high percentage of epicardial implantation and the high complication rate in ICD Group (approximately 6%) While the impact of percutaneous coronary revascularization was not evaluated, this negative trial is the primary reason why current guidelines do not recommend ICD implantation for patients who have recently undergone coronary revascularization [9].

While not designed as a randomized ICD trial, the Multicenter Unsustained Tachycardia Trial (MUSTT) utilized EPS in the management of high-risk patients enrolling 704 patients with prior MI (4 days to >3 years), LVEF ≤ 40%, asymptomatic NSVT (at least 4 days post MI or post revascularization but within 6 months of enrollment), no history of sustained ventricular tachyarrhythmia or syncope with inducible sustained VT during EPS to standard medical therapy or EPS guided antiarrhythmic therapy, or an ICD (if at least one antiarrhythmic medication was ineffective). After a median follow-up of 39 months, the 2 year (12% vs 18%) and 5 year (25% vs 32%) rates for arrhythmic death or resuscitated SCA were significantly lower for the EPS-guided patients. The reduction in the primary endpoint was largely attributable to ICD therapy and at 5 years, arrhythmic death or resuscitated SCA occurred in 9% of patients with an ICD and 37% of those treated with an antiarrhythmic drug [10]. A subsequent analysis of the MUSST trial in patients with an LVEF 30–40% showed the rate of arrhythmic death at 5 years was significantly increased for those with inducible VT suggesting EP testing may have predictive value in this group [11].

The Sudden Cardiac Death in Heart Failure Trial (SCD-HeFT) randomized 2521 patients with both ischemic (52%) or nonischemic (48%) cardiomyopathy, LVEF ≤ 35% with NYHA Class II or III HF treated with beta-blocker and ACE inhibitor for at least 3 months prior to enrollment to ICD implantation, amiodarone, or placebo with a median follow-up of 46 months. ICD therapy significantly reduced total mortality at 5 years (29% vs 36% with placebo). The benefit of an ICD was comparable for patients with either ischemic or nonischemic cardiomyopathy while amiodarone provided no benefit compared to placebo [12].

9.2.1.1 Early Post-MI Trials

The Defibrillator in Acute Myocardial Infarction Trial (DINAMIT) randomized 674 patients with prior MI (6–40 days, mean of 18 days), LVEF ≤ 35%, and reduced heart rate variability or elevated resting heart rate (≥80 bpm) to either prophylactic ICD or standard medical therapy. With a mean follow-up of 30 months, there was no significant difference in annual all-cause mortality. Arrhythmic deaths were more frequent in the medical therapy group while nonarrhythmic deaths were more frequent in the ICD group [13]. This negative trial provides rationale for the current guidelines that ICD implantation is not recommended until at least 40 days following a MI.

The Immediate Risk Stratification Improves Survival (IRIS) trial randomized 898 patients with a MI in the prior 5–31 days and at least one of the following: LVEF ≤ 40% and resting HR ≥ 90 bpm, NSVT ≥ 150 bpm, or both to ICD therapy or standard medical therapy. With an average follow-up of 37 months, there was no difference in all-cause mortality. As seen in DINAMIT, SCD was higher in the medical therapy group while nonarrhythmic deaths were more frequent in the ICD group [14].

The lack of benefit in the early post-MI trials were likely due to: recovery of LV function, SCD in the early post-MI period due to recurrent ischemia or mechanical complications that an ICD would not effectively treat, and additional risk of ICD implantation immediately following MI [15]. Higher resting HR and reduced HR variability may identify a group of patients with higher mortality from non-arrhythmic causes [16].

9.2.2 Nonischemic Cardiomyopathy

Patients with nonischemic cardiomyopathy are at increased risk for sudden cardiac death from ventricular arrhythmias. While smaller trails suggested no benefit of ICD therapy to these patients, larger trials and meta-analyses have demonstrated mortality benefit from prophylactic ICD implantation. Current guidelines recommend ICD implantation for patients with nonischemic cardiomyopathy with LVEF $\leq$ 35%, NYHA Class II-III, treated with a beta-blocker and ACE inhibitor for at least 3 months prior to implantation.

The Cardiomyopathy Trial (CAT) enrolled 104 patients with $\leq$9 months of nonischemic dilated CM with LVEF $\leq$ 30% to ICD implantation versus medical therapy. The Amiodarone Versus Implantable Cardioverter-Defibrillator trial (AMIOVIRT) randomized 103 patients with nonischemic dilated CM with LVEF $\leq$ 35%, Class I to III CHF, and asymptomatic NSVT to ICD vs amiodarone therapy. Both showed no significant benefit to ICD therapy for all-cause mortality but both were limited by small patient numbers and unexpectedly low mortality rate; also there was no placebo control group in AMIOVIRT [16, 17].

The Defibrillators in Non Ischemic Cardiomyopathy Treatment Evaluation (DEFINITE) randomized 458 patients with NICM, LVEF $\leq$ 35%, NSVT or premature ventricular contractions (PVCs) to ICD or medical therapy. There was a trend towards a reduction in all-cause mortality with an ICD (7.9% vs 14.1% with medical therapy) with a significant reduction in patients with NYHA Class III CHF. While fewer sudden deaths occurred in the ICD group (3 deaths vs 14 deaths in the medication group), the mortality rate in the medical arm was lower than anticipated during study design leading to the trial being underpowered for its primary endpoint [18].

As discussed earlier, SCD-HeFT randomized patients with both ischemic and non-ischemic CM to ICD therapies, amiodarone, or placebo and a significant reduction in overall mortality was seen with ICD therapy with comparable benefit in ischemic and nonischemic patients [12]. ICD therapy was also associated with a short term improvement in psychological wellbeing [19]. There was no survival benefit with amiodarone over placebo [12].

9.2.3 ICD Therapy Is NOT Recommended

ICD therapy is not indicated: ventricular arrhythmias are due to completely reversible conditions (metabolic abnormalities, drugs, trauma) in the absence of structural heart disease; life expectancy less than 1 year; incessant VT or VF; significant psychiatric illness that could be aggravated by ICD therapies or limit follow-up; NYHA Class IV HF refractory to GDMT who are not candidates for transplantation, LVAD, or CRT; syncope without inducible VT or structural heart disease; and patients with structurally normal heart amenable to ablation [6].

9.2.4 ICD System

The transvenous ICD system includes pace-sense and defibrillation electrodes on a single ventricular lead and a pulse generator. Pacing and sensing functions require a pair of electrodes (bipolar): a distal electrode at the tip of the lead and a second ring electrode several millimeters back from the tip. Bipolar leads provide high amplitude, narrow electrograms for more accurate sensing and reduce the risk of sensing extracardiac signals, which could lead to inappropriate device function. With the vast majority of new ICD implantations, the ICD lead is placed transvenously via the cephalic, axillary, or subclavian vein with the distal electrode at the right ventricular apical endocardium.

The defibrillation electrode is a "coil" of wire along the distal lead body that provides a relatively large surface area to maximize the density of current flow through the ventricular myocardium. In addition to the distal shock coil in RV, some leads have a second proximal coil (SVC coil) to reduce the amount of energy for defibrillation. The metal housing of the pulse generator can also serve as a shock electrode but requires pectoral location. The ICD system should achieve a minimum energy for successful defibrillation (defibrillation threshold) that is at least 10 J less than the maximum output of the device. The pulse generator contains the high voltage capacitors, battery, and sensing circuitry and will typically last 8–10 years or more.

In rare cases (due to prior infection, lack of venous access, high defibrillation energy requirements, or concurrent cardiac surgery), electrodes and defibrillation patches can be placed on the epicardium. In patients with normal sinus and AV nodal function (who do not have a pacemaker indication), a single chamber ICD is implanted. Some devices utilize an ICD lead with electrodes incorporated on the lead for atrial sensing for detection of atrial arrhythmias. A dual chamber ICD has an additional right atrial lead for atrial sensing and pacing in patients where bradycardia support is indicated. A subcutaneous ICD (S-ICD) has a lead that is placed subcutaneously (no lead within the vasculature or the heart) for defibrillation only.

The device categorizes any detected heart rate above programmed cut-offs as a ventricular arrhythmia. Current ICDs offer multiple programming and therapeutic options including multiple detection zones, arrhythmia discrimination (ventricular vs supraventricular), and multiple therapies (antitachycardia pacing, cardioversion, and defibrillation). The ICD can be programmed to provide different therapies (also known as tiered therapy) in up to 3 different heart rate zones so that therapies can be tailored in each zone. Slower VTs may not lead to loss of consciousness and may be terminated with antitachycardia pacing (ATP) while faster VTs are more likely to be poorly tolerated, unstable, and may become more difficult to treat if definitive therapy (defibrillation) is delayed. In each zone, multiple sequential therapies can be delivered (ATP, then cardioversion, defibrillation); following each therapy, the device will reevaluate the rhythm and if it persists or accelerates, the next therapy in the appropriate zone is delivered.

Patients at risk for ventricular arrhythmias are also at risk for supraventricular arrhythmias and if the ICD interprets a SVT incorrectly as VT, the patient may experience inappropriate shocks which occur in up to 20–25% of patients [20–23]. ICDs utilize additional features to improve discrimination between ventricular and supraventricular arrhythmias. With a dual chamber device also detecting the atrial rhythm, the primary discriminator remains heart rate. If the atrial rate is faster than the ventricular rate (A > V), the arrhythmia is classified as a SVT, most commonly atrial fibrillation or atrial flutter and therapy is withheld. An arrhythmia with a faster ventricular than atrial rate (V > A) is consistent with atrioventricular dissociation with VT and therapy is delivered.

The device will also record a template of the ventricular electrogram during sinus rhythm which it then compares to the electrogram seen during a tachyarrhythmia. Changes in morphology, duration, polarity from baseline increase the likelihood of categorizing it as ventricular arrhythmia. The device will also detect the stability (lack of R- R variability) of the tachycardia; VT will typically be more regular while AF will not be. It also utilizes an onset criterion since VT will tend to be sudden onset while sinus tachycardia will have more gradual onset. Of course, SVTs can also be sudden onset and stable, this is one of the reasons why patients may receive inappropriate shocks.

While the discriminators are designed to prevent an SVT being incorrectly categorized as VT or VF and limit inappropriate shocks, no combination of discriminators is 100% specific for SVT. Also, for persistent tachyarrhythmias, the discriminators have a "time out" so that the ICD will treat the arrhythmia as VT or VF.

Once criteria for delivering a shock are met, the capacitors charge which take several seconds; after charging, the ICD will take a "second look" to determine if the arrhythmia has spontaneously terminated. If the tachycardia persists, the shock will be delivered. If the first shock fails, the defibrillator will deliver up to five more shocks in an attempt to terminate the arrhythmia.

9.2.5 Antitachycardia Pacing (ATP)

Reentrant arrhythmias can be terminated by pacing at a rate faster than the arrhythmia. The reason for termination is an antegrade and retrograde collision of the pacing wave front within the VT circuit that leads to termination of the arrhythmia. ATP refers to the delivery of short bursts of rapid ventricular pacing (typically 8/10 beats) to terminate VT. It is typically programmed to be delivered 10–20% faster than the rate of the tachycardia. Several prospective randomized and observational studies have shown that up to 95% of spontaneous VTs can be successfully terminated with ATP with similar efficacy to low energy (≤10 J) cardioversions [24–28].

ATP has also been shown to be effective with more rapid VTs. In the PainFREE Rx II trial, 634 patients were randomly assigned to empiric ATP or ICD shock for initial therapy of rapid VT (188–250 bpm). With mean follow-up of 11 months, 98 patients experienced 431 episodes of rapid VT and 81% were successfully pace terminated. There was no difference in the incidence of VT acceleration, syncope, sudden death, or median VT duration between the ATP and ICD shock arms [29].

Unfortunately, ATP tends to be less successful in patients with multiple VT morphologies. In one cohort of 52 patients with 833 episodes over mean follow-up of 30 months, ATP terminated 95% of VT episodes in patients with 1 morphology, 85% with 2 morphologies, and 70% with ≥3 morphologies [30].

9.2.6 Cardioversion

A shock that is delivered at the peak of the R wave (synchronized) is referred to as a cardioversion. If a shock is not synchronized and delivered during the vulnerable period of repolarization, this can cause VT to degenerate into VF.

9.2.7 Defibrillation & Threshold Testing

A shock delivered randomly during the cardiac cycle (unsynchronized) is defibrillation. Since VF is an unorganized rhythm, synchronized cardioversion is not necessary or possible. The amount of energy that is necessary to defibrillate the heart is the defibrillation threshold (DFT).

Historically, DFT was tested at device implant and generator changeout but recent studies have shown, in left sided implants, this is not necessary with modern ICDs. When performing DFTs at implant, VF is induced by a programmed shock on the T wave or with high frequency (50 Hz) pacing. The ICD should appropriately detect VF, charge, and deliver a shock. If the shock defibrillates the heart, the testing is repeated after a 5 min delay with a lower energy shock (step-down). Testing is repeated until defibrillation does not occur and the patient is rescued with a maximum output shock or external defibrillation. The DFT is defined as the lowest successful energy. Current clinical practice is one induction of VF and successful defibrillation occurs at 17 J or 2 inductions and successful defibrillation at 21 J occurs [31], an appropriate safety margin is confirmed. Early ICDs had a monophasic shock waveform while current ICDs have a biphasic waveform with an initial positive phase followed by a negative phase which is significantly more effective. With modern ICD systems with biphasic shocks, the DFT is typically $\leq$15 J.

Given clinical variations (CHF, ischemia, autonomic tone) and probabilistic nature of defibrillation, a shock at the energy level of the DFT may not always successfully defibrillate [32]; thus, an ICD must be able to deliver a shock at a higher energy than the DFT and a safety margin of at least 10 J is typically recommended. If DFTs have been performed at implant, the 1st shock is typically programmed 10 J above the threshold allowing a shorter charge time prior to therapy. If this shock is unsuccessful, subsequent shocks are delivered at higher energies, typically at the maximum output of the ICD.

As ICD technology has improved, DFTs have substantially decreased and it is uncommon for adjustments to be required at implant to ensure an adequate safety margin. Several studies have shown that DFT testing at implant may not be necessary for most patients. A small study of 145 patients undergoing ICD implant with or without CRT randomized patients to DFTs or no DFT. All patients in the DFT arm were successfully defibrillated and only 4% required any system modifications and there were no differences in outcomes between the 2 groups [33]. In the Shockless Implant Evaluation (SIMPLE) [34] and NORDIC [35] ICD trials, patients undergoing initial ICD implant were randomized to DFTs or no DFTs; no DFT testing was non-inferior to DFT testing (with a trend towards superiority). Based on these studies, DFTs are not routinely performed at implantation and ICD shocks are programmed at maximum output.

There are patients where DFTs are still performed (those with known elevated DFTs, on antiarrhythmic drug therapy that may raise the DFT, and those with right sided devices). Current recommendations also encourage performing DFTs in patients undergoing implantation of a S-ICD.

9.2.8 Programming to Minimize Right Ventricular Pacing

RV pacing is associated with an increased incidence of HF hospitalizations, AF, and death [36–38] by causing ventricular dyssynchrony due to functional LBBB. Whenever possible, both ICDs and pacemakers are programmed in modes to minimize RV pacing. For single chamber ICDs, the lower rate limit is typically programmed to 40 bpm (VVI 40 bpm). Dual chamber ICDs have algorithms that allow for intrinsic AVN conduction (AAI-DDD) and only provide ventricular pacing when AV block occurs. CRT is currently recommended for patients on GDMT with LVEF $\leq$ 35% undergoing new implantation or device replacement with anticipated requirement for significant (>40%) ventricular pacing [6].

9.2.9 Optimal ICD Programming

Historically the goal of ICD programming was to deliver ICD therapies with minimal possible delay for any ventricular arrhythmia. Many times, ICD therapies were delivered for arrhythmias that were non-sustained and may have spontaneously terminated if longer detection times prior to therapy were present [39]. Both appropriate and inappropriate ICD shocks are painful, psychologic stressful, and adversely affecting quality of life [40, 41], myocardial function [42], and are associated with increased mortality [40, 43, 44].

Several trials have investigated the impact of extended VT/VF detection intervals. In the Pooled Analysis of the IDE Study and EFFORTLESS a time to therapy of 19.2 ± 5.3 s was associated with spontaneous termination of 37% of all ventricular arrhythmias [45].

9.2.10 MADIT–RIT

The aims of this study were to evaluate the effect of device programming on inappropriate therapy and mortality. 1500 patients undergoing primary prevention ICD implantation were randomized to three different programming strategies: conventional (2.5 s delay at rates of 170–199 bpm with 1 s delay at rates of >200 bpm), delayed (60 s delay at rates of 170–199 bpm with 12 s delay at rates 200–249 bpm, and 2.5 s delay at rates >250 bpm), and high-rate (no therapy for 170–199 bpm, 2.5 s delay at rates of >200 bpm).

With delayed and high rate programming, inappropriate therapies were lower; all-cause mortality was lower in the high-rate group with a trend toward lower mortality in the delayed therapy group. The risk of mortality was higher in patients who received appropriate or inappropriate therapies, including ATP, regardless of programming strategy [46].

The ADVANCE III Trial randomized 1902 patients undergoing primary or secondary ICD implantation to one of two detection strategies (ATP and ICD shock programming was the same in both groups) for ventricular tachycardia >187 bpm. The two groups were: standard detection intervals 18/24 (5.4–7.2 s for detection with VT 200 bpm) and long detection intervals 30/40 (9–12 s for detection with VT 200 bpm).

Patients in the long detection group had fewer delivered therapies, lower likelihood of receiving ATP and near significant trend towards lower likelihood of delivered shock, and no significant change in mortality between the 2 groups [47]. Both MADIT-RIT and ADVANCE III showed that longer detection intervals prior to ICD therapies is both safe and effective in both primary and secondary prevention patients. It is important to notice that the increase in time to therapy or higher detection rates were not associated with increase in syncopal episodes. A meta-analysis of 4 studies showed that patients programmed with longer detection intervals had significantly fewer inappropriate shocks and lower mortality [48].

9.2.11 ICDs in Patients with LVADs

Ventricular arrhythmias are common in patients with left ventricular assist devices (LVADs) and are often better tolerated due to the hemodynamic support from the LVAD. Patients may remain in rapid ventricular arrhythmias for prolonged periods of times and SCD is an uncommon method of death in LVAD patients. The role of ICDs and optimal programming in LVAD patients has been uncertain. Recent meta-analyses have shown ICD use is associated with a significant mortality reduction in LVAD patients. In those with continuous-flow LVADs, there was a nonsignificant trend for improved survival in those with an ICD [49, 50]. Further randomized clinical trial data is needed to fully address this issue. It has been uncertain if ICD programming should be adjusted in LVAD patients to allow ventricular arrhythmias (permissive programming) or maintain traditional programming to avoid the complications of sustained ventricular arrhythmias. With permissive programming, VT/VF detections limits are increased to only treat faster HRs with prolonged detection intervals and increased use of ATP prior to delivering a shock. In a small study, permissive ICD programming lead to a non-significant trend toward fewer ICD shocks with no change in mortality or time to first hospitalization [51]. Larger studies are needed to define optimal ICD programming in LVAD patients.

9.2.12 Ambulatory Monitoring

ICDs allow for remote monitoring that allow physicians to interrogate the ICD, evaluate device and lead parameters and event EGMs over the telephone or internet without requiring the patient to come to the office or hospital. Programming changes cannot be made remotely but require in person interrogations. Multiple parameters may trigger an alert on remote monitoring (Table 9.1).

In a study assessing the clinical impact of remote monitoring, (TRUST-trial [34]) randomized patients with single and dual chamber defibrillators to remote monitoring or routine office visits. Remote monitoring reduced in-hospital device interrogation visits by 45% with no increase in adverse events and problems were identified 30 days earlier with remote monitoring [52]. In the Clinical Evaluation of Remote Notification to Reduce Time to Clinical Decision (CONNECT), a decreased length of stay was seen with remote monitoring of patients with ICDs or CRT-Ds [53]. In the ALTITUDE study, 185,778 patients with ICD or CRT-D were randomized to remote monitoring 3–4 times per month with office visits twice a year or to routine office visits only. A 50% reduction in mortality was seen at 1 and 5 years and the lowest mortality was seen in patients who reported weight and BP readings, suggesting that improved survival may be attributable to better patient self-care rather than remote monitoring alone [54]. The above benefits were seen across all manufacturers.

Remote monitoring also offers data that may assist in the treatment of HF patients. As a surrogate for pulmonary vascular fluid status, intrathoracic impedance can be measured

Table 9.1 Remote monitoring parameters triggering patient alerts

New onset, duration of SVTs, AF
RV pacing over programmable percentage
BiV pacing under programmable percentage
Significant change in lead function (impedances, capture thresholds)
NSVT, VT, ICD therapies
Generator at recommended replacement interval

between the tip of ICD lead and the pulse generator. The Medtronic OptiVol system is a measurement of the difference between the daily and reference impedances plotted against a programmable threshold and when crossed an alert will trigger. Figure OptiVol Fluid Trends (Dec-2014 to Feb-2016) shows an Optivol trend seen on remote monitoring for a patient with an acute exacerbation of HF. An alert should lead to patient evaluation not reflexive medication adjustment since the transthoracic impedance can be affected by pneumonia, pleural effusion, pocket edema, or inflammation.

In one study of 532 patients, CHF hospitalizations were significantly reduced in patients with OptiVol monitored turned "on" [55]. However, in the Diagnostic Outcome Trial for Heart Failure (DOT-HF), an audible alert was emitted by the device when the Optivol threshold was crossed; leading to increased outpatient visits and admissions for CHF with no change in mortality [56]. In the OptiLink HF Study, OptiVol monitoring did not reduce CV hospitalizations or mortality [57].

Devices can also monitor patient activity and heart rate variability; decreased levels of both may predict heart failure exacerbation. The use of multiple clinical variables may assist the predictive value of impedance measurements. In the Program to Access and Review Trending Information and Evaluate Correlation to Symptoms in Patients with Heart Failure (PARTNERS HF) trial, 694 patients with CRT-Ds were evaluated. Patients with a fluid index >100 and any 2 of the following: long duration of AF, AF with RVR, low patient activity, high nocturnal HR, low HR variability, low CRT-pacing, or ICD shocks had a 5.5-fold increased risk of CHF admission in the next 30 days [58].

One important advance in device follow up is the development of remote monitoring (fig see the one I sent you). In the Influence of Home Monitoring on Mortality and Morbidity in HF Patients with Impaired LV function (IN-TIME), all-cause mortality in the tele-monitoring group was 3.4% versus 8.7% in the control group [59]. Similarly, in a "big-data" Registry analysis of 269,471 US patients, remote monitoring was associated with improved survival and survival was associated to the level of adherence to remote monitoring [60].

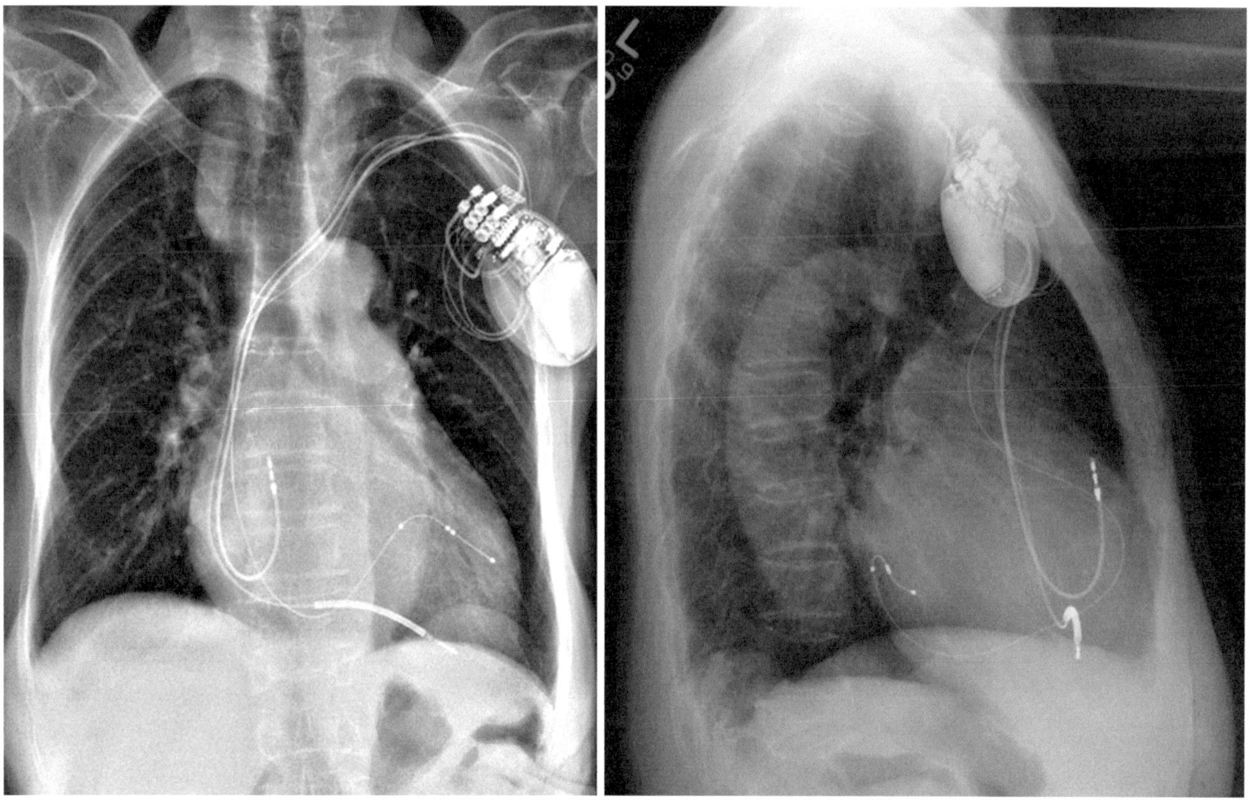

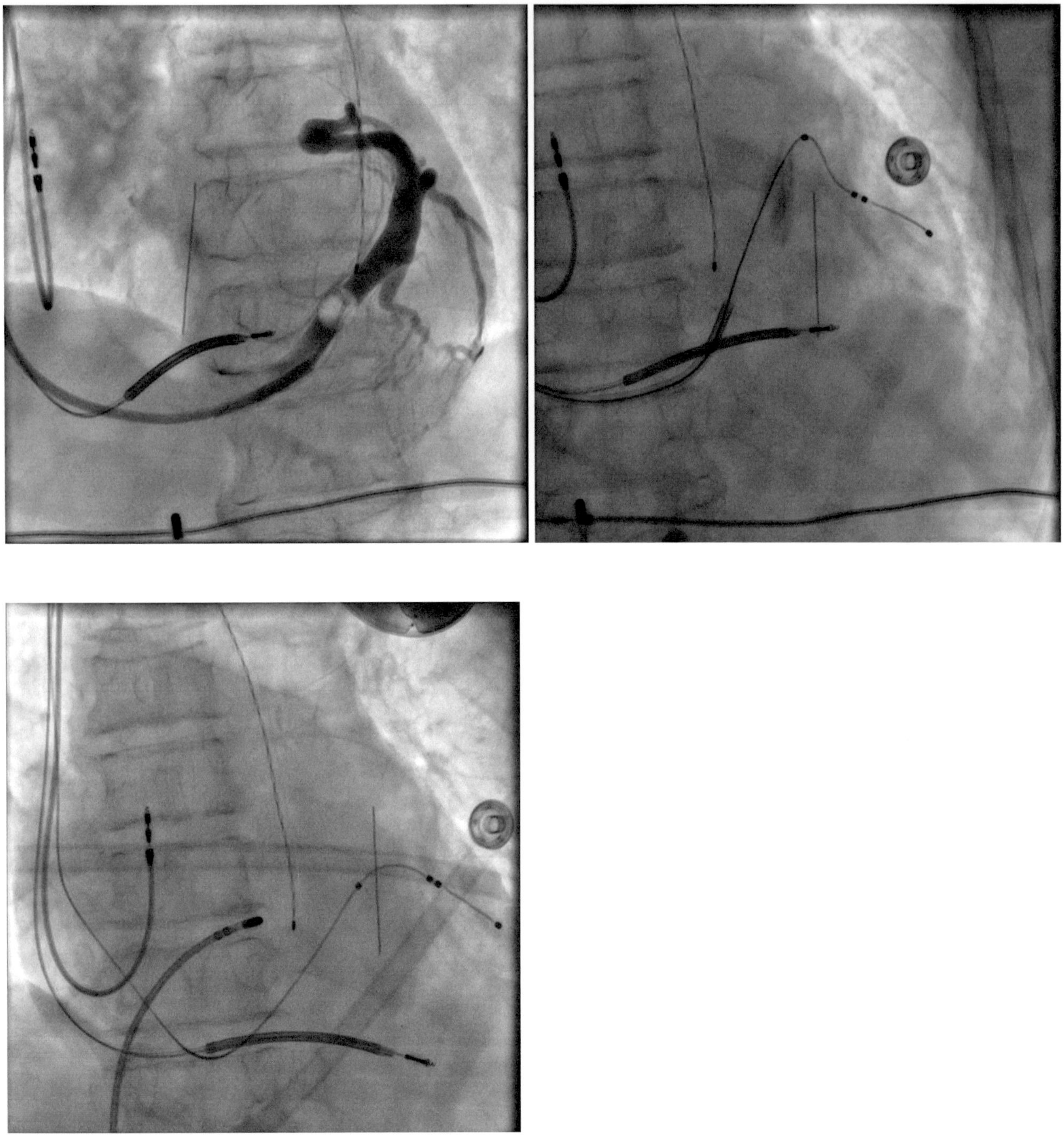

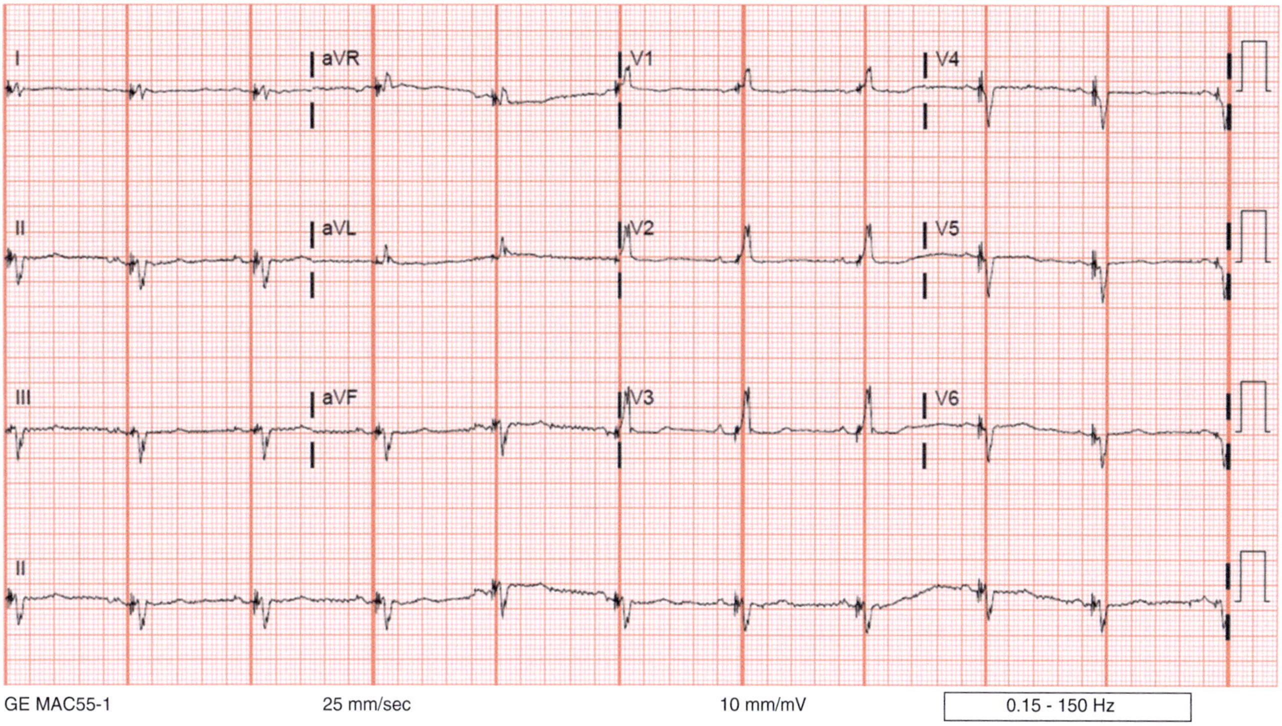
I
aVR
V1
V4
II
aVL
V2
V5
III
aVF
V3
V6
II
GE MAC55-1
25 mm/sec
10 mm/mV
0.15 - 150 Hz

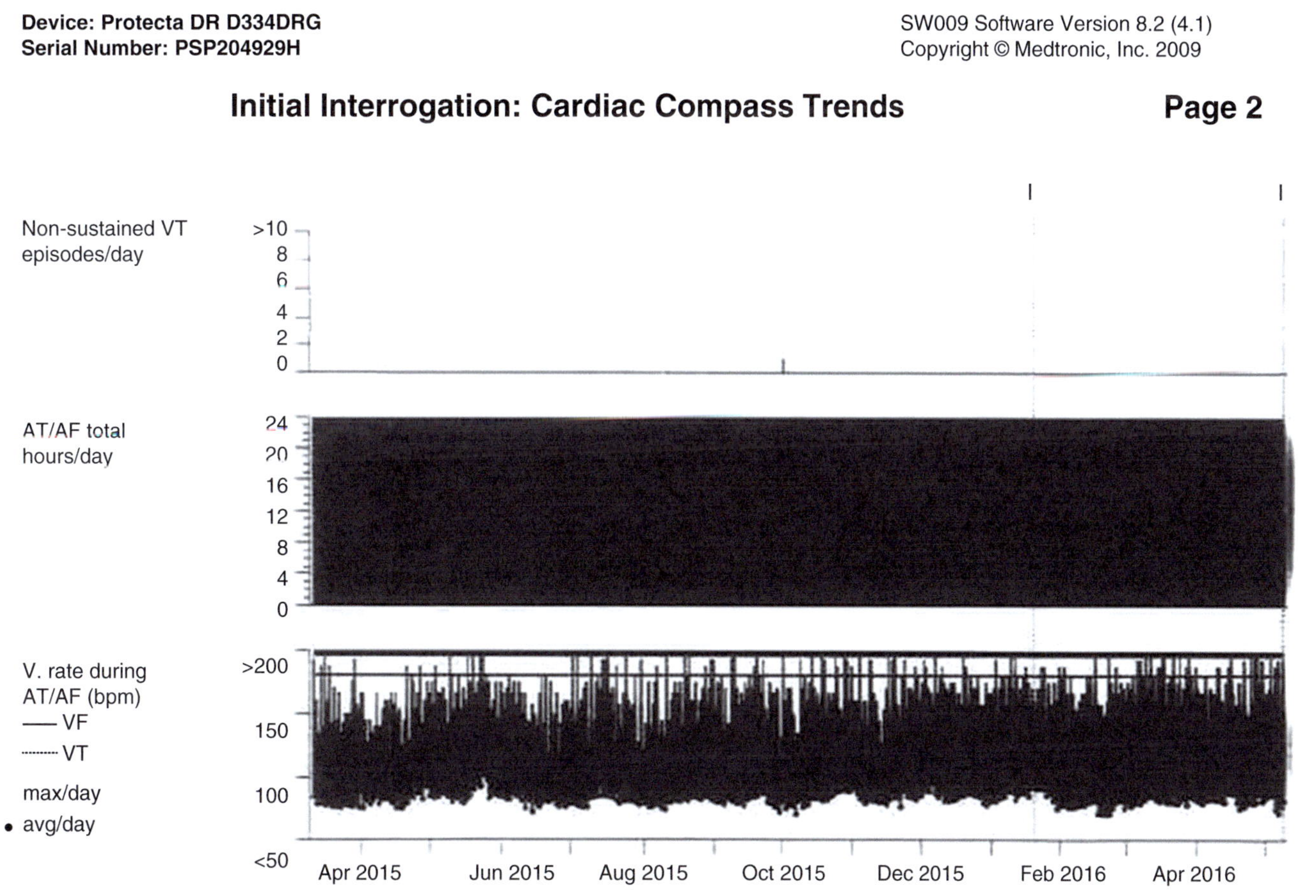
Device: Protecta DR D334DRG
Serial Number: PSP204929H
SW009 Software Version 8.2 (4.1)
Copyright © Medtronic, Inc. 2009
Initial Interrogation: Cardiac Compass Trends
Page 2
Non-sustained VT episodes/day
>10
8
6
4
2
0
AT/AF total hours/day
24
20
16
12
8
4
0
V. rate during AT/AF (bpm)
VF
VT
max/day
avg/day
>200
150
100
<50
Apr 2015
Jun 2015
Aug 2015
Oct 2015
Dec 2015
Feb 2016
Apr 2016

OptiVol Fluid Trends (Dec-2014 to Feb-2016)

OptiVol fluid index is an accumulation of the difference between the daily and reference impedance.

The OptiVol feature is an additional source of information for patient management and does not replace assessments that are part of standard clinical practice. Note: The OptiVol threshold and observations are not available from the Medtronic CareLink Network.

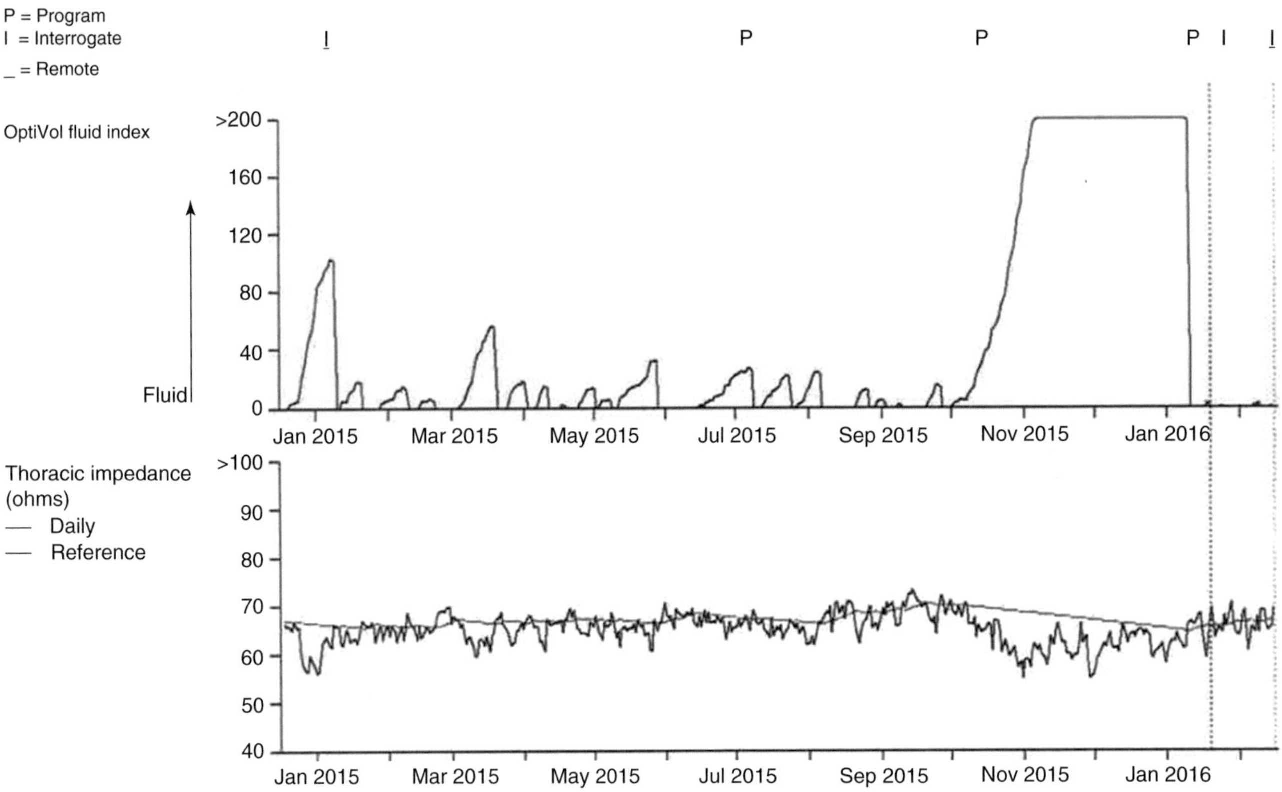

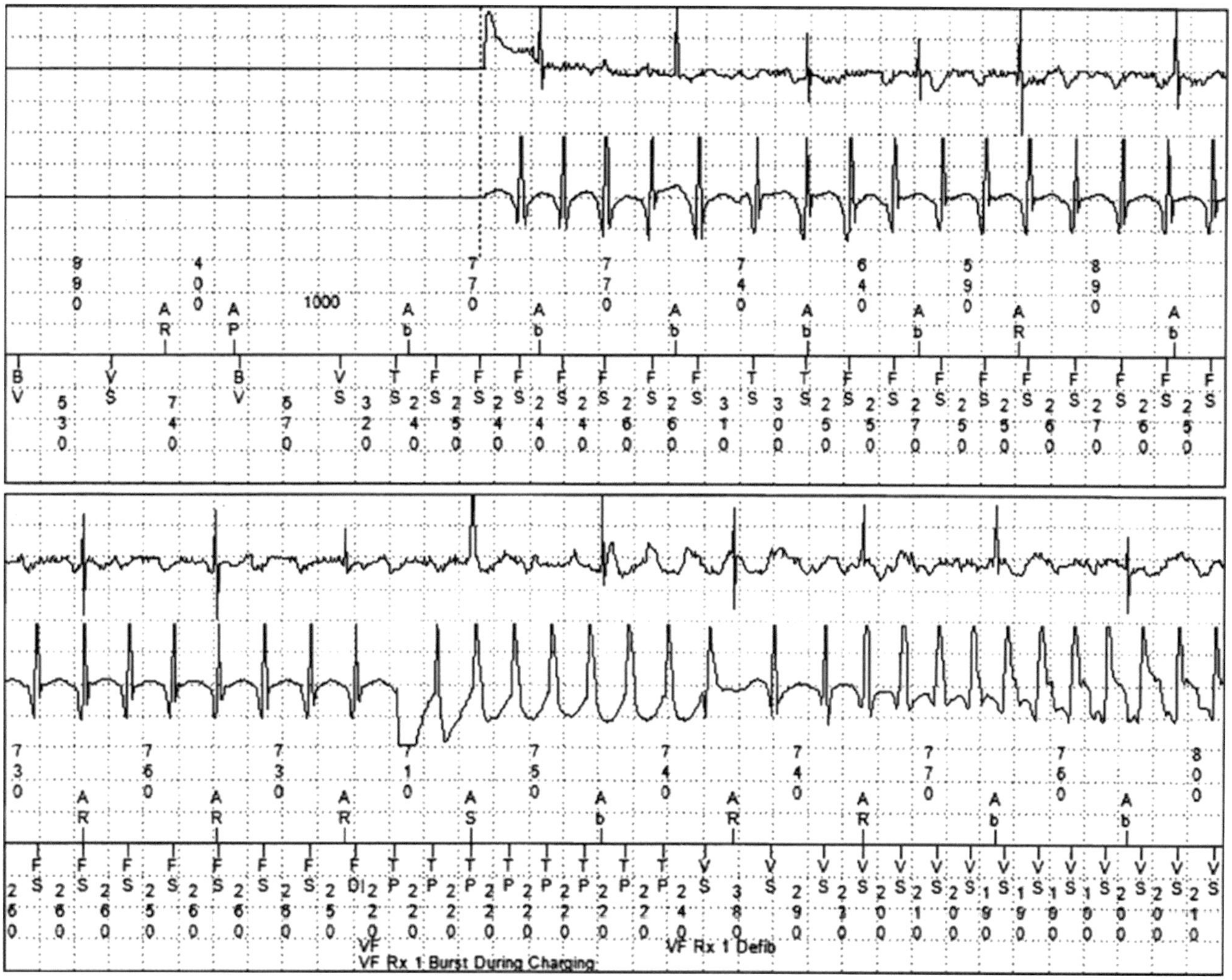
VF
VF Rx 1 Burst During Charging
VF Rx 1 Defib

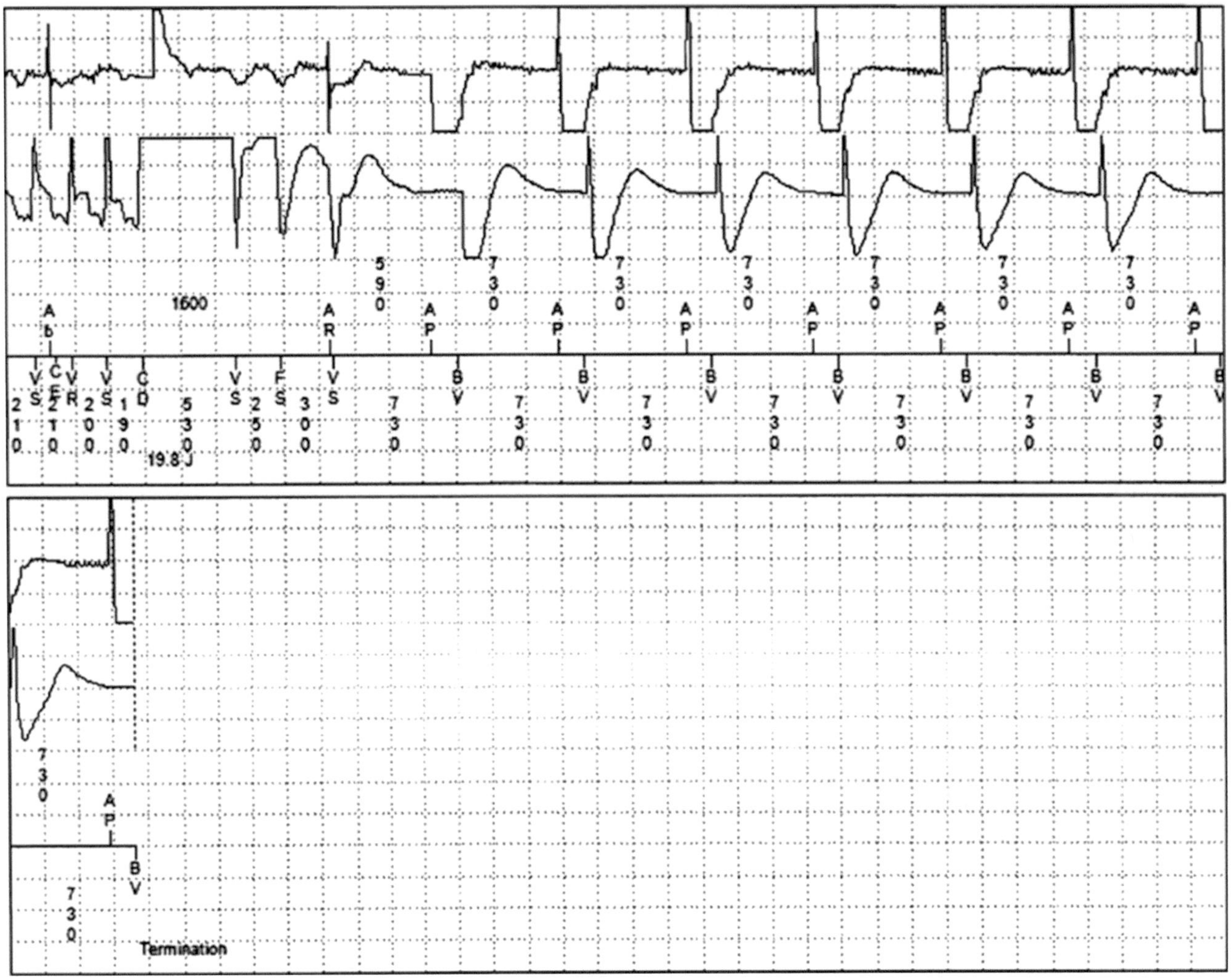
1600
19.8 J
Termination

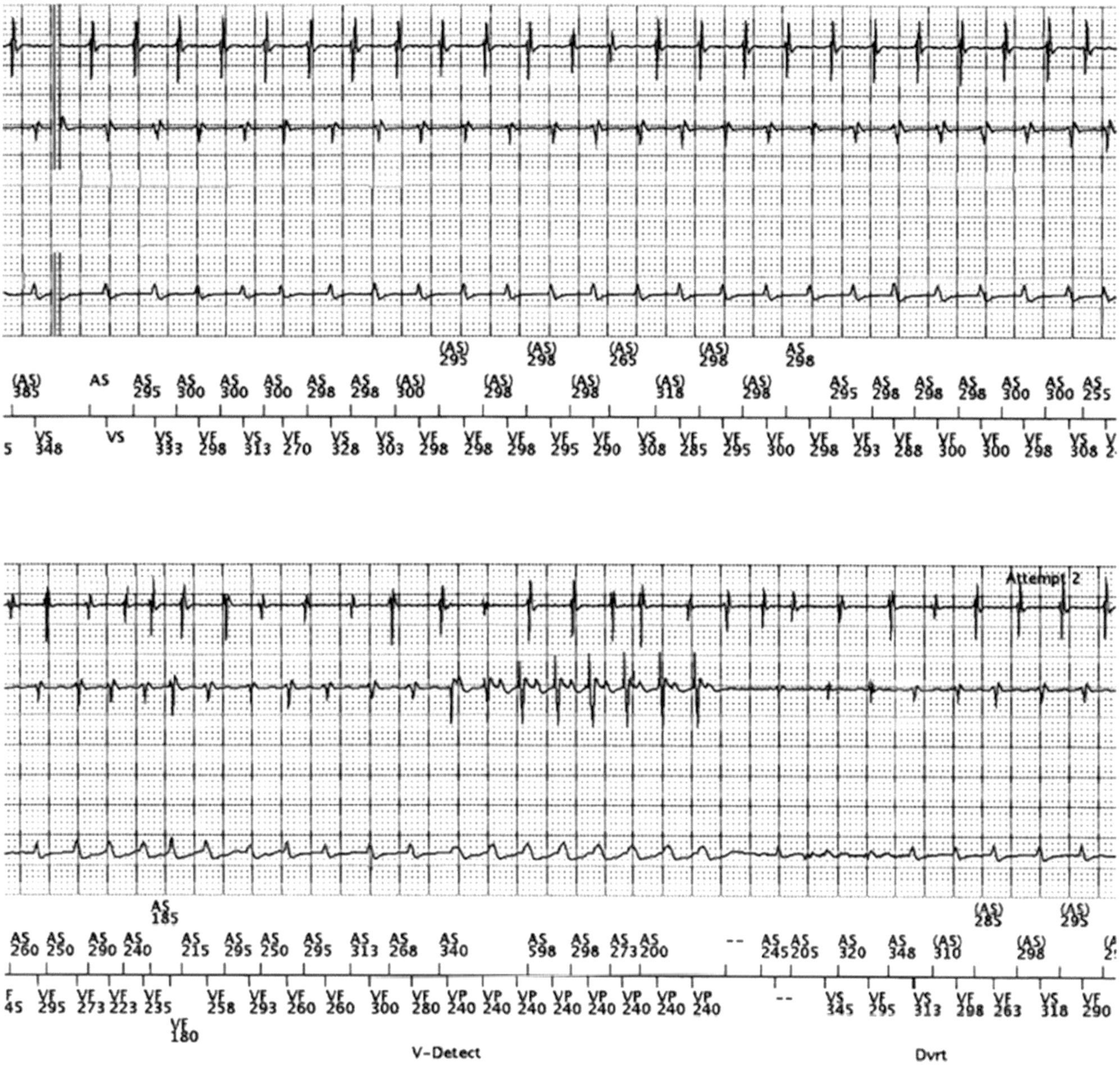
Attempt 2
V-Detect
Dvrt

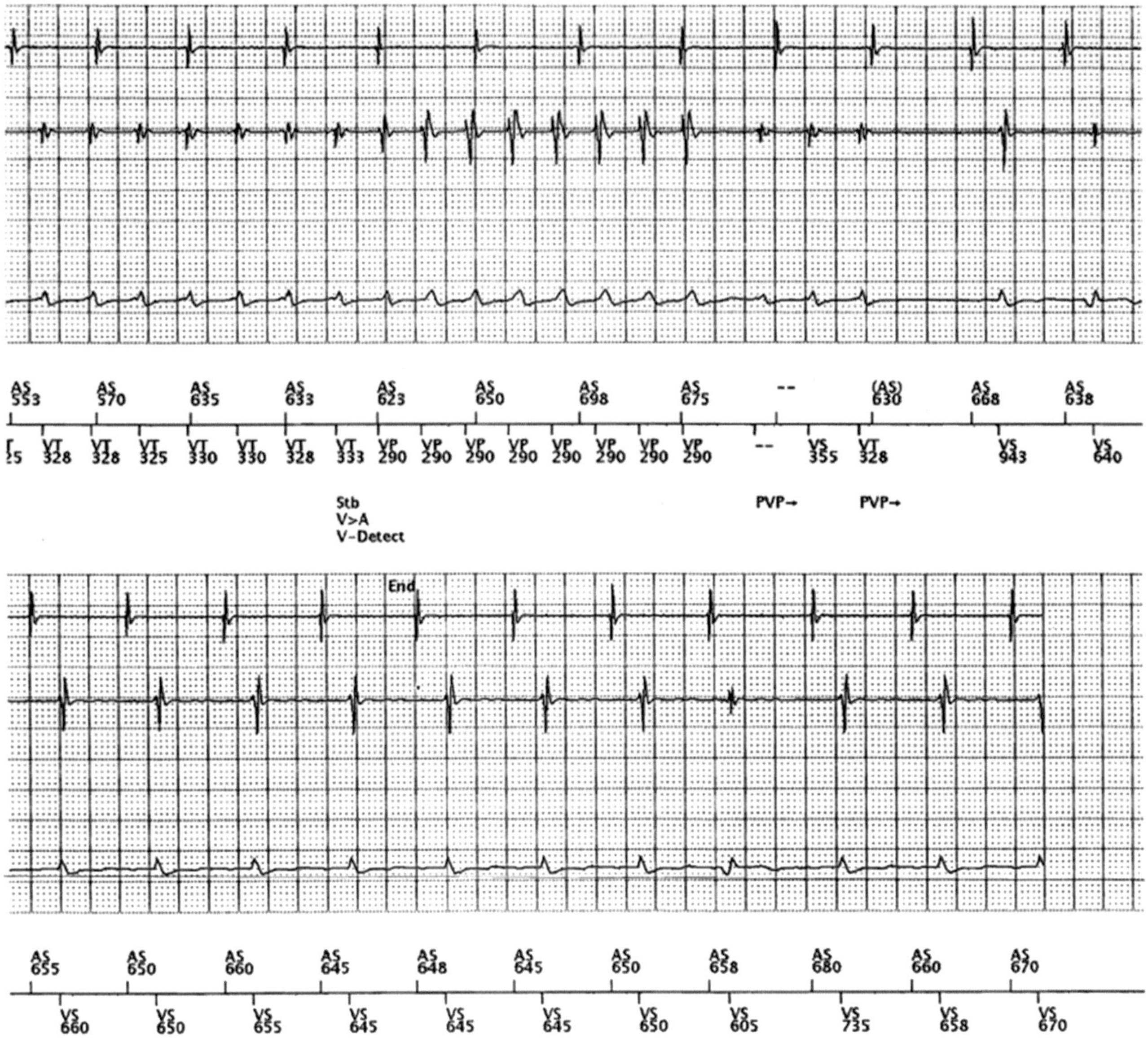
AS 553 AS 570 AS 635 AS 633 AS 623 AS 650 AS 698 AS 675 -- (AS) 630 AS 668 AS 638
VT 25 VT 328 VT 328 VT 325 VT 330 VT 330 VT 328 VT 333 VP 290 VP 290 VP 290 VP 290 VP 290 VP 290 VP 290 VP 290 -- VS 355 VT 328 VS 943 VS 640
Stb
V>A
V-Detect
PVP→ PVP→
End
AS 655 AS 650 AS 660 AS 645 AS 648 AS 645 AS 650 AS 658 AS 680 AS 660 AS 670
VS 660 VS 650 VS 655 VS 645 VS 645 VS 645 VS 650 VS 605 VS 735 VS 658 VS 670

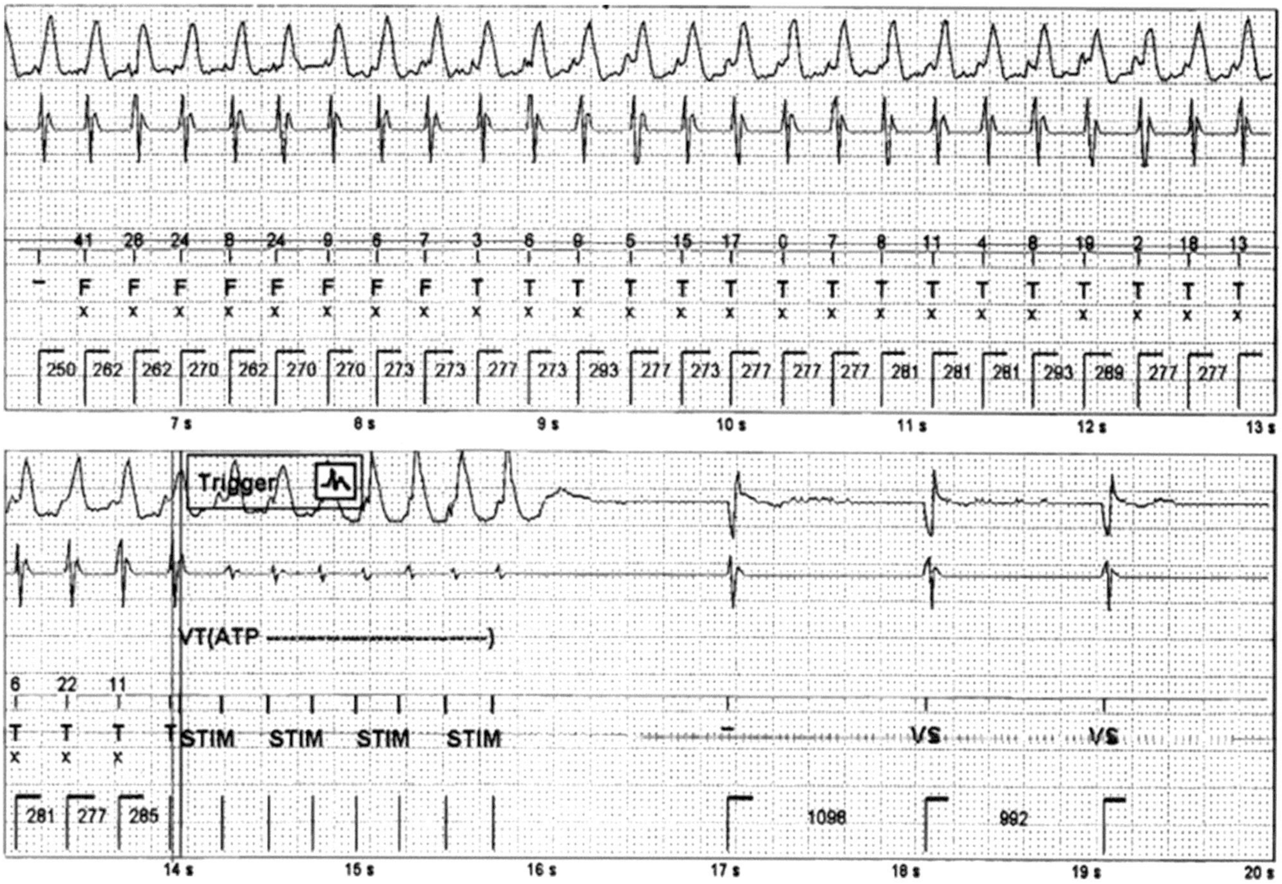
Trigger
VT(ATP)
STIM STIM STIM STIM
VS VS
1098
992
7 s 8 s 9 s 10 s 11 s 12 s 13 s
14 s 15 s 16 s 17 s 18 s 19 s 20 s

Type	ATP Seq	Shocks	Success	ID#	Date	Time hh:mm	Duration hh:mm:ss	Avg bpm A/V
VF	ATP: 1		Yes	#54	04-Jan-2016	20:21	:16	102/222

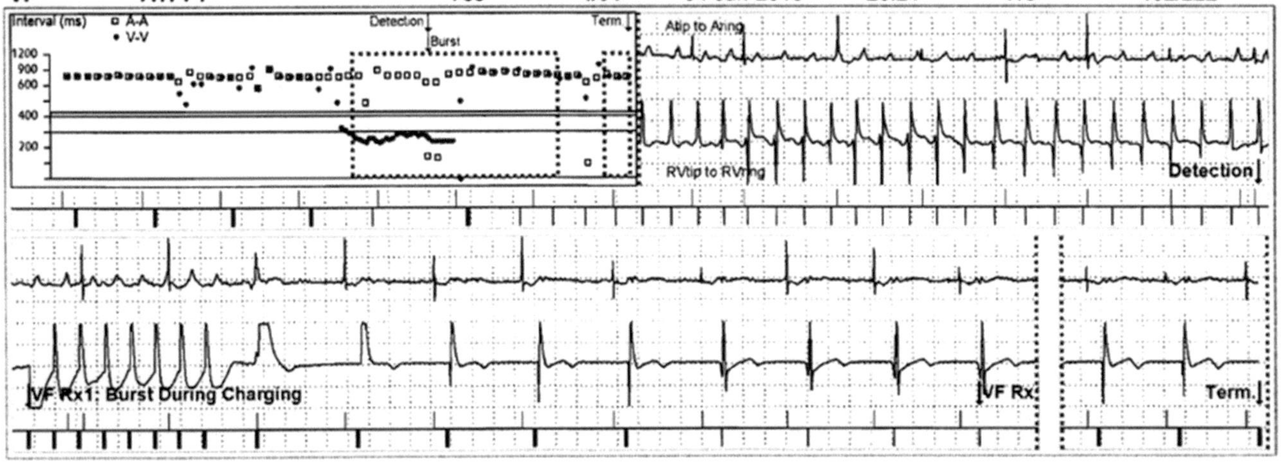

VF	ATP: 1	20J	Yes	#53	03-Jan-2016	15:54	:13	78/240

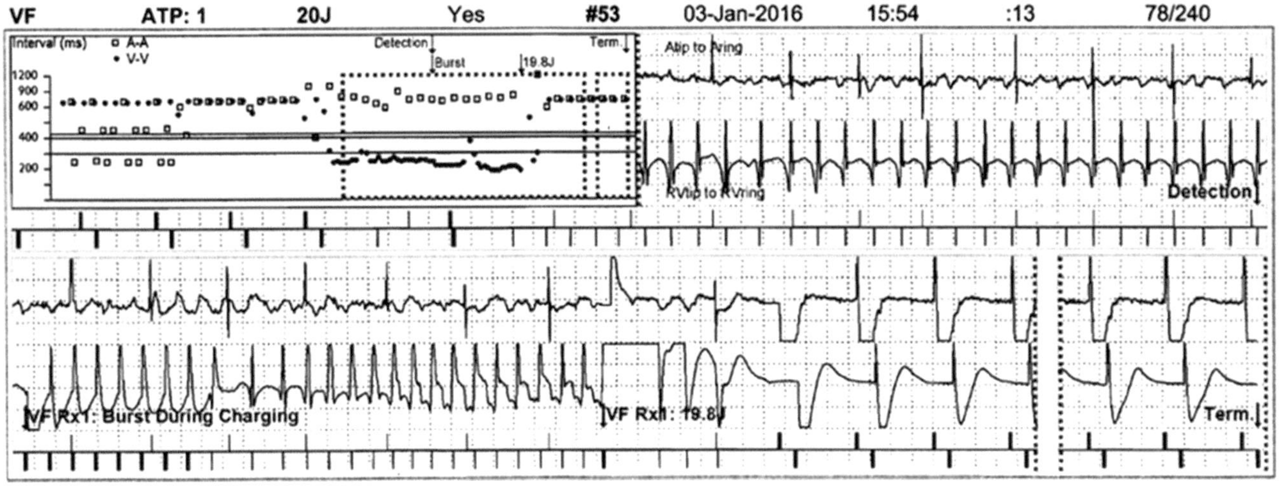

VF		20J, 30J	Yes	#51	23-Dec-2015	18:39	:23	88/316

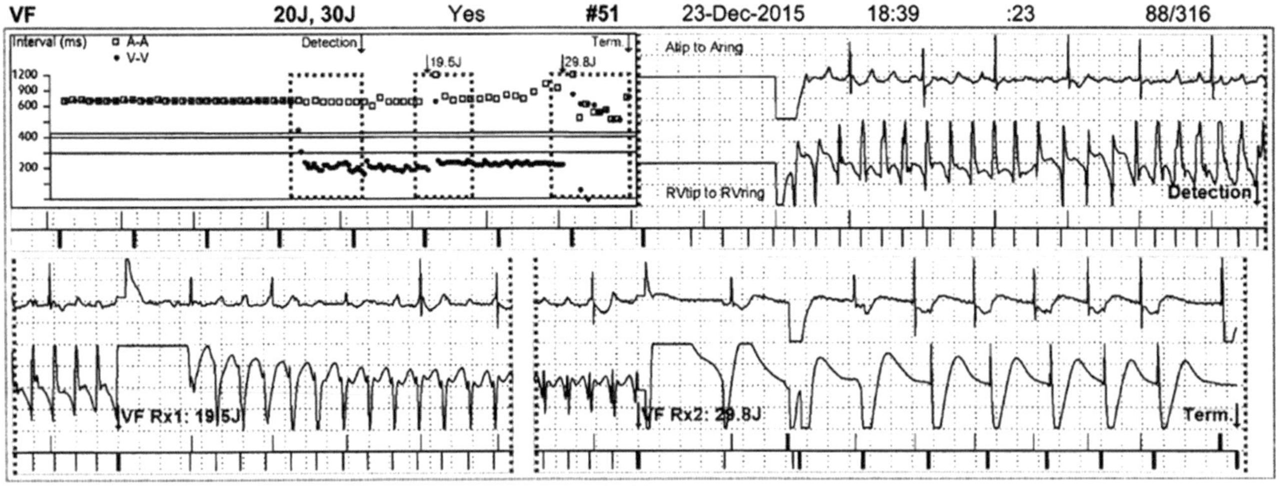

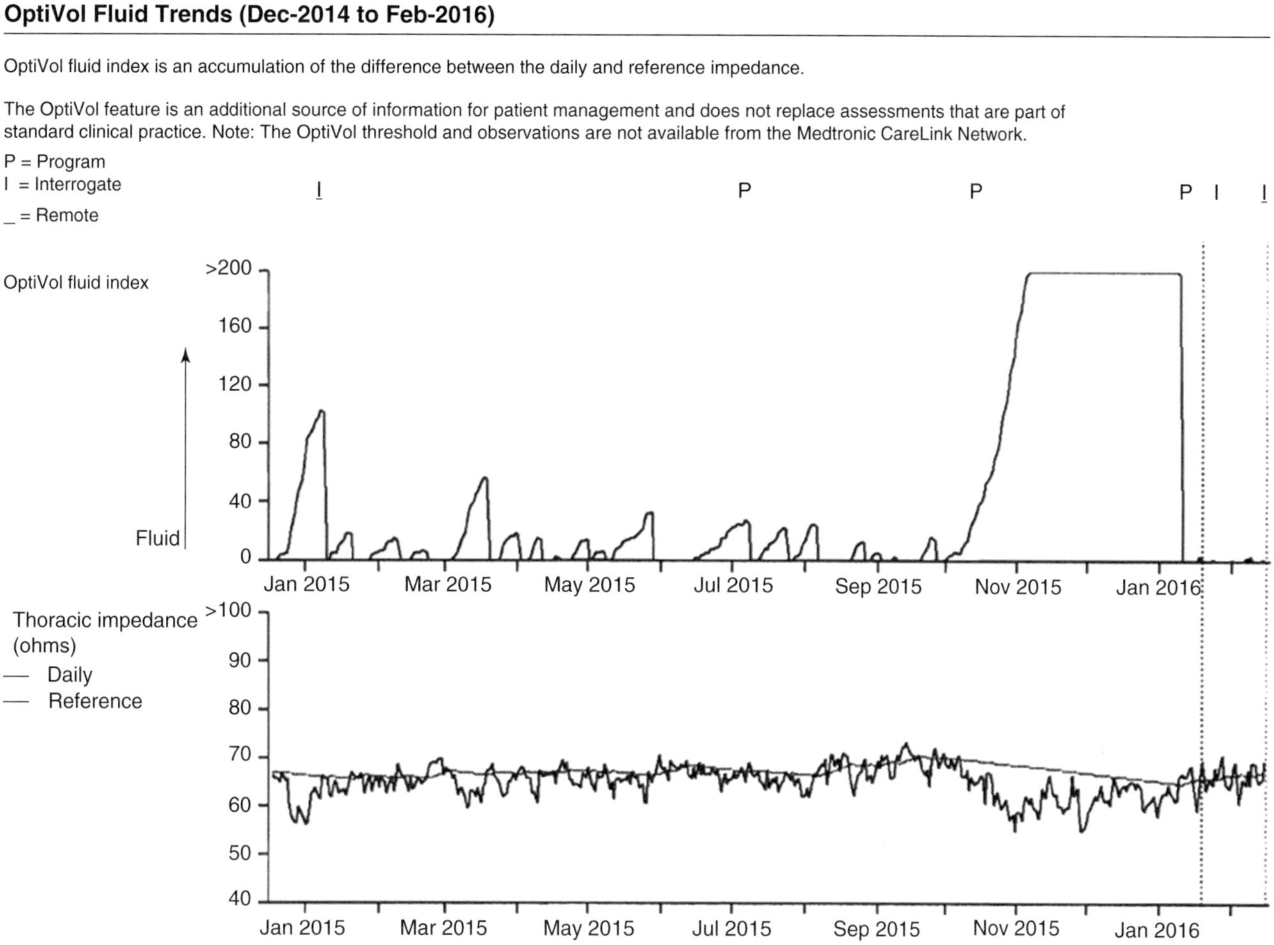

9.2.13 ICD System Integrity

In addition to notification that the pulse generator has reached the recommended replacement time (RRT), the device monitors for early lead failure. An insulation break or inner conductor fracture can lead to failure to capture or oversensing with inhibition of pacing which could be catastrophic in pacemaker dependent patients. Inner conductor fracture of an ICD lead can lead to oversensing and inappropriate ICD shocks. An alert for a sudden change in lead impedance can result in earlier identification and management to reduce the chance for inappropriate shocks. Remote monitoring has shown that lead malfunctions are identified 54 days earlier and inappropriate shocks from lead fracture were reduced by 50% (53–27%) [61, 62].

9.2.14 Approach to the Patient Presenting with Suspected ICD Therapies

Reported ICD shocks are due to 3 possible situations: appropriate shock, inappropriate shock, or a phantom shock. Within 2 years of ICD implantation, one-third of patients will experience an appropriate ICD therapy for a ventricular tachyarrhythmia that satisfied programmed detection criteria [63]. Inappropriate therapies can occur due to SVTs that satisfied VT/VF criteria, oversensing of environmental electrical noise, or ICD malfunction due to sensing of noise (i.e., ICD lead fracture). A phantom shock is the sensation of an ICD shock in the absence of an arrhythmia or ICD therapy [64].

Some patients may receive multiple ICD therapies within minutes to hours following the initial shock. VT storm is defined as 3 or more sustained episodes of VT, VF, or appropriate ICD shocks within 24 h [65]. Patients who receive more than 1 ICD therapy, require emergent evaluation for persistent arrhythmia not adequately treated by the ICD, concomitant illnesses such as myocardial infarction, decompensated HF, metabolic derangements, or ICD malfunction [66]. Prompt device interrogation should be performed to assess the nature of the arrhythmias and device therapies, and ensure appropriate device function. Patients with ongoing arrhythmias should be treated according to advanced cardiac life support (ACLS) guidelines.

In the event of device malfunction causing repeated inappropriate ICD therapies, VT/VF detection and therapies can be disabled by placing a magnet directly over the ICD. Magnet placement still allows backup bradycardia pacing but will not cause asynchronous pacing (DOO or VOO) as seen with pacemakers. With a magnet in place, the patient must remain on continuous monitoring with preparations for external cardioversion-defibrillation since neither SVTs, VT, of VF will be detected or treated by the ICD. Once the magnet is removed, normal ICD function will resume [64].

9.2.15 Management of VT & ICD Therapies

ICD shocks are associated with decreased quality of life [67] and lead to increased risk of hospitalization, HF, and death. While ICDs therapies effectively terminate VT-VF, they do prevent them and concomitant antiarrhythmic drug (AAD) therapy is frequently necessary. In the first year of treatment, amiodarone reduced recurrent arrhythmias by 71% [68] and the rate of arrhythmic death [69] but with long term use is associated with significant side effects that often lead to discontinuation [70]. If VT recurs despite AAD therapy, either escalation of AAD therapy or catheter ablation of VT are the next steps [71]. Randomized trials of catheter ablation in patients with ischemic cardiomyopathy reduced the rate of VT recurrence [72, 73] and observational studies have shown increased survival [74]. The Ventricular Tachycardia Ablation versus Escalated Antiarrhythmic Drug Therapy in Ischemic Heart Disease (VANISH) trial randomized 259 patients to VT ablation or escalated AAD therapy with a significantly lower rate of appropriate ICD shocks, VT storm, and death in those undergoing catheter ablation [75]. Current guidelines recommend catheter ablation when AAD therapy is ineffective [65, 71, 76] but this trial supports catheter ablation over escalation of AAD therapy in patients with ischemic VT [75]. Unfortunately, VT ablation in patients with nonischemic CM have not been as successful likely due to the differences in arrhythmic substrate [77].

9.2.16 Driving with ICDs

Patients with ICDs are at risk for syncope secondary to VT/VF and incapacitation due to surprise and pain from ICD shocks and therefore, driving restrictions should be recommended. Primary prevention patients may drive 1 week following device implantation. Secondary prevention patients (at implant) and those who receive appropriate ICD therapies for VT and VF, should be restricted from driving for 6 months from their last ICD therapy [78]. These recommendations differ among countries.

9.2.17 Wearable Cardioverter-Defibrillator

For patients at risk for SCD but do not meet accepted criteria for ICD implantation, those with infectious issues awaiting device re-implantation or awaiting cardiac transplantation, a wearable cardioverter-defibrillator (WCD) offers short term protection. The WCD also plays a role for protection of newly diagnosed HF patients to allow time for medical therapy with potential recovery of LV systolic function so permanent ICD implantation is unnecessary. In a recent 10 year, single center, retrospective study of newly diagnosed ischemic and non-ischemic CM patients treated with WCDs, no appropriate therapies were seen in patients with NICM. Additional prospective studies are needed, but newly diagnosed ischemic CM patients may benefit from WCD more than NICM patients [79].

9.3 Cardiac Resynchronization Therapy

Ventricular dyssynchrony can worsen heart failure symptoms by impairing pump function. Cardiac resynchronization therapy (CRT) involves pacing both ventricles (biventricular or BiV pacing) to reduce dyssynchrony, improve pump function, reduce functional mitral regurgitation, and reverse ventricular remodeling. In randomized controlled trials, CRT reduces mortality, HF symptoms and hospitalizations.

The Comparison of Medical Therapy, Pacing, and Defibrillation in Heart Failure (COMPANION) trial randomized 1520 patients with LVEF $\leq$ 35%, NYHA Class III-IV HF, and QRS $\geq$ 120 ms to CRT with a defibrillator (CRT-D), CRT without a defibrillator (CRT-P), or optimal HF medical therapy. CRT-D was better than optimal medical therapy at all QRS durations ($\leq$147 ms, 148–168 ms, and >168 ms) but the greatest effect was seen with increasing QRS duration and CRT-P benefited those with QRS $\geq$ 150 ms [80]. A subsequent analysis using QRS cutoffs of <150 ms and $\geq$150 ms showed a reduction in death and all-cause hospitalization for those with a QRS $\geq$ 150 ms.

The Cardiac Resynchronization Heart Failure trial (CARE-HF) randomized 813 patients with QRS ≥ 120 ms, LVEF ≤ 35%, and NYHA III-IV to CRT-P or optimal medical therapy (no ICD arm) with the primary endpoint of mortality and unplanned cardiovascular hospitalization reported according to QRS intervals above or below 160 ms. Echocardiographic evidence of ventricular dyssynchrony was required for patients with QRS 120–149 ms. As seen in COMPANION, CRT was better than medical therapy for all QRS durations but the greatest benefit was in those with QRS ≥ 160 ms [81].

Three trials investigated the benefit of CRT in predominantly NYHA II patients: REVERSE (Resynchronization Reverses Remodeling in Systolic Left Ventricular Dysfunction), MADIT-CRT (Multicenter Automatic Defibrillator Implantation Trial with Cardiac Resynchronization Trial), and RAFT (Resynchronization-Defibrillation for Ambulatory Heart Failure Trial).

REVERSE enrolled 610 patients with NYHA I-II HF, EF ≤ 40%, and QRS duration ≥ 120 ms were enrolled to either CRT-P or CRT-D based on clinical indications and were then randomized to active CRT On or Off for 12 month follow-up with a clinical composite score as the primary endpoint. Remodeling, as measured by change in LV index volume, progressively improved with increasing QRS duration with shortest QRS cutpoint of 134 ms [82] while a further analysis showed progressive CRT benefit when QRS duration > 120 ms was evaluated as a continuous variable for each 10 ms increase in QRS duration [83]. No CRT benefit was seen with QRS < 120 ms [82].

MADIT-CRT enrolled 1820 patients with EF < 30%, NYHA Class I-II, and QRS duration ≥ 130 ms to CRT-D or ICD alone and the benefit of CRT-D on death or nonfatal HF event was only seen in those patients with QRS duration ≥ 150 ms [84]. While female patients benefited across all QRS durations, male patients received benefit mainly when the QRS duration was at least 160 ms [85]. Nonetheless, with long term follow-up, CRT-D improved all-cause mortality in the 1281 patients with LBBB QRS morphology, regardless of the QRS duration [86].

In RAFT, 1798 patients with NYHA I-II, EF ≤ 30%, and QRS durations ≥ 120 ms were randomized to CRT-D or ICD alone with a primary endpoint of all cause death or HF hospitalization. CRT benefit was only observed in patients with QRS duration ≥ 150 ms compared with patients with QRS < 150 ms or a paced QRS duration ≥ 200 ms [87].

Meta-analyses of these CRT trials have added further support that QRS duration is a useful surrogate for electromechanical dyssynchrony but is not the sole determinant of CRT response [88, 89].

9.3.1 AV Block and CRT

In BLOCK HF trials, 691 patients with high grade AV block, NYHA Class I-III HF, and LVEF ≤ 50% were randomized to BiV pacing or RV pacing. With mean follow-up of 37 months, the combined primary endpoint of all-cause mortality, urgent HF visit requiring intravenous therapy, or ≥15% increase in LV end-systolic volume index was significantly less likely to occur in the BiV pacing group [90]. Similarly, in the PACE trial, 177 pacemaker candidates with LVEF ≥ 45% underwent implant of a CRT system were then randomized to either BiV pacing or RV pacing. At 12 months follow-up, those receiving RV pacing had significantly lower LVEF and higher LV end-systolic volume than those with BiV pacing [38]. Current guidelines recommend CRT in patients with LVEF ≤ 35% with significant (>40%) anticipated or present RV pacing at implant or device replacement, respectively. Based upon BLOCK HF, FDA approved CRT for patients with LVEF ≤ 50%, NYHA I-III, and AV block with significant RV pacing.

9.3.2 CRT & Narrow QRS

In patients with a QRS duration ≤ 120 ms, 20–40% have evidence of mechanical dyssynchrony by echocardiography and is a predictor of mortality. Four trials have investigated patients with normal or near normal QRS durations (<130 ms) and echocardiographic mechanical dyssynchrony who then underwent implantation of CRT-D with randomization to CRT on or off.

EchoCRT (Echocardiography Guided Cardiac Resynchronization Therapy) was stopped early due to futility and showed a nonsignificant trend towards harm in patients with an EF < 35% a NYHA III-IF HF and QRS durations < 130 ms who received CRT-D [91]. Similarly, the LESSER EARTH (Evaluation of Resynchronization Therapy in Heart Failure) Trial was terminated early due to safety concerns and futility [92]. NARROW CRT (Narrow QRS Ischemic Patients Treated with Cardiac Resynchronization Therapy) trial enrolled 120 patients with echocardiographic dyssynchrony to CRT-D or dual chamber ICD. At 1 year, CRT was associated with an improved HF clinical composite response (primary endpoint) and at 16 months, improved survival from the combined endpoint of HF hospitalization, HF death, and spontaneous VF [93]. Differences in the results between the three trials are likely due to variable patient populations, endpoints, and follow-up intervals [94].

RethinQ (Resynchronization Therapy in Normal QRS or slightly prolonged QRS (130 ms) enrolled 85 patients prior to study termination with 27% of patients with QRS duration of 120–130 ms showing an improvement in NYHA functional class and maximal oxygen consumption but no benefit for the primary endpoint of an increase of peak oxygen consumption >1.0 ml/kg during cardiopulmonary testing at 6 months. Symptoms improved in all QRS duration groups but exercise capacity increased significantly only in those with QRS duration > 120 [95].

9.3.3 QRS Morphology & CRT Response

While patients were not enrolled in randomized controlled CRT trials on the basis of QRS morphology, important observations have been obtained from post hoc analyses. The majority of patients enrolled had a LBBB or nonspecific IVCD and those with LBBB have shown the greatest response to CRT whereas those with non-LBBB have responded poorly. Overall, trial data support CRT for LBBB patients when the QRS duration is at least 120 ms but the greater response to CRT is seen as the QRS duration lengthens [94].

While few patients with RBBB were enrolled, it is clear that patients with RBBB received little to no benefit from CRT. A meta-analysis of 5 trials (MIRACLE, CONTAK CD, CARE-HR, RAFT, and MADIT-CRT) identified 259 patients with RBBB and there was no benefit from CRT [96]. In predominantly NYHA Class II HF patients with non-LBBB, IVCD, or RBBB morphologies (REVERSE, MADIT-CRT, and RAFT) reduced or no CRT benefit was seen [82, 84, 87].

Using data from the Medicare ICD Registry in 14,946 patients who underwent CRT-D implantation with RBBB, decreased survival was seen compared to those with LBBB [97]. Among 24,169 patients who underwent CRT-D implantation in the National Cardiovascular Data Registry ICD Registry, 1 year hospital readmission rates and 3 year mortality were higher in those with non-LBBB and LBBB <150 ms [98]. In another study, the benefit of CRT only emerged in non-LBBB patients, once the QRS $\geq$ 160 ms [96].

In MADIT-CRT, seven factors were associated with reverse remodeling (reduced LV end-diastolic volume): female sex, nonischemic CM, LBBB $\geq$ 150 ms, prior admission for HF, LVEDV $\geq$ 125 ml/m^2, and left atrial volume <40 ml/m^2. All factors were worth 2 points except 3 points for left atrial volume. The response score predicted CRT response with a 13% increase per each point in the response score and correlated with reduced risk of HF or death [99].

9.3.4 Other Factors Affecting CRT Response

While the optimal LV lead position is not fully defined; the lateral and posterolateral wall have been the preferred location since it is often the last segment to contract in dyssynchronous LV. Reverse remodeling was significantly greater in patients where the LV lead was placed at the site of maximal delay [100]. Unfortunately, placing a transvenous lead at this site may be limited by coronary sinus anatomy, diaphragmatic stimulation, or scar burden. A lower CRT response rate has been seen in patients with transmural posterolateral scar by cardiac magnetic resonance imaging [101].

A meta-analysis of five CRT trials involving 3872 patients showed a similar mortality benefit in men and women [102] which was in contrast to a subset analysis of MADIT-CRT showing that both the mortality benefit and adverse event rate were higher in women [84, 103].

Clinical trials have not specifically addressed the benefit of CRT in elderly patients. A meta-analysis of five randomized CRT trials (median age 66, range 58–73 years) found no significant interaction between age and CRT effect on all-cause mortality or heart failure hospitalization [102].

AF is common in patients with HF affecting 10–25% of patients with NYHA Class II-III and 50% of patients with NYHA Class IV [104]. Studies have suggested that CRT may not be as effective for patients with AF. Randomized, controlled clinical trials have almost always excluded patients with AF. With AF, there is loss of atrioventricular synchrony and rapid ventricular rates lead to electrical fusion and reduced true biventricular pacing capture. AV nodal agents have been the main treatments for controlling ventricular response while atrioventricular junction ablation (AVJA) has also been used as an alternative to drug therapy to control the ventricular rates in patients with permanent AF. In patients with HF and permanent AF undergoing CRT, AVJA is associated with a significant reduction in all-cause mortality, cardiovascular mortality, and improvements in NYHA functional class compared to those treated with AV nodal agents [105].

The majority of patients enrolled in CRT trials were NYHA HF Class III while some had NYHA Class IV HF. There has been concern that NYHA Class IV HF patients may not benefit from CRT or CRT-D since implantation may destabilize their HF and their life expectancy would limit long term benefits. In the COMPANION trial, 217 patients had NYHA Class IV HF but this represented a relatively stable patient group ("Ambulatory Class IV") since patients were excluded if cardiac transplantation was expected within 6 months and no HF hospitalizations within 30 days of enrollment. In this group, CRT and CRT-D significantly reduced the time to hospitalization or death with a trend towards reduced all-cause mortality in both arms [106].

9.3.5 CRT Impact on Ventricular Tachyarrhythmias

The reverse remodeling seen in CRT responders is associated with a reduced risk of ventricular tachyarrhythmias (VTA).

In MADIT-CRT, the risk of first VTA was lowest among high CRT responders and highest for low responders [107]. Continued CRT following LVAD lead to significant reduction in VTA burden and ICD shocks [108].

9.3.6 Interruption of CRT

Loss of CRT due to malfunction or cessation typically leads to rapid deterioration with subsequent HF exacerbation. In a report of 20 patients who underwent temporary cessation of BiV pacing, there was a significant decline in the maximal rate of rise of LV systolic pressure (711–442 mm Hg) with a twofold increase in mitral regurgitation at 72 h [109].

9.3.7 Alternatives to Coronary Sinus Lead

Unfortunately, a large number of patients do not receive CRT due to inability of deploying a lead via the coronary sinus or receive a suboptimal position of the left ventricular epicardial lead related to anatomic constraints. This is likely a contributing factor to the high non-responder rate to CRT [110].

In these cases, the leads can be implanted epicardially via a thoracotomy or thoracoscopically [111, 112]. This approach, due to it higher morbidity and mortality, is mainly reserved for patients that failed the transvenous CS approach. A variant to the surgical approach, is the implantation of epicardial lead with via percutaneous subxiphoid approach. This less invasive technique has been already validated in animal studies [113].

More recently, an in an attempt to prevent extensive surgical procedures in patients with compromised hemodynamic parameters, LV endocardial pacing have been attempted. This technique has been described in a small number of patients, mainly single center experiences and lack the large randomized clinical trial that support the transvenous coronary sinus approach. Endocardial LV-pacing appears to have hemodynamic advantage to CS-epicardial pacing [114] and have the disadvantage of exposing the lead to the systemic circulation, increasing the risk for thromboembolic stroke and the need for lifelong anticoagulation [115]. There are descriptions of LV lead deployment via a transseptal puncture [116, 117] or even a transventricular septal puncture [118].

9.3.8 Assessing CRT Response at Follow-up

In the MIRACLE trial, clinical and QOL improvement was seen at 1 month [119] while in CARE-HF & COMPANION, benefit was assessed at 3 months [120, 121]. Multiple criteria have been used to assess CRT response at follow-up: one level improvement in NYHA class, improved 6 min walk, quality of life measures, and decreased HF admissions. Up to one third of patients do not have a clinical response to CRT and over 40% do not show evidence of reverse remodeling [122]. For those patients who do not show clinical improvement following CRT, the following considerations are recommended:

9.3.9 Evaluation of Non-Responders at 3 Month Follow-up

1. Does 12 lead ECG show evidence of BiV pacing?
2. Is patient in sinus rhythm or AF
3. Device interrogation, capture thresholds
4. What is the percentage of BiV pacing?
5. CXR evaluation for lead position (stable, lateral position)?
6. 6 min walk time (if done pre-implant)
7. Repeat echocardiogram to assess LVEF and LVESV

Some patients exhibit a super-response to CRT defined as a two-fold or more increase in LVEF or LVEF > 45%, a decrease in LV end-systolic volume, and a decrease in NYHA HF functional class ≥1. Super-responders had significantly smaller mitral regurgitation and LV end-diastolic diameter (LVEDD) and mitral regurgitation jet, and heart failure symptoms for <12 months prior to implant [123]. In MADIT-CRT, 6 factors predicted super-response: female sex, no prior myocardial infarction, QRS duration ≥ 150 ms, left bundle branch block, body mass index <30 kg/m^2, and smaller baseline left atrial volume index. Super-response was associated with significantly reduced risk of HF or all-cause death [124] prompting the question if these patients should be changed to a CRT-P system at subsequent generator replacement.

References

1. Kannel WB, Wilson PW, D'Agostino RB, Cobb J. Sudden coronary death in women. Am Heart J. 1998;136(2):205–12.
2. MERIT-HF Study Group. Effect of metoprolol CR/XL in chronic heart failure: metoprolol CR/XL randomised intervention trial in congestive heart failure (MERIT-HF). Lancet (London, England). 1999;353(9169):2001–7.
3. Narang R, Cleland JG, Erhardt L, Ball SG, Coats AJ, Cowley AJ, et al. Mode of death in chronic heart failure. A request and proposition for more accurate classification. Eur Heart J. 1996;17(9):1390–403.
4. Mirowski M, Mower MM, Staewen WS, Tabatznik B, Mendeloff AI. Standby automatic defibrillator. An approach to prevention of sudden coronary death. Arch Intern Med. 1970;126(1):158–61.
5. Mirowski M, Reid PR, Mower MM, Watkins L, Gott VL, Schauble JF, et al. Termination of malignant ventricular arrhythmias with an implanted automatic defibrillator in human beings. N Engl J Med. 1980;303(6):322–4.

6. Tracy CM, Epstein AE, Darbar D, Dimarco JP, Dunbar SB, Estes NA 3rd, et al. 2012 ACCF/AHA/HRS focused update of the 2008 guidelines for device-based therapy of cardiac rhythm abnormalities: a report of the American College of Cardiology Foundation/ American Heart Association Task Force on Practice Guidelines. J Am Coll Cardiol. 2012;60(14):1297–313.
7. Moss AJ, Hall WJ, Cannom DS, Daubert JP, Higgins SL, Klein H, et al. Improved survival with an implanted defibrillator in patients with coronary disease at high risk for ventricular arrhythmia. Multicenter automatic defibrillator implantation trial investigators. N Engl J Med. 1996;335(26):1933–40.
8. Moss AJ, Zareba W, Hall WJ, Klein H, Wilber DJ, Cannom DS, et al. Prophylactic implantation of a defibrillator in patients with myocardial infarction and reduced ejection fraction. N Engl J Med. 2002;346(12):877–83.
9. Bigger JT Jr. Prophylactic use of implanted cardiac defibrillators in patients at high risk for ventricular arrhythmias after coronary-artery bypass graft surgery. Coronary artery bypass graft (CABG) patch trial investigators. N Engl J Med. 1997;337(22):1569–75.
10. Buxton AE, Lee KL, Fisher JD, Josephson ME, Prystowsky EN, Hafley G. A randomized study of the prevention of sudden death in patients with coronary artery disease. Multicenter unsustained tachycardia trial investigators. N Engl J Med. 1999;341(25):1882–90.
11. Buxton AE, Lee KL, Hafley GE, Wyse DG, Fisher JD, Lehmann MH, et al. Relation of ejection fraction and inducible ventricular tachycardia to mode of death in patients with coronary artery disease: an analysis of patients enrolled in the multicenter unsustained tachycardia trial. Circulation. 2002;106(19):2466–72.
12. Bardy GH, Lee KL, Mark DB, Poole JE, Packer DL, Boineau R, et al. Amiodarone or an implantable cardioverter-defibrillator for congestive heart failure. N Engl J Med. 2005;352(3):225–37.
13. Hohnloser SH, Kuck KH, Dorian P, Roberts RS, Hampton JR, Hatala R, et al. Prophylactic use of an implantable cardioverter-defibrillator after acute myocardial infarction. N Engl J Med. 2004;351(24):2481–8.
14. Steinbeck G, Andresen D, Seidl K, Brachmann J, Hoffmann E, Wojciechowski D, et al. Defibrillator implantation early after myocardial infarction. N Engl J Med. 2009;361(15):1427–36.
15. Orn S, Cleland JG, Romo M, Kjekshus J, Dickstein K. Recurrent infarction causes the most deaths following myocardial infarction with left ventricular dysfunction. Am J Med. 2005;118(7): 752–8.
16. Strickberger SA, Hummel JD, Bartlett TG, Frumin HI, Schuger CD, Beau SL, et al. Amiodarone versus implantable cardioverter-defibrillator:randomized trial in patients with nonischemic dilated cardiomyopathy and asymptomatic nonsustained ventricular tachycardia – AMIOVIRT. J Am Coll Cardiol. 2003;41(10):1707–12.
17. Bansch D, Antz M, Boczor S, Volkmer M, Tebbenjohanns J, Seidl K, et al. Primary prevention of sudden cardiac death in idiopathic dilated cardiomyopathy: the Cardiomyopathy Trial (CAT). Circulation. 2002;105(12):1453–8.
18. Kadish A, Dyer A, Daubert JP, Quigg R, Estes NA, Anderson KP, et al. Prophylactic defibrillator implantation in patients with nonischemic dilated cardiomyopathy. N Engl J Med. 2004;350(21):2151–8.
19. Mark DB, Anstrom KJ, Sun JL, Clapp-Channing NE, Tsiatis AA, Davidson-Ray L, et al. Quality of life with defibrillator therapy or amiodarone in heart failure. N Engl J Med. 2008;359(10):999–1008.
20. Wood MA, Stambler BS, Damiano RJ, Greenway P, Ellenbogen KA. Lessons learned from data logging in a multicenter clinical trial using a late-generation implantable cardioverter-defibrillator. The Guardian ATP 4210 Multicenter Investigators Group. J Am Coll Cardiol. 1994;24(7):1692–9.
21. Nunain SO, Roelke M, Trouton T, Osswald S, Kim YH, Sosa-Suarez G, et al. Limitations and late complications of third-generation automatic cardioverter-defibrillators. Circulation. 1995;91(8):2204–13.
22. Grimm W, Flores BF, Marchlinski FE. Electrocardiographically documented unnecessary, spontaneous shocks in 241 patients with implantable cardioverter defibrillators. Pacing Clin Electrophysiol. 1992;15(11 Pt 1):1667–73.
23. Klein RC, Raitt MH, Wilkoff BL, Beckman KJ, Coromilas J, Wyse DG, et al. Analysis of implantable cardioverter defibrillator therapy in the Antiarrhythmics Versus Implantable Defibrillators (AVID) trial. J Cardiovasc Electrophysiol. 2003;14(9):940–8.
24. Schaumann A, von zur Muhlen F, Herse B, Gonska BD, Kreuzer H. Empirical versus tested antitachycardia pacing in implantable cardioverter defibrillators: a prospective study including 200 patients. Circulation. 1998;97(1):66–74.
25. Saksena S, Chandran P, Shah Y, Boccadamo R, Pantopoulos D, Rothbart ST. Comparative efficacy of transvenous cardioversion and pacing in patients with sustained ventricular tachycardia: a prospective, randomized, crossover study. Circulation. 1985;72(1):153–60.
26. Bardy GH, Poole JE, Kudenchuk PJ, Dolack GL, Kelso D, Mitchell R. A prospective randomized repeat-crossover comparison of antitachycardia pacing with low-energy cardioversion. Circulation. 1993;87(6):1889–96.
27. Saksena S. Clinical outcome of patients with malignant ventricular tachyarrhythmias and a multiprogrammable implantable cardioverter-defibrillator implanted with or without thoracotomy: an international multicenter study. PCD Investigator Group. Journal of the American College of Cardiology. 1994;23(7):1521–30.
28. Sullivan RM, Russo AM, Berg KC, Stolen KQ, Seth M, Perschbacher D, et al. Arrhythmia rate distribution and tachyarrhythmia therapy in an ICD population: results from the INTRINSIC RV trial. Heart Rhythm. 2012;9(3):351–8.
29. Wathen MS, DeGroot PJ, Sweeney MO, Stark AJ, Otterness MF, Adkisson WO, et al. Prospective randomized multicenter trial of empirical antitachycardia pacing versus shocks for spontaneous rapid ventricular tachycardia in patients with implantable cardioverter-defibrillators: Pacing Fast Ventricular Tachycardia Reduces Shock Therapies (PainFREE Rx II) trial results. Circulation. 2004;110(17):2591–6.
30. Clemens M, Nagy-Balo E, Herczku C, Kun C, Edes I, Csanadi Z. Long-term arrhythmia variability after monomorphic ventricular tachycardia in patients with an implantable cardioverter defibrillator. Pacing Clin Electrophysiol. 2011;34(10):1185–91.
31. Healey JS, Dorian P, Mitchell LB, Talajic M, Philippon F, Simpson C, et al. Canadian Registry of ICD Implant Testing procedures (CREDIT): current practice, risks, and costs of intraoperative defibrillation testing. J Cardiovasc Electrophysiol. 2010;21(2):177–82.
32. Venditti FJ Jr, John RM, Hull M, Tofler GH, Shahian DM, Martin DT. Circadian variation in defibrillation energy requirements. Circulation. 1996;94(7):1607–12.
33. Healey JS, Gula LJ, Birnie DH, Sterns L, Connolly SJ, Sapp J, et al. A randomized-controlled pilot study comparing ICD implantation with and without intraoperative defibrillation testing in patients with heart failure and severe left ventricular dysfunction: a substudy of the RAFT trial. J Cardiovasc Electrophysiol. 2012;23(12):1313–6.
34. Healey JS, Hohnloser SH, Glikson M, Neuzner J, Mabo P, Vinolas X, et al. Cardioverter defibrillator implantation without induction of ventricular fibrillation: a single-blind, non-inferiority, randomised controlled trial (SIMPLE). Lancet (London, England). 2015;385(9970):785–91.

35. Bansch D, Bonnemeier H, Brandt J, Bode F, Svendsen JH, Taborsky M, et al. Intra-operative defibrillation testing and clinical shock efficacy in patients with implantable cardioverter-defibrillators: the NORDIC ICD randomized clinical trial. Eur Heart J. 2015;36(37):2500–7.
36. Wilkoff BL, Cook JR, Epstein AE, Greene HL, Hallstrom AP, Hsia H, et al. Dual-chamber pacing or ventricular backup pacing in patients with an implantable defibrillator: the dual chamber and VVI implantable defibrillator (DAVID) trial. JAMA. 2002;288(24):3115–23.
37. Sweeney MO, Hellkamp AS, Ellenbogen KA, Greenspon AJ, Freedman RA, Lee KL, et al. Adverse effect of ventricular pacing on heart failure and atrial fibrillation among patients with normal baseline QRS duration in a clinical trial of pacemaker therapy for sinus node dysfunction. Circulation. 2003;107(23):2932–7.
38. Yu CM, Chan JY, Zhang Q, Omar R, Yip GW, Hussin A, et al. Biventricular pacing in patients with bradycardia and normal ejection fraction. N Engl J Med. 2009;361(22):2123–34.
39. Madhavan M, Friedman PA. Optimal programming of implantable cardiac-defibrillators. Circulation. 2013;128(6):659–72.
40. Poole JE, Johnson GW, Hellkamp AS, Anderson J, Callans DJ, Raitt MH, et al. Prognostic importance of defibrillator shocks in patients with heart failure. N Engl J Med. 2008;359(10): 1009–17.
41. Sweeney MO, Wathen MS, Volosin K, Abdalla I, DeGroot PJ, Otterness MF, et al. Appropriate and inappropriate ventricular therapies, quality of life, and mortality among primary and secondary prevention implantable cardioverter defibrillator patients: results from the Pacing Fast VT Reduces Shock Therapies (PainFREE Rx II) trial. Circulation. 2005;111(22):2898–905.
42. Tokano T, Bach D, Chang J, Davis J, Souza JJ, Zivin A, et al. Effect of ventricular shock strength on cardiac hemodynamics. J Cardiovasc Electrophysiol. 1998;9(8):791–7.
43. Goldenberg I, Moss AJ, Hall WJ, McNitt S, Zareba W, Andrews ML, et al. Causes and consequences of heart failure after prophylactic implantation of a defibrillator in the multicenter automatic defibrillator implantation trial II. Circulation. 2006;113(24):2810–7.
44. Daubert JP, Zareba W, Cannom DS, McNitt S, Rosero SZ, Wang P, et al. Inappropriate implantable cardioverter-defibrillator shocks in MADIT II: frequency, mechanisms, predictors, and survival impact. J Am Coll Cardiol. 2008;51(14):1357–65.
45. Burke MC, Gold MR, Knight BP, Barr CS, Theuns DA, Boersma LV, et al. Safety and efficacy of the totally subcutaneous implantable defibrillator: 2-year results from a pooled analysis of the IDE study and EFFORTLESS registry. J Am Coll Cardiol. 2015;65(16):1605–15.
46. Moss AJ, Schuger C, Beck CA, Brown MW, Cannom DS, Daubert JP, et al. Reduction in inappropriate therapy and mortality through ICD programming. N Engl J Med. 2012;367(24): 2275–83.
47. Gasparini M, Proclemer A, Klersy C, Kloppe A, Lunati M, Ferrer JB, et al. Effect of long-detection interval vs standard-detection interval for implantable cardioverter-defibrillators on antitachycardia pacing and shock delivery: the ADVANCE III randomized clinical trial. JAMA. 2013;309(18):1903–11.
48. Scott PA, Silberbauer J, McDonagh TA, Murgatroyd FD. Impact of prolonged implantable cardioverter-defibrillator arrhythmia detection times on outcomes: a meta-analysis. Heart Rhythm. 2014;11(5):828–35.
49. Vakil K, Kazmirczak F, Sathnur N, Adabag S, Cantillon DJ, Kiehl EL, et al. Implantable cardioverter-defibrillator use in patients with left ventricular assist devices: a systematic review and meta-analysis. JACC Heart Fail. 2016;4(10):772–9.
50. Patel D, Hasselblad V, Patel C, Pokorney S, Zeitler E, Rogers J, et al. The role of implantable cardioverter defibrillators (ICDS) in patients with a left ventricular assist device (LVAD): a systematic review and meta-analysis. J Am Coll Cardiol. 2016;67(13_S):700.
51. Williams D, Rao P, Nassif M, Novak E, Sandberg S, LaRue S, et al. Permissive ICD programming for LVAD patients. J Card Fail. 2015;21(8):S105.
52. Varma N, Epstein AE, Irimpen A, Schweikert R, Love C. Efficacy and safety of automatic remote monitoring for implantable cardioverter-defibrillator follow-up: the lumos-T safely reduces routine office device follow-up (TRUST) trial. Circulation. 2010;122(4):325–32.
53. Crossley GH, Boyle A, Vitense H, Chang Y, Mead RH. The CONNECT (clinical evaluation of remote notification to reduce time to clinical decision) trial: the value of wireless remote monitoring with automatic clinician alerts. J Am Coll Cardiol. 2011;57(10):1181–9.
54. Saxon LA, Hayes DL, Gilliam FR, Heidenreich PA, Day J, Seth M, et al. Long-term outcome after ICD and CRT implantation and influence of remote device follow-up: the ALTITUDE survival study. Circulation. 2010;122(23):2359–67.
55. Catanzariti D, Lunati M, Landolina M, Zanotto G, Lonardi G, Iacopino S, et al. Monitoring intrathoracic impedance with an implantable defibrillator reduces hospitalizations in patients with heart failure. Pacing Clin Electrophysiol. 2009;32(3):363–70.
56. van Veldhuisen DJ, Braunschweig F, Conraads V, Ford I, Cowie MR, Jondeau G, et al. Intrathoracic impedance monitoring, audible patient alerts, and outcome in patients with heart failure. Circulation. 2011;124(16):1719–26.
57. Brachmann J, Bohm M, Rybak K, Klein G, Butter C, Klemm H, et al. Fluid status monitoring with a wireless network to reduce cardiovascular-related hospitalizations and mortality in heart failure: rationale and design of the OptiLink HF study (Optimization of Heart Failure Management using OptiVol Fluid Status Monitoring and CareLink). Eur J Heart Fail. 2011;13(7):796–804.
58. Whellan DJ, Ousdigian KT, Al-Khatib SM, Pu W, Sarkar S, Porter CB, et al. Combined heart failure device diagnostics identify patients at higher risk of subsequent heart failure hospitalizations: results from PARTNERS HF (program to access and review trending information and evaluate correlation to symptoms in patients with heart failure) study. J Am Coll Cardiol. 2010;55(17):1803–10.
59. Hindricks G, Taborsky M, Glikson M, Heinrich U, Schumacher B, Katz A, et al. Implant-based multiparameter telemonitoring of patients with heart failure (IN-TIME): a randomised controlled trial. Lancet (London, England). 2014;384(9943):583–90.
60. Varma N, Piccini JP, Snell J, Fischer A, Dalal N, Mittal S. The relationship between level of adherence to automatic wireless remote monitoring and survival in pacemaker and defibrillator patients. J Am Coll Cardiol. 2015;65(24):2601–10.
61. Neuzil P, Taborsky M, Holy F, Wallbrueck K. Early automatic remote detection of combined lead insulation defect and ICD damage. Europace. 2008;10(5):556–7.
62. Spencker S, Coban N, Koch L, Schirdewan A, Muller D. Potential role of home monitoring to reduce inappropriate shocks in implantable cardioverter-defibrillator patients due to lead failure. Europace. 2009;11(4):483–8.
63. Schron EB, Exner DV, Yao Q, Jenkins LS, Steinberg JS, Cook JR, et al. Quality of life in the antiarrhythmics versus implantable defibrillators trial: impact of therapy and influence of adverse symptoms and defibrillator shocks. Circulation. 2002;105(5):589–94.
64. Stevenson WG, Chaitman BR, Ellenbogen KA, Epstein AE, Gross WL, Hayes DL, et al. Clinical assessment and management of patients with implanted cardioverter-defibrillators presenting to nonelectrophysiologists. Circulation. 2004;110(25):3866–9.

65. Zipes DP, Camm AJ, Borggrefe M, Buxton AE, Chaitman B, Fromer M, et al. ACC/AHA/ESC 2006 guidelines for management of patients with ventricular arrhythmias and the prevention of sudden cardiac death: a report of the American College of Cardiology/American Heart Association Task Force and the European Society of Cardiology Committee for Practice Guidelines (writing committee to develop guidelines for management of patients with ventricular arrhythmias and the prevention of sudden cardiac death). J Am Coll Cardiol. 2006;48(5):e247–346.
66. Exner DV, Pinski SL, Wyse DG, Renfroe EG, Follmann D, Gold M, et al. Electrical storm presages nonsudden death: the antiarrhythmics versus implantable defibrillators (AVID) trial. Circulation. 2001;103(16):2066–71.
67. Dunbar SB, Dougherty CM, Sears SF, Carroll DL, Goldstein NE, Mark DB, et al. Educational and psychological interventions to improve outcomes for recipients of implantable cardioverter defibrillators and their families: a scientific statement from the American Heart Association. Circulation. 2012;126(17):2146–72.
68. Connolly SJ, Dorian P, Roberts RS, Gent M, Bailin S, Fain ES, et al. Comparison of beta-blockers, amiodarone plus beta-blockers, or sotalol for prevention of shocks from implantable cardioverter defibrillators: the OPTIC study: a randomized trial. JAMA. 2006;295(2):165–71.
69. Piccini JP, Berger JS, O'Connor CM. Amiodarone for the prevention of sudden cardiac death: a meta-analysis of randomized controlled trials. Eur Heart J. 2009;30(10):1245–53.
70. Bokhari F, Newman D, Greene M, Korley V, Mangat I, Dorian P. Long-term comparison of the implantable cardioverter defibrillator versus amiodarone: eleven-year follow-up of a subset of patients in the Canadian implantable defibrillator study (CIDS). Circulation. 2004;110(2):112–6.
71. Pedersen CT, Kay GN, Kalman J, Borggrefe M, Della-Bella P, Dickfeld T, et al. EHRA/HRS/APHRS expert consensus on ventricular arrhythmias. Heart Rhythm. 2014;11(10):e166–96.
72. Reddy VY, Reynolds MR, Neuzil P, Richardson AW, Taborsky M, Jongnarangsin K, et al. Prophylactic catheter ablation for the prevention of defibrillator therapy. N Engl J Med. 2007;357(26):2657–65.
73. Kuck KH, Schaumann A, Eckardt L, Willems S, Ventura R, Delacretaz E, et al. Catheter ablation of stable ventricular tachycardia before defibrillator implantation in patients with coronary heart disease (VTACH): a multicentre randomised controlled trial. Lancet (London, England). 2010;375(9708):31–40.
74. Tung R, Vaseghi M, Frankel DS, Vergara P, Di Biase L, Nagashima K, et al. Freedom from recurrent ventricular tachycardia after catheter ablation is associated with improved survival in patients with structural heart disease: an International VT Ablation Center Collaborative Group study. Heart Rhythm. 2015;12(9):1997–2007.
75. Sapp JL, Wells GA, Parkash R, Stevenson WG, Blier L, Sarrazin JF, et al. Ventricular tachycardia ablation versus escalation of antiarrhythmic drugs. New Engl J Med. 2016;375(2):111–21.
76. Aliot EM, Stevenson WG, Almendral-Garrote JM, Bogun F, Calkins CH, Delacretaz E, et al. EHRA/HRS expert consensus on catheter ablation of ventricular arrhythmias: developed in a partnership with the European Heart Rhythm Association (EHRA), a registered branch of the European Society of Cardiology (ESC), and the Heart Rhythm Society (HRS); in collaboration with the American College of Cardiology (ACC) and the American Heart Association (AHA). Heart Rhythm. 2009;6(6):886–933.
77. Dinov B, Arya A, Schratter A, Schirripa V, Fiedler L, Sommer P, et al. Catheter ablation of ventricular tachycardia and mortality in patients with nonischemic dilated cardiomyopathy: can noninducibility after ablation be a predictor for reduced mortality? Circ Arrhythm Electrophysiol. 2015;8(3):598–605.
78. Epstein AE, Baessler CA, Curtis AB, Estes NA 3rd, Gersh BJ, Grubb B, et al. Addendum to "personal and public safety issues related to arrhythmias that may affect consciousness: implications for regulation and physician recommendations. A medical/scientific statement from the American Heart Association and the North American Society of Pacing and Electrophysiology". Public safety issues in patients with implantable defibrillators. A scientific statement from the American Heart Association and the Heart Rhythm Society. Heart Rhythm. 2007;4(3):386–93.
79. Singh M, Wang NC, Jain S, Voigt AH, Saba S, Adelstein EC. Utility of the wearable cardioverter-defibrillator in patients with newly diagnosed cardiomyopathy: a decade-long single-center experience. J Am Coll Cardiol. 2015;66(23):2607–13.
80. Bristow MR, Saxon LA, Boehmer J, Krueger S, Kass DA, De Marco T, et al. Cardiac-resynchronization therapy with or without an implantable defibrillator in advanced chronic heart failure. N Engl J Med. 2004;350(21):2140–50.
81. Cleland JG, Daubert JC, Erdmann E, Freemantle N, Gras D, Kappenberger L, et al. Longer-term effects of cardiac resynchronization therapy on mortality in heart failure [the CArdiac REsynchronization-Heart Failure (CARE-HF) trial extension phase]. Eur Heart J. 2006;27(16):1928–32.
82. Linde C, Abraham WT, Gold MR, St John Sutton M, Ghio S, Daubert C. Randomized trial of cardiac resynchronization in mildly symptomatic heart failure patients and in asymptomatic patients with left ventricular dysfunction and previous heart failure symptoms. J Am Coll Cardiol. 2008;52(23):1834–43.
83. Gold MR, Thebault C, Linde C, Abraham WT, Gerritse B, Ghio S, et al. Effect of QRS duration and morphology on cardiac resynchronization therapy outcomes in mild heart failure: results from the resynchronization reverses remodeling in systolic left ventricular dysfunction (REVERSE) study. Circulation. 2012;126(7):822–9.
84. Moss AJ, Hall WJ, Cannom DS, Klein H, Brown MW, Daubert JP, et al. Cardiac-resynchronization therapy for the prevention of heart-failure events. N Engl J Med. 2009;361(14):1329–38.
85. Zareba W, Klein H, Cygankiewicz I, Hall WJ, McNitt S, Brown M, et al. Effectiveness of cardiac resynchronization therapy by QRS morphology in the multicenter automatic defibrillator implantation trial-cardiac resynchronization therapy (MADIT-CRT). Circulation. 2011;123(10):1061–72.
86. Goldenberg I, Kutyifa V, Klein HU, Cannom DS, Brown MW, Dan A, et al. Survival with cardiac-resynchronization therapy in mild heart failure. N Engl J Med. 2014;370(18):1694–701.
87. Tang AS, Wells GA, Talajic M, Arnold MO, Sheldon R, Connolly S, et al. Cardiac-resynchronization therapy for mild-to-moderate heart failure. N Engl J Med. 2010;363(25):2385–95.
88. Sipahi I, Carrigan TP, Rowland DY, Stambler BS, Fang JC. Impact of QRS duration on clinical event reduction with cardiac resynchronization therapy: meta-analysis of randomized controlled trials. Arch Intern Med. 2011;171(16):1454–62.
89. Stavrakis S, Lazzara R, Thadani U. The benefit of cardiac resynchronization therapy and QRS duration: a meta-analysis. J Cardiovasc Electrophysiol. 2012;23(2):163–8.
90. Curtis AB, Worley SJ, Adamson PB, Chung ES, Niazi I, Sherfesee L, et al. Biventricular pacing for atrioventricular block and systolic dysfunction. N Engl J Med. 2013;368(17):1585–93.
91. Ruschitzka F, Abraham WT, Singh JP, Bax JJ, Borer JS, Brugada J, et al. Cardiac-resynchronization therapy in heart failure with a narrow QRS complex. N Engl J Med. 2013;369(15):1395–405.
92. Thibault B, Harel F, Ducharme A, White M, Ellenbogen KA, Frasure-Smith N, et al. Cardiac resynchronization therapy in patients with heart failure and a QRS complex <120 milliseconds: the Evaluation of Resynchronization Therapy for Heart Failure (LESSER-EARTH) trial. Circulation. 2013;127(8):873–81.
93. Muto C, Solimene F, Gallo P, Nastasi M, La Rosa C, Calvanese R, et al. A randomized study of cardiac resynchronization therapy defibrillator versus dual-chamber implantable cardioverter-defibrillator in ischemic cardiomyopathy with narrow QRS: the NARROW-CRT study. Circ Arrhythm Electrophysiol. 2013;6(3):538–45.

94. Poole JE, Singh JP, Birgersdotter-Green U. QRS duration or QRS morphology: what really matters in cardiac resynchronization therapy? J Am Coll Cardiol. 2016;67(9):1104–17.
95. Beshai JF, Grimm RA, Nagueh SF, Baker JH 2nd, Beau SL, Greenberg SM, et al. Cardiac-resynchronization therapy in heart failure with narrow QRS complexes. N Engl J Med. 2007;357(24):2461–71.
96. Nery PB, Ha AC, Keren A, Birnie DH. Cardiac resynchronization therapy in patients with left ventricular systolic dysfunction and right bundle branch block: a systematic review. Heart Rhythm. 2011;8(7):1083–7.
97. Bilchick KC, Kamath S, DiMarco JP, Stukenborg GJ. Bundle-branch block morphology and other predictors of outcome after cardiac resynchronization therapy in Medicare patients. Circulation. 2010;122(20):2022–30.
98. Peterson PN, Greiner MA, Qualls LG, Al-Khatib SM, Curtis JP, Fonarow GC, et al. QRS duration, bundle-branch block morphology, and outcomes among older patients with heart failure receiving cardiac resynchronization therapy. JAMA. 2013;310(6):617–26.
99. Goldenberg I, Moss AJ, Hall WJ, Foster E, Goldberger JJ, Santucci P, et al. Predictors of response to cardiac resynchronization therapy in the multicenter automatic defibrillator implantation trial with cardiac resynchronization therapy (MADIT-CRT). Circulation. 2011;124(14):1527–36.
100. Murphy RT, Sigurdsson G, Mulamalla S, Agler D, Popovic ZB, Starling RC, et al. Tissue synchronization imaging and optimal left ventricular pacing site in cardiac resynchronization therapy. Am J Cardiol. 2006;97(11):1615–21.
101. Bleeker GB, Kaandorp TA, Lamb HJ, Boersma E, Steendijk P, de Roos A, et al. Effect of posterolateral scar tissue on clinical and echocardiographic improvement after cardiac resynchronization therapy. Circulation. 2006;113(7):969–76.
102. Cleland JG, Abraham WT, Linde C, Gold MR, Young JB, Claude Daubert J, et al. An individual patient meta-analysis of five randomized trials assessing the effects of cardiac resynchronization therapy on morbidity and mortality in patients with symptomatic heart failure. Eur Heart J. 2013;34(46):3547–56.
103. Arshad A, Moss AJ, Foster E, Padeletti L, Barsheshet A, Goldenberg I, et al. Cardiac resynchronization therapy is more effective in women than in men: the MADIT-CRT (multicenter automatic defibrillator implantation trial with cardiac resynchronization therapy) trial. J Am Coll Cardiol. 2011;57(7):813–20.
104. Maisel WH, Stevenson LW. Atrial fibrillation in heart failure: epidemiology, pathophysiology, and rationale for therapy. Am J Cardiol. 2003;91(6a):2d–8d.
105. Ganesan AN, Brooks AG, Roberts-Thomson KC, Lau DH, Kalman JM, Sanders P. Role of AV nodal ablation in cardiac resynchronization in patients with coexistent atrial fibrillation and heart failure a systematic review. J Am Coll Cardiol. 2012;59(8):719–26.
106. Lindenfeld J, Feldman AM, Saxon L, Boehmer J, Carson P, Ghali JK, et al. Effects of cardiac resynchronization therapy with or without a defibrillator on survival and hospitalizations in patients with New York Heart Association class IV heart failure. Circulation. 2007;115(2):204–12.
107. Barsheshet A, Wang PJ, Moss AJ, Solomon SD, Al-Ahmad A, McNitt S, et al. Reverse remodeling and the risk of ventricular tachyarrhythmias in the MADIT-CRT (multicenter automatic defibrillator implantation trial-cardiac resynchronization therapy). J Am Coll Cardiol. 2011;57(24):2416–23.
108. Schleifer JW, Mookadam F, Kransdorf EP, Nanda U, Adams JC, Cha S, et al. Effect of continued cardiac resynchronization therapy on ventricular arrhythmias after left ventricular assist device implantation. Ame J Cardiol. 2016;118:556–9.
109. Brandt RR, Reiner C, Arnold R, Sperzel J, Pitschner HF, Hamm CW. Contractile response and mitral regurgitation after temporary interruption of long-term cardiac resynchronization therapy. Eur Heart J. 2006;27(2):187–92.
110. St John Sutton MG, Plappert T, Abraham WT, Smith AL, Delurgio DB, Leon AR, et al. Effect of cardiac resynchronization therapy on left ventricular size and function in chronic heart failure. Circulation. 2003;107(15):1985–90.
111. Mair H, Jansens JL, Lattouf OM, Reichart B, Dabritz S. Epicardial lead implantation techniques for biventricular pacing via left lateral mini-thoracotomy, video-assisted thoracoscopy, and robotic approach. Heart Surg Forum. 2003;6(5):412–7.
112. Gabor S, Prenner G, Wasler A, Schweiger M, Tscheliessnigg KH, Smolle-Juttner FM. A simplified technique for implantation of left ventricular epicardial leads for biventricular re-synchronization using video-assisted thoracoscopy (VATS). European J Cardiothorac Surg. 2005;28(6):797–800.
113. John RM, Morgan K, Brennecke LH, Benser ME, Jais P. Acute and chronic performance evaluation of a novel epicardial pacing lead placed by percutaneous subxiphoid approach in a canine model. Circ Arrhythm Electrophysiol. 2015;8(3):659–66.
114. Bordachar P, Derval N, Ploux S, Garrigue S, Ritter P, Haissaguerre M, et al. Left ventricular endocardial stimulation for severe heart failure. J Am Coll Cardiol. 2010;56(10):747–53.
115. Morgan JM, Biffi M, Geller L, Leclercq C, Ruffa F, Tung S, et al. ALternate Site Cardiac ResYNChronization (ALSYNC): a prospective and multicentre study of left ventricular endocardial pacing for cardiac resynchronization therapy. Eur Heart J. 2016;37(27):2118–27.
116. van Gelder BM, Scheffer MG, Meijer A, Bracke FA. Transseptal endocardial left ventricular pacing: an alternative technique for coronary sinus lead placement in cardiac resynchronization therapy. Heart Rhythm. 2007;4(4):454–60.
117. Elencwajg B, Lopez Cabanillas N, Cardinali EL, Barisani JL, Trainini J, Fischer A, et al. The Jurdham procedure: endocardial left ventricular lead insertion via a femoral transseptal sheath for cardiac resynchronization therapy pectoral device implantation. Heart Rhythm. 2012;9(11):1798–804.
118. Betts TR, Gamble JH, Khiani R, Bashir Y, Rajappan K. Development of a technique for left ventricular endocardial pacing via puncture of the interventricular septum. Circ Arrhythm Electrophysiol. 2014;7(1):17–22.
119. Ermis C, Seutter R, Zhu AX, Benditt LC, VanHeel L, Sakaguchi S, et al. Impact of upgrade to cardiac resynchronization therapy on ventricular arrhythmia frequency in patients with implantable cardioverter-defibrillators. J Am Coll Cardiol. 2005;46(12):2258–63.
120. Cleland JG, Daubert JC, Erdmann E, Freemantle N, Gras D, Kappenberger L, et al. The effect of cardiac resynchronization on morbidity and mortality in heart failure. N Engl J Med. 2005;352(15):1539–49.
121. Fantoni C, Raffa S, Regoli F, Giraldi F, La Rovere MT, Prentice J, et al. Cardiac resynchronization therapy improves heart rate profile and heart rate variability of patients with moderate to severe heart failure. J Am Coll Cardiol. 2005;46(10):1875–82.
122. Mullens W, Grimm RA, Verga T, Dresing T, Starling RC, Wilkoff BL, et al. Insights from a cardiac resynchronization optimization clinic as part of a heart failure disease management program. J Am Coll Cardiol. 2009;53(9):765–73.
123. Antonio N, Teixeira R, Coelho L, Lourenco C, Monteiro P, Ventura M, et al. Identification of 'super-responders' to cardiac resynchronization therapy: the importance of symptom duration and left ventricular geometry. Europace. 2009;11(3):343–9.
124. Hsu JC, Solomon SD, Bourgoun M, McNitt S, Goldenberg I, Klein H, et al. Predictors of super-response to cardiac resynchronization therapy and associated improvement in clinical outcome: the MADIT-CRT (multicenter automatic defibrillator implantation trial with cardiac resynchronization therapy) study. J Am Coll Cardiol. 2012;59(25):2366–73.

Interpretation of Clinical Trials in the Context of Personalized/Individualized Medicine and End of Life Issues

10

Georg Ertl

Randomized controlled trials (RCT) provide evidence based medicine that has substantially improved prognosis, symptoms and quality of life of patients with chronic heart failure (Fig. 10.1). Most importantly, negative RCT have stopped super fluent or even harmful therapies [1–3]. Recent trials have however required thousands of patients to achieve statistical significance. In heart failure, variable etiologies, the manifestation as systolic or diastolic heart failure, chronic stable or acute decompensated heart failure, multiple comorbidities and complications pose a major challenge to clinical studies [4] (Fig. 10.2). For good reasons, many patients have been excluded from trials since their prognosis was foreseeable too good or too fatal. Studies focus on patients with coronary heart disease or non-coronary etiology with variant results. So far, no drug has provided benefit in studies with diastolic heart failure [5]. Nevertheless, most patients with diastolic heart failure are treated with drugs used in systolic heart failure mostly since they are hypertensive. Diuretics are used without evidence of benefit in large trials simply since considered essential for re-compensation in acute heart failure and for fluid control in chronic stable heart failure. The age of our heart failure patients in daily practice is well beyond 70 years, on average 75 years in our INH-registry, and thus older than in most clinical studies [6–8]. But they are treated as recommended in guidelines based on substantially younger samples. Older patients may have other requirements of therapy. Quality of life out of hospital may be a primary end-point for an aged patient rather than mortality. This may be true also for patients with severe comorbidities, mostly excluded from clinical trials. Standard therapy of diseases failed when they occurred as a comorbidity of heart failure. But can therapy of heart failure be the same in the presence or absence of comorbidity? In a patient with advanced cancer and chemotherapy-induced cardiomyopathy, we would probably be reluctant to recommend an Implantable Cardioverter Defibrillator (ICD). However, heart failure itself may have a similar morbidity and mortality. So what does the mega-trials mean for the individual patient? [9].

10.1 Various Etiologies

Coronary Heart Disease (CHD) and hypertension are the most frequent etiologies of heart failure. Hypertension is the most frequent reason for Heart Failure with preserved Ejection Fraction (HFpEF) which will be discussed below. In studies on Heart Failure with reduced Ejection Fraction (HFrEF), the most frequent etiology is CHD, information on patients with other etiologies of HFrEF is comparably sparse, and therapy relies in part on extrapolation from CHD. But prophylactic ICD therapy for example has revealed different results in patients with HF of ischemic versus HF of non-ischemic etiology [10]. Thus, a specific etiology may request a different therapy. In addition, large HF trials have not included the therapy of underlying diseases, which require an individual treatment. In fact, correction of the underlying disorder may cure patients with heart failure of certain etiologies like valve disease, hyperthyroid disease, tachyarrhythmia or anemia. The combination of standard medical therapy with etiologically oriented therapy is not widely represented in clinical studies. Nevertheless, we frequently continue standard medical care in patients after correction of the condition underlying heart failure. It remains an individual decision when to stop heart failure therapy in these patients.

G. Ertl (✉)
University Hospital and Comprehensive Heart Failure Center
(Deutsches Zentrum für Herzinsuffizienz), Würzburg, Germany
e-mail: ertl_g@ukw.de

D. S. Feldman, P. Mohacsi (eds.), *Heart Failure*, Cardiovascular Medicine, https://doi.org/10.1007/978-3-319-98184-0_10

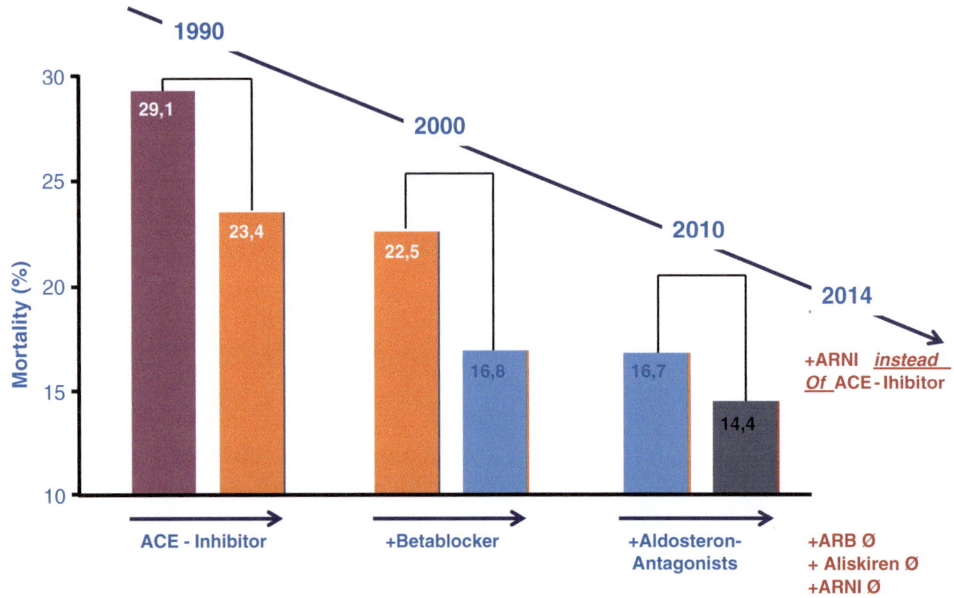

Fig. 10.1 Reduction of mortality by drug therapy in Randomized Controlled Trials (RCT)

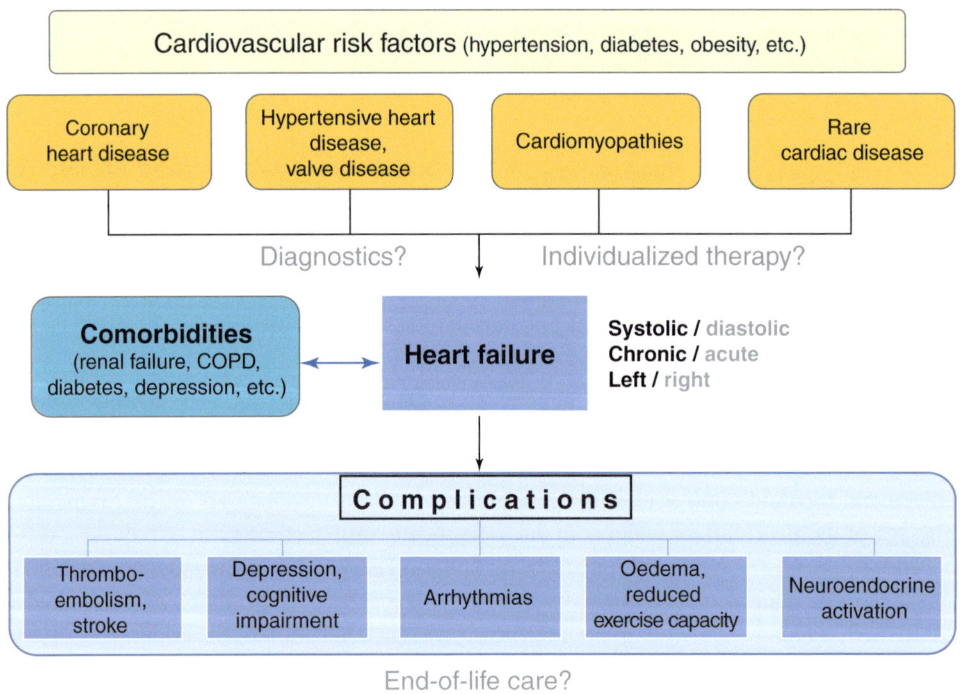

Fig. 10.2 Complex etiology and complications, comorbidities and the manifestation as systolic or diastolic heart failure challenge the methods of evidence-based medicine, which rely on randomized controlled mega trials [4]

10.2 Risk Factors and Comorbidities

Most risk factors for heart disease persist through the development of heart failure and present then as comorbidities. Diabetes remains as a strong risk factor in patients with heart failure, and recent studies testing effects of empagliflozin have opened new perspectives on therapy of heart failure [11]. In contrast, hypercholesterolemia and hypertension predict a rather better prognosis in patients with heart failure at least when it is advanced or acutely decompensated [12]. These patients require individual consideration whether treatment of risk factors is still adequate. Statins have not shown beneficial effects in patients with or without coronary artery disease and heart failure [13, 14]. Most patients with HFrEF are no longer hypertensive after up-titration of heart failure drugs. In contrast, patients with HFpEF may remain hypertensive and may need additional anti-hypertensive drugs.

The fact that prognosis is worse in presence of comorbidities has driven studies on therapy of comorbidities in heart failure. The hypothesis was that treating comorbidities would improve the course of heart failure. The results of these studies were devastating. The MOOD-HF study failed to prove the hypothesis that the antidepressant escitalopram in depressive patients with heart failure would improve heart failure related cardiovascular endpoints [15]. Patients treated with placebo and patients treated with escitalopram received the same high level of care by heart failure nurses and physicians. Depression scores significantly improved over time in both groups, but escitalopram did not improve scores of depression more than placebo. The SERVE-HF trial on patients with heart failure and central sleep apnea tested the hypothesis that CPAP therapy would reduce vascular events in patients with heart failure [16]. However, patients with CPAP treatment reached more cardiovascular end-points than control patients did. Thus, standard treatment failed when the diseases occurred as conditions comorbid to heart failure. It is left to the decision of the treating physician how to treat the comorbidity as well as heart failure in patients with comorbidities.

10.3 HFrEF Versus HFpEF

Good evidence has accumulated for the medical therapy of patients with HFrEF [5]. In fact, ejection fraction below 40 or 35% is obviously a fair measure to select patients for clinical studies on heart failure. However, "normal values" of EF range above 55%. By using the lower values as inclusion criteria, the investigators tempted to avoid including patients with normal left ventricular function. This does not imply that patients with a LVEF above 40 or 35% and symptoms of HF have diastolic HF. It does also not imply that patients with an ejection fraction below 40 or 35% do not have diastolic HF. It is likely that most patients with HFrEF have a diastolic component of heart failure due to large left ventricular volumes and increased wall stress, an infarct scar or diffuse left ventricular fibrosis and thus increased wall stiffness.

Rather artificial is the definition of "diastolic" heart failure as HFpEF or normal systolic left ventricular function in the presence of symptoms of HF. Adding Doppler echocardiographic parameters of left ventricular diastolic dysfunction or left ventricular hypertrophy may help in an individual patient for diagnosis. Even more a product than the basis of study design is the new definition of HFmrEF, Heart Failure with mid-range Ejection Fraction, i. e. a LVEF in the range of 40–49%, which represents the echocardiographic 'grey zone' between HFrEF and HFpEF [5]. These patients have been systematically left out of clinical studies on systolic heart failure.

Thus, our definition today of systolic heart failure bases on requirements of study design and technical reasons to measure EF in large patient populations rather than on pathophysiology. It may well be questioned whether this definition applies to the individual patient. EF is clearly not a good measure for LV function since it depends on afterload and may well decay and recover during acute decompensation and after recompensation, respectively [17]. On the other hand, many patients with HFpEF and HFmrEF are probably hypertensive and may fare well if their hypertension is well treated [5]. At least their symptoms may be controlled by diuretics and vasodilators even if they don't live longer. In studies on patients at risk, ACE inhibitors prevented HF [18]. Thus, therapy of patients with HFpEF and HFmrEF does not rest on evidence for improved survival; it is in the hands of an experienced therapist nevertheless helpful.

10.4 Acute Versus Chronic Heart Failure

Recent studies have dashed our hopes on new (classes of) drugs for the treatment of acute decompensated heart failure (ADHF). The situation is complex since some studies were positive others negative. The hypothesis of the RELAX studies was that a specific treatment with the pregnancy hormone serelaxin may prevent the damage by ADHF which results in later decay of prognosis. The endpoint varies among studies. The strongest, the RELAX-HF-2 study, randomly assigned patients to either serelaxin 30 μg/kg per day (n = 3274) or placebo (n = 3271) and was negative in its primary endpoint "cardiovascular mortality" at 6 month and showed only a trend in reducing worsening HF (serelaxin vs. placebo: 6.9% vs. 7.7%, p = 0.10). Secondary endpoints all cause mortality and length of stay in the hospital were negative as well. The results of this study prompted the immediate and all-encompassing stop of further development of serelaxin although results of other, albeit weaker studies were positive. One difficulty of research on ADHF may be that reasons for acute decompensation are variable requiring specific treatment: tachyarrhythmia, acute ischemia, exacerbation of hypertension, pneumonia, drugs, and perioperative complications. A major fraction of patients with ADHF is hypertensive and/or hydropic and the use of diuretics and vasodilators is justified for relieving symptoms. Predefined diuretic strategies were not superior to the usual symptom oriented regimen [19]. Thus, again, we are left with the individual, symptom-guided decision how to treat our patient with ADHF. Prevention of decompensation by comprehensive care remains a main objective in heart failure therapy.

10.5 Complications

Arrhythmias and sudden death, and hydropic decompensation are the major acute complications of heart failure. The incidence varies, however, greatly among patients and studies, depending on inclusion criteria and length of follow up. The number needed to treat with ICD is still high especially in primary prevention of sudden death. It remains unsettled whether patients with non-ischemic cardiomyopathy profit of ICD therapy [10]. Should we withhold the ICD from a young patient with non-ischemic cardiomyopathy and a low ejection fraction? Again, a difficult question, and we probably will include "soft" clinical information in our individual decision.

Other more chronic complications, like cognitive dysfunction, anxiety, depression and central sleep apnea, may be due to direct or indirect effects of heart failure on the central nervous system. The mechanisms are unclear but probably vary from patient to patient. Drugs used in heart failure, chronic hypoperfusion of the brain, inflammation and activation of neurohumoral systems may contribute. Specific drugs like antidepressants [15] are probably ineffective in these patients, as well as adaptive servo-ventilation in patients with heart failure and sleep apnea (see above) [16]. It seems that consequent and guideline driven therapy of heart failure supported by a structured disease management and by skilled personnel is the best available therapy for these complications [20].

10.6 Therapy in the Elderly

Heart failure is prominent in the older population. Several obstacles hamper therapy in older patients. The problems of one comorbidity are potentiated by multimorbidity [21]. Prevalence of cognitive impairment increases with age and interferes with regular therapy and status control. Frailty and social isolation contribute further to the unstable condition. Therapeutic objectives may differ in older patients from that of younger patients. Prolongation of life may have less priority than quality of life, days out of hospital or independence. Symptoms of comorbidities like pain in rheumatic disease or arthrosis may dominate and require therapy, which interferes with heart failure therapy. Finally, clinical studies do not generally apply to the older population. Most early trials have excluded patients older than 75 or 80 years and even in studies with no upper limit of age, the average age is much lower in most studies than in a general population of heart failure patients [6, 7]. Thus, therapy in the elderly relies on extrapolation from studies on younger populations. Taking all this imponderability into account, heart failure therapy for the older patient must be adapted to individual needs without a clear guidance by guidelines. This includes in particular the indication for an ICD and end of life care.

10.7 End of Life Care

Heart failure is a chronic in most instances progressive disease, increasingly symptomatic, with a poor prognosis [22]. ICD protects against sudden death and the lifetime with illness has increased steadily in patients with heart failure [23]. Table 10.1 shows the respective data of the Multicenter Automatic Defibrillator Implantation Trial II (MADIT-II). The ICD reduces total mortality by 9%, but non-sudden death increases by 29%. Thus, patients suffer and die of heart failure or comorbid conditions. Most therapeutic concepts of care do not include the psychosocial situation of the patient. Sub-specialization in cardiology and reimbursement focus on procedures rather than comprehensive care. The therapy plan is not regularly "chosen wisely" together with the patient and his family. However, comprehensive concepts are required including end of life care for the patient with advanced heart failure. There is experience and research in palliative care of patients with cancer but little in cardiovascular diseases. Prognosis is similarly poor in patients with heart failure as in many types of cancer, but requirements of the patients differ in many other respects [24]. Thus, palliative care of patients with cardiovascular disease needs definitely more research.

Three quarters of the patients with heart failure suffer from the typical symptoms: dyspnea and fatigue. Nearly half of the patients report pain, sleep disturbances, inappetence or indigestions, one third admit depression, one quarter anxiety [25]. In the INH study most spontaneously reported problems were non-cardiac. Gastrointestinal disturbance and alimentary disorders 44%, musculoskeletal problems 31%, depressive and cognitive disorders 37% of the patients (Fig. 10.3) [20]. The systemic involvement of all organ systems in chronic heart failure and the frequency of comorbidities probably contribute to this complex syndrome of symptoms. On an average, the patients in the INH-registry had four, 52% had more than six comorbidities. Comorbidities obviously co-determine quality of life and prognosis [21]. Hospitalizations are frequent, but in 50% of patients the reason for admission was not heart failure but comorbidities or infections [26]. Thus, heart failure patients meet the World Health Organization (WHO) Definition of Palliative Care 2002: "Palliative care is an approach that improves the quality of life of patients and their families facing the problems

Table 10.1 Effect of implantation[a] of an ICD[b] in patients with reduced ejection fraction (EF < 30%) [23]

	ICD (%)	No CD (%)	Difference (%)
Total Mortality	22	31	−9
Sudden Death	35	61	−26
Non Sudden Death	55	26	+29

[a]At least 4 weeks after a myocardial infarction
[b]*ICD* Implantable Cardioverter-Defibrillator

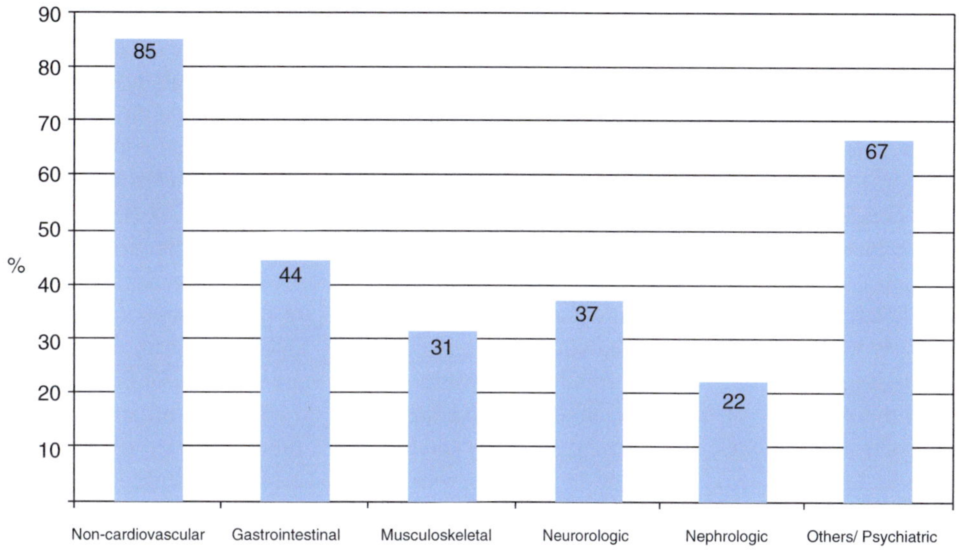

Fig. 10.3 Non-cardiovascular problems and comorbidities reported by patients with heart failure to a specialized heart failure nurse [20]

associated with life-threatening illness, through the prevention and relief of suffering by means of early identification and impeccable assessment and treatment of pain and other problems, physical, psychosocial and spiritual" [27].

Palliative care was initiated for patients with oncologic disease; in 2003 in Germany 98% of patients in palliative care had cancer [28]. There are some basic differences between the palliative requirements in oncology and cardiology [29]. Most drugs used in heart failure for reducing mortality also improve quality of life and reduce hospitalizations [30]. In contrast, side effects are frequent in oncologic therapy and quality of life may be sacrificed for a longer life. In public, palliative care is sometimes conceived as an ethical and political issue [31] but not recognized that there is very little data for specific palliative concepts. This is even more the case in patients with advanced heart failure or cardiac disease. Indirect conclusions may be drawn from studies on disease management in patients with heart failure.

The European Society of Cardiology published in 2009 a Position Statement of the European Heart Failure Association on palliative care in heart failure, based on a workshop of the Heart Failure As- sociation of the European Society of Cardiology [32]. The Position Statement tended to

1. draw attention to palliative care of patients with heart failure,
2. provide access and improve quality of palliative care,
3. further develop palliative care in Europe.

The Position Statement adapts standards of palliative care to cardiovascular disease and elaborates the differences to cancer diseases. It lays major emphasis on research since recommendations so far lack a scientific basis.

10.8 The Project of the German Cardiac Society

In 2013, the German Cardiac Society established a Project Group "Ethics in Cardiology" for the discussion of relevant ethical topics [33]. A core group of cardiologists, ethicists, jurists, theologians and nursing specialists consults specialists of other fields for specific objects. The first project was a "Statement of the German Society of Cardiology and sister societies. Responsible handling of ICDs." In the paper, the group discusses the problems, "when patients approach the end of life independent of their concomitant heart disease. In such cases, often many years after the initial implantation, ICDs may burden patients by unwanted shocks and by prolonging the process of dying." The statement discusses the legal and ethical considerations of deactivation of ICD and pacemakers in detail. It is emphasized that the situation needs deeper knowledge on the technical capabilities of the ICD, which may not be present in those who are the caregivers at the end of life of the heart failure patient. It is the physicians' responsibility to inform patients and their relatives about potential hazards of the ICD and the option to stop the function of the ICD in a palliative situation.

It is important to challenge adequacy of each therapy in patients in an advanced stage of their disease or at the end of their life. Future research needs to address diagnostic and therapeutic algorithms rather than only individual drugs or interventions.

10.9 Deficits in Patient Care

One deficit in care for patients with advanced heart failure is the already discussed ICD therapy. The ICD prevents sudden death (see above and Table 10.1). However, sudden death may be preferential in an advanced stage of the disease with no quality of life. Guidelines recommend discussing the adequate procedures for an advanced stage with the patient [34]. However, in a telephone survey of 278 ICD patients, 86% declare that they never had thought of it and 42% rejected to decide in advance, while 28% wanted to deactivate their ICD and 11% to maintain function [35]. Numerous deficits in communication became apparent in this study, 95% of the patients would have wished a discussion of the end of life situation earlier. In a survey of 417 representatives of hospices in USA, 97% reported that they took care of ICD patients, 58% had experienced a defibrillation in the last year of their life. Although only 10% of the hospices had standards for deactivation of an ICD, 42% of the patients had their ICD deactivated [36]. A survey in 47 large European centers revealed that only 4% of the centers discussed systematically deactivation of the ICD [37]. Guidelines remain vague and stress the granted patient's right on self-determination but also the right of the physician to refuse deactivation of the ICD [38]. Nurses in general prefer and request planning ahead [39].

Palliative care requires comprehensive care of patients with heart failure in a multidisciplinary disease management program proven to be effective in heart failure [20, 40]. The German health care system has special problems with care of patients with chronic and severe diseases. The sectoral organization, with strict separation of in and out patient care, requires special programs to provide a secure transfer [20]. Such programs can be very successful as shown in controlled studies, and may reduce mortality and morbidity, on a long term also hospitalizations, and substantially improve quality of life and depression [20]. They include home visits by specialized nurses, which could help integrating palliative care in a comprehensive therapy.

10.10 Research Requirements

Palliative care urgently needs basic research on mechanisms of multi-morbidity, frailty and cachexia. Animal models need to be developed on pathophysiology of heart failure symptoms, interactions between the cardiovascular system and the central nervous system, and on interactions of drugs in advanced age and heart failure.

Registries are important on advanced and end-stage heart failure, to better define the requirements and adequate endpoints for clinical studies on palliative care. Prospective studies should include patients with advanced cardiovascular disease and address pharmacotherapy in multimobide patients. Models of comprehensive care including holistic, psychologic, sociocultural, spiritual and legal aspects for the end of life phase would represent a new type of research in medical care. Specific interventions in heart failure like ICD or cardiac support systems need evaluation in this context. Interdisciplinary research groups including various faculties are required for this type of research.

Methods of healthcare research are able to evaluate algorithms for care of patients with advanced heart failure. To achieve evidence in this type of studies, special research tools need to include standardized assessment of quality of life and care in patients at the end of their life. First approaches with an innovative research methodology understanding palliative care on the heart failure care team have been published [40]. A recent small study on 150 patients with advanced HF has shown that palliative care improved quality of life, anxiety, depression, and spiritual well-being more than usual care [41].

10.11 Conclusions

The "Gaps in Evidence" listed in the ESC-Guidelines leave room for individualized medicine in diagnostics and therapy of heart failure.

Heart failure research of the last decades was driven by hard end-points and focused on reduction of mortality.

This approach was very successful and substantially reduced mortality of patients with heart failure.

An increasing number of older patients live with heart failure and multiple comorbidities.

Advanced and terminal heart failure need comprehensive palliative concepts, which may differ from that for patients in earlier stages or with other diseases like cancer.

Research is urgently needed on the principles of multimorbidity and symptoms as well as on out and in-patient care for the advanced and terminal stage of heart failure.

References

1. Echt DS, Liebson PR, Mitchell LB, Peters RW, Obias-Manno D, Barker AH, Arensberg D, Baker A, Friedman L, Greene HL, Huther ML, Richardson DW. Mortality and morbidity in patients receiving encainide, flecainide, or placebo. The Cardiac Arrhythmia Suppression Trial. N Engl J Med. 1991;324:781–8.
2. Køber L, Torp-Pedersen C, McMurray JJV, Gøtzsche O, Le'vy S, Crijns H, Amlie J, Carlsen J. Increased mortality after dronedarone therapy for severe heart failure. N Engl J Med. 2008;358:2678–87.
3. Packer M, Carver JR, Rodeheffer RJ, Ivanhoe RJ, DiBianco R, Zeldis SM, Hendrix GH, Bommer WJ, Elkayam U, Kukin ML, et al. Effect of oral milrinone on mortality in severe chronic heart

failure. The PROMISE Study Research Group. N Engl J Med. 1991;325:1468–75.
4. Ertl G, Ruschitzka F. The year in cardiology 2013: heart failure. Eur Heart J. 2014;35:470–3.
5. Ponikowski P, Voors AA, Anker SD, et al. 2016 ESC guide lines for the diagnosis and treatment of acute and chronic heart failure: the Task Force for the diagnosis and treatment of acute and chronic heart failure of the European Society of Cardiology (ESC). Developed with the special contribution of the Heart Failure Association (HFA) of the ESC. Eur J Heart Fail. 2016;37:2129–200.
6. Kitzman DW, Rich MW. Age disparities in heart failure research. JAMA. 2010;304:1950–1.
7. Heiat A, Gross CP, Krumholz HM. Representation of the elderly, women, and minorities in heart failure clinical trials. Arch Intern Med. 2002;162:1682–8.
8. Störk S, Hense HW, Zentgraf C, Uebelacker I, Jahns R, Ertl G, Angermann CE. Pharmacotherapy according to treatment guidelines is associated with lower mortality in a community-based sample of patients with chronic heart failure. A prospective cohort study. Eur J Heart Fail. 2008;10:1236–45.
9. Ertl G, Jugdutt B. ACE inhibition after myocardial infarction: can megatrials provide answers? Lancet. 1994;344:1068–9.
10. Køber L, Thune JJ, Nielsen JC, Haarbo J, Videbæk L, Korup E, Jensen G, Hildebrandt P, Steffensen FH, Bruun NE, Eiskjær H, Brandes A, Thøgersen AM, Gustafsson F, Egstrup K, Videbæk R, Hassager C, Svendsen JH, Høfsten DE, Torp-Pedersen C, Pehrson S, DANISH Investigators. Defibrillator implantation in patients with nonischemic systolic heart failure. N Engl J Med. 2016;375:1221–30.
11. Zinman B, Wanner C, Lachin JM, Fitchett D, Bluhmki E, Hantel S, Mattheus M, Devins T, Johansen OE, Woerle HJ, Broedl UC, Inzucchi SE. Empagliflozin, cardiovascular outcomes, and mortality in type 2 diabetes. N Engl J Med. 2015;373:2117–28.
12. Güder G, Frantz S, Bauersachs J, Allolio B, Wanner C, Koller MT, Ertl G, Angermann CA, Störk S. Reverse epidemiology in systolic and non-systolic heart failure: cumulative prognostic benefit of classical cardiovascular risk factors. Circ Heart Fail. 2009;2:563–71.
13. Tavazzi L, Maggioni AP, Marchioli R, Barlera S, Franzosi MG, Latini R, Lucci D, Nicolosi GL, Porcu M, Tognoni G; Gissi-HF Investigators. Effect of rosuvastatin in patients with chronic heart failure (the GISSI-HF trial): a randomised, double-blind, placebo-controlled trial. Lancet. 2008,372:1231–9.
14. Ertl G. Statine bei Herzinsuffizienz. Sinnvoll oder überflüssig? Cardiovasc. 2017;17:37–40.
15. Angermann CE, Gelbrich G, Störk S, Gunold H, Edelmann F, Wachter R, Schunkert H, Graf T, Kindermann I, Haass M, Blankenberg S, Pankuweit S, Prettin C, Gottwik M, Böhm M, Faller H, Deckert J, Ertl G. Effect of escitalopram on all-cause mortality and hospitalization in patients with heart failure and depression: the MOOD-HF randomized clinical trial. JAMA. 2016;315:2683–93.
16. Cowie MR, Woehrle H, Wegscheider K, Angermann C, d'Ortho MP, Erdmann E, Levy P, Simonds AK, Somers VK, Zannad F, Teschler H. Adaptive servo-ventilation for central sleep apnea in systolic heart failure. N Engl J Med. 2015;373:1095–105.
17. Wallenborn J, Marx A, Störk S, Güder G, Brenner S, Ertl G, Angermann CE. Prognostic significance of serial high-sensitivity troponin I measurements following acute cardiac decompensation-correlation with longer-term clinical outcomes and reverse remodelling. Int J Cardiol. 2017;232:199–207.
18. Arnold JM, Yusuf S, Young J, Mathew J, Johnstone D, Avezum A, Lonn E, Pogue J, Bosch J; HOPE Investigators. Prevention of heart failure in patients in the Heart Outcomes Prevention Evaluation (HOPE) study. Circulation. 2003;107:1284–90.
19. Felker GM, Lee KL, Bull DA, Redfield MM, Stevenson LW, Goldsmith SR, LeWinter MM, Deswal A, Rouleau JL, Ofili EO, Anstrom KJ, Hernandez Ad F, McNulty SE, Velazquez EJ, Kfoury AG, Chen HH, Givertz MM, Semigran MJ, Bart BA, Mascette AM, Braunwald E, O'Connor CMfor the NHLBI Heart Failure Clinical Research Network. Diuretic strategies in patients with acute decompensated heart failure. N Engl J Med. 2011;364:797–805.
20. Angermann CA, Stoerk S, Gelbrich G, Faller H, Jahns R, Frantz S, Loeffler M, Ertl G. Mode of action and effects of standardized collaborative disease management on mortality and morbidity in patients with systolic heart failure: the interdisciplinary network for heart failure (INH) study. Circ Heart Fail. 2012;5:25–35.
21. Braunstein JB, Anderson GF, Gerstenblith G, Weller W, Niefeld M, Herbert R, Wu AW. Noncardiac comorbidity increases preventable hospitalizations and mortality among medicare beneficiaries with chronic heart failure. J Am Coll Cardiol. 2003;42:1226–33.
22. Murray CJL, Lopez AD. Alternative projections of mortality and disability by cause: Global Burden of Disease Study. Lancet. 1997;349:1498–504.
23. Moss AJ, Zareba W, Hall WJ, Klein H, Wilber DJ, Cannom DS, Daubert JP, Higgins SL, Brown MW, Andrews ML; Multicenter Automatic Defibrillator Implantation Trial II Investigators. Prophylactic implantation of a defibrillator in patients with myocardial infarction and reduced ejection fraction. N Engl J Med. 2002;346:877–83.
24. Stewart S, MacIntyre K, Hole DJ, Capewell S, McMurray JJ. More 'malignant' than cancer? Five-year survival following a first admission for heart failure. Eur J Heart Fail. 2001;3:315–22.
25. Bekelman DB, Hutt E, Masoudi FA, Kutner JS, Rumsfeld JS. Defining the role of palliative care in older adults with heart failure. Int J Cardiol. 2008;25:183–90.
26. Dunlay SM, Redfield MM, Weston SA, Therneau TM, Hall Long K, Shah ND, Roger VL. Hospitalizations after heart failure diagnosis a community perspective. J Am Coll Cardiol. 2009;54:1695–702.
27. Weltgesundheitsorganisation (WHO). WHO definition of palliative care. http://www.who.int/cancer/palliative/definition/en/ (27.03.2013).
28. Radbruch L, Nauck F, Ostgathe C, Elsner F, Bausewein C, Fuchs M, Lindena G, Neuwöhner K, Schulenberg D. What are the prob lems in palliative care? Results from a represen- tative survey. Support Care Cancer. 2003;11:442–51.
29. Goodlin SJ. Palliative care in congestive heart failure. J Am Coll Cardiol. 2009;54:386–96.
30. Garg R, Yusuf S. Overview of randomized trials of angiotensin converting enzyme inhibitors on mortality and morbidity in patients with heart failure. Collaborative Group on ACE Inhibitor Trials. JAMA. 1995;273:1450–6.
31. Ertl G. Klinischer Fortschritt: Forschung muss beim Patienten ankommen. Dtsch Med Wochenschr. 2011;136:1993.
32. Jaarsma T, Beattie JM, Ryder M, Rutten FH, McDonagh T, Mohacsi P, Murray SA, Grodzicki T, Bergh I, Metra M, Ekman I, Angermann C, Leventhal M, Pitsis A, Anker SD, Gavazzi A, Ponikowski P, Dickstein K, Delacretaz E, Blue L, Strasser F, McMurray J. Advanced Heart Failure Study Group of the HFA of the ESC palliative care in heart failure: a position statement from the palliative care workshop of the Heart Failure Association of the European Society of Cardiology. Eur J Heart Fail. 2009;11:433–43.
33. Waltenberger J, Schöne-Seifert B, Friedrich DR, Alt-Epping B, Bestehorn M, Dutzmann J, Ertl G, Fateh-Moghadam B, Israel CW, Maase A. Verantwortlicher Umgang mit ICDs. Stellungnahme der Deutschen Gesellschaft für Kardiologie und ihrer Schwester-Gesellschaften. © Deutsche Gesellschaft für Kardiologie – Herz- und Kreislaufforschung e.V. Published by Springer Medizin Verlag GmbH – all rights reserved 2017. Kardiologe. https://doi.org/10.1007/s12181-017-0185-6.
34. Hunt SA, Abraham WT, Chin MH, Feldman AM, Francis GS, Ganiats TG, Jessup M, Konstam MA, Mancini DM, Michl K, Oates JA, Rahko PS, Silver MA, Stevenson LW, Yancy CW, Antman EM, Smith SC Jr, Adams CD, Anderson JL, Faxon

DP, Fuster V, Halperin JL, Hiratzka LF, Jacobs AK, Nishimura R, Ornato JP, Page RL, Riegel B. ACC/AHA 2005 guideline update for the diagnosis and management of chronic heart failure in the adult: a report of the American College of Cardiology/American Heart Association Task Force on Practice Guidelines (Writing Committee to Update the 2001 Guidelines for the Evaluation and Management of Heart Failure), developed in collaboration with the American College of Chest Physicians and the International Society for Heart and Lung Transplantation, endorsed by the Heart Rhythm Society. Circulation. 2005;112:e154–235.
35. Kirkpatrick JN, Gottlieb M, Sehgal P, Patel R, Verdino RJ. Deactivation of implantable cardioverter defibrillators in terminal illness and end of life care. Am J Cardiol. 2012;109:91–4.
36. Goldstein N, Carlson M, Livote E, Kutner JS. Brief communication: management of implantable cardioverter- defibrillators in hospice: a nationwide survey. Ann Intern Med. 2010;152:296–9.
37. Marinskis G, van Erven L on behalf of the EHRA Scientific Initiatives Committee. Deactivation of implanted cardioverter-defibrillators at the end of life: results of the EHRA survey. Europace. 2010;12:1176–7.
38. Padeletti L, Arnar DO, Boncinelli L, Brachman J, Camm JA, Daubert JC, Hassam SK, Deliens L, Glikson M, Hayes D, Israel C, Lampert R, Lobban T, Raatikainen P, Siegal G, Vardas P; Reviewers: Kirchhof P, Becker R, Cosio F, Loh P, Cobbe S, Grace A, Morgan J; European Heart Rhythm Association; Heart Rhythm Society. EHRA Expert Consensus Statement on the management of cardiovascular implantable electronic devices in patients nearing end of life or requesting withdrawal of therapy. Europace. 2010;12:1480–89.
39. Kramer DB, Ottenberg AL, Gerhardson S, Mueller LA, Kaufman SR, Koenig BA, Mueller PS. "Just Because We Can Doesn't Mean We Should": views of nurses on deactivation of pacemakers and implantable cardioverter-defibrillators. J Interv Card Electrophysiol. 2011;32:243–52.
40. Lingard LA, McDougall A, Schulz V, Shadd J, Marshall D, Strachan PH, Tait GR, Arnold JM, Kimel G. Understanding palliative care on the heart failure care team, an innovative research methodology. J Pain Symptom Manag. 2013;45:901–11.
41. Rogers JG, Patel CB, Mentz RJ, Granger BB, Steinhauser KE, Fiuzat M, Adams PA, Speck A, Johnson KS, Krishnamoorthy A, Yang H, Anstrom KJ, Dodson GC, Taylor DH Jr, Kirchner JL, Mark DB, O'Connor CM, Tulsky JA. Palliative care in heart failure: the PAL-HF randomized, controlled clinical trial. J Am Coll Cardiol. 2017;70:331–41.

Part VI

Hospitalized Patients and Comorbidities

Inpatient Therapeutic Options

11

Michael M. Kreusser and Philip W. Raake

11.1 General Considerations

Patients with acute dyspnea resulting from acute heart failure should be rapidly assessed and stabilized. First, patients should be put in a seated posture and, if necessary, supplemental oxygen and ventilatory support (noninvasive or invasive, see below) should be provided [1]. After that, therapeutic aims should be focused on the correction of hemodynamic and intravascular volume abnormalities. Therapy has to be tailored to the individual situation, however, diuretics are the mainstay of therapy in the acute setting. Early intravenous vasodilator therapy is important for selected patients with the need of targeting systemic vascular resistance and left ventricular overload. This includes patients with severe hypertension, acute mitral regurgitation, or acute aortic regurgitation. The patient's hemodynamic and volume status determines how aggressive diuretic and vasodilator therapy has to be initiated. Acute heart failure therapy may be guided differentially in three stages of treatment: urgent/emergent care, hospitalization, and pre-discharge [2]. Therapies can be necessary to be used during any of these stages and are discussed in the following in detail. Monitoring and diagnostics in acute heart failure are discussed above.

11.2 Pharmacotherapy

11.2.1 Diuretics

Diuretics are the primary pharmacologic treatment for volume overload in patients with acute heart failure [3]. Patients presenting with volume overload usually receive intravenous loop diuretics (e.g. furosemide, torasemide, bumetanide) with a dose equivalent to 20–40 mg furosamide for patients without prior loop diuretic therapy. The dose should be adjusted/increased in the setting of renal dysfunction and chronic oral diuretic use. Loop diuretics should be administered intravenous, and if there is little or no response to the initial dose, the dose should be doubled at two-hour intervals as needed up to the maximum recommended dose.

In patients treated intravenously with loops diuretics, urine output needs to be carefully monitored, often by using a bladder catheter. In case of a significant volume overload (>5–10 l) or diuretic resistance, a continuous intravenous infusion is often necessary, usually furosemide 5–40 mg/h. In the recent DOSE trial Felker et al. found no differences in acute heart failure patients treated with loop diuretics as bolus or continuous infusion at low or high doses [3].

As noted below, vasodilators may increase diuresis and lower the need for high dose diuretics. Moreover, loop diuretics may be combined with another type of diuretics, such as thiazides (intravenous chlorothiazide or oral metolazone) or aldosteron antagonists (oral spironolactone, eplerenone) to increase diuresis. Patients under diuretic therapy have to be carefully monitored for hypotension, worsening renal function and electrolyte disturbances. Non-steroidal anti-inflammatory drugs should be avoided, because they can greatly reduce the efficiacy of diuretic drugs and can negatively influence kidney function. Patients with hypotension (<90 mmHg systolic blood pressure), severe hyponatremia and/or acidosis have to be carefully treated with diuretics and may not respond to diuretic therapy. If volume redistribution is more than volume overload the case of acute heart failure, e.g. in the case of hypertensive acute heart failure, aggressive diuretic therapy may be rather harmful.

M. M. Kreusser · P. W. Raake (✉)
University Hospital of Heidelberg, University of Heidelberg, Heidelberg, Germany
e-mail: Philip.Raake@med.uni-heidelberg.de

D. S. Feldman, P. Mohacsi (eds.), *Heart Failure*, Cardiovascular Medicine, https://doi.org/10.1007/978-3-319-98184-0_11

11.2.2 Vasodilators

Vasolidators are first line therapy for patients with acute heart failure, if hypotension is absent, and are recommended for patients with a systolic blood pressure >90 mmHg and the absence of serious obstructive valve disease [1]. Vasodilators have dual benefit by decreasing venous tone (to optimize preload) and arterial tone (decrease afterload), and thereby may increase stroke volume. Three types of vasodilators are currently available, all of which cause vasodilation by increasing intracellular cGMP, but each with distinct characteristics and indications.

Nitrates Nitrates are used for medical treatments since the 1870s, and the organic nitrates are one of the oldest treatments for acute heart failure. At low doses, nitrates dilate veins, produce rapid decrease in pulmonary venous and ventricular filling pressures and improve pulmonary congestion, dyspnoea and myocardial oxygen demand. At higher doses and in the presence of vasoconstriction, nitrates also dilate arteries and reduce afterload, and increase cardiac output.

Nitrates are preferentially used in patients with coronary artery disease and can be easily and immediately administered orally, sublingually or by spray. In a randomized study of 110 patients with fulminant pulmonary edema, patients treated with high dose nitrates were compared to low dose nitrate combined with high dose furosemid, and latter group were in disadvantage in terms of myocardial infactions and the need for mechanical ventilation [4]. Other studies provided evidence for beneficial effects of nitroglycerin on hemodynamics [5].

Nitroglycerine may be acutely administered sublingually (0.25–0.5 mg), buccally (isosorbide dinitrate 1–3 mg) or spray (0.4 mg or 2 puffs). Intravenous nitroglycerine is usually initially dosed 10–20 μg/min with up-titration in increments of 5–10 μg/min to blood pressure or symptom target. Inadequate up-titration is a common reason for failure of therapeutic efficacy. Nitroglycerine tolerance can develop within 24 h, and headache and symptomatic hypotension, the latter usually resolves within minutes, are fairly common adverse effect.

Sodium Nitroprusside Sodium nitroprusside induces a balanced vasodilation in veins and arteries and is easily titratable due to a very short half-life (seconds to a few minutes). It is intravenously administered and should be monitored by continuous blood pressure monitoring, or at least with automated blood pressure cuffs to guide dosage. Sodium nitroprusside very potently induces a dramatic decrease of left ventricular filling pressures and therefore is one of the most efficiant therapies, especially in the setting of elevated afterload (e.g., hypertensive acute heart failure). There are no randomized trials of nitroprusside in acute heart failure patients, but multiple studies demonstrated a dramatic reduction in pulmonary capillary wedge pressure and increases in cardiac output, as well as beneficial increases of diuresis, natriuresis and decreased neurohumoral activation [6] and also reduced mortality [7].

The initial dose of sodium nitroprusside is 0.3 μg/Kg/min with titration every 5 min up to 5 μg/Kg/min, a fast up-titration can cause profound hypotension. Nitroprosside is a prodrug and is rapidly metabolized to oxide and cyanide. Possible side effects are related to the cyanide metabolite and include nausea, abdominal dyscomfort, dissociative feelings and dysphoria. Cyanide rarely accumulates in patients, but physician discomfort with the potentially toxic metabolites may be the cause that nitroprusside is markedly underutilized (<1% of acute heart failure patients in Europe and the United States [8]). However, it has no arrhythmogenic properties, may improve myocardial oxygen demand by reducing afterload and wall stress and creates no significant electrolyte disturbancies.

Nesiritide B-type natriuretic peptide (BNP) may also be used for the treatment of acute heart failure. Nesiritide (recombinant human BNP) reduces venous and verntricular filling pressures by potent venous and arterial vasodilation and thereby mildly increases cardiac output, with subsequent improvement in symptoms of dyspnea. In one randomized trial with 489 patients with decompensated heart failure and dyspnoe at rest, patients were treated with placebo, nitroglycerin, or nesiritide for 3 h [5]. Patients receiving nesiritide had a significantly greater decrease in left ventricular filling pressure compared to nitroglycerine and placebo, and improvement in dyspnea compared with placebo.

Nesiritide may be administered with or without a bolus followed by an infusion of 0.015–0.03 μg/Kg/min. Hypotension more often occurs in patients with volume depletion, and consequently, nesiritide is indicated for patients with congestive signs and symptoms. Headache occurs less frequent as with nitroglycerin, and nesiritide is with limited need for frequent dose adjustments and an absence of tolerance. However, its high costs and lack of clear clinical benefit beyond other less expensive agents, and potential safety concerns, including higher mortality in some studies [9], have limited its use. Nesiritide is not available in many European countries.

11.2.3 Inotropes

Inotropes include agents that stimulate adrenergic receptors and thereby have varied effects on the vasculature, but all increase cardiac pump function (inotropy) and are reserved for selected situations of hypoperfusion or decreased blood flow when other interventions are inappropriate or have failed. The concept of intermittend infusions of inotropes, or "inotrope holidays", cannot be recommended due to lacking supportive data.

Dobutamine Dobutamine is the most commonly used positive inotrope in the United States and Europe [2]. However, there are data that dobutamine may be associated with increased mortality. Dobutamine increases cardiac output through direct inotropy, decreasing afterload and increasing heart rate. It is indicated for patients with acute heart failure due to low output. Dobutamine is administered as an infusion without a loading dose starting at 2–3 μg/Kg/min and can be up-titrated to doses of 15–20 μg/Kg/min. A need for increasing doses may occur with infusions over 24–28 h. Adverse effects of dobutamine include tachycardia, increasing occurrence of atrial and ventricular arrhythmias, myocardial ischemia and possible direct toxic effects on the myocardium inducing necrosis. Lower doses of dobutamine improve renal perfusion and in general, dobutamine (or dopamine) is the preferred inotrope in patients with hypotension and in the setting of renal dyfunction, given the renal excretion of milrinone. Beta-blocker therapy results in competitive antagonism of the effects of dobutamine and may require higher doses of dobutamine and/or the substitution of milrinone. Dobutamine should be gradually weaned off under carefully clinical re-evaluation and adaption of co-medication with each dose adjustment.

Dopamine Dopamine was in both the United States and Europe as often used as dobutamine, especially for patients with renal insufficiency because of its renal vasodilation effect. However, a meta-analysis suggested that dopamine may only mildly increase urinary output on the first day with no effect on creatinine clearance and a trend toward increased adverse events [10]. In the initial phase of titration, dopamine can induce tachycardia and atrial and/or ventricular arrhythmias. Intermediate to high doses can cause significant vasoconstricion, leading to worsening of heart failure and poor perfusion.

Epinephrine and Norepinephrine Epinephrine is a potent inotropic agent with balanced vasodilator and vasoconstrictor effects. Norepinephrine is also a potent inotropic agent, but can also cause marked vasoconstriction, potentially inducing end-organ hypoperfusion and tissue necrosis. Both of these agents are given to raise blood pressure and redistribute blood to the vital organs at the expense of an increase in left ventricular afterload and therefore are reserved for profound hypotension or for cardiac resuscitation.

Phosphodiesterase Inhibitors (PDEI) Phosphodiesterase III is found in cardiac and smooth muscle and degrades the signaling molecule cAMP to AMP. cAMP increases inotropy (contractile function), chronotropy (heart rate) and lusitropy (myocardial relaxation). This signaling pathway being downstream of adrenergic receptors bypasses beta-adrenergic receptor desensitization and antagonism by betablockers in heart failure patients. PDEI cause significant peripheral and pulmonary vasodilation, reduce afterload and preload and increase inotropy.

Milrinone is the most commonly used PDEI, but only used in 1–3% of acute heart failure patients [8, 11]. Milrinone has adverse effects as marked hypotension, as well as atrial and ventricular arrhythmias. In one study, 951 patients with acute heart failure not requiring intravenous inotropic support were randomized to receive milrinone or placebo [12]. In the milrinone-treated group, there were found increased sustained hypotension and new atrial arrhythmias, as well as increased mortality in a post-hoc sub-group analysis for patients with ischemic heart disease who received milrinone [13]. Therefore, administration, titration, and withdrawal of milrinone has to be done very carefully.

Enoximone is a PDEI that is available in Europe and is metabolized by the liver into renally cleared active metabolites and needs to be reduced in the setting of either renal or hepatic insufficiency.

Calcium Sensitizers The calcium sensitizer levosimendan acts via multiple mechanisms, including cardiac myofilament calcium sensitization by calcium-dependent binding of troponin C, activation of ATP-sensitive vascular smoth muscle potassium channels and mild PDEI activity. These actions increase myocardial contractility and produce peripheral vasodilation. Levosimendan is used in about 4% of acute heart failure patients [8], mainly for patients with reduced left ventricular systolic function and the absence of severe arterial hypotension. Clinical trials demonstrated beneficial hemodynamic effects and relief of dyspnea [14]. However, randomized trials found more episodes of atrial fibrillation in levosimendan-treated patients and ambiguous effects on survival [15]. Levosimendan has gained popularity in Europe, were it is used as an alternative to adrenergic agens, preferably to reverse the effect of beta-blockade if beta-blocker is thought to be contributing to hypoperfusion in acute heart failure. Levosimendan may be administered with an initial loading dose of 3–12 μg/Kg during 10 min, although many clinicians avoid a loading dose to prevent hypotension. Levosimendan is then continuously given with a rate of 0.1 μg/Kg/min and may be up- or down-titrated between 0.05 and 0.2 μg/Kg/min, adjusted to the clinical need. Levosimendan has a half-life of over 80 h, and has hemodynamic effects even days after discontinuation of the infusion.

Relaxin Relaxin is a naturally occurring peptide vasodilator. Serelaxin, recombinant human relaxin-2 was investigated in the RELAX-HF trial that included 1161 patients with acute heart failure and included patients with decreased and preserved left ventricular ejection fraction [16]. Serelaxin improved one measure of dyspnea and reduced the length of index hospital stay. Interestingly the serelaxin group displayed a lower rate of cardiovascular death and all-cause mortality. However, additional studies are required to confirm efficiacy and safety of this new agent.

11.2.4 Others

Morphine Opiate therapy in patients with acute heart failure should be avoided, because observational studies suggested that morphine and its analogs may increase the likelihood of admission to the intensive care unit and intubation, and may prolong hospital stay [17]. However, to relieve anxiety, distress, and dyspnoea it may be recommended for selected patients under careful monitoring.

Anxiolytics and Sedatives Anxiolytics or sedatives may be needed in patients with agitation or delirium. Cautious use of benzodiazepines (diazepam, lorazepam) is recommended as the safest approach.

Venous Thromboembolism Prophylaxis Thromboembolism prophylaxis is recommended for hospitalized patients with heparin or other anticoagulant agents unless contraindicated or unnecessary.

Sodium Restriction Sodium restriction is suggested for all patients with heart failure.

Vasopressor Receptor Antagonists Vasopressin receptor antagonists such as tolvaptan block the action of arginine vasopressin (AVP) at the V2 receptor in renal tubules and promote aquaresis. These agents are a rarely used option for patients with volume overload and severe hyponatremia (i.e. serum sodium <120 mmol/l). The EVEREST (The Efficacy of Vasopressin Antagonism in Heart Failure Outcome Study With Tolvaptan) trial showed no benefit regarding long-term mortality or heart failure morbidity related to tolvaptan treatment in patients hospitalized for worsening of heart failure [18].

11.3 Renal Replacement

Ultrafiltration involves the removal of plasma water across a semipermeable membrane in response to a transmembrane pressure gradient. In the UNLOAD trial ultrafiltration was related to an intensified weight loss and fewer rehospitaltisations in patients with acute heart failure [19]. However, renal insfficiency and/or diuretics resistance were not a prerequisite for study inclusion. In the CARRESS-HF trial only patients with acute decompensated heart failure, worsening renal function and congestion were included. In this trial ultrafiltratrion was even inferior to pharmacologic therapy regarding change in serum creatinine level and body weight and was associated with more adverse events [20]. As such, there is no evidence favouring ultrafiltration over intensification of diuretics as first-line therapy in the setting of acute heart failure [20] and therefore ultrafiltration is not recommended in general and should be restricted to patients who fail to respond to diuretic-based therapies. Current guidelines recommend the following criteria to indicate the need for renal replacement therapy in patients with refractory volume overload: severe hyperkalaemia ($K^+ > 6.5$ mmol/l), severe acidaemia (pH < 7.2), serum urea level >25 mmol/l (150 mg/dl) and serum creatinine >300 µmol/l (>3.4 mg/dl) [1]. Renal replacement will be further discussed below (see chapter on cardiorenal syndrome).

11.4 Non-Invasive Ventilation (and Oxygen Supplementation)

In the presence of decreased oxygen in the blood (hypoxemia; $SaO_2 < 95\%$ or $SaO_2 < 90\%$ in patients with chronic obstructive pulmonary disease (COPD) to avoid ventilation-perfusion mismatch and suppressing of ventilation), administration of oxygen is recommended, although it has not been studied rigorously. In the absence of hypoxemia, supplemental oxygen may cause hyperoxia-induced vasoconstriction and thereby may worsen acute heart failure [21].

Non-invasive ventilation has further developed in recent years and provides the possibility to relieve symptoms of dyspnoe and improve oxygenation of the blood without intubation by using multiple different face-mask based modalities such as continuous positive airway pressure (CPAP) and bi-level positive pressure ventilation (PPV). Meta-analyses have suggested that non-invasive ventilation reduced the need for invasive ventilation and short-term mortality. However, a randomized, controlled clinical trial of 1069 patients with acute cardiogenic edema demonstrated no effect on short-term mortality, but improved symptoms and the associated metabolic and hemodynamic abnormalities [22]. In Europe, over 30% of patients with pulmonary edema received non-invasive ventilation [8]. Mechanical ventilation needs to be performed in about 4–5% of all patients, with a high risk for patients with muscle fatigue and myocardial infarction [8].

11.5 Temporary Mechanical Support

For patients with acute heart failure and INTERMACS (The Interagency Registry for Mechanically Assisted Circulatory support level 1 or 2), short-term mechanical support systems include percutaneous cardiac support devices, extracorporal life support (ECLS) and extracorporal membrane oxygenation (ECMO). These systems can be used to support patients with left or biventricular failure until cardiac and other organ functions have recovered, but typically are restricted to a few days or weeks. In addition, these mechanical support systems can be used as a "bridge to decision".

Intra-Aortic Ballon Pump The intra-aortic ballon pump (IABP) was originally used for temporary left ventricular support before surgical corrections of specific acute mechanical problems (e.g., acute mitral regurgitation or interventricular septal rupture), during severe acute myocarditis and in selected patients with acute myocardial infaction before, during and after percutaneous or surgical revascularization. Benefits of IABP support were found in the era of thrombolysis of acute myocardial infarction [23] In this regards, the recent SHOCK II (The Intraaortic Balloon Pump in Cardiogenic Shock II) trial found no additional benefit in IABP treatment in paitents in cardiogenic shock due to myocardial infarction undergoing percutaneous revascularization [24, 25].

Percutaneous Microxial and Centrifugal Pumps Two different systems may be distinguished: microaxial (e.g. Impella pump Abiomed) and centrifugal pumps (e.g. Tandem Heart, Tandem Life). All systems can be placed percutenously, except the Impella 5 l/min requires surgical cutdown in the groin. The Impella pump draws blood in the left ventricle and via a microxial pump the blood is transported into the ascending aorta above the aortic valve; it performs according to size 2.5–5.0 l/min. The centrifugal Tandem Heart consists of a transseptal cannula introduced blood in the left atrium for suction, a centrifugal pump and an arterial femoral cannula for return of oxygenized blood. Both systems are capable of unloading the left heart. The efficiency of the Impella microaxial pump and the centrifugal Tandem Heart were shown in smaller studies [26, 27]. However, a meta-analysis collecting these smaller studies found no advantage of these two systems over IABP usage in cardiogenic shock [28]. Larger multicenter, controlled, randomized studies are certainly needed to provide more solid data and finally draw conclusions. However, in situations of refractoy cardiogenic shock these systems may provide temporary support for decision making. Due to lacking data it should only be used on an individual basis.

Extracorporal Life Support Extracorporal life support systems (ECLS) allow full cardiopulmonary support including oxygenation. Access is veno-arterial. A venous suction cannula is placed in or close to the right atrium via inferior or superior caval vein. The venous blood is accelerated via a roller pump, oxygenized and returned via a femoral artery cannula. First single center studies could show safety and effectiveness in infarct-related cardiogenic shock [29]. Still evidence is more than weak to support general usage in cardiogenic shock, particularly, as ECLS treatment does not unload the left heart and instead increases left ventricular afterload. It is considered as a rescue strategy in individual patients with refractory cardiogenic shock [1]. Chen et al. could demonstrate that ECLS supported resuscitation was superior to standard of care in inhospital cardiac arrest regarding outcome [30]. However, more evidence is needed and larger multicenter, prospective, randomized studies are still pending.

11.6 Other Interventions

In patients with acute heart failure and pleural effusion, pleurocentesis and fluid evacuation may be considered in order to alleviate dyspnea. In patients with ascites, ascites paracentesis with fluid evacuation may be considered to alleviate symptoms and may also, by decreasing intra-abdominal pressure, partially normalize the transrenal pressure gradient and thereby improve renal function.

References

1. Ponikowski P, Voors AA, Anker SD, Bueno H, Cleland JGF, Coats AJS, et al. 2016 ESC guidelines for the diagnosis and treatment of acute and chronic heart failure: the task force for the diagnosis and treatment of acute and chronic heart failure of the European Society of Cardiology (ESC)developed with the special contribution of the Heart Failure Association (HFA) of the ESC. Eur Heart J. 2016:ehw128. https://doi.org/10.1093/eurheartj/ehw128.
2. Gheorghiade M, Zannad F, Sopko G, Klein L, Piña IL, Konstam MA, et al. Acute heart failure syndromes: current state and framework for future research. Vol 112, p 3958–3968. Presented at the Circulation, Lippincott Williams & Wilkins. https://doi.org/10.1161/CIRCULATIONAHA.105.590091.
3. Felker GM, Lee KL, Bull DA, Redfield MM, Stevenson LW, Goldsmith SR, et al. Diuretic strategies in patients with acute decompensated heart failure. N Engl J Med. 2011;364(9):797–805. https://doi.org/10.1056/NEJMoa1005419.
4. Cotter G, Metzkor E, Kaluski E, Faigenberg Z, Miller R, Simovitz A, et al. Randomised trial of high-dose isosorbide dinitrate plus low-dose furosemide versus high-dose furosemide plus low-dose isosorbide dinitrate in severe pulmonary oedema. Lancet. 1998;351(9100):389–93. https://doi.org/10.1016/S0140-6736(97)08417-1.
5. Publication Committee for the VMAC Investigators (Vasodilatation in the Management of Acute CHF). Intravenous nesiritide vs nitro-

glycerin for treatment of decompensated congestive heart failure: a randomized controlled trial. JAMA. 2002;287(12):1531–40.
6. Johnson W, Omland T, Hall C, Lucas C, Myking OL, Collins C, et al. Neurohormonal activation rapidly decreases after intravenous therapy with diuretics and vasodilators for class IV heart failure. J Am Coll Cardiol. 2002;39(10):1623–9.
7. Mullens W, Abrahams Z, Francis GS, Skouri HN, Starling RC, Young JB, et al. Sodium nitroprusside for advanced low-output heart failure. J Am Coll Cardiol. 2008;52(3):200–7. https://doi.org/10.1016/j.jacc.2008.02.083.
8. Nieminen MS, Brutsaert D, Dickstein K, Drexler H, Follath F, Harjola V-P, et al. EuroHeart Failure Survey II (EHFS II): a survey on hospitalized acute heart failure patients: description of population. Eur Heart J. 2006;27(22):2725–36. https://doi.org/10.1093/eurheartj/ehl193.
9. Aaronson KD, Sackner-Bernstein J. Risk of death associated with nesiritide in patients with acutely decompensated heart failure. JAMA. 2006;296(12):1465–6. https://doi.org/10.1001/jama.296.12.1465.
10. Friedrich JO, Adhikari N, Herridge MS, Beyene J. Meta-analysis: low-dose dopamine increases urine output but does not prevent renal dysfunction or death. Ann Intern Med. 2005;142(7):510–24.
11. Kociol RD, Hammill BG, Fonarow GC, Klaskala W, Mills RM, Hernandez AF, Curtis LH. Generalizability and longitudinal outcomes of a national heart failure clinical registry: comparison of Acute Decompensated Heart Failure National Registry (ADHERE) and non-ADHERE Medicare beneficiaries. Am Heart J. 2010;160(5):885–92. https://doi.org/10.1016/j.ahj.2010.07.020.
12. Cuffe MS, Califf RM, Adams KF, Benza R, Bourge R, Colucci WS, et al. Short-term intravenous milrinone for acute exacerbation of chronic heart failure: a randomized controlled trial. JAMA. 2002;287(12):1541–7.
13. Felker GM, Benza RL, Chandler AB, Leimberger JD, Cuffe MS, Califf RM, et al. Heart failure etiology and response to milrinone in decompensated heart failure: results from the OPTIME-CHF study. J Am Coll Cardiol. 2003;41(6):997–1003.
14. Teerlink JR. Overview of randomized clinical trials in acute heart failure syndromes. Am J Cardiol. 2005;96(6A):59G–67G. https://doi.org/10.1016/j.amjcard.2005.07.022.
15. Cleland JGF, Freemantle N, Coletta AP, Clark AL. Clinical trials update from the American Heart Association: REPAIR-AMI, ASTAMI, JELIS, MEGA, REVIVE-II, SURVIVE, and PROACTIVE. Eur J Heart Fail. 2006;8(1):105–10. https://doi.org/10.1016/j.ejheart.2005.12.003.
16. Teerlink JR, Cotter G, Davison BA, Felker GM, Filippatos G, Greenberg BH, et al. Serelaxin, recombinant human relaxin-2, for treatment of acute heart failure (RELAX-AHF): a randomised, placebo-controlled trial. Lancet. 2013;381(9860):29–39. https://doi.org/10.1016/S0140-6736(12)61855-8.
17. Peacock WF, Hollander JE, Diercks DB, Lopatin M, Fonarow G, Emerman CL. Morphine and outcomes in acute decompensated heart failure: an ADHERE analysis. Emerg Med J. 2008;25(4):205–9. https://doi.org/10.1136/emj.2007.050419.
18. Konstam MA, Gheorghiade M, Burnett JC, Grinfeld L, Maggioni AP, Swedberg K, et al. Effects of oral tolvaptan in patients hospitalized for worsening heart failure: the EVEREST outcome trial. JAMA. 2007;297(12):1319–31. https://doi.org/10.1001/jama.297.12.1319.
19. Costanzo MR, Guglin ME, Saltzberg MT, Jessup ML, Bart BA, Teerlink JR, et al. Ultrafiltration versus intravenous diuretics for patients hospitalized for acute decompensated heart failure. J Am Coll Cardiol. 2007;49(6):675–83. https://doi.org/10.1016/j.jacc.2006.07.073.
20. Bart BA, Goldsmith SR, Lee KL, Givertz MM, O'Connor CM, Bull DA, et al. Ultrafiltration in decompensated heart failure with cardiorenal syndrome. N Engl J Med. 2012;367(24):2296–304. https://doi.org/10.1056/NEJMoa1210357.
21. Park JH, Balmain S, Berry C, Morton JJ, McMurray JJV. Potentially detrimental cardiovascular effects of oxygen in patients with chronic left ventricular systolic dysfunction. Heart. 2010;96(7):533–8. https://doi.org/10.1136/hrt.2009.175257.
22. Gray AJ, Goodacre S, Newby DE, Masson MA, Sampson F, Dixon S, et al. A multicentre randomised controlled trial of the use of continuous positive airway pressure and non-invasive positive pressure ventilation in the early treatment of patients presenting to the emergency department with severe acute cardiogenic pulmonary oedema: the 3CPO trial. Health Technol Assess (Winchester, England). 2009;13(33):1–106. https://doi.org/10.3310/hta13330.
23. Thiele H, Allam B, Chatellier G, Schuler G, Lafont A. Shock in acute myocardial infarction: the Cape Horn for trials? Eur Heart J. 2010;31(15):1828–35. https://doi.org/10.1093/eurheartj/ehq220.
24. Thiele H, Zeymer U, Neumann F-J, Ferenc M, Olbrich H-G, Hausleiter J, et al. Intraaortic balloon support for myocardial infarction with cardiogenic shock. N Engl J Med. 2012;367(14):1287–96. https://doi.org/10.1056/NEJMoa1208410.
25. Thiele H, Zeymer U, Neumann F-J, Ferenc M, Olbrich H-G, Hausleiter J, et al. Intra-aortic balloon counterpulsation in acute myocardial infarction complicated by cardiogenic shock (IABP-SHOCK II): final 12 month results of a randomised, open-label trial. Lancet. 2013;382(9905):1638–45. https://doi.org/10.1016/S0140-6736(13)61783-3.
26. Thiele H. Treatment of cardiogenic shock: what is proven? Dtsch Med Wochenschr. 2013;138(39):1960–5. https://doi.org/10.1055/s-0033-1349457.
27. Thiele H, Ohman EM, Desch S, Eitel I, de Waha S. Management of cardiogenic shock. Eur Heart J. 2015;36(20):1223–30. https://doi.org/10.1093/eurheartj/ehv051.
28. Cheng JM, den Uil CA, Hoeks SE, van der Ent M, Jewbali LSD, van Domburg RT, Serruys PW. Percutaneous left ventricular assist devices vs. intra-aortic balloon pump counterpulsation for treatment of cardiogenic shock: a meta-analysis of controlled trials. Eur Heart J. 2009;30(17):2102–8. https://doi.org/10.1093/eurheartj/ehp292.
29. Sheu J-J, Tsai T-H, Lee F-Y, Fang H-Y, Sun C-K, Leu S, et al. Early extracorporeal membrane oxygenator-assisted primary percutaneous coronary intervention improved 30-day clinical outcomes in patients with ST-segment elevation myocardial infarction complicated with profound cardiogenic shock. Crit Care Med. 2010;38(9):1810–7. https://doi.org/10.1097/CCM.0b013e3181e8acf7.
30. Chen Y-S, Lin J-W, Yu H-Y, Ko W-J, Jerng J-S, Chang W-T, et al. Cardiopulmonary resuscitation with assisted extracorporeal life-support versus conventional cardiopulmonary resuscitation in adults with in-hospital cardiac arrest: an observational study and propensity analysis. Lancet. 2008;372(9638):554–61. https://doi.org/10.1016/S0140-6736(08)60958-7.

12 Anemia and Iron Deficiency in Heart Failure

Otmar Pfister

12.1 Anemia in Heart Failure

12.1.1 Prevalence and Pathophysiology of Anemia in CHF

Estimates of the prevalence of anemia in CHF patients vary broadly due to the use of inconsistent definitions of anemia in different studies. In a meta-analysis derived from 34 published studies, involving more than 150′000 CHF patients, the mean prevalence of anemia was estimated 37.2% with lower prevalence in mild and higher prevalence in severe CHF [1]. Consistent with these data, a recent observational study involving 4456 consecutive patients referred to a cardiology outpatient clinic in the UK reported a prevalence of anemia of 33%, if defined according to the World Health Organization (WHO) criteria as hemoglobin (Hb) concentration <12 g/dl in women and <13 g/dl in men [2]. Anemia is equally prevalent in patients with heart failure with reduced ejection fraction (HFrEF) and those with preserved ejection fraction (HFpEF) [1].

Factors associated with anemia include older age, chronic kidney disease, volume overload, diabetes mellitus, advanced myocardial remodelling, chronic inflammation and most predominantly iron deficiency (ID) [2, 3]. Other nutritional deficits such as Vitamin B12 or folate acid deficiency are uncommon [2]. The pathophysiology of anemia in HF is complex and multifactorial (Fig. 12.1). The predominant mechanisms that contribute to anemia in HF patients are listed below.

Iron Deficiency ID is the major cause of anemia in HF patients. Parameters of ID (e.g. serum iron, transferrin saturation) are strongly associated with anemia in newly diagnosed HF patients [2]. ID in HF may occur in the context of anemia of chronic disease (functional iron deficiency) or as a consequence of depletion of iron stores (absolute iron deficiency).

Inflammatory Cytokines and Erythropoietin (EPO) Resistance CHF is a chronic inflammatory condition with chronic elevation of various inflammatory cytokines [4]. This chronic inflammatory state mitigates EPO production in the kidneys and reduces EPO sensitivity in the bone marrow. EPO resistance in the bone marrow may contribute to anemia in HF. Indeed, there is the phenomenon of a veritable bone marrow dysfunction in patients with CHF [5]. In some anemic CHF patients EPO serum levels are inadequately high, suggestive of profound EPO resistance of the bone marrow. Inadequately high EPO levels are inversely correlated with the prognosis in CHF patients [6].

From the inflammatory perspective, anemia in CHF shares many mechanisms seen in anemia of chronic diseases (e.g. inflammatory bowel disease, chronic rheumatoid diseases).

Chronic Kidney Disease (CKD) CKD affects 30–50% of patients with CHF. Renal hypoxia constitutes the main stimulus for EPO production in the kidneys. In CKD the capacity of appropriate EPO production in response to hypoxia is impaired. Also reduced renal perfusion due to low cardiac output may lead to inappropriately low EPO levels, if corrected to hemoglobin levels. Therefore, reduced synthesis of EPO in the context of CKD or low cardiac output are important causes of anemia [7].

Hemodilution In most patients with CHF hemodilution is a contributing factor to anemia. However, a true red cell deficit is found in the majority of anemic CHF patients on top of hemodilution [8].

O. Pfister (✉)
Internal Medicine/Cardiology, University Hospital Basel, University of Basel, Basel, Switzerland
e-mail: Otmar.Pfister@usb.ch

D. S. Feldman, P. Mohacsi (eds.), *Heart Failure*, Cardiovascular Medicine, https://doi.org/10.1007/978-3-319-98184-0_12

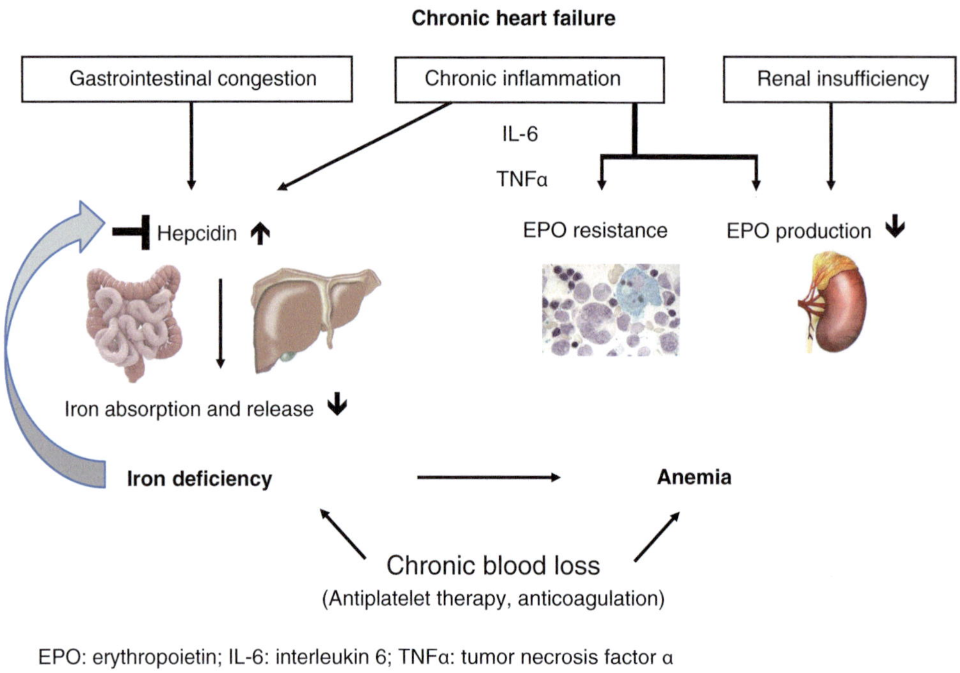

Fig. 12.1 Chronic heart failure

Malabsorption Altered intestinal function due to redistribution of blood away from the splanchnic region or increased bowel wall thickness due to edema may affect iron absorption in the gut thereby contributing to iron deficient anemia.

12.1.2 Diagnostic Work-Up of Anemia in CHF

According to the WHO criteria, anemia is defined as Hb < 120 g/l in women and Hb < 130 g/l in men. Regardless of erythrocyte size (microcytosis vs. normocytosis vs. macrocytosis) evaluation of iron stores (ferritin) should be performed in all cases of anemia to exclude iron deficient anemia (see diagnosis of ID below). The reticulocyte count helps to distinguish hyporegenerative anemia (e.g. renal anemia, anemia of chronic disease, myelodysplastic syndrome) from hyperregenerative anemia (hemolysis, blood loss). In general, any unexplained anemia or ID should be regarded as a potential sign of chronic bleeding and should trigger screening for occult gastrointestinal blood loss. Anemia due to vitamin B12 or folic acid deficiency is rare and of secondary importance in patients with CHF.

12.1.3 Prognostic Impact of Anemia in CHF

Anemia in patients with CHF is an independent risk factor for reduced exercise tolerance, low quality of life, HF hospitalizations and all-cause mortality with an inverse and linear association between Hb values and the risk of death [9]. The risk of hospitalization for HF was increased by 43% in anemic patients compared to non-anemic patients ($p < 0.0001$) in the COMET trial [10]. Even relatively mild degrees of anemia (Hb < 116 g/l for women, and Hb < 126 g/l for men) may confer increased morbidity and mortality [11], such that each 1 g/dl decrease in Hb was associated with a 16% increase in mortality. In terms of mode of death, the presence of anemia is a predictor of both progressive HF-related death and sudden cardiac death [2].

12.1.4 Treatment of Anemia in CHF

Treating anemia in CHF is a clinical challenge due to the fact that its main driver is chronic inflammation. Because the inflammatory process interferes with the production of EPO, the sensitivity of the bone marrow to EPO and the delivery of iron to the bone marrow, protocols for the treatment of anemia in HF have focused primarily on the chronic substitution of erythropoiesis-stimulating agents (ESAs) and the administration of intravenous (i.v.) iron.

Although single-centre, open-label studies have suggested an improvement of exercise capacity and reduced rehospitalisation rates with ESAs in CHF patients with anemia, big randomized trials failed to reproduce these findings [12, 13]. In STAMINA-HeFT administration of the EPO derivate darbepoetin-alpha every 2 weeks for 1 year did not result in any benefit in terms of exercise tolerance, NYHA class or quality of life. There was, however, a trend towards lower risk of all-cause mortality and first HF hospitalization in the darbepoetin-treated group compared to the placebo group [12]. In the RED-HF trial darbepoietin-alpha could increase hemoglobin concentration with only modest improvement in quality of life and no reduction in hospitalization and mortality [13].

Moreover, concerns have emerged regarding the safety of chronic ESA treatment in patients with cardiovascular diseases. Two studies in patients with CKD (CHOIR, CREATE), where EPO was administered to reach either a higher (up to 15.0 g/dl) or a lower (up to 11.5 g/dl) target Hb showed that EPO administration aiming at higher Hb level may be associated with increased risk of morbidity and mortality [14, 15]. The results of the TREAT study, which randomized 4044 patients with type 2 diabetes, CKD, and anemia to treatment with darbepoietin-alpha or placebo with a target Hb of 13.0 mg/dl was neutral in terms of overall mortality but revealed an excess rate of stroke in the darbepoietin treated group (101 versus 53) [16]. Therefore, current international guidelines do not recommend therapy with ESAs in CHF patients with anemia [17].

12.2 Iron Deficiency in Heart Failure

12.2.1 Definition and Diagnosis

Serum ferritin reflects total body iron stores. Transferrin is a transport protein that circulates iron in a nonreactive state. A widely established cut-off value for the diagnosis of ID in the general population is a serum ferritin level <30 ug/l [18]. Being an acute phase protein, ferritin is increased in chronic inflammatory states such as CHF, independently of iron stores. Therefore, the diagnostic threshold to diagnose ID in CHF is already met at higher ferritin levels. Current international guidelines utilise ferritin and transferrin saturation (Tsat) for the diagnosis of ID, with the following cut-off values: ferritin <100 ug/l (absolute ID = depleted iron stores); or ferritin 100–299 ug/l and Tsat < 20% (functional ID = sufficient iron stores but impaired mobilization to target tissues), Table 12.1 [17].

The ratio of soluble transferrin receptor (sTfR) to log serum ferritin has been proposed to be a sensitive predictor of functional ID in patients with chronic inflammation [19]. sTfR reflects the cellular iron demand and therefore might be a more sensitive indicator of ID than ferritin. However, to date, no cut-off levels of sTfR have been defined for CHF patients. The gold standard for the diagnosis of absolute ID remains bone marrow aspiration. Due to its invasiveness, bone marrow aspiration is, however, not suitable for diagnosing ID in clinical practice.

Table 12.1 Definition of iron deficiency in chronic heart failure

	Ferritin (ug/l)	Transferrin-saturation (Tsat), %
Absolute iron deficiency (depleted iron stores)	<100	
Functional iron deficiency (iron sequestration)	100–299	20

12.2.2 Prevalence

Depending on the definition and diagnostic algorithm the prevalence of ID in CHF patients varies between 37% and 73%, with higher prevalence in more advanced CHF patients (Table 12.2). In anemic patients admitted to the hospital because of advanced CHF (NYHA IV), absolute ID was present in 73% as assessed by the absence of iron staining in bone marrow biopsies (gold standard diagnosis of absolut ID) [20]. In a pooled analysis of five European CHF Cohorts (n = 1506), the prevalence of ID defined according to the ESC-criteria was 61.2% in anemic and 45.6% in non-anemic patients [21]. According to current European registry data, 50% of in- and outpatients with reduced left ventricular ejection fraction (LVEF < 40%) fulfil the ESC-criteria for ID [21, 22]. Independent clinical predictors of ID include female sex, higher NYHA functional class, higher NT-pro BNP, unstable disease and presence of anemia. As for anemia, the prevalence of ID is similar in patients with HFrEF and HFpEF [2].

12.2.3 Etiology and Pathophysiology

ID in CHF is characterized by impaired gastrointestinal iron uptake and impaired mobilization of existing iron stores. In some patients chronic blood loss also contributes to ID, particularly in the context of chronic anti-platelet therapy or oral anticoagulation. The liver protein hepcidin is a key regulator of iron hemostasis (Fig. 12.1). Hepcidin inhibits ferroportin, a protein that is responsible for the transport of

Table 12.2 Prevalence of iron deficiency in selected registries and cohorts

	RAID-HF [22] 2016 (n = 923)	Klip et al. [21] 2013 (n = 1506)	Jankowska et al. [30] 2010 (n = 546)
LVEF %	27	33	26
NYHA ≥ III %	71	54	49
Women %	25	26	12
Age (years)	70	64	55
Anemia %	44	28	ND
ID %	**55**	**50**	**37**

LVEF left ventricular ejection fraction, *NYHA* New York Heart Association Class, *ID* iron deficiency iron from enterocytes, macrophages and hepatocytes to circulating transferrin. Thus, by blocking ferroportin, hepcidin blocks gastrointestinal iron absorption and the release of iron from its storage sites. As a result, high levels of hepcidin "trap" iron in storage cells [23]. HF-associated inflammatory cytokines and hepatic congestion both increase hepcidin serum levels resulting in decreased availability of functional iron, despite adequate total iron stores (iron sequestration). This type of ID is referred to as "functional ID". High levels of circulating hepcidin typically characterize early stages of HF with predominant functional ID [24]. As the severity of CHF progresses chronic mucosal edema and reduced gastrointestinal blood flow may impair iron uptake from the gut resulting in vanishing iron stores and the development of absolute ID [25]. Also, poor nutritional state may further contribute to absolute ID. Therefore, in advanced CHF, hepcidin levels may be low in order to facilitate iron uptake. Low hepcidin levels have been shown to be associated with poor outcome in CHF [24].

Iron is a vital element involved in many physiologic processes. Iron is crucial for hematopoiesis and plays a pivotal role in oxygen transport (hemoglobin), oxygen storage (myoglobin) and oxygen-dependent ATP generation in the mitochondria (element of the respiratory chain). ID leads to a decrease in the number of mitochondria and their cristae, thereby promoting energy deprivation of muscle tissue [26]. Normal cardiac and skeletal muscle function is thus dependent on sufficient iron uptake and proper intracellular iron handling. The effects of ID in CHF are manifold. (1) Impairment of oxygen delivery; (2) impairment of energy (ATP) generation; (3) impairment of skeletal and cardiac muscle function. These pathophysiolgical mechanisms add to the inherent exercise intolerance of the HF syndrome.

12.2.4 Impact on Morbidity and Mortality

The impact of ID on morbidity and mortality in CHF patients has been evaluated in various studies. These studies provide solid evidence that patients with CHF and ID suffer from lower exercise capacity, impaired quality of life and increased mortality. Cardiopulmonary exercise testing (CPET) demonstrated lower mean peak oxygen consumption (PVO2) and steeper VE/VCO2 slopes in patients with ID versus those without ID [27]. This relationship was independent from Hb levels or NYHA class, suggesting that ID alone may impair exercise capacity. There is also good evidence that ID is independently associated with lower quality of life [28, 29]. Jankowska et al. provided first evidence that ID, independently of anemia, might exert detrimental effects on prognosis, including hospitalizations and mortality. In a large cohort of patients with HFrEF the presence of ID was associated with a 12% increase in mortality within 3 years of follow up ($p = 0.0006$) [30]. The independent association of ID with mortality was further substantiated in an international pooled analysis of a mixed population of 1506 HF patients. In this analysis, patients with ID exhibited a more than twofold higher mortality (8.7% versus 3.6%) at 6 months follow up, independently of the presence of anemia [21]. Taken together these observational data suggest that ID is a stronger prognostic marker than anemia in patients with CHF.

12.2.5 Treatment of Iron Deficiency

Oral Iron Oral iron is inexpensive and widely used to treat iron deficient states in various clinical situations. However, oral iron therapy might have important shortcomings in the context of ID and CHF. (1) Due to impaired gastrointestinal absorption in CHF patients, oral iron therapy might have limited efficacy to increase storage iron and Hb. (2) Treatment adherence for oral iron therapy might be limited due to its propensity for gastrointestinal side effects. (3) Oral iron therapy is inadequate to achieve rapid treatment effects or might be insufficient to overcome the rate of chronic iron loss in CHF patients.

Data about oral iron therapy in CHF patients is scarce. A small retrospective analysis of HFrEF patients taking oral iron supplementation suggested similar improvement of iron stores as previously reported with the use of intravenous iron therapy [31]. To date, randomized controlled multicenter trials exploring the efficacy of oral iron in CHF patients are still lacking. The National Institute of Health-sponsored IRONOUT HF trial (NCT02188784) will be the first to address this important question [32].

Intravenous Iron In contrast to oral iron, intravenous (i.v.) iron therapy bypasses the problem of malabsorption and malcompliance. At present, the safety and efficacy of i.v. iron administration for the treatment of ID in CHF patients was evaluated in nine studies (Table 12.3) [33–41]. Five studies were double-blinded, randomized and placebo-controlled by design [34, 38, 40–42]. In these trials, i.v. iron was administrated in the form of iron sucrose or iron carboxymaltose. Both formulations were well tolerated without evidence of serious adverse effects compared to placebo. Anemic CHF patients exhibited a significant increase in Hb levels. The magnitude of Hb increase across the studies seems dependent on the total iron dose administered, suggesting a possible dose-response relationship. In addition to Hb correction, i.v. iron administration resulted in significant improvement in NYHA class [33–36, 38], exercise tolerance and quality of life [33–35, 38], LVEF [34, 36], N-terminal pro BNP [34] and renal

Table 12.3 Clinical trials of intravenous iron in patients with heart failure

Study	Design	Population	N	Treatment	Follow-up	Outcomes: Functional Capacity/NYHA Class	QoL	Mortality/ hospitalization	Specific outcomes
Bolger et al. [33] 2006	Uncontrolled	Hb < 120 g/L Ferritin ≤ 400 ug/L LVEF < 30%	16	Iron sucrose 1000 mg (cumulative) over 12 days	3 months	6MWT↑ NYHA Class↓	QoL↑	ND	Hb↑ Ferritin↑ Tsat↑
Toblli et al. [34] 2007	Randomized, double-blind, placebo-controlled	Hb < 125 g/L Ferritin < 100 ug/L Tsat < 20% LVEF ≤ 35%	40	Iron sucrose 200 mg/week for 5 weeks	6 months	6MWT↑ NYHA class↓	QoL↑	ND	Hb↑ Ferritin↑ Tsat↑ NTproBNP↓ CrCl↑ LVEF↑
Usmanov et al. [36] 2008	Uncontrolled	Hb < 110 g/L NYHA class III/IV	32	Iron sucrose	6 months	NYHA class↓ (only in NYHA III)	ND	ND	Hb↑ Ferritin↑ Tsat↑ LVEF↑ Creatinin (NS)
FERRIC-HF [35] 2008	Randomized, controlled, observer-blinded	Hb < 145 g/L Ferritin < 100 ug/L or Ferritin 100–299 ug/L and Tsat < 20% LVEF ≤ 45%	35	Iron sucrose 200 mg/week until ferritin>500 ug/L 200 mg/months thereafter	18 weeks	ΔPVO2↑ NYHA Class↓	NS	ND	Hb (NS) Ferritin↑ Tsat↑ LVEF (NS) Creatinin (NS)
FAIR-HF [38] 2009	Randomized, double-blind, placebo-controlled	Hb ≥ 95,≤135 g/L Ferritin < 100 ug/L or Ferritin 100–299 ug/L and Tsat < 20% LVEF ≤ 40–45%	459	Iron carboxymaltose 200 mg/week until iron repletion	24 weeks	6MWT↑ NYHA Class↓	QoL↑ PGA↑	NS	
Gaber et al. [39] 2011	Uncontrolled	Hb > 120 g/L Ferritin < 100 ug/L and Tsat < 20% LVEF < 40%	40	Iron dextran 200 mg/week until iron repletion	12 weeks	6MWT↑ NYHA Class↓	ND	ND	Echo-parameters S′↑ E'↑ E/E'↓ LVEF (NS) E/A ratio (NS)
IRON-HF [40] 2013	Randomized, double-blind, placebo-controlled	Hb ≥ 90,≤120 g/L Ferritin<500ug/L and Tsat<20% LVEF<40%	23	i.v. iron versus oral iron	3 months	ΔPVO2↑	ND	ND	

(continued)

Table 12.3 (continued)

Study	Design	Population	N	Treatment	Follow-up	Outcomes			
						Functional Capacity/NYHA Class	QoL	Mortality/ hospitalization	Specific outcomes
CONFIRM-HF [42] 2014	Randomized, double-blind, placebo-controlled	Hb ≤ 150 g/L Ferritin<100ug/L or ferritin 100–299 ug/L and Tsat<20% LVEF≤45%	304	Iron carboxymaltose bolus 500–1000 mg Until iron repletion	1 year	6MWT↑ NYHA class↓	QoL↑ PGA↑	Hospitalization↓ Mortality (NS)	
Toblli et al. [41] 2015	Randomized, double-blind, placebo-controlled	Hb < 125 g/L (men) Hb < 115 g/L (women) Ferritin<1 00ug/L or Tsat<20% LVEF≤35%	60		6 months	ND	ND		CrCl↑ NT-proBNP↓ Heart rate↓ LVEF↑

BMC bone marrow cells, *MSC* mesenchymal stem cells, *CSC* cardiac stem cells, *CMR* cardiac magnetic resonance tomography, *ICMP* ischemic cardiomyopathy, *ECHO* echocardiography, *SPECT* single-photon emission computed tomography, *CCT* contrast-enhanced computer tomography, *LVA* left ventricular angiogram, *LVEF* left ventricular ejection fraction, *RNA* radionuclide angiogram, *ND* not determined, *NS* non significant function [38]. There was also a trend towards less cardiovascular events. Importantly, the CONFIRM-HF trial was the first study to show a significant reduction in the number of hospital admissions secondary to worsening HF, although the reductions in all hospital admissions was not significant [42]. The simplified i.v. administration scheme used in CONFIRM-HF is particularly attractive for application in clinical practice. In this study, an undiluted bolus of ferric-carboxymaltose (500–1000 mg) was injected intravenously over 1 min. Interestingly, clinical improvements occurred rapidly within the first month of treatment. Subgroup analyses demonstrated that not only anemic patients benefited from i.v. iron but also iron deficient patients without anemia, suggesting that part of the treatment efficacy is Hb-independent. Two meta-analyses including around 600 patients have evaluated the treatment efficacy of i.v. iron in CHF patients with HFrEF [43, 44]. They consistently show improvement of NYHA class, 6-minute walking test and quality of life and reduced rehospitalisation rates. Neither meta-analysis demonstrated a mortality benefit, possibly due to the short follow-ups and inadequate patient numbers in included studies. The results of a number of randomized controlled trials of i.v. iron in different CHF populations are still pending (IRON-MAN, EFFECT-HF, ICHF, FAIR-HF-HFpEF, PRACTICEASIAHF).

12.2.6 Recommendations for Clinical Practice

Current international HF guidelines recommend checking for Hb, ferritin and Tsat in all patients with CHF as part of the initial work-up [17]. These measurements should be repeated every 6–12 months. The ESC Guidelines recommend i.v. iron substitution if ferritin is <100 ug/l or 100–299 ug/l if Tsat < 20% (Table 12.1) [17]. In order to prevent potentially deleterious iatrogenic iron overload, it is mandatory to estimate the total iron dose required to restore iron stores. The total cumulative iron dose can be calculated according to the Ganzoni formula (Table 12.4). In most cases, 1000 mg of iron will be a good starting dose to replenish iron stores [45]. As shown in CONFIRM-HF, 1000 mg can be administered as a single bolus or divided in two boli of 500 mg that are administered within 2–4 weeks. Except for a history of allergic reaction to components of the iron preparation used and the absence of iron deficiency, there are no contraindications to i.v. iron therapy. If Hb levels exceed 15 g/l, iron substitution is not recommended. Because of the possibility of longstanding skin "tattooing" in cases of transcutaneous iron infusion, a solid intravenous access is absolutely mandatory for the administration of i.v. iron. The patient should be observed for at least 30 min following each injection and the administration staff must be trained to diagnose and manage possible anaphylactic reactions. Iron therapy should be stopped if ferritin levels exceed 500 ug/l or Hb levels reach 15 g/dl. Because serum ferritin levels are not representative for total iron stores within the first 3 months after i.v. iron administration, serum ferritin and Tsat should only be measured at least 3 months after the last iron administration in order to document successful repletion of iron stores.

Table 12.4 Estimation of required total iron dose according to the Ganzoni formula

Body weight (kg) × (15 – Hb (g/dL)) × 2.4 + 500 = iron dose (mg)
Example: Patient 80 kg with Hb 12 g/dl:
→ 80 × 3 × 2.4 + 500 mg = 1076 mg

References

1. Groenveld HF, Januzzi JL, Damman K, van Wijngaarden J, Hillege HL, van Veldhuisen DJ, et al. Anemia and mortality in heart failure patients a systematic review and meta-analysis. J Am Coll Cardiol. 2008;52(10):818–27.
2. Cleland JG, Zhang J, Pellicori P, Dicken B, Dierckx R, Shoaib A, et al. Prevalence and outcomes of anemia and hematinic deficiencies in patients with chronic heart failure. JAMA Cardiol. 2016;1(5):539–47.
3. O'Meara E, Rouleau JL, White M, Roy K, Blondeau L, Ducharme A, et al. Heart failure with anemia: novel findings on the roles of renal disease, interleukins, and specific left ventricular remodeling processes. Circ Heart Fail. 2014;7(5):773–81.
4. Deswal A, Petersen NJ, Feldman AM, Young JB, White BG, Mann DL. Cytokines and cytokine receptors in advanced heart failure: an analysis of the cytokine database from the Vesnarinone trial (VEST). Circulation. 2001;103(16):2055–9.
5. Westenbrink BD, Voors AA, de Boer RA, Schuringa JJ, Klinkenberg T, van der Harst P, et al. Bone marrow dysfunction in chronic heart failure patients. Eur J Heart Fail. 2010;12(7):676–84.
6. van der Meer P, Lok DJ, Januzzi JL, de la Porte PW, Lipsic E, van Wijngaarden J, et al. Adequacy of endogenous erythropoietin levels and mortality in anaemic heart failure patients. Eur Heart J. 2008;29(12):1510–5.
7. van der Putten K, Braam B, Jie KE, Gaillard CA. Mechanisms of disease: erythropoietin resistance in patients with both heart and kidney failure. Nat Clin Pract Nephrol. 2008;4(1):47–57.
8. Abramov D, Cohen RS, Katz SD, Mancini D, Maurer MS. Comparison of blood volume characteristics in anemic patients with low versus preserved left ventricular ejection fractions. Am J Cardiol. 2008;102(8):1069–72.
9. O'Meara E, Clayton T, McEntegart MB, McMurray JJ, Lang CC, Roger SD, et al. Clinical correlates and consequences of anemia in a broad spectrum of patients with heart failure: results of the candesartan in Heart Failure: Assessment of Reduction in Mortality and Morbidity (CHARM) program. Circulation. 2006;113(7):986–94.
10. Komajda M, Anker SD, Charlesworth A, Okonko D, Metra M, Di Lenarda A, et al. The impact of new onset anaemia on morbidity and mortality in chronic heart failure: results from COMET. Eur Heart J. 2006;27(12):1440–6.
11. Horwich TB, Fonarow GC, Hamilton MA, MacLellan WR, Borenstein J. Anemia is associated with worse symptoms, greater impairment in functional capacity and a significant increase in mortality in patients with advanced heart failure. J Am Coll Cardiol. 2002;39(11):1780–6.

12. Ghali JK, Anand IS, Abraham WT, Fonarow GC, Greenberg B, Krum H, et al. Randomized double-blind trial of darbepoetin alfa in patients with symptomatic heart failure and anemia. Circulation. 2008;117(4):526–35.
13. Swedberg K, Young JB, Anand IS, Cheng S, Desai AS, Diaz R, et al. Treatment of anemia with darbepoetin alfa in systolic heart failure. N Engl J Med. 2013;368(13):1210–9.
14. Singh AK, Szczech L, Tang KL, Barnhart H, Sapp S, Wolfson M, et al. Correction of anemia with epoetin alfa in chronic kidney disease. N Engl J Med. 2006;355(20):2085–98.
15. Drueke TB, Locatelli F, Clyne N, Eckardt KU, Macdougall IC, Tsakiris D, et al. Normalization of hemoglobin level in patients with chronic kidney disease and anemia. N Engl J Med. 2006;355(20):2071–84.
16. Solomon SD, Uno H, Lewis EF, Eckardt KU, Lin J, Burdmann EA, et al. Erythropoietic response and outcomes in kidney disease and type 2 diabetes. N Engl J Med. 2010;363(12):1146–55.
17. Ponikowski P, Voors AA, Anker SD, Bueno H, Cleland JG, Coats AJ, et al. 2016 ESC guidelines for the diagnosis and treatment of acute and chronic heart failure: the Task Force for the diagnosis and treatment of acute and chronic heart failure of the European Society of Cardiology (ESC). Developed with the special contribution of the Heart Failure Association (HFA) of the ESC. Eur J Heart Fail. 2016;18(8):891–975.
18. Goodnough LT, Nemeth E, Ganz T. Detection, evaluation, and management of iron-restricted erythropoiesis. Blood. 2010;116(23):4754–61.
19. Punnonen K, Irjala K, Rajamaki A. Serum transferrin receptor and its ratio to serum ferritin in the diagnosis of iron deficiency. Blood. 1997;89(3):1052–7.
20. Nanas JN, Matsouka C, Karageorgopoulos D, Leonti A, Tsolakis E, Drakos SG, et al. Etiology of anemia in patients with advanced heart failure. J Am Coll Cardiol. 2006;48(12):2485–9.
21. Klip IT, Comin-Colet J, Voors AA, Ponikowski P, Enjuanes C, Banasiak W, et al. Iron deficiency in chronic heart failure: an international pooled analysis. Am Heart J. 2013;165(4):575–82. e3
22. Wienbergen H, Pfister O, Hochadel M, Michel S, Bruder O, Remppis BA, et al. Usefulness of iron deficiency correction in management of patients with heart failure [from the Registry Analysis of Iron Deficiency-Heart Failure (RAID-HF) registry]. Am J Cardiol. 2016;118:1875–80.
23. Weiss G, Goodnough LT. Anemia of chronic disease. N Engl J Med. 2005;352(10):1011–23.
24. Jankowska EA, Malyszko J, Ardehali H, Koc-Zorawska E, Banasiak W, von Haehling S, et al. Iron status in patients with chronic heart failure. Eur Heart J. 2013;34(11):827–34.
25. Sica DA. Pharmacotherapy in congestive heart failure: drug absorption in the management of congestive heart failure: loop diuretics. Congest Heart Fail. 2003;9(5):287–92.
26. Stugiewicz M, Tkaczyszyn M, Kasztura M, Banasiak W, Ponikowski P, Jankowska EA. The influence of iron deficiency on the functioning of skeletal muscles: experimental evidence and clinical implications. Eur J Heart Fail. 2016;18(7):762–73.
27. Okonko DO, Mandal AK, Missouris CG, Poole-Wilson PA. Disordered iron homeostasis in chronic heart failure: prevalence, predictors, and relation to anemia, exercise capacity, and survival. J Am Coll Cardiol. 2011;58(12):1241–51.
28. Comin-Colet J, Enjuanes C, Gonzalez G, Torrens A, Cladellas M, Merono O, et al. Iron deficiency is a key determinant of health-related quality of life in patients with chronic heart failure regardless of anaemia status. Eur J Heart Fail. 2013;15(10):1164–72.
29. Enjuanes C, Klip IT, Bruguera J, Cladellas M, Ponikowski P, Banasiak W, et al. Iron deficiency and health-related quality of life in chronic heart failure: results from a multicenter European study. Int J Cardiol. 2014;174(2):268–75.
30. Jankowska EA, Rozentryt P, Witkowska A, Nowak J, Hartmann O, Ponikowska B, et al. Iron deficiency: an ominous sign in patients with systolic chronic heart failure. Eur Heart J. 2010;31(15):1872–80.
31. Niehaus ED, Malhotra R, Cocca-Spofford D, Semigran M, Lewis GD. Repletion of iron stores with the use of oral iron supplementation in patients with systolic heart failure. J Card Fail. 2015;21(8):694–7.
32. Lewis GD, Semigran MJ, Givertz MM, Malhotra R, Anstrom KJ, Hernandez AF, et al. Oral iron therapy for heart failure with reduced ejection fraction: design and rationale for oral iron repletion effects on oxygen uptake in heart failure. Circ Heart Fail. 2016;9(5):e000345.
33. Bolger AP, Bartlett FR, Penston HS, O'Leary J, Pollock N, Kaprielian R, et al. Intravenous iron alone for the treatment of anemia in patients with chronic heart failure. J Am Coll Cardiol. 2006;48(6):1225–7.
34. Toblli JE, Lombrana A, Duarte P, Di Gennaro F. Intravenous iron reduces NT-pro-brain natriuretic peptide in anemic patients with chronic heart failure and renal insufficiency. J Am Coll Cardiol. 2007;50(17):1657–65.
35. Okonko DO, Grzeslo A, Witkowski T, Mandal AK, Slater RM, Roughton M, et al. Effect of intravenous iron sucrose on exercise tolerance in anemic and nonanemic patients with symptomatic chronic heart failure and iron deficiency FERRIC-HF: a randomized, controlled, observer-blinded trial. J Am Coll Cardiol. 2008;51(2):103–12.
36. Usmanov RI, Zueva EB, Silverberg DS, Shaked M. Intravenous iron without erythropoietin for the treatment of iron deficiency anemia in patients with moderate to severe congestive heart failure and chronic kidney insufficiency. J Nephrol. 2008;21(2):236–42.
37. Drakos SG, Anastasiou-Nana MI, Malliaras KG, Nanas JN. Anemia in chronic heart failure. Congest Heart Fail. 2009;15(2):87–92.
38. Anker SD, Comin Colet J, Filippatos G, Willenheimer R, Dickstein K, Drexler H, et al. Ferric carboxymaltose in patients with heart failure and iron deficiency. N Engl J Med. 2009;361(25):2436–48.
39. Gaber R, Kotb NA, Ghazy M, Nagy HM, Salama M, Elhendy A. Tissue Doppler and strain rate imaging detect improvement of myocardial function in iron deficient patients with congestive heart failure after iron replacement therapy. Echocardiography. 2012;29(1):13–8.
40. Beck-da-Silva L, Piardi D, Soder S, Rohde LE, Pereira-Barretto AC, de Albuquerque D, et al. IRON-HF study: a randomized trial to assess the effects of iron in heart failure patients with anemia. Int J Cardiol. 2013;168(4):3439–42.
41. Toblli JE, Di Gennaro F, Rivas C. Changes in echocardiographic parameters in iron deficiency patients with heart failure and chronic kidney disease treated with intravenous iron. Heart Lung Circ. 2015;24(7):686–95.
42. Ponikowski P, van Veldhuisen DJ, Comin-Colet J, Ertl G, Komajda M, Mareev V, et al. Beneficial effects of long-term intravenous iron therapy with ferric carboxymaltose in patients with symptomatic heart failure and iron deficiencydagger. Eur Heart J. 2015;36(11):657–68.
43. Avni T, Leibovici L, Gafter-Gvili A. Iron supplementation for the treatment of chronic heart failure and iron deficiency: systematic review and meta-analysis. Eur J Heart Fail. 2012;14(4):423–9.
44. Kapoor M, Schleinitz MD, Gemignani A, Wu WC. Outcomes of patients with chronic heart failure and iron deficiency treated with intravenous iron: a meta-analysis. Cardiovasc Hematol Disord Drug Targets. 2013;13(1):35–44.
45. Filippatos G, Farmakis D, Colet JC, Dickstein K, Luscher TF, Willenheimer R, et al. Intravenous ferric carboxymaltose in iron-deficient chronic heart failure patients with and without anaemia: a subanalysis of the FAIR-HF trial. Eur J Heart Fail. 2013;15(11):1267–76.

Psychological Comorbidities in Heart Failure

13

Christiane E. Angermann and Julia Wallenborn

13.1 Incidence and Symptoms of Psychological Comorbidities

Depression can be easily overlooked during routine clinical care of heart failure patients because symptoms of the two conditions are similar and may, therefore, be misinterpreted by physicians and also by the patients themselves. For example, fatigue, difficulty concentrating, listlessness and sleep disorders can be associated with both heart failure and depression.

The rate of depression increases in parallel with increasing heart failure severity [1]. Available data suggest that depression occurs in 10% of clinically asymptomatic outpatients up to 40–70% in hospitalized patients with New York Heart Association (NYHA) class III–IV symptoms [1–3]. Similar to the general population, depression in heart failure patients is more common in women and younger individuals [1, 4, 5]. At least a quarter of patients with heart failure exhibit symptoms of both anxiety and depression [6]. According to the literature, severe anxiety is also associated with increased mortality, independent of coexisting depression, particularly when cardiac output is markedly reduced [7].

Several studies have demonstrated a close interrelation between the intensity of cardiac and depressive symptoms and anxiety disorders [2, 8]. Independent of objective findings such as cardiac output or blood levels of heart failure biomarkers, heart failure patients with depression or anxiety more often experience severe dyspnoea and impaired quality of life. Intensified perception of symptoms may result from misjudgement or overestimation, but also from psychological strain or genetic disposition [9].

C. E. Angermann (✉) · J. Wallenborn
Department of Internal Medicine I and Comprehensive Heart Failure Center, University and University Hospital of Würzburg, Würzburg, Germany
e-mail: Angermann_C@ukw.de

Memory disorders (cognitive dysfunction) are also more common in cardiac patients than in the general population. Cognitive dysfunction limits patients' ability to cope with heart failure (e.g. underestimate or misinterpret signs of worsening disease), meaning that recognition of this comorbidity is of clinical relevance. Furthermore, patients with cognitive dysfunction may be unable to cope with more complex treatment plans. Reports on the frequency of cognitive dysfunction in heart failure vary between 25% and 75% [10, 11]. It is clinically relevant to discriminate between mild cognitive impairment (MCI) and dementia. In more advanced stages, cognitive dysfunction may be associated with the loss of cerebral grey matter [12]. In the early stages, patients may be able to compensate for cognitive deficits so that these are not readily recognized during regular communication with their physicians. Poor adherence to treatment recommendations may be the first indicator of cognitive dysfunction.

In particular, discrepancy between subjective symptoms and objective findings indicate that the possibility of psychiatric comorbidities must be considered. Standardized and validated screening tools, which are easy to apply (often by the patients themselves) are helpful to identify such conditions, better understand their symptoms and lead to more targeted management and therapeutic interventions.

13.2 Pathogenesis and Interactions

To date, interrelations between affective disorders and increased cardiac risk have primarily been studied in patients with coronary disease. Twin data indicate that genetically determined pathophysiological mechanisms play a role in the development of both coronary disease and depression [13]. Interestingly, own investigations demonstrated that a functional sequence variant of the neuropeptide S receptor-1 gene may modulate clinical outcomes and healthcare utilization in patients with systolic heart failure undergoing telephone-based disease management. Consistent with the

D. S. Feldman, P. Mohacsi (eds.), *Heart Failure*, Cardiovascular Medicine, https://doi.org/10.1007/978-3-319-98184-0_13

previous observation of an association between the T-allele [9] and higher anxiety sensitivity index scores in response to bodily symptoms [14], we found that homozygous carriers of the gain-of-function T-allele were rehospitalized following cardiac decompensation for systolic heart failure significantly more often than those with the AT or AA genotype [9]. This gene x treatment interaction was not observed in patients undergoing usual care, and we therefore assumed that TT genotype carriers exaggerated self-assessed somatic symptoms during telephone contacts. This could have led nurses and physicians to more often recommend closer assessment of problems they perceived as potentially dangerous when reported by patients with increased anxiety and a tendency to over-interpret physical symptoms. In summary, this proof-of-principle study suggested the possibility of psychogenetic determinants of clinical outcomes and healthcare utilization in patients with heart failure that, in the case of the neuropeptide S receptor-1 gene, was modulated by the type of care.

Figure 13.1 provides a simplified schematic of possible complex interrelations between mental and somatic factors that may lead to the development and progression of cardiovascular disease, and/or depression, anxiety and cognitive dysfunction. Negative emotions may have adverse effects on the neurohormonal system in a similar way to external stress. Dysregulation of autonomic nervous control leads to increased sympathetic tone and higher circulating levels of stress hormones, including cortisol and proinflammatory cytokines, thus increasing the risk for cardiovascular events [16–19]. Autonomic dysregulation and systemic inflammation may also induce a procoagulant state by potentiating platelet activation, altering the coagulation cascade and inducing endothelial dysfunction, all of which contribute to the development and progression of atherosclerosis [15, 20–22]. Other relevant pathogenic mechanisms include abnormal lipid metabolism and insulin resistance. Thus, there are complex interrelations between depressive symptoms and increased anxiety levels and multiple somatic facets of

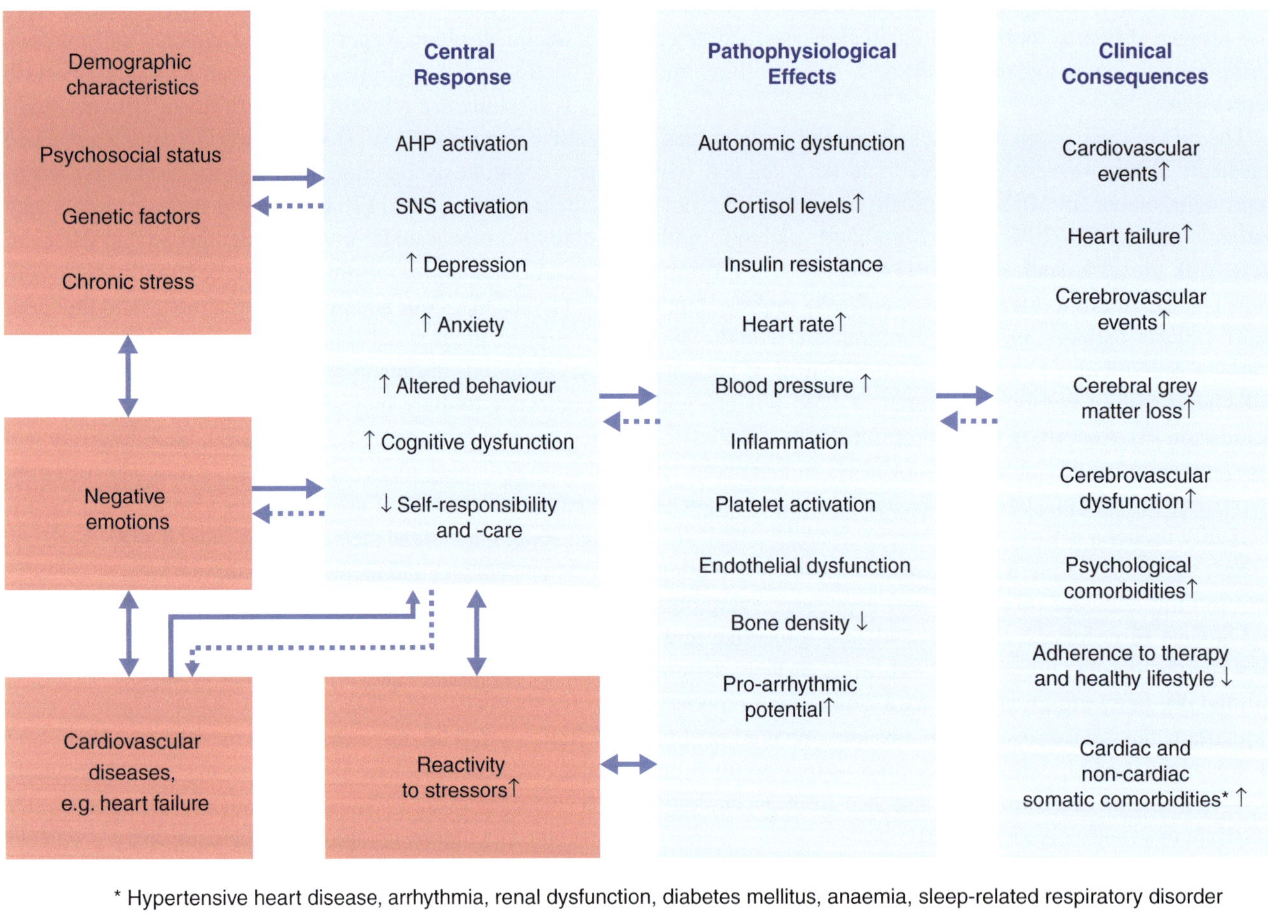

Fig. 13.1 Interrelations and pathophysiological mechanisms with possible bidirectional impact that may contribute to the development of depressive symptoms and other negative emotions in cardiovascular disease and/or that may increase the likelihood of psychological comorbidities in chronic somatic diseases such as heart failure. AHP: adrenal-hypothalamic-pituitary axis; SNS: sympathetic nervous system. (Modified from [15])

cardiovascular diseases that may accelerate disease progression.

The pathogenesis of cognitive dysfunction is also likely to be multifactorial. Trigger mechanisms include diminished perfusion of the brain and dysfunction of the blood-brain barrier due to reduced oxygen supply as a consequence of low cardiac output or embolic events [23]. The complex consequences of diminished oxygen supply include altered cerebral metabolism, a proinflammatory state, augmented oxidative stress and neuronal dysfunction [24]. Frequent heart failure comorbidities and complications could also play a role, including diabetes, anaemia, arteriosclerosis, atrial fibrillation, renal dysfunction, electrolyte imbalance, coagulopathies, ischaemic cerebral events, malnutrition, and drug-induced side effects [24, 25]. Moreover, depression and anxiety tend to augment cognitive dysfunction. Loss of retentiveness, diminished ability to concentrate and memory decline further reduce logical and emotional functions.

All of the described biological pathophysiological mechanisms occur in addition to behavioural factors that are also modulated by depression and anxiety. Patients with depression and/or anxiety tend to not take their medicine regularly and often show inadequate adherence to non-pharmacological treatment recommendations regarding life style issues such as nicotine abstinence, healthy nutrition or, in particular, physical activity [26]. In additional to psychosocial components, demographic and genetic factors, and personal life circumstances multiply the manifold losses that patients may experience as a consequence of the somatic disease (e.g. a decline of health, functional capacity, independence and sexual activity, and loss of employment or financial security), which all together might also help to explain the interrelation between heart failure and depressive symptoms.

Depression, anxiety and cognitive dysfunction may share several principal somatic risks and disease mechanisms. However, since the significance of each contributing factor as well as personal resilience may differ considerably between individuals, the pathogenesis, disease profile and clinical phenotype of psychological comorbidities may be heterogeneous, and therefore treatment requirements may differ between individuals, also depending on whether affected patients are physically healthy or suffer from chronic somatic illness. Why depression, anxiety and cognitive dysfunction are invariably associated with a significantly increased mortality risk und more frequent hospital admissions in all affected patients with cardiovascular diseases and whether psychological comorbidities are true mediators or only markers of increased risk in cardiac patients is still poorly understood [27].

13.3 Diagnosis

Depression is defined based on subjective symptoms [28, 29]; there is no biological test for diagnosis verification. Severity is an important characteristic of major depression and also an 'episode specifier' in the 5th revised edition of the *Diagnostic and Statistical Manual of Mental Disorders* (DSM-V), where depressive episodes are classified as 'mild', 'moderate' or 'severe' [29]. These severity subtypes rely on three different criteria: the number of symptoms present, symptom severity and the degree of functional disability resulting from the symptoms. Criteria have been proposed to estimate depression severity (Table 13.1) [29]: Mild: >1 major symptom plus 1–2 additional symptoms or 5–6 symptoms of mild severity and functional impairment; Moderate: >1 major symptom plus 2–3 additional symptoms, or 7–8 symptoms with moderate functional impairment; Severe: All 3 major symptoms plus >3 additional symptoms, or fewer symptoms but any of the following: severe functional impairment, psychotic symptoms, recent suicide attempt, or specific suicide plan or clear intent. Several validated questionnaires allow for standardised depression screening according to the DSM criteria.

Our working group has often used the self-administered nine-item Patient Health Questionnaire (PHQ-9) in patients with heart failure. The PHQ-9 is validated in different languages and freely accessible online (http://www.phqscreeners.com, Fig. 13.2) [30]. Patients are asked how often nine of the most important symptoms have been present in the past 2 weeks. Possible answers are "not at all", "several days", "more than half the days "and "nearly every day". Each item of the PHQ-9 yields a score of 0–3 resulting in an overall sum-score from 0 to 27, with higher values indicating more severe depression. Usual cut-off points are: 0–5, normal;

Table 13.1 Symptoms required to be present for the diagnosis of a depressive episode according to DSM [28, 29]

Major symptoms	Additional symptoms
Depressed mood Loss of interest and/or pleasure in activities that are normally pleasurable Loss of energy or increased fatigability	Loss of confidence and self-esteem Unreasonable feelings of self-reproach or excessive and inappropriate guilt Recurrent thoughts of death or suicide, or any suicidal behaviour Complaints or evidence of diminished ability to think or concentrate, such as indecisiveness or vacillation Change in psychomotor activity, with agitation or retardation (either subjective or objective) Sleep disturbance of any type Change in appetite (decrease or increase) with corresponding weight change

	Over the last **last 2 weeks,** how often have you been bothered by any of the following problems?	Not at all	Several days	More than half the days	Nearly every day
1.	Little interest or pleasure in doing things	**0**	**1**	**2**	**3**
2.	Feeling down, depressed, or hopeless	**0**	**1**	**2**	**3**
3.	Trouble falling or staying asleep, or sleeping too much	**0**	**1**	**2**	**3**
4.	Feeling tired or having little energy	**0**	**1**	**2**	**3**
5.	Poor appetite or overeating	**0**	**1**	**2**	**3**
6.	Feeling bad about yourself–or that you are a failure or have let yourself or your family down	**0**	**1**	**2**	**3**
7.	Trouble concentrating on things, such as reading the newspaper or watching television	**0**	**1**	**2**	**3**
8.	Moving or speaking so slowly that other people could have noticed? Or the opposite–being so figety or restless that you have been moving around a lot more than usual	**0**	**1**	**2**	**3**
9.	Thoughts that you would be better off dead or of hurting yourself in some way	**0**	**1**	**2**	**3**

PHQ-9 / PHQ-2 Questionnaire for the diagnosis of depression **PHQ-2**

Fig. 13.2 Original form of the 9-item Patient Health Questionnaire (PHQ-9). The two questions of the abbreviated version (PHQ-2) are shaded. Sum-scores of 10 points or higher (PHQ-9) and 2 points or higher (PHQ-2) support the diagnosis of depression [35]. PHQ-9 and PHQ-2 are freely accessible online: www.phqscreeners.com

6–10, mild depression; 11–15, moderate depression; 16–20, moderately severe depression; >20, severe depression. Compared with a Structured Clinical Interview and using DSM diagnostic criteria [29], a sum-score of >9 had a sensitivity (specificity) of 88% (88%) for the diagnosis of major depressive disorder (likelihood ratio 7.1). Corresponding values for a sum-score > 11 were 83% (92%), likelihood ratio 10.2 [31]. The abbreviated version of the questionnaire, the PHQ-2 (Fig. 13.2, shaded fields), depicts the most important symptoms (loss of interest or pleasure, melancholia, depression and hopelessness) [32]. In patients with heart failure, the PHQ-2 has proven adequate for risk assessment of depression similar to the PHQ-9 [33], and the American Heart Association recommends its use as a screening tool in patients with cardiovascular diseases [34]. Patients scoring 2 or more points in the PHQ-2 should undergo an extended diagnostic work-up [29]. Yearly follow-ups are recommended.

The 7-Item Questionnaire on Generalized Anxiety Disorder (GAD-7) [36] or its abbreviated version the GAD-2 [37] are suitable for the diagnosis of anxiety, and are also freely available online (http://www.phqscreeners.com, Fig. 13.3). The GAD has a similar structure to the PHQ and includes the most relevant diagnostic criteria for generalized anxiety disorders. Each item of the GAD-7 yields a score of 0–3 resulting in an overall sum-score from 0–21, with higher values indicating more severe anxiety. Usual cut-off points are: 0–5, normal; 6–10, mild anxiety; 11–15, moderate anxiety; >15, severe anxiety. Using a threshold score of 10, the GAD-7 has a sensitivity of 89% and a specificity of 82% for diagnosing generalized anxiety disorders. GAD sum-scores of ≥10 require further diagnostic evaluation [36]. The items

Over the last **last 2 weeks,** how often have you been bothered by any of the following problems?	Not at all	Several days	More than half the days	Nearly every day
1. Feeling nervous, anxious or on edge	0	1	2	3
2. Not being able to stop or control worrying	0	1	2	3
3. Worrying too much about different things	0	1	2	3
4. Trouble relaxing	0	1	2	3
5. Being so restless that it is hard to sit still	0	1	2	3
6. Becoming easily annoyed or irritable	0	1	2	3
7. Feeling afraid as if something awful might happen	0	1	2	3

GAD-7 / GAD-2 Questionnaire for the diagnosis of anxiety disorders **GAD-2**

Fig. 13.3 Original form of the 7-item Questionnaire (GAD-7) that can be used for general anxiety disorder screening. The abbreviated version GAD-2 (shaded fields) includes the first two questions. Scores of 10 points or higher (GAD-7) and 3 points or higher (GAD-2) support the diagnosis of an at least moderate anxiety disorder [36]. GAD-7 and GAD-2 are freely accessible online: www.phqscreeners.com

of the abbreviated version GAD-2 (Fig. 13.3, shaded fields) include the most important diagnostic criteria (anxiety and worries concerning particular events and actions, difficulty in controlling these worries). Sum-scores of 3 points or higher support the diagnosis of an anxiety disorder.

Cognitive dysfunction can be diagnosed using neurophysiological tests. For example, the Mini Mental State Examination (MMSE) examines 11 domains of orientation with regard to short-term memory, attentiveness and visual spatial perception using a 30-point-scale [38]. The Montreal Cognition Assessment has a better sensitivity especially when assessing Mild Cognitive Impairment [39, 40]. Serial examinations are recommended.

13.4 Prognostic Relevance

Depression is a significant predictor of poor survival and higher hospitalization rates in patients with heart failure [1, 2, 4, 5, 41–44]. Even mild depressive symptoms worsen the prognosis and increase healthcare costs [1, 43]. Analyses from the Interdisciplinary Network Heart Failure (INH) program demonstrated a proportional relationship between the severity of depressive symptoms measured by the PHQ-9 and the risk of mortality and rehospitalization (Fig. 13.4) [5, 33]. The relationship between depression and more frequent heart failure decompensations and visits to the emergency ward has been repeatedly demonstrated and confirmed by meta-analysis [1, 43].

Similarly, physically healthy but depressed people have a 2- to 3-fold increased risk of developing cardiac diseases during their lifetime [45]. Depression and heart failure are common diseases, and therefore could occur independently in the same patient by chance, without any actual relationship between the two conditions. However, the information above indicates that bidirectional pathophysiological inter relations rather than mere coincidence are likely. When anxiety and depression coexist, the risk of adverse clinical outcomes appears to increase in a cumulative fashion [7]. Poor treatment adherence due to psychological disorders has a negative effect on disease progression and prognosis, and cognitive dysfunction is likely to play a major causal role [46].

13.5 Therapy

Heart failure guidelines do not provide specific recommendations about the treatment of psychological comorbidities [47]. Various antidepressants are known to have unfavourable side effects and should only be prescribed in heart failure patients after careful consideration of possible benefits and risks. For example, tricyclic antidepressants have been shown to have significant pro-arrhythmic effects [48].

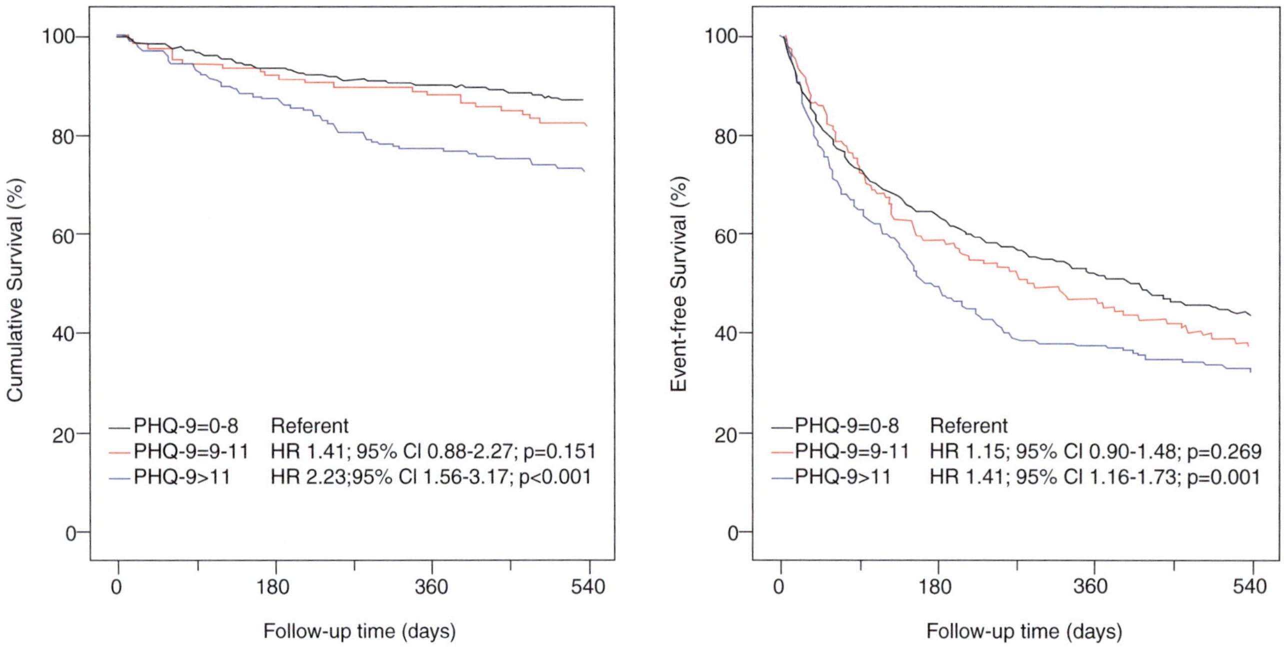

Fig. 13.4 Kaplan-Meier curves depicting cumulative survival and event-free survival (i.e., freedom of all-cause death and rehospitalization) in participants of Interdisciplinary Network Heart Failure (INH) program (n = 852) according to 9-item Patient Health Questionnaire (PHQ-9) results. PHQ-9 sum-scores were categorized as 0–8 (no depression, n = 519), 9–11 (minor depression, n = 127) und >11 (major depression, n = 206). The observation period was 18 months. Left: Cumulative survival; Right: Event-free survival. Compared to non-depressed patients, significantly lower survival rates and event-free survival rates were found in patients with suspected major depression according to the PHQ-9 result [5]

Selective serotonin reuptake inhibitors (SSRIs) are the antidepressant agents of choice in cardiovascular patients due to a relatively favourable safety profile. However, there are also contraindications with these agents, including co-medication with substances prolonging the QT interval (e.g. amiodarone or several beta-blockers). In addition to antidepressant pharmacotherapy, psychotherapy, exercise training, disease management programmes, and other multimodal strategies have been applied with the aim of improving comorbid depression [49, 50]. An overview of some important randomized controlled trials and meta-analyses evaluating different treatment modalities in patients with depressive symptoms and cardiovascular diseases is summarized in Table 13.2 and discussed briefly below. A comprehensive overview of various therapeutic approaches is available [51].

13.5.1 Safety and Efficacy of Antidepressants

To date, use of antidepressants has not been shown to improve prognosis in patients with depression and cardiovascular diseases. Two randomized controlled trials have evaluated the SSRIs sertraline and escitalopram in patients with symptomatic heart failure. The 12-week *Sertraline Against Depression and Heart Disease in Chronic Heart Failure* (SADHART-CHF) study and the 24-month *Morbidity, Mortality and Mood in Depressed Heart Failure Patients* (MOOD-HF) study did not detect any beneficial effects of antidepressant therapy [56, 57]. However, the heart failure disease management with optimization of pharmacotherapy, monitoring, and patient empowerment for all participants offered to all MOOD-HF participants was associated with significant improvement of depressive symptoms and low overall mortality in both study arms. In addition, exploratory analyses from MOOD-HF suggested that escitalopram had an unfavourable effect on cardiac function, quality of life and clinical outcomes, especially in elderly patients with more compromised cardiac function and more severe depressive symptoms [57].

Currently available evidence does not necessarily prove that antidepressants have no benefit and are potentially harmful in all patients with cardiovascular disease and depressive symptoms because depression is a heterogeneous condition and patients with several depression subtypes (e.g. bipolar

Table 13.2 Important randomized controlled trials on various treatment approaches in patients with cardiovascular diseases and depression (modified from [49])

Trials and meta-analyses	Study population	RCT groups (Treatment period)	Outcome
Antidepressant pharmacotherapy			
SADHART [52]	n = 369 post-ACS (57 y, 71% m)	Sertraline vs. placebo (24 weeks)	Safety of the SSRI sertraline Antidepressant efficacy No effect on cardiac function No improvement of mortality
ENRICHD [53]	n = 2481 post-AMI (61 y, 66% m)	CBT +/– SSRI vs. UC (24 weeks)	Antidepressant efficacy of CBT +/– SSRI No effect on event rate (death or recurrent MI)
CREATE [54]	n = 284 chronic CAD (58 y, 75% m)	1) IPT + UC vs. UC only 2) Citalopram vs. placebo (12 weeks)	Antidepressant efficacy of SSRI + UC No benefit of IPT over UC
MIND-IT [55]	n = 331 post-AMI (58 y, 75% m)	Mirtazapin (1. Choice) or SSRI vs. placebo (18 months)	No improvement of depression or cardiac prognosis
SADHART-CHF [56]	n = 469 CHF (62 y, 69% m)	Sertraline vs. placebo; simultaneous nurse-based care in both study groups (12 weeks)	No improvement of depression compared to placebo No effect on cardiac status No effect on event rate (cardiovascular death or hospitalization)
MOOD-HF [57]	n = 372 CHF (62 y, 76% m)	Escitalopram vs. placebo (24 months)	No improvement of depression compared to placebo Clinical suspicion of unfavourable effects of escitalopram on cardiac status No effect on event rate (all-cause death or hospitalization)
Cognitive behavioural therapy			
Freedland KE et al. [58]	n = 158 CHF (54 y, 56% m)	CBT vs. UC (6 months)	CBT improved depression, not HF self-management or functioning of the body
MOSAIC [59]	n = 183 CAD and CHF (60 y, 47% m)	Telephone-based CBT / Disease Management vs. enhanced UC (6 months)	Multimodal care based on the patient's needs improved psychiatric dimensions and quality of life
Physical Exercise			
HF- ACTION [60]	n = 2322 CHF (61 y, 69% m)	Aerobic training vs. UC (12 months)	Physical exercise reduced depressive symptoms and improves prognosis
Tu et al. [61]	n = 3226 CHF	Training alone or as part of cardiac rehabilitation programme vs. UC or education only control group	Training decreased symptoms of depression

ACS acute coronary syndrome, *AMI* acute myocardial infarction, *CAD* coronary artery disease, *CBT* cognitive behavioural therapy, *CHF* chronic heart failure, *IPT* interpersonal psychotherapy, *m* male, *SSRI* selective serotonin reuptake inhibitors, *UC* usual care, *vs.* versus, *y* years

disorders or suicidal ideations) were excluded from the clinical trials. Nevertheless, a reliable specialist diagnosis of depression should be obtained before introducing any specific antidepressant pharmacotherapy. In populations as those investigated in MOOD-HF [57] and SADHART-CHF [56] the use of antidepressants cannot not generally be recommended and a treatment decision should always be made on a case-by-case basis.

A secondary analysis from the SADHART-CHF trial investigated the prognostic value of omega-3 polyunsaturated fatty acids in patients with heart failure and major depression and showed that low levels were a significant predictor of reduced survival [62]. Meta-analysis findings suggest that omega-3 fatty acid supplementation might be beneficial for depressed patients with heart failure [63]. In addition, the large Gruppo Italiano per lo Studio della Sopravvivenza nella Insufficienza Cardiaca-Heart Failure (GISSI-HF) trial demonstrated that omega-3 fatty acid supplementation improved survival and reduced cardiovascular re-hospitalization rates compared with placebo [64]. Whether supplementing omega-3 fatty acids could improve depression as well as survival and other cardiovascular outcomes in patients with heart failure needs to be further addressed in prospective studies.

The question whether depressive symptoms in heart failure patients represent a truly independent *causal* risk factor or rather a risk *marker* for adverse prognosis has so far remained unanswered. Future research needs to focus on mechanisms that may account for the adverse prognostic significance of depressive symptoms. Observations from the MOOD-HF and the SADHART-CHF trial support the concept of alternative pathophysiological pathways for mood disorders in somatic illnesses, with depressive symptoms less responsive or even unresponsive to sertraline or escitalopram in patients with advanced heart diseases [56, 57]. Results from the recent *Chronic Kidney Disease Antidepressant Sertraline* (CAST) trial evaluating the effects of sertraline on depressive symptoms in patients with major depression and chronic kidney disease, who also suffered from multiple other conditions such as diabetes, coronary disease or heart failure, strengthen this theory [65, 66]. In the 12-week CAST study, antidepressant treatment was no more effective than placebo and was associated with unfavourable side effects [65]. Placebo-controlled trials for marketing authorization of antidepressants tend to exclude patients with severe chronic somatic illnesses. As becomes more and more apparent, the efficacy results of such studies are not necessarily transferable to many individuals with advanced chronic somatic illnesses in whom antidepressants are often prescribed in clinical practice.

13.5.2 Psychotherapy

Psychotherapy as an interactive process to influence psychological comorbidities includes a variety of treatment modalities. None of these has so far been shown to have any significant beneficial effect on prognosis in heart failure patients. However, although relevant effects on event rates could not be identified, patients did benefit from cognitive behavioural therapy (CBT) in some studies in terms of improved mood, anxiety and quality of life, especially when CBT was combined with physical activity [58, 67].

13.5.3 Physical Exercise

The effects of exercise on depression in patients with heart failure have been determined in a systematic review and meta-analysis of randomized controlled clinical trial data [61]. Data from 19 studies in 3447 patients showed that exercise training significantly decreased depressive symptoms. Obviously, physical exercise can improve the perfusion of the frontal cortex and cognitive functions [68–70]. Positive systemic effects with improvement of endothelial function, inflammation, neurohumoral activity and function of the skeletal muscle further modulate biological mechanisms of depression [68, 71].

In the HF-ACTION trial [60], exercise three times per week over 3 months significantly decreased depressive symptoms, and reduced mortality and hospitalization rates, compared with guideline-based usual care. The results of a meta-analysis of physical exercise in middle-aged and elderly women demonstrated that low to moderate intensity exercise reduces depressive symptoms [72]. In addition to the positive biological effects of exercise [68, 71], the psychosocial effects of the training situation should not be underestimated. Individualized physical training may restore confidence in the body and training in groups may be experienced as socially supportive. In the real-world setting, motivation to adhere to physical exercise is often the greatest problem. However, physical training should be recommended and prescribed as much as possible to help break the vicious cycle of dyspnoea-anxiety-inactivity.

13.5.4 Comprehensive Care

Depression has many somatic correlates [4] and its prevalence, incidence and severity are closely related to the severity of heart failure symptoms and quality of life [4, 5]. Therefore, comprehensive care addressing the multifaceted heart failure syndrome appears to be a meaningful primary therapeutic approach. This includes effective management of physical symptoms alongside standard disease-modifying treatment of heart failure and associated comorbidities (Fig. 13.5). The goal of multidisciplinary collaborative disease management is to integrate patients' medical and social surroundings, thereby improving psychosocial functioning, health care competence and self-empowerment [73]. This approach has proven efficacious in patients with heart failure and was associated with improved quality of life and survival [73], although hospitalization rates are not always reduced in randomized trials that included patients early after a hospitalization for cardiac decompensation [73, 74]. As health care competence and symptoms improve, depression, anxiety and cognitive dysfunction are reduced. Management of heart failure patients using a multidisciplinary approach incorporating psychosomatic factors should play a key role in the care of heart failure patients, and is central to managing psychological comorbidities (Fig. 13.5).

References

1. Rutledge T, Reis VA, Linke SE, Greenberg BH, Mills PJ. Depression in heart failure a meta-analytic review of prevalence, intervention effects, and associations with clinical outcomes. J Am Coll Cardiol. 2006;48(8):1527–37.
2. Vaccarino V, Kasl SV, Abramson J, Krumholz HM. Depressive symptoms and risk of functional decline and death in patients with heart failure. J Am Coll Cardiol. 2001;38(1):199–205.

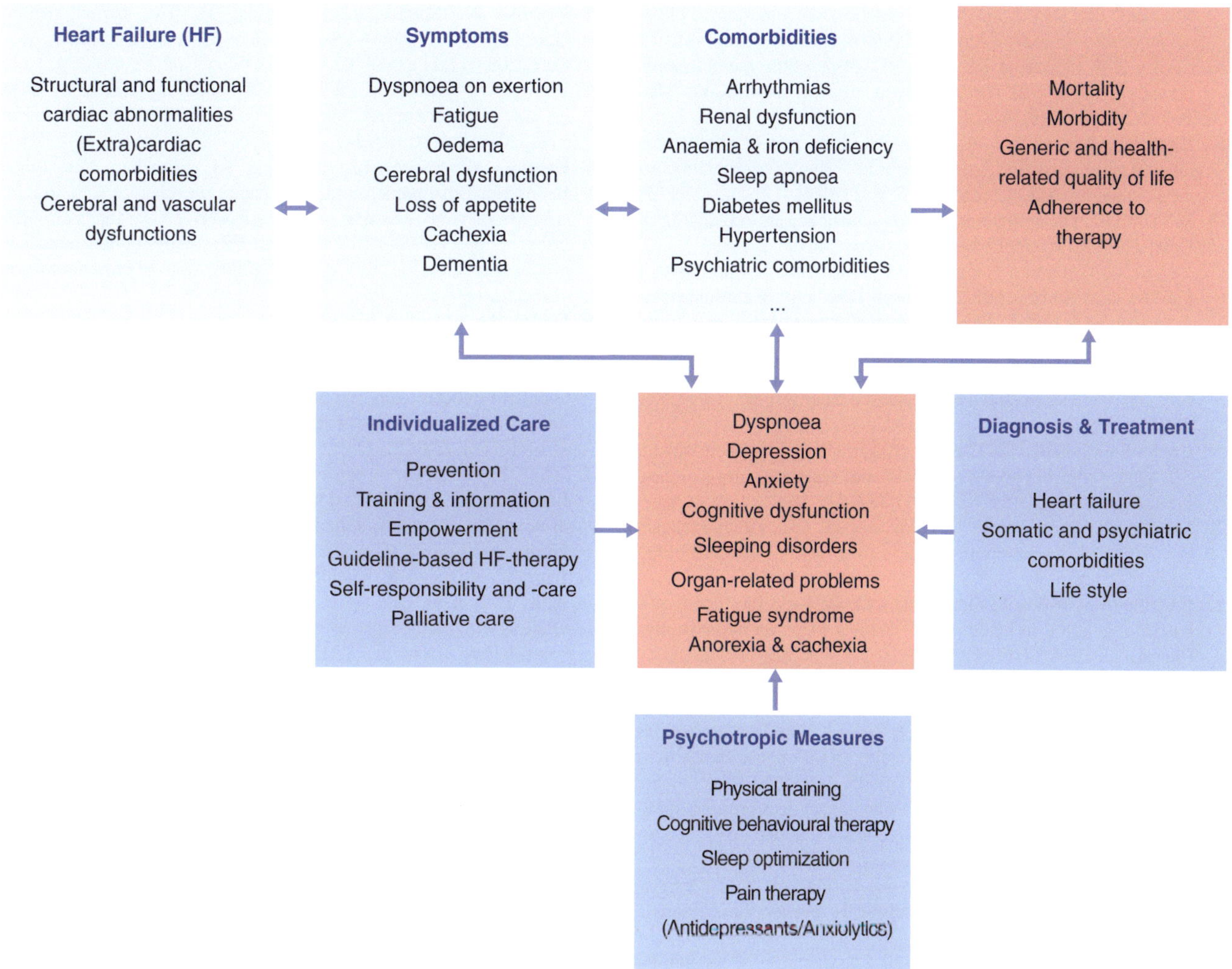

Fig. 13.5 Multimodal holistic therapy of the heart failure syndrome. Somatic and psychological problems, and subjective symptoms of heart failure and its complications and comorbidities require an individualized approach to care. (Modified from [75])

3. Konstam V, Moser DK, De Jong MJ. Depression and anxiety in heart failure. J Card Fail. 2005;11(6):455–63.
4. Angermann CE, Gelbrich G, Stork S, Schowalter M, Deckert J, Ertl G, et al. Somatic correlates of comorbid major depression in patients with systolic heart failure. Int J Cardiol. 2011;147(1):66–73.
5. Faller H, Stork S, Schowalter M, Steinbuchel T, Wollner V, Ertl G, et al. Depression and survival in chronic heart failure: does gender play a role? Eur J Heart Fail. 2007;9(10):1018–23.
6. Dekker RL, Lennie TA, Doering LV, Chung ML, Wu JR, Moser DK. Coexisting anxiety and depressive symptoms in patients with heart failure. Eur J Cardiovasc Nurs. 2014;13(2):168–76.
7. Suzuki T, Shiga T, Kuwahara K, Kobayashi S, Suzuki S, Nishimura K, et al. Impact of clustered depression and anxiety on mortality and rehospitalization in patients with heart failure. J Cardiol. 2014;64(6):456–62.
8. Chapa DW, Akintade B, Son H, Woltz P, Hunt D, Friedmann E, et al. Pathophysiological relationships between heart failure and depression and anxiety. Crit Care Nurse. 2014;34(2):14–24. quiz 5
9. Angermann CE, Kaspar M, Marx A, Kittel-Schneider S, Menhofer D, Stork S, et al. A functional variant of the neuropeptide S receptor-1 gene modulates clinical outcomes and healthcare utilization in patients with systolic heart failure: results from the Interdisciplinary Network Heart Failure (INH) Study. Eur J Heart Fail. 2017;19(3):314–23.
10. Alosco ML, Spitznagel MB, Raz N, Cohen R, Sweet LH, Colbert LH, et al. Obesity interacts with cerebral hypoperfusion to exacerbate cognitive impairment in older adults with heart failure. Cerebrovasc Dis Extra. 2012;2(1):88–98.
11. Gure TR, Blaum CS, Giordani B, Koelling TM, Galecki A, Pressler SJ, et al. Prevalence of cognitive impairment in older adults with heart failure. J Am Geriatr Soc. 2012;60(9):1724–9.
12. Almeida OP, Garrido GJ, Beer C, Lautenschlager NT, Arnolda L, Flicker L. Cognitive and brain changes associated with ischaemic heart disease and heart failure. Eur Heart J. 2012;33(14):1769–76.
13. McCaffery JM, Frasure-Smith N, Dube MP, Theroux P, Rouleau GA, Duan Q, et al. Common genetic vulnerability to depressive symptoms and coronary artery disease: a review and development of candidate genes related to inflammation and serotonin. Psychosom Med. 2006;68(2):187–200.
14. Domschke K, Reif A, Weber H, Richter J, Hohoff C, Ohrmann P, et al. Neuropeptide S receptor gene – converging evidence for a role in panic disorder. Mol Psychiatry. 2011;16(9):938–48.
15. Rozanski A, Blumenthal JA, Davidson KW, Saab PG, Kubzansky L. The epidemiology, pathophysiology, and management of psy-

chosocial risk factors in cardiac practice: the emerging field of behavioral cardiology. J Am Coll Cardiol. 2005;45(5):637–51.
16. Carney RM, Freedland KE, Veith RC. Depression, the autonomic nervous system, and coronary heart disease. Psychosom Med. 2005;67(Suppl 1):S29–33.
17. Kliks BR, Burgess MJ, Abildskov JA. Influence of sympathetic tone on ventricular fibrillation threshold during experimental coronary occlusion. Am J Cardiol. 1975;36(1):45–9.
18. Schwartz PJ. The autonomic nervous system and sudden death. Eur Heart J. 1998;19(Suppl F):F72–80.
19. Yamaji M, Tsutamoto T, Kawahara C, Nishiyama K, Yamamoto T, Fujii M, et al. Serum cortisol as a useful predictor of cardiac events in patients with chronic heart failure: the impact of oxidative stress. Circ Heart Fail. 2009;2(6):608–15.
20. Grippo AJ, Johnson AK. Biological mechanisms in the relationship between depression and heart disease. Neurosci Biobehav Rev. 2002;26(8):941–62.
21. Kop WJ, Gottdiener JS. The role of immune system parameters in the relationship between depression and coronary artery disease. Psychosom Med. 2005;67(Suppl 1):S37–41.
22. Mahmoudi M, Curzen N, Gallagher PJ. Atherogenesis: the role of inflammation and infection. Histopathology. 2007;50(5):535–46.
23. Engelhardt S, Patkar S, Ogunshola OO. Cell-specific blood-brain barrier regulation in health and disease: a focus on hypoxia. Br J Pharmacol. 2014;171(5):1210–30.
24. Ampadu J, Morley JE. Heart failure and cognitive dysfunction. Int J Cardiol. 2015;178:12–23.
25. Fan H, Yu W, Zhang Q, Cao H, Li J, Wang J, et al. Depression after heart failure and risk of cardiovascular and all-cause mortality: a meta-analysis. Prev Med. 2014;63:36–42.
26. Bane C, Hughes CM, McElnay JC. The impact of depressive symptoms and psychosocial factors on medication adherence in cardiovascular disease. Patient Educ Couns. 2006;60(2):187–93.
27. Hare DL, Toukhsati SR, Johansson P, Jaarsma T. Depression and cardiovascular disease: a clinical review. Eur Heart J. 2014;35(21):1365–72.
28. World Health Organization. ICD-10 Classification of mental and behavioural disorders: clinical descriptions and diagnostic guidelines. Geneva: World Health Organization; 1992.
29. American Psychiatric Association. Diagnostic and statistical manual of mental disorders, fifth edition (DSM-5). Arlington: American Psychiatric Publishing; 2013.
30. Lowe B, Grafe K, Zipfel S, Witte S, Loerch B, Herzog W. Diagnosing ICD-10 depressive episodes: superior criterion validity of the Patient health questionnaire. Psychother Psychosom. 2004;73(6):386–90.
31. Spitzer RL, Williams JB, Gibbon M, First MB. The structured clinical interview for DSM-III-R (SCID). I: history, rationale, and description. Arch Gen Psychiatry. 1992;49(8):624–9.
32. Lowe B, Kroenke K, Grafe K. Detecting and monitoring depression with a two-item questionnaire (PHQ-2). J Psychosom Res. 2005;58(2):163–71.
33. Piepenburg SM, Faller H, Gelbrich G, Stork S, Warrings B, Ertl G, et al. Comparative potential of the 2-item versus the 9-item patient health questionnaire to predict death or rehospitalization in heart failure. Circ Heart Fail. 2015;8(3):464–72.
34. Lichtman JH, Bigger JT Jr, Blumenthal JA, Frasure-Smith N, Kaufmann PG, Lesperance F, et al. Depression and coronary heart disease: recommendations for screening, referral, and treatment: a science advisory from the American Heart Association prevention committee of the council on cardiovascular nursing, council on clinical cardiology, council on epidemiology and prevention, and interdisciplinary council on quality of care and outcomes research: endorsed by the American Psychiatric Association. Circulation. 2008;118(17):1768–75.
35. Kroenke K, Spitzer RL, Williams JB. The patient health Questionnaire-2: validity of a two-item depression screener. Med Care. 2003;41(11):1284–92.
36. Spitzer RL, Kroenke K, Williams JB, Lowe B. A brief measure for assessing generalized anxiety disorder: the GAD-7. Arch Intern Med. 2006;166(10):1092–7.
37. Kroenke K, Spitzer RL, Williams JB, Monahan PO, Lowe B. Anxiety disorders in primary care: prevalence, impairment, comorbidity, and detection. Ann Intern Med. 2007;146(5):317–25.
38. Folstein MF, Folstein SE, McHugh PR. "Mini-mental state". A practical method for grading the cognitive state of patients for the clinician. J Psychiatr Res. 1975;12(3):189–98.
39. Dodson JA, Chaudhry SI. Geriatric conditions in heart failure. Curr Cardiovasc Risk Rep. 2012;6(5):404–10.
40. Harkness K, Demers C, Heckman GA, McKelvie RS. Screening for cognitive deficits using the Montreal cognitive assessment tool in outpatients >/=65 years of age with heart failure. Am J Cardiol. 2011;107(8):1203–7.
41. Jiang W, Alexander J, Christopher E, Kuchibhatla M, Gaulden LH, Cuffe MS, et al. Relationship of depression to increased risk of mortality and rehospitalization in patients with congestive heart failure. Arch Intern Med. 2001;161(15):1849–56.
42. Jiang W, Krishnan R, Kuchibhatla M, Cuffe MS, Martsberger C, Arias RM, et al. Characteristics of depression remission and its relation with cardiovascular outcome among patients with chronic heart failure (from the SADHART-CHF Study). Am J Cardiol. 2011;107(4):545–51.
43. Moraska AR, Chamberlain AM, Shah ND, Vickers KS, Rummans TA, Dunlay SM, et al. Depression, healthcare utilization, and death in heart failure: A community study. Circ Heart Fail. 2013;6(3):387.
44. Sayers SL, Hanrahan N, Kutney A, Clarke SP, Reis BF, Riegel B. Psychiatric comorbidity and greater hospitalization risk, longer length of stay, and higher hospitalization costs in older adults with heart failure. J Am Geriatr Soc. 2007;55(10):1585–91.
45. Wulsin LR, Singal BM. Do depressive symptoms increase the risk for the onset of coronary disease? A systematic quantitative review. Psychosom Med. 2003;65(2):201–10.
46. De Jong MJ, Chung ML, Wu JR, Riegel B, Rayens MK, Moser DK. Linkages between anxiety and outcomes in heart failure. Heart Lung. 2011;40(5):393–404.
47. Ponikowski P, Voors AA, Anker SD, Bueno H, Cleland JG, Coats AJ, et al. ESC guidelines for the diagnosis and treatment of acute and chronic heart failure: the task force for the diagnosis and treatment of acute and chronic heart failure of the European Society of Cardiology (ESC). Developed with the special contribution of the Heart Failure Association (HFA) of the ESC. Eur J Heart Fail. 2016;18(8):891–975.
48. Cohen HW, Gibson G, Alderman MH. Excess risk of myocardial infarction in patients treated with antidepressant medications: association with use of tricyclic agents. Am J Med. 2000;108(1):2–8.
49. Piepenburg SM, Ertl G, Angermann CE. Depression und Herzinsuffizienz – eine gefährliche Kombination. Dtsch Med Wochenschr. 2016;141(17):1222–7. (im Druck)
50. Wallenborn J, Angermann CE. Comorbid depression in heart failure. Herz. 2013;38(6):587–96.
51. Woltz PC, Chapa DW, Friedmann E, Son H, Akintade B, Thomas SA. Effects of interventions on depression in heart failure: a systematic review. Heart Lung. 2012;41(5):469–83.
52. Glassman AH, O'Connor CM, Califf RM, Swedberg K, Schwartz P, Bigger JT Jr, et al. Sertraline treatment of major depression in patients with acute MI or unstable angina. JAMA. 2002;288(6):701–9.
53. Berkman LF, Blumenthal J, Burg M, Carney RM, Catellier D, Cowan MJ, et al. Effects of treating depression and low perceived social support on clinical events after myocardial infarction: the Enhancing Recovery in Coronary Heart Disease Patients (ENRICHD) randomized trial. JAMA. 2003;289(23):3106–16.

54. Lesperance F, Frasure-Smith N, Koszycki D, Laliberte MA, van Zyl LT, Baker B, et al. Effects of citalopram and interpersonal psychotherapy on depression in patients with coronary artery disease: the Canadian Cardiac Randomized Evaluation of Antidepressant and Psychotherapy Efficacy (CREATE) trial. JAMA. 2007;297(4):367–79.
55. van den Brink RH, van Melle JP, Honig A, Schene AH, Crijns HJ, Lambert FP, et al. Treatment of depression after myocardial infarction and the effects on cardiac prognosis and quality of life: rationale and outline of the Myocardial INfarction and Depression-Intervention Trial (MIND-IT). Am Heart J. 2002;144(2):219–25.
56. O'Connor CM, Jiang W, Kuchibhatla M, Silva SG, Cuffe MS, Callwood DD, et al. Safety and efficacy of sertraline for depression in patients with heart failure: results of the SADHART-CHF (Sertraline Against Depression and Heart Disease in Chronic Heart Failure) trial. J Am Coll Cardiol. 2010;56(9):692–9.
57. Angermann CE, Gelbrich G, Stork S, Gunold H, Edelmann F, Wachter R, et al. Effect of Escitalopram on all-cause mortality and hospitalization in patients with heart failure and depression: The MOOD-HF randomized clinical trial. JAMA. 2016;315(24):2683–93.
58. Freedland KE, Carney RM, Rich MW, Steinmeyer BC, Rubin EH. Cognitive behavior therapy for depression and self-care in heart failure patients: a randomized clinical trial. JAMA Intern Med. 2015;175(11):1773–82.
59. Huffman JC, Mastromauro CA, Beach SR, Celano CM, Dubois CM, Healy BC, et al. Collaborative care for depression and anxiety disorders in patients with recent cardiac events: the Management of Sadness and Anxiety in Cardiology (MOSAIC) randomized clinical trial. JAMA Intern Med. 2014;174(6):927–35.
60. Blumenthal JA, Babyak MA, O'Connor C, Keteyian S, Landzberg J, Howlett J, et al. Effects of exercise training on depressive symptoms in patients with chronic heart failure: the HF-ACTION randomized trial. JAMA. 2012;308(5):465–74.
61. Tu RH, Zeng ZY, Zhong GQ, Wu WF, Lu YJ, Bo ZD, et al. Effects of exercise training on depression in patients with heart failure: a systematic review and meta-analysis of randomized controlled trials. Eur J Heart Fail. 2014;16(7):749–57.
62. Jiang W, Oken H, Fiuzat M, Shaw LK, Martsberger C, Kuchibhatla M, et al. Plasma omega-3 polyunsaturated fatty acids and survival in patients with chronic heart failure and major depressive disorder. J Cardiovasc Transl Res. 2012;5(1):92–9.
63. Appleton KM, Rogers PJ, Ness AR. Updated systematic review and meta-analysis of the effects of n-3 long-chain polyunsaturated fatty acids on depressed mood. Am J Clin Nutr. 2010;91(3):757–70.
64. Tavazzi L, Maggioni AP, Marchioli R, Barlera S, Franzosi MG, Latini R, et al. Effect of n-3 polyunsaturated fatty acids in patients with chronic heart failure (the GISSI-HF trial): a randomised, double-blind, placebo-controlled trial. Lancet. 2008;372(9645):1223–30.
65. Hedayati SS, Gregg LP, Carmody T, Jain N, Toups M, Rush AJ, et al. Effect of sertraline on depressive symptoms in patients with chronic kidney disease without dialysis dependence: the CAST randomized clinical trial. JAMA. 2017;318(19):1876–90.
66. Walther CP, Shah AA, Winkelmayer WC. Treating depression in patients with advanced CKD: beyond the generalizability frontier. JAMA. 2017;318(19):1873–4.
67. Gary RA, Dunbar SB, Higgins MK, Musselman DL, Smith AL. Combined exercise and cognitive behavioral therapy improves outcomes in patients with heart failure. J Psychosom Res. 2010;69(2):119–31.
68. Groot C, Hooghiemstra AM, Raijmakers PG, van Berckel BN, Scheltens P, Scherder EJ, et al. The effect of physical activity on cognitive function in patients with dementia: A meta-analysis of randomized control trials. Ageing Res Rev. 2016;25:13–23.
69. Smith PJ, Blumenthal JA, Hoffman BM, Cooper H, Strauman TA, Welsh-Bohmer K, et al. Aerobic exercise and neurocognitive performance: a meta-analytic review of randomized controlled trials. Psychosom Med. 2010;72(3):239–52.
70. Zheng G, Xia R, Zhou W, Tao J, Chen L. Aerobic exercise ameliorates cognitive function in older adults with mild cognitive impairment: a systematic review and meta-analysis of randomised controlled trials. Br J Sports Med. 2016;50(23):1443–50.
71. Wenger NK. Current status of cardiac rehabilitation. J Am Coll Cardiol. 2008;51(17):1619–31.
72. Perez-Lopez FR, Martinez-Dominguez SJ, Lajusticia H, Chedraui P. Health outcomes systematic analyses P. Effects of programmed exercise on depressive symptoms in midlife and older women: A meta-analysis of randomized controlled trials. Maturitas. 2017;106:38–47.
73. Angermann CE, Stork S, Gelbrich G, Faller H, Jahns R, Frantz S, et al. Mode of action and effects of standardized collaborative disease management on mortality and morbidity in patients with systolic heart failure: the Interdisciplinary Network for Heart Failure (INH) study. Circ Heart Fail. 2012;5(1):25–35.
74. Jaarsma T, van der Wal MH, Lesman-Leegte I, Luttik ML, Hogenhuis J, Veeger NJ, et al. Effect of moderate or intensive disease management program on outcome in patients with heart failure: Coordinating Study Evaluating Outcomes of Advising and Counseling in Heart Failure (COACH). Arch Intern Med. 2008;168(3):316–24.
75. Gunold H, Angermann CE. Kognitive Dysfunktion, Depression und Angst bei Herzinsuffizienz. Aktuel Kardol. 2015,4:379–86.

Part VII

Cardiac Surgery in HF

14 Surgical Intervention on the Mitral and Tricuspid Valves in Patients with Left Ventricular Dysfunction and Heart Failure

Vivek Rao

14.1 Introduction

Patients with left ventricular dysfunction due to either an ischemic or non-ischemic etiology often present with mitral insufficiency, usually in the setting of a structurally normal valve. This "functional" mitral insufficiency has been previously described by Carpentier as Type III insufficiency whereby restricted leaflet motion during either diastole (IIIa) or systole (IIIb) renders the valve incompetent [1]. The former is usually seen in rheumatic heart disease while the latter is a hallmark of ischemic mitral regurgitation. The management of Type IIIb mitral insufficiency remains controversial and two recent trials sponsored by the NIH have only partially improved our understanding of the surgical management of this pathology [2, 3]. In addition, patients with left ventricular dysfunction and severe mitral insufficiency may also present with pulmonary hypertension and secondary tricuspid insufficiency. Again, the management of functional tricuspid insufficiency remains controversial [4, 5].

14.2 Preoperative Assessment

Most patients with functional valvular insufficiency have significant left ventricular dysfunction and a proportion will also present with significant right ventricular dysfunction [6]. As such, these patients require a careful preoperative assessment of their comorbidities and an optimal assessment of their valvular disease. All patients with significant left ventricular dysfunction should have coronary angiography to detect underlying coronary artery disease. In those patients who present in decompensated heart failure, a pre-operative period of optimization including potential intraaortic balloon pump support should be considered [7]. Importantly, an echocardiographic reassessment of valvular pathology should be performed after adequate normalization of volume status as often regurgitant lesions may resolve after appropriate diuresis. Lastly, where appropriate, a consultation with the advanced heart failure team is advised in order to determine surgical options in the event of inadequate myocardial performance. The choice of mechanical circulatory support device may depend upon the patient's transplant eligibility and thus, these assessments should be performed preoperatively when possible.

14.2.1 Key Preoperative Notes

- *Complete angiographic assessment in all patients with significant left ventricular dysfunction*
- *Preoperative optimization with diuresis, inotropic +/− IABP support*
- *Re-evaluation of valvular pathology after preoperative optimization*
- *Consultation with advanced heart failure service*

14.3 Intraoperative Decision Making

Subsequent to the two NIH trials in ischemic mitral regurgitation (MR), the surgical paradigm for the management of functional mitral insufficiency has been redefined. In the moderate MR trial, no difference was found in those patients who received mitral repair versus those who underwent isolated surgical revascularization [2]. Despite this finding, many surgeons feel that persistent moderate MR will lead to subsequent ventricular dilatation and poorer clinical outcomes. There are several intraoperative findings that may influence the decision to proceed with mitral repair. In patients with profound left ventricular dysfunction, especially those who may

V. Rao (✉)
Munk Professor in Advanced Cardiac Therapeutics, Peter Munk Cardiac Centre, Toronto General Hospital, University of Toronto, Toronto, ON, Canada
e-mail: Vivek.rao@uhn.ca

D. S. Feldman, P. Mohacsi (eds.), *Heart Failure*, Cardiovascular Medicine, https://doi.org/10.1007/978-3-319-98184-0_14

undergo surgical ventricular reconstruction (SVR), the additive risk of a mitral procedure may lead one to pursue a more conservative approach [8–10]. Indeed, a subanalysis of the STICH trial demonstrated that the performance of an SVR had a similar effect as mitral repair, but the combination of the two procedures was associated with inferior outcome [9].

The presence of transmural infarction in the inferolateral territory may lead to either a posterior left ventricular reconstruction or mitral repair since this territory is unlikely to improve after revascularization [7]. Similarly, where the coronary target is diffusely diseased or non-bypassable one may pursue mitral repair. However, based upon the NIH results, patients with viable myocardium and good coronary targets may be well served by isolated revascularization alone.

In patients with severe MR, surgeons have tended to prefer mitral repair with an undersized annuloplasty band as popularized by Bolling et al. [11] The prevailing sentiment prior to the NIH trial was that mitral replacement was associated with a prohibitive mortality risk and mitral repair was a reasonable compromise. The NIH trial comparing repair versus replacement (MVR) in patients with severe ischemic MR (admittedly a different population than non-ischemic heart failure) demonstrated that there was a minimal, non-significant, increase in mortality associated with MVR; however, the rates of recurrent MR in patients undergoing repair were 33% in year one and 59% by year two [3]. Again, despite no significant differences in clinical outcomes between groups, the high rates of recurrent MR leave many surgeons concerned that additional followup will demonstrate adverse outcomes after repair. An important consideration is that surgeons who replaced the valve in these trials were advised to preserve as much of the subvalvular apparatus as possible. It is likely that the lower mortality rate compared to historical series may in part be due to the preservation of chordal structures.

The most recent American Association of Thoracic Surgery (AATS) surgical guidelines have adopted the findings of the two NIH trials and suggest that isolated CABG may suffice for those patients suffering from moderate MR (particularly if their presenting complaint is angina) and that MVR provides more durable therapy for MR in those patients with severe insufficiency [12].

Interestingly, Kron et al. demonstrated that there are also intraoperative factors that can determine the success of mitral repair even in patients with severe MR [13, 14]. The presence of an inferobasal aneurysm (Fig. 14.1) was highly predictive of recurrent MR as was the ratio of LV size to ring size. In these patients, the authors suggest the addition of subvalvular repair techniques to ring annuloplasty.

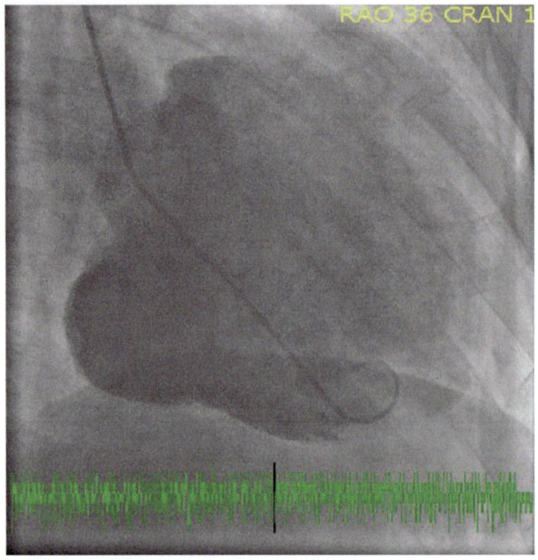

Fig. 14.1 Left ventricular angiogram demonstrating an inferobasal aneurysm

14.3.1 Key Intraoperative Decisions

1. *Assess for the presence of viable myocardium and the quality of coronary revascularization. In patients with excellent targets and potentially viable myocardium, isolated revascularization may suffice for the treatment of moderate MR.*
2. *Identify inferobasal aneurysms, which if present should favour formal MV replacement.*
3. *When proceeding to formal MVR, ensure complete preservation of all subvalvular structures to reduce perioperative mortality.*

14.4 Subvalvular Interventions

Due to the high rate of recurrent MR in patients treated with an isolated ring annuloplasty, several surgeons have introduced subvalvular interventions in an attempt to address the "ventricular" aspect of this disease [15].

Based upon pre-clinical work by Levine et al., our group reported on 44 patients who underwent chordal-cutting procedures at the time of valve repair [16, 17]. The theory behind this approach was to eliminate the tethering forces of the secondary chordae, while preserving the primary leading edge structures (Fig. 14.2, reproduced with permission). While this technique appeared to lower the rates of recurrent MR, a subsequent analysis revealed that perioperative mortality was higher in those patients with extremely large ventricles (>65 mm) [8].

Another approach to restrict the tethering forces is to approximate papillary muscles or to resuspend them to the

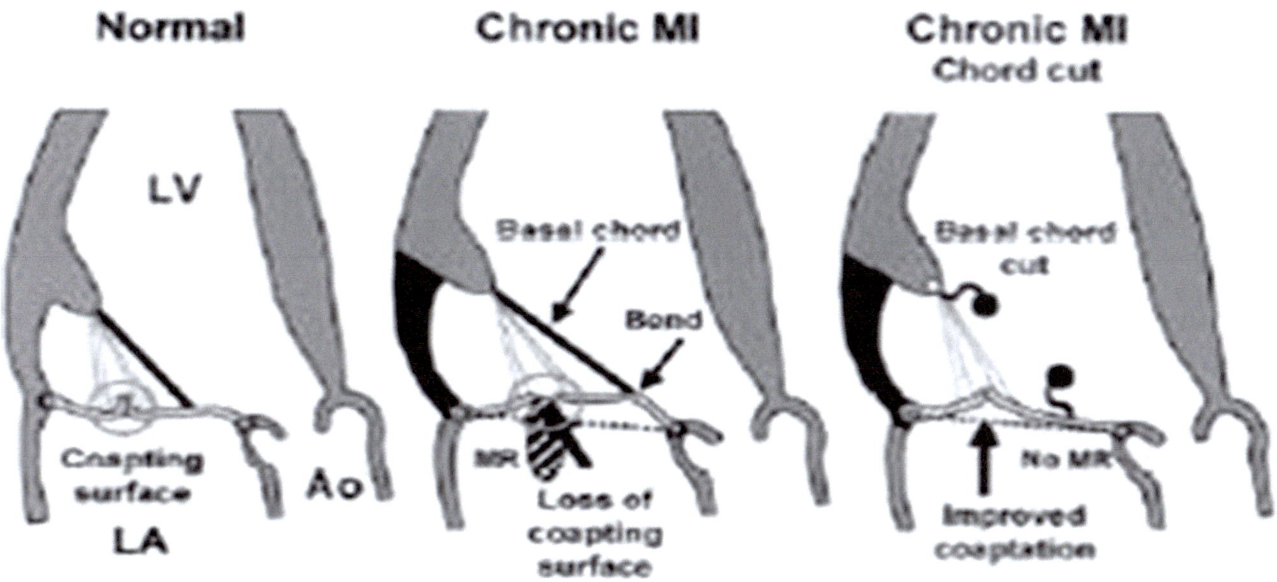

Fig. 14.2 The concept of division of secondary chords to the mitral valve. (Reproduced with permission from Messass et al.; Circulation 2003)

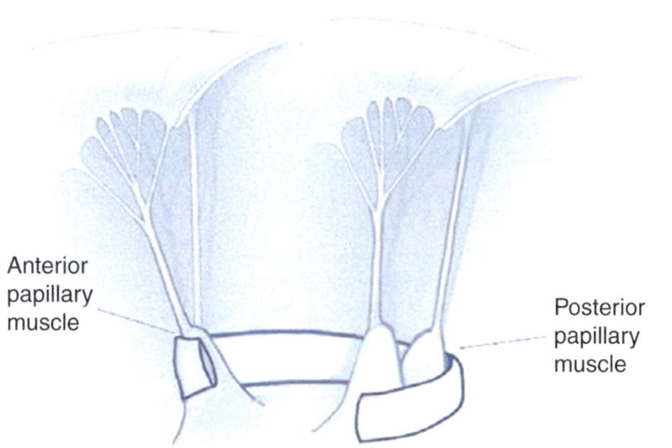

Fig. 14.3 Papillary muscle sling for surgical management of functional mitral insufficiency. (Reproduced with permission from Napi et al.; JTCVS 2016)

mitral annulus [18–20]. Again, the premise of papillary muscle approximation is to relieve the tethering forces on the mitral valve by reducing the displacement of the papillary muscles caused by adverse left ventricular remodeling (Fig. 14.3, reproduced with permission). A recently reported clinical trial randomizing patients to isolated restrictive annuloplasty versus annuloplasty plus papillary muscle approximation demonstrated improvements in mitral morphology and reverse remodeling, but failed to impact on mortality or functional status [18]. A subsequent morphologic analysis of this study suggested that this technique was more useful in patients with inferior wall motion abnormalities, but less effective in those patients with anterior dyskinesia [19].

A technique for posterior papillary muscle relocation was described by Kron et al. as early as 2002 [20]. In this simple procedure, a single prolene suture is passed through the fibrous tip of the posterior papillary muscle and then sewn to the mitral annulus. By "relocating" the papillary muscle head, the surgeons effectively diminished the tethering forces.

The use of a multitude of valvular (i.e. – leaflet augmentation) and subvalvular techniques to augment restrictive annuloplasty will likely lead to improved surgical results of mitral repair for severe ischemic MR; however, it is important to point out that in patients with profound left ventricular dysfunction and severe functional MR long term survival may be poor and a durable surgical result such as that afforded by formal MVR may be a preferred approach.

14.4.1 Tricuspid Valve Repair

As controversial as the topic of mitral repair is for functional MR, the debate over tricuspid repair is ongoing and is currently the subject of another CTSnet trial. Unfortunately, the management of "secondary" tricuspid insufficiency is complicated by the heterogeneous nature of the patient population. By far, the most studied patient population are those who undergo mitral valve repair for degenerative disease and present with either concomitant tricuspid insufficiency or annular dilatation. Even in this relatively homogeneous group, management options are controversial with some advocating for near uniform tricuspid valve repair while others adopting a more conservative approach restricting TV repair to those patients with severe TR, atrial fibrillation and evidence of RV dysfunction [21–23].

For functional tricuspid insufficiency, most surgeons favour a non-planar rigid ring (i.e. – Edwards Physio II; Edwards LifeSciences, Irvine, CA). Simple suture repair, such as a DeVega annuloplasty, has been shown repeatedly to be inferior to an annuloplasty band. The management of pacemaker lead-induced TR is dependent upon the findings at surgery. If the lead passes freely through the tricuspid valve, simple reduction annuloplasty will usually suffice. However, if the lead is adherent to a leaflet (commonly the anterior or septal), then the lead must be separated from the leaflet and usually placed in the commissure between the posterior and septal leaflet. Our institution prefers to exclude the lead by placing annuloplasty sutures in such a manner as to "bicuspidize" the valve as described originally by Kay et al. [24] Fig. 14.4 illustrates the Kay repair. When a pacer lead is present, we often exclude the lead external to the annuloplasty band which is placed over the "excluded" posterior leaflet.

Provided that there is adequate leaflet tissue, simple undersized annuloplasty of the tricuspid valve (with or without bicuspidization) suffices for functional TR. In cases where the anterior leaflet tissue is insufficient, either leaflet augmentation or formal valve replacement is required.

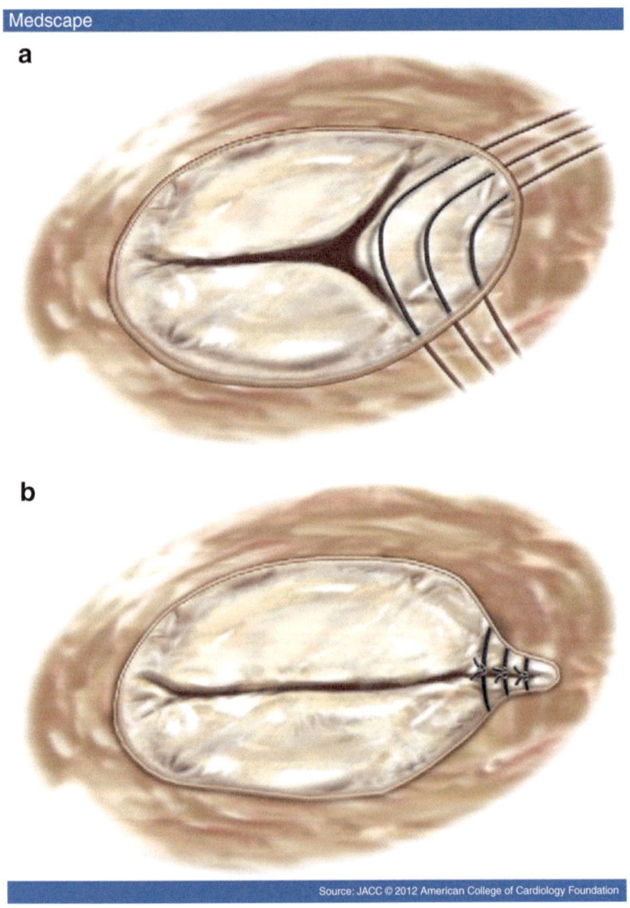

Fig. 14.4 Kay bicuspidization repair of the tricuspid valve

14.4.2 Key Surgical Points

1. *Moderate or more TR should be addressed at the time of surgery, especially in the setting of pulmonary hypertension, RV dysfunction and/or chronic atrial fibrillation.*
2. *If TV repair is to be performed, a non-planar rigid annuloplasty device is preferred.*
3. *If there is an obstructive pacer lead, consideration should be given to a bicuspidization procedure and exclusion of the lead.*

References

1. Carpentier A. Cardiac valve surgery (the French correction). J Thorac Cardiovasc Surg. 1983;86:323–37.
2. Michler RE, Smith PK, Parides MK, et al. Two year outcomes of surgical treatment of moderate ischemic mitral regurgitation. N Engl J Med. 2016;374:1932–41.
3. Goldstein DJ, Moskowitz AJ, Gelijns AC, et al. Two year outcomes of surgical treatment of severe ischemic mitral regurgitation. N Engl J Med. 2016;374:344–53.
4. Redondo Palancios A, Lopez Menendez J, Miguelena Hycka J, et al. Which type of valve should we use in tricuspid position? Long term comparison between mechanical and biological valves. J Cardiovasc Surg. 2016;58(5):739–46. epub ahead of print.
5. Teman NR, Huffman LC, Krajacic M, Pagani FD, Haft JW, Bolling SF. Prophylactic tricuspid repair for functional tricuspid insufficiency. Ann Thor Surg. 2014;97:1520–4.
6. Haddad F, Denault A, Couture P, et al. Right ventricular performance index predicts perioperative mortality or circulatory failure in high risk valvular surgery. J Am Soc Echocardiogr. 2007;20:1065–72.
7. Pilarczyk K, Boening A, Jakob H, et al. Preoperative intra-aortic counterpulsation in high-risk patients undergoing cardiac surgery: a meta-analysis of randomized controlled trials. Eur J Cardiothorac Surg. 2016;49:5–17.
8. Jeganathan R, Maganti M, Badiwala MV, Rao V. Concomitant mitral valve surgery in patients undergoing surgical ventricular reconstruction for ischemic cardiomyopathy. Eur J Cardiothorac Surg. 2013;43:1000–5.
9. Deja MA, Grayburn PA, Sun B, et al. Influence of mitral regurgitation repair on survival in the surgical treatment for ischemic heart failure trial. Circulation. 2012;125:2639–48.
10. Maganti M, Badiwala MV, Sheikh A, et al. Predictors of low output syndrome after isolated mitral valve surgery. J Thorac Cardiovasc Surg. 2010;140:790–6.
11. Romano MA, Bolling SF. Update on mitral repair in dilated cardiomyopathy. J Card Surg. 2004;19:396–400.
12. Kron IL, Acker MA, Adams DH, for the AATS Ischemic Mitral Regurgitation Consensus Guidelines Writing Committee. 2015 the American Association for Thoracic Surgery consensus guidelines: ischemic mitral valve regurgitation. J Thorac Cardiovasc Surg. 2016;151:940–56.

13. Kron IL, Hung J, Overbey JR, et al. Predicting recurrent mitral regurgitation after mitral valve repair for severe ischemic mitral regurgitation. J Thorac Cardiovasc Surg. 2015;149:752–61.
14. Capoulade R, Zeng X, Overbey JR, et al. Impact of left ventricular to mitral valve ring mismatch on recurrent ischemic mitral regurgitation after ring annuloplasty. Circulation. 2016;134:1247–56.
15. Badiwala MV, Verma S, Rao V. Surgical management of ischemic mitral regurgitation. Circulation. 2009;120:1287–93.
16. Messas E, Pouzet B, Touchot B, et al. Efficacy of chordal cutting to relieve chronic persistent ischemic mitral regurgitation. Circulation. 2003;108(Suppl1):I-111-115.
17. Borger MA, Murphy PM, Alam A, et al. Initial results of the chordal-cutting operation for ischemic mitral regurgitation. J Thorac Cardiovasc Surg. 2007;133:1483–92.
18. Nappi F, Lusini M, Spadaccio C, et al. Papillary muscle approximation versus restrictive annuloplasty alone for severe ischemic mitral regurgitation: a randomized trial. J Am Coll Cardiol. 2016;24:2334–46.
19. Nappi F, Spadaccio C, Nenna A, et al. Is subvalvular repair worthwhile in severe ischemic mitral regurgitation? Subanalysis of the papillary muscle approximation trial. J Thorac Cardiovasc Surg 2016.; epub ahead of print.
20. Kron IL, Green GR, Cope JT. Surgical relocation of the posterior papillary muscle in chronic ischemic mitral regurgitation. Ann Thorac Surg. 2002;74:600–1.
21. Chikwe J, Itagaki S, Anyanwu A, Adams DH. Impact of concomitant tricuspid annuloplasty on tricuspid regurgitation, right ventricular function and pulmonary hypertension after repair of mitral valve prolapse. J Am Coll Cardiol. 2015;65:1931–8.
22. Pfannmuller B, Doenst T, Eberhard K, Seeburger J, Borger MA, Mohr FW. Increased risk of dehiscence after tricuspid valve repair with rigid annuloplasty rings. J Thorac Cardiovasc Surg. 2012;143:1050–5.
23. Tang GH, David TE, Singh SK, Maganti MD, Armstrong S, Borger MA. Tricuspid valve repair with an annuloplasty ring results in improved long-term outcomes. Circulation. 2006;114(suppl 1):577–81.
24. Kay JH, Maselli-Campagna G, Tsuji H. Surgical treatment of tricuspid insufficiency. Ann Surg. 1965;162:53–8.

Myocardial Revascularization in Patients with Left Ventricular Dysfunction

15

D. Reineke and T. Carrel

Do patients with ischemic cardiomyopathy benefit from surgical revascularization? This question has been studied extensively over the last 20–30 years and needs to be analyzed from different viewpoints. What is the evidence concerning surgical revascularization of patients with an ejection fraction of 35%? What is the role of percutaneous coronary interventions (PCI) and optimal medical therapy (OMT). What do the guidelines tell us? And are current strategies still timely in view of new developments in the field of end-stage heart failure?

15.1 What Is the Evidence Concerning Surgical Revascularization?

Surgical revascularization has, for the last 30 years, been regarded as primary management strategy when coronary disease impairs left ventricular function. Most evidence supporting coronary artery bypass grafting (CABG) for patients with ischemic cardiomyopathy comes from nonrandomized retrospective studies, anecdotal clinical experience and has for quite some time been driven by a more or less intuitive approach [1–4]. These landmark clinical trials established coronary-artery bypass grafting (CABG) as an effective treatment for patients with ischemic cardiomyopathy avoiding further myocardial loss and arrhythmias. They associated CABG with longer survival compared to medical therapy alone among subgroups with more extensive coronary artery disease and worse left ventricular dysfunction. These trials, however, were conducted up to 40 years ago, without the availability of today's guideline-based medical therapy for coronary artery disease and heart failure and they did not include populations with severe left ventricular dysfunction.

The Surgical Treatment of Ischemic Heart Failure (STITCH) trial was the first trial designed to answer this question in a prospective randomized manner [5]. This multicenter international trial was designed to examine the effect of CABG, with or without left ventricular reconstruction (LVR), on patients with an ischemic cardiomyopathy presenting with an ejection fraction of 35% and less. To date, it is the only randomized trial that looked at the impact of surgical revascularization on outcomes in patients with ischemic cardiomyopathy.

The primary outcome was defined as mortality from any cause. Secondary endpoints were hospitalizations and mortality from cardiovascular causes. In the arm of our main focus (hypothesis: CABG with medical therapy would improve mortality and decrease cardiovascular hospitalization when compared with medical therapy alone) there was no significant difference between the two study groups with respect to the primary end point of all cause mortality over 5 years of follow-up.

Secondary combinations of endpoints (cardiovascular death, cardiovascular hospitalization, heart failure hospitalization) were decreased by the addition of CABG to OMT. Those who underwent CABG independent of randomization had lower rates of hospitalization and cardiovascular death.

The most rigorous interpretation of this well designed study would suggest, that in the setting of clinical equality and in view of future strategies CABG should not be first line treatment when taking into account the 5 year STITCH data, even when secondary endpoints like death from cardiovascular cause see a benefit in surgical revascularization [6].

The most compelling data published comes from the STICH Extension Study (STICHES), which was constructed to evaluate the long-term (10-year) effects of CABG in patients with ischemic cardiomyopathy [1]. Death from any cause over 10 years was lower by 16% among patients who underwent CABG in addition to receiving medical therapy than among those who received medical therapy alone. It

D. Reineke (✉) · T. Carrel
Department of Cardiovascular Surgery, University Hospital Bern, Bern, Switzerland
e-mail: david.reineke@insel.ch

D. S. Feldman, P. Mohacsi (eds.), *Heart Failure*, Cardiovascular Medicine, https://doi.org/10.1007/978-3-319-98184-0_15

appears that the operative risk associated with CABG is overpowered by the durable effect that translates into clinical benfit in the long-term.

15.2 The Role of Optimal Medical Therapy

Alternatives to surgery in the form of optimal medical therapy (OMT) exist and have in the last decades challenged surgical therapy substantially. OAT [7] and COURAGE [8], both prospective randomized studies, have shown that the justification to accept upfront morbidity and mortality with surgical revascularization in these high risk patients must include a demonstrable long-term benefit in survival and quality of life.

The Occluded Artery Trial (OAT) had the purpose to determine whether opening an occluded infarcted artery 3–28 days after an acute myocardial infarction in high-risk asymptomatic patients reduce the composite endpoint of mortality, recurrent myocardial infarction and hospitalization due to heart failure compared to optimal medical therapy alone. Although the study showed high rates of procedural success and sustained patency, no clinical benefit was seen during a 3 year follow-up. A trend toward an excess risk of re-infarction in the PCI-group was the cause for concern [7].

The Clinical Outcomes Utilizing Revascularization and Aggressive Drug Evaluation (COURAGE) trial was to determine whether PCI and optimal therapy reduces the risk of death and nonfatal myocardial infarction in patients with stable coronary artery disease compared to isolated optimal medical therapy. During a follow-up of 2.5–7 years, PCI did not reduce the risk of death, myocardial infarction, or other major cardiovascular events when added to optimal medical therapy [8].

Extended follow-up from OAT and COURAGE to determine whether late trends would favor either treatment group confirmed earlier results [9, 10].

Two other randomized strategies for the management of ischemic cardiomyopathy have been conducted. In the Heart Failure Revascularisation trial (HEART), patients with ischemic cardiomyopathy (EF 35%) and substantial viability were randomized either to coronary angiography with an intent to revascularize (percutaneous or surgically) or conservative medical management [11]. Due to slow enrolment the study was halted and unfortunately stayed underpowered. Nonetheless a follow-up of 138 patients over 59 month showed no difference between invasive therapy and conservative medical treatment.

The Carvedilol Hibernating Reversible Ischaemia trial (Christmas) was able to demonstrate that medical treatment with carvedilol might even be an alternative to revascularization for patients with hibernating myocardium. Patients with more myocardium affected by hibernation or by hibernation and ischaemia had a greater increase in LVEF on carvedilol compared to placebo [12]. All these studies provide further reassurance, that medical therapy is not inferior and has its place. A large metanalysis by Kunadia et al. comparing PCI and CABG in patients with left ventricular systolic dysfunction showed that neither intervention may improve outcome compared with pharmacological therapy alone [13].

15.3 Role of PCI

Several studies have focused on the role of surgical revascularisation in heart failure patients. Limited reports exist regarding the role of percutaneous coronary intervention (PCI) in patients with low LV systolic dysfunction especially in complex cases of 3-vessel or left main disease. Most large observational studies where able to demonstrate the benefit of CABG relative to PCI in patients with ischemic cardiomyopathy.

The CREDO-Kyoto PCI/CABG Registry Cohort-2 Investigators compared the 5 years outcomes between PCI and CABG in Japanese patients with LV systolic dysfunction in the drug eluting stent (DES) era having 3-vessel and or/left main disease. CABG was associated with better 5-year survival outcomes than PCI in patients with impaired LV systolic function (LVEF <50%) with complex coronary disease. In both patients with moderate (LVEF <50%) and severe (LVEF <35%) LV systolic dysfunction, CABG tended to have better survival outcomes than PCI [14]. Hannan and colleagues reported from the New York Registry database that CABG relative to PCI reduced the risk of death and MI in patients with LVEF<40% [15]. Hlatky et al. showed that 5-year after CABG risk of death proved to be significantly lower compared to the PCI group in patients with heart failure [16]. Survival benefits in CABG patients with an EF < 35% were also demonstrated by the sub analysis of the APPROACH database [17].

A soon as study populations include less complex coronary lesions such as single- or double vessel disease long-term survival benefits of surgical treatment becomes less evident. Meta-analyses of Hlatky and Kunadian could not demonstrate the long-term survival benefits of CABG compared with PCI [13, 18]. An observational study by Yang and collegues compared DES with CABG in patients with LV dysfunction showing comparable long-term clinical outcomes, except for repeat revascularization [19].

This phenomenom is also comfirmed by the SYNTAX trial in the final 5-year outcomes. The advantage of CABG is more evident in complex lesions such as 3-vessels disease and left main stem involvement.

15.4 What Do the Guidelines Tell Us?

Existing guidelines recommend revascularization for prognostic purposes in patients with LV dysfunction and suitable coronary anatomy [20–23]. The latest European Society of Cardiology Guidelines (ESC) guidelines on myocardial revascularization recommend CABG in patients with LV dysfunction and left main stem disease with class one level evidence C. If the anatomy is suitable and there is proof of viable myocardium PCI may be considered in case surgery is no option (class IIb evidence level C). For prognostic purposes revascularization in stable coronary artery disease in patients with a LVEF <40% is given class I level evidence A [21]. The most recent American Heart Association (AHA) heart failure guidelines recommend CABG to be undertaken in patients with operable anatomy and ischemic cardiomyopathy (ICM), irrespective of the presence of viability (class IIb level evidence B) [22].

Guidelines concerning myocardial revascularization in patients with LV dysfunction are predominantly based on the above cited observational studies and the STITCH trial. Whether the compelling data of the study's extension [1] will considerably change guidelines, has to be seen.

It has to be stated that especially American Guidelines have, over the years, advocated myocardial revascularization in heart failure patients less enthusiastically than their European counterparts (Table 15.1).

15.5 Modern Strategies

Finally the question has to be asked whether it is wise to focus on a therapeutical option that shows its profit in the form of superior all-cause mortality only after 10 years [1]. It has to be emphasized that STITCH Patients had a significant overall mortality of 40% at 6 years. 10 years after STICH more definite surgical options exist for patients with advanced symptoms and poor survival.

A cardiac surgical therapy such as CABG that provides a marginal symptomatic or survival benefit could complicate future options such as the use of LVADS and transplantation. The big picture and concept of the virgin chest with several anticipated re-operations should not be sacrificed for a therapy with has its effect when half of the population has died.

The above mentioned studies and strategies might also support modern strategies of low risk therapy first and move to more invasive options in the form of left ventricular assist device (LVAD implantation) and/or transplantation.

The STICH data also reveals that CABG was associated with a risk of death within the initial 30 days after randomization that was triple the risk of medical therapy alone [5].

Looking at the ROADMAP study, a prospective randomized, controlled observational study comparing a second generation LVAD to OMT in INTERMACS 4–6 (ambulatory setting), the 30 day mortality is 1% in both groups with a 25% survival benefit in the LVAD group after 12 months [24].

Although there now is substantial data showing that CABG has its role in the treatment of ischemic cardiomy-

Table 15.1 Summary of existing international guidelines on revascularization in patients with ICM

Society	Guideline	Year	Recommendation	Class	Level
AHA	CABG	2011	CABG is reasonable in patients with EF 35–50% and significant multivessel CAD or proximal LAD stenosis where viable myocardium is present	IIa	B
AHA	CABG	2011	CABG is reasonable in patients without significant left main CAD with EF <35%, irrespective of viability	IIb	B
AHA	Heart Failure	2013	CABG should be considered in patients with ICM and operable anatomy irrrespective of viable myocardium	IIb	B
ESC	Heart Failure	2016	Myocardial revascularization is recommended in patients with reduced EF and persistent angina despite medical treatment	I	A
ESC	Myocardial revascularization	2014	Revascularisation for prognosis in 2–3 vessel coronary artery disease (stenosis >50%) and EF <40%	I	A
ESC	Myocardial revascularization	2014	CABG is recommended in left main stenosis in patients with severe LV dysfunction	I	C

opathy [1] we have to ask ourselves whether this role is still timely?

References

1. Velazquez E, Lee L, Jones R, Al-Khalidi H, Hill J, Panza J, et al. Coronary-artery bypass surgery in patients with ischemic cardiomyopathy. N Engl J Med. 2016;374(16):1511–20.
2. Aldermann EL, Fisher LD, Litwin P, et al. Results of coronary artery surgery in patients with poor left ventricular function (CASS). Circulation. 1983;68:785–95.
3. The Veterans Administration Coronary Artery Bypass Surgery Cooperative Study Group. Eleven-year survival in the veterans administration randomized trial of coronary bypass surgery for stable angina. N Engl J Med. 1984;311:1333–9.
4. Varnauskas E, the European Coronary Surgery Study Group. Twelve-year follow-up of survival in the randomized European Coronary Surgery Study. N Engl J Med. 1988;319:332–7.
5. Velazquez E, Lee K, Deja M, et al. Coronary-artery bypass surgery in patients with left ventricular dysfunction. N Engl J Med. 2011;364(17):1607–16.
6. Elamm C, Fang J. The world post-STITCH: is this a "game changer?" A non-invasive cardiologist's perspective – revascularisation is the treatment of choice only in patients who fail medical therapy. Prog Cardiovasc Dis. 2013;55:466–9.
7. Hochman J, Lamas G, Buller C, et al. Coronary intervention for persistent occlusion after myocardial infarction. N Engl J Med. 2006;355:2395–407.
8. Boden WE, O'Rourke RA, Teo KK, et al. Optimal medical therapy with or without PCI for stable coronary disease. N Engl J Med. 2007;356:1503–16.
9. Hochmann J, Reynolds H, Dzavik V, et al. Long-term effects of percutaneous coronary intervention of the totally occluded infarct-related artery in the subacute phase after myocardial infarction. Circulation. 2011;124(21):2320–8.
10. Sedlis S, Hartigan P, Teo K, et al. Effect of PCI on long-term survival in patients with stable ischemic heart disease. N Engl J Med. 2015;373(20):1937–46.
11. Cleland JG, Calvert M, Freemantle N, et al. The heart failure revascularization trial (HEART). Eur J Heart Fail. 2011;13:227–33.
12. Cleland JG, Pennell DJ, Ray SG, Coats AJ, Macfarlane PW, Murray GD, et al. Myocardial viability as a determinant of the ejection fraction response to carvedilol in patients with heart failure (CHRISTMAS trial): randomized controlled trial. Lancet. 2003;362:14–21.
13. Kunadian V, Pugh A, Zaman AG, Qiu W. Percutaneous coronary intervention among patients with left ventricular systolic dysfunction: a review and meta-analysis of 19 clinical studies. Coron Artery Dis. 2012;23:469–79.
14. Marui A, Kimura T, Nishiwaki N, et al. Comparison of five-year outcomes of coronary artery bypass grafting versus percutaneous coronary intervention in patients with left ventricular ejection fractions≤50% versus >50% (from the CREDO-Kyoto PCI/CABG Registry Cohort-2). Am J Cardiol. 2014;114:988–96.
15. Hannan EL, Wu C, Walford G, Culliford AT, Gold JP, Smith CR, Higgins RS, Carlson RE, Jones RH. Drug-eluting stents vs. coronary artery bypass grafting in multivessel coronary disease. N Engl J Med. 2008;358:331–41.
16. Hlatky MA, Boothroyd DB, Baker L, Kazi DS, Solomon MD, Chang TI, Shilane D, Go AS. Comparative effectiveness of multivessel coronary bypass surgery and multivessel percutaneous coronary intervention a cohort study. Ann Intern Med. 2013;158:727–35.
17. Nagendran J, Norris CM, Graham MM, Ross DB, Macarthur RG, Kieser TM, Maitland AM, Southern D, Meyer SR. Coronary revascularization for patients with severe left ventricular dysfunction. Ann Thorac Surg. 2013;96:2038–44.
18. Hlatky M, Boothroyd D, Bravata D, et al. Coronary artery bypass surgery compared with percutaneous coronary interventions for multivessel disease: a collaborative analysis of individual patient data from ten randomised trials. Lancet. 2009;373:1190–7.
19. Yang JH, Choi SH, Song YB, Hahn JY, Choi JH, Jeong DS, Sung K, Kim WS, Lee YT, Gwon HC. Long-term outcomes of drug-eluting stent implantation versus coronary artery bypass grafting for patients with coronary artery disease and chronic left ventricular systolic dysfunction. Am J Cardiol. 2013;112:623–9.
20. Hillis LD, Smith PK, Anderson JL, et al. 2011 ACCF/AHA guideline for coronary artery bypass graft surgery: a report of the American College of Cardiology Foundation/American Heart Association Task Force on practice guidelines. Circulation. 2011;124(23):e652–735.
21. Windecker S, Kolh P, Alfonso F, et al. 2014 ESC/EACTS guidelines on myocardial revascularization: the Task Force on Myocardial Revascularization of the European Society of Cardiology (ESC) and the European Association for Cardio-Thoracic Surgery (EACTS). Eur Heart J. 2014;35:2541–619.
22. Yancy CW, Jessup M, Bozkurt B, et al. 2013ACCF/AHAguideline for the management of heart failure: a report of the American College of Cardiology Foundation/American Heart Association Task Force on practice guidelines. Circulation. 2013;128(16):e240–327.
23. Ponikowski P, Voors AA, Anker SD, et al. 2016 ESC Guidelines for the diagnosis and treatment of acute and chronic heart failure: The Task Force for the diagnosis and treatment of acute and chronic heart failure of the European Society of Cardiology (ESC)Developed with the special contribution of the Heart Failure Association (HFA) of the ESC. Eur Heart J. 2016;37:2129–200.
24. Estep J, Starling R, Horstmanshof D. Risk assessment and comparative effectiveness of left ventricular assist device and medical management in ambulatory heart failure patients: results from the ROADMAP study. J Am Coll Cardiol. 2015;66:1747–61.

Part VIII

Heart Transplantation (I, Surgical)

Early Postoperative Management

16

Balthasar Eberle and Heiko Kaiser

Key Points

Despite progressive shortage of donor organs and higher perioperative risks of recipients, early postoperative mortality of heart transplant recipients has decreased over the decades to about 5% after 30 days [1, 2]. Risk depends not only on recipient and donor age, etiology of heart failure, size mismatch and preoperative condition, but also on the incidence of early postoperative complications [3, 4]. Primary graft failure contributes 2–3%, multiorgan failure 1–2%, infection about 1%, and acute rejection, less than 0.5% [4]. Postoperative care after heart transplantation is basically similar to that after other cardiac surgery. Specific features to be addressed are primary graft failure due to right or left heart dysfunction, complications of extensive surgery and prolonged extracorporeal perfusion, immunosuppression, rejection and infection.

Mainstays of early postoperative management are

- close monitoring by invasive hemodynamic assessment, echocardiography and point-of-care laboratory methods
- diagnosis and treatment of surgical complications, coagulopathy and bleeding
- identification of risk factors and early signs of RV dysfunction
- maintenance of adequate biventricular preload, heart rate, contractility and systemic blood pressure by inotropes, rate and rhythm control and judicious fluid titration.
- reduction of PVR with oxygenation, hyperventilation and inhaled pulmonary vasodilators
- with deteriorating graft function, early initiation of MCS (ECMO)
- immunosuppression, rejection monitoring, and protection from nosocomial infection
- early weaning from ventilator support
- prevention and early treatment of acute kidney injury
- early physiotherapy, mobilization and nutrition

16.1 Background

Short-term survival after cardiac transplantation in adults has continued to improve over time, to more than 95% at 30 days after transplantation [5]. This is not only due to continuous improvement in pre-transplantation optimization and support, but also to progress in perioperative management, immunosuppressive therapy and early detection of allograft rejection. Graft failure (31–42%) and multiorgan failure (15–22%) remain the most frequent causes of early postoperative mortality [5] Fig. 16.1.

16.2 Perioperative Implications of Pre-Transplantation Issues

16.2.1 Pre-Anesthetic Recipient Assessment

Within any cardiac transplantation program, close cooperation between the heart failure team and the cardiac anesthesia group is required. Potential recipients of a heart transplant undergo a well-defined program of pre-transplant diagnostic procedures and optimized medical therapy. As soon as candidates are put on the waiting list, perioperative teams should make themselves familiar with the condition of recipients,

B. Eberle (✉) · H. Kaiser
Universitätsklinik für Anästhesiologie und Schmerztherapie, Universitätsspital Bern | INSELSPITAL, Bern, Switzerland
e-mail: balthasar.eberle@insel.ch

D. S. Feldman, P. Mohacsi (eds.), *Heart Failure*, Cardiovascular Medicine, https://doi.org/10.1007/978-3-319-98184-0_16

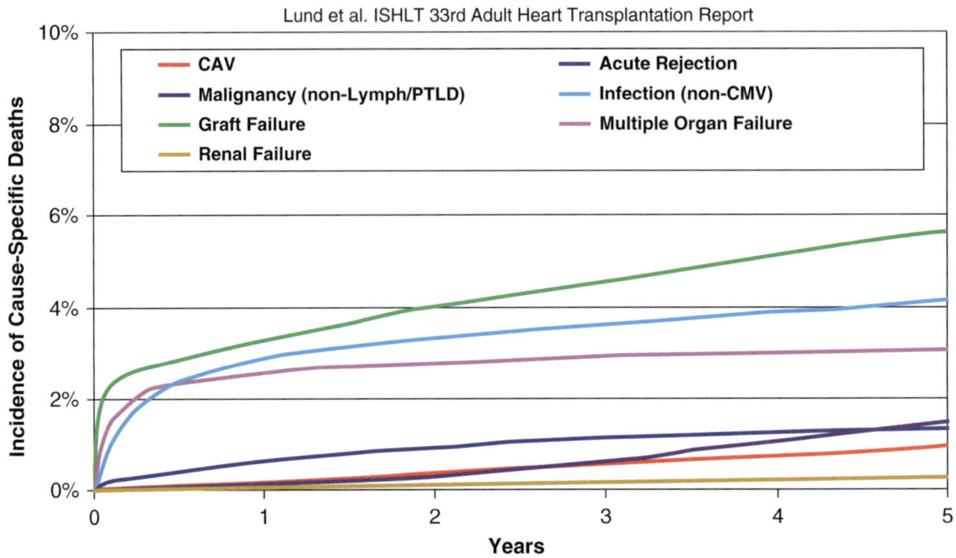

Fig. 16.1 The leading causes of death after adult HTX (cumulative incidence) [5]

e.g., in pre-anesthesia clinics. Patients awaiting urgent transplantation on critical or intermediate care units should be evaluated there as early as possible. All pertinent information should be accessible for anesthesiology and intensivists anytime in the hospital information system.

16.2.2 Preoperative Preparation

Heart transplantation is urgent surgery. Current heart failure therapy allows that today most candidates present for transplantation with end-organ functions maintained. They are on potent medications, and frequently have had a previous sternotomy and implanted devices. Implications for the peri- and early postoperative period are:

- Oral anticoagulation (e.g., vitamin K antagonists, oral Factor Xa inhibitors) or antiplatelet therapy: These agents are usually stopped on admission in order to reduce coagulopathic bleeding after weaning from CPB.
  - Vitamin K should be substituted (5 mg slowly IV) with the aim to correct INR to ≤1.5. Its onset of action occurs within the 2–3 h of preparatory time. During the preoperative waiting period, IV bridging with unfractionated heparin can be initiated anytime when INR < 2.0, since UFH does not usually interfere with cardiac surgery. Alternatives are FFP or prothrombin complex concentrates (PCC). These have a faster onset of action, but carry the risks of volume overload (FFP) or thrombotic complications (PCC). Their domain is emergent anticoagulant reversal, which is usually not needed during the waiting period between admission and incision.
  - Oral Factor Xa inhibitor action requires 24–48 h to wear off; after weaning from CPB, bleeding complications may therefore necessitate emergent replacement with 4-factor PCC (F. II, VII, IX, X, Protein S and C), or reversal with recombinant agents which may be available in the near future (Andexanet alfa).
  - For recipients with a history of heparin-induced thrombocytopenia (HIT) and with IgG antibodies to the platelet factor 4-heparin complex still present, an alternative perioperative non-heparin anticoagulation strategy must be selected [6].
- Renin-Angiotensin-Aldosterone System (RAAS) inhibitors: Active treatment with angiotensin converting enzyme inhibitors or angiotensin II receptor antagonists is associated with a propensity for intraoperative and post-transplantation vasoplegic syndrome. Anesthesiologists and intensivists should be aware of the risk of severe hypotension, and prepare for increased vasopressor requirement.
- Cardiac Implantable Electronic Devices (CIED): Surgical electrocautery will interfere with CIED. Reprogramming and ICD inactivation is necessary in the OR, and external defibrillator/pacing pads must be in place. Transvenous CIED leads may cause mechanical obstruction and/or thrombosis of central venous access routes. Sonography, alternative access routes and additional time may be needed for invasive instrumentation.
- Previous sternotomy and "hostile chest": Repeat sternotomy, dissection of adhesions and device removal prolong pre-implantation surgery. There is a substantial risk of mechanically or cautery-induced ventricular fibrillation, right ventricular perforation or coronary artery bypass graft laceration. Capabilities for external defibrillation and shed blood salvage (cell saver) must be in place. Cross-matched red cell concentrate (CMV negative) must be immediately available in the OR. Emergency access for CPB may be prepared or even fully established via

femoral vessels or subclavian artery. Peripheral arterial access will need postoperative surveillance for limb ischemia.

Mechanical Circulatory Support (MCS): More than 50% of candidate recipients now come to transplantation bridged with MCS, i.e., on a ventricular assist device (VAD) or on extracorporeal life support (ECLS, or ECMO) [5]. Additional time needed for device explantation must be factored into the preoperative time schedule of all teams involved. Device extraction will often require red cell salvage or allogeneic transfusion already prior to CPB. Large wound surfaces will also increase postoperative blood loss.

16.3 Intraoperative Recipient Management

16.3.1 Anesthesia

Meticulous timing with close communication between anesthesiologist, surgeon and transplant coordinator is paramount to minimize donor organ ischemic time.

NPO status prior to anesthesia induction is frequently uncertain in transplant recipients. The risk of pulmonary aspiration of gastric contents is reduced by premedication with proton pump inhibitors and antacids, and by a "rapid-sequence" induction of anesthesia, which ensures endotracheal intubation immediately after the patient has lost protective airway reflexes.

General anesthesia is induced in the OR with surgical and CPB stand-by, with the goal to maintain hemodynamic stability (preload, contractility, afterload, heart rate and rhythm) within the narrow limits typical for patients in end-stage heart failure with LV ejection fraction of less than 20% and fixed stroke volume. Induction of patients on mechanical circulatory support is, in comparison, less demanding due to the robust maintenance of an adequate pump flow.

A typical induction sequence combines short-acting opioids (fentanyl, sufentanil, remifentanil) and hypnotics (etomidate, midazolam or ketamine) followed by a rapid-acting neuromuscular blocker (e.g., rocuronium) to facilitate orotracheal intubation. Propofol is a hypnotic suitable for stable patients on LVAD support.

Maintenance of anesthesia is usually based on continuous opioid infusion (e.g. sufentanil) combined with either a volatile anesthetic agent (e.g. sevoflurane), or continuous infusion of propofol.

16.3.2 Monitoring and Instrumentation

General policies of perioperative hygiene apply, in particular strict compliance with maximum barrier precautions during central line insertion. Immunosuppression renders recipients highly vulnerable by infection. Whether pre- or postoperatively in ICU, vascular access for invasive monitoring should be established using ultrasound guidance, which reduces puncture risk in anticoagulated patients.

Monitoring and instrumentation of a recipient for cardiac transplantation routinely includes

- non-invasive standard monitors, i.e., pulse oximetry, five-lead ECG, oscillometric blood pressure, respiratory gas analysis with capnography, core and nasopharyngeal temperatures, and urinary output (Foley catheter with urimeter).
- invasive arterial pressure monitoring, i.e., radial and frequently also femoral arterial pressure (preferably on the left, to save the right femoral artery for IABP and MCS cannula insertion);
- large-bore peripheral and central venous access (e.g., 8.5–9.0 French multi-access catheters)
- invasive central venous and pulmonary arterial pressures via a multi-lumen balloon-tipped pulmonary artery catheter (PAC), which provides continuous thermodilution cardiac index and mixed venous oxygen saturation measurement, and allows calculation of systemic and pulmonary vascular resistance indices (SVRI, PVRI).
- The PAC/introducer is inserted preferably via the left jugular vein to save the right internal jugular vein for later endomyocardial biopsy access. Its distal tip must be withdrawn high into the SVC prior to venous cannulation for CPB. It is re-floated into the pulmonary artery after coming off CPB but prior to chest closure. This facilitates management of any complications (arrhythmia, malposition).
- perioperative transesophageal echocardiography (TEE). TEE is indispensable to monitor biventricular and valvular function, volume status, deairing maneuvers and reperfusion, and to diagnose aortic atheromatosis, pleural effusion, intracardiac thrombus or shunting, anastomotic problems, and early graft failure.
- external defibrillator-pacemaker electrodes and temporary pacemaker generator.

Depending on institutional policies, additional monitoring includes

- processed EEG monitoring of cerebrocortical function, anesthetic drug effect, and hypothermia.
- cerebral oximetry monitoring, using near-infrared spectroscopy (NIRS). This appears useful to monitor cerebral oxygen delivery during non-pulsatile circulation (LVAD, CPB, ECMO) or circulatory instability. Use during heart transplantation is recommended by several national societies [7].

– point-of-care laboratory monitoring (hemoximetry, blood gases, glucose and lactate; unfractionated heparin anticoagulation using activated coagulation time (ACT) or heparin concentration monitoring (HepCon® HMS); viscoelastic monitoring of clot function (ROTEM®, TEG®) and aggregometric platelet function testing.

16.3.3 Perioperative Antibiotic Prophylaxis

Perioperative antibiotic prophylaxis is given according to guidelines [8]. Preoperatively, topical mupirocin is recommended in the absence of a documented negative testing for staphylococcal colonization. Within 30–60 min prior to incision, a weight-adapted first dose of a second-generation cephalosporine is administered iv and repeated after 3–6 h (two elimination half-times), depending on renal function and blood loss, and is maintained for 48 h. Most centers add a single dose of vancomycin (15 mg/kg infused over at least 1 h prior to incision), since immunosuppression and resternotomy increase the risk of postoperative sternal wound infection [9].

16.3.4 Induction of Immunosuppression

With the decision to accept the donor heart, immunosuppressive therapy is started according to institutional transplant team orders, e.g., with azathioprine (5 mg/kg iv, dose adapted to renal function). During CPB just prior to opening of the aortic cross-clamp and donor heart reperfusion, a bolus dose of methylprednisolon (1 g iv) is given in order to reduce the risk of hyperacute rejection. Additional induction immunosuppressives may be given as devised by the transplant cardiologist.

16.3.5 Perioperative Transfusion Issues

Throughout the perioperative period, anesthesia and intensivist teams must be prepared for volume and blood product administration, including intraoperative autologous red cell salvage and postoperative massive transfusion. Adequate amounts of cross-matched leukodepleted, CMV-negative allogeneic blood products must be available in the OR/ICU, and replenishable on short notice. This includes packed red cell concentrates, fresh frozen plasma, platelet concentrates and stable coagulation factor concentrates (i.e., prothrombin complex concentrate, fibrinogen concentrate, recombinant F-VIIa, antithrombin III, F-XIII concentrate).

Cellular blood products nowadays undergo routine leukodepletion. This reduces the risk of HLA exposure. Many recipients have had contact to allogeneic HLA in their past, e.g., during transfusion (VAD insertion, other cardiac surgery) or pregnancies. Particularly platelet transfusion exposes to a substantial amount of MHC Class I antigen and increases the risk of developing anti-MHC Class I antibodies [10]. Also, since CMV infection promotes HLA expression on platelets and leukocytes, CMV-negative blood should be preferred regardless of the recipient's CMV status [10].

Routine leukodepletion also makes irradiation of allogeneic blood products for and after solid organ transplantation disposable (unless on anti-CD52 agents) [11]. A recent survey finds that in this context, only 37% of institutions still routinely irradiate red cell and platelet concentrate to avoid potential transfusion-associated graft-versus-host disease [12]. This facilitates blood product logistics in scenarios of massive transfusion.

Significant hemodilution occurs on CPB due to the asanguineous circuit prime (800–1200 ml). Allogeneic transfusion should be avoided or minimized by processing of shed blood, autologous retransfusion and ultrafiltration with the goal to maintain hematocrit at 25% or higher. Nadir hematocrit levels below 25% as well as allogeneic transfusion are associated with an increased incidence of postoperative acute kidney injury [13].

16.3.6 Anticoagulation for CPB

Anticoagulation for CPB is established using unfractionated heparin (UFH, 400–500 IU/kg iv). Despite full UFH anticoagulation, intense shed-blood suction, blood-air and blood-surface contact activate inflammation, complement, coagulation, and fibrinolysis. Antifibrinolytic prophylaxis using tranexamic acid is nowadays routine in all major cardiac surgery. It has been proven to reduce postoperative chest drain loss and red cell transfusion in standard cardiac surgery [14].

UFH anticoagulation is monitored, point-of-care, using the Activated Clotting Time bedside test (ACT, normal value 100–120 s, target during CPB of 480–600 s). Heparin regimens and ACT targets vary considerably between institutions. Despite its universal use, ACT is not very specific for UFH effect. It is also prolonged in response to hemodilution, hypothermia or loss of coagulation factors and platelets, and may underestimate high UFH levels in the presence of AT III deficiency. Therefore many institutions do not rely on ACT alone during and after high-risk cardiac surgery, but also use direct point-of-care monitoring of UFH concentration in whole-blood samples (e.g., Hepcon® HMS system, Medtronic Inc.). After successful weaning from CPB and postoperatively, heparin anticoagulation is routinely reversed with protamine until ACT has returned to its pre-CPB level and/or free UFH concentration is zero.

16.3.7 Weaning from CPB

16.3.7.1 De-Airing of the Heart

Prior to opening of the aortic cross clamp the left heart is meticulously deaired. Efficacy of deairing is assessed by TEE to reduce the risk of gaseous (micro-) embolism to brain and coronaries (preferably to the non-dependent right ostium). Right coronary air, when detected macroscopically and by ST-segment analysis, will predict at least transient impairment of right ventricular performance.

16.3.7.2 Reperfusion

During graft reperfusion after cross-clamp removal, cardioplegic preservation solution, byproducts of ischemic metabolism and gaseous microemboli are cleared from the post-ischemic myocardium. Aerobic energy metabolism resumes; grafted organ and patient are rewarmed slowly and homogeneously. Electrical activity may resume with a slow rhythm or with initial ventricular fibrillation. Overdistension of a fibrillating heart must be prevented until internal defibrillation is successful. Recurrent reperfusion arrhythmia may indicate substantial ischemia-reperfusion injury. Immediate spontaneous return of a regular rhythm on reperfusion indicates good myocardial preservation.

Cardiac grafts usually undergo an extended reperfusion period on CPB, compared to reperfusion after routine cardiac surgery. The grafted heart is decompressed by venting, remains on full extracorporeal support and is thus unloaded from external work. The duration of this reperfusion period is about half the ischemic time of the donor organ (e.g., 45–120 min, with institutional variation).

Preparations for weaning the transplanted heart from CPB include routine measures and some specifics:

The patient is rewarmed, usually from moderate hypothermia, to a core temperature of 36.5 °C, keeping nasopharyngeal temperature strictly below 37 °C. Post-CPB hyperthermia above 37° has been associated with an increased risk of cognitive dysfunction [15].

Hematocrit is adjusted to 26–28%, preferably with salvaged autologous red cell concentrate to minimize the risk of acute kidney injury [13]. However, depending on the patient's preoperative volemic state, the blood turnover during pre-CPB dissection, and risk of post-CPB coagulopathy, additional allogeneic red cell transfusion may be indicated.

Acid-base balance and electrolyte status should be corrected during rewarming. High-normal potassium levels (4.5–5.0 mmol/L) stabilize cardiac rhythm during adrenergic stimulation. Mild alkalosis helps to reduce pulmonary vascular resistance (PVR) and thus right ventricular (RV) afterload. Bicarbonate infusion is useful to produce a mildly positive base excess (± 0 to +5 meq/L), since CO_2 elimination on CPB is nearly unrestricted.

Mechanical ventilation is resumed after re-institution of pulmonary blood flow, i.e., after the pulmonary artery anastomosis has been completed. A recruitment maneuver (inspiratory hold) followed by PEEP will help to aerate previously compressed, atelectatic lung. Low tidal volume (6–7 ml/kg ideal body weight) ventilation is started and continuously adapted to spontaneous (transaortic) cardiac output. Re-expansion of atelectasis without alveolar overdistension is important. First, pulmonary vascular resistance (PVR) is lowest when alveolar space is at its functional residual capacity; and second, inhaled pulmonary vasodilator drugs are effective in ventilated alveoli only. In many centers, inhaled pulmonary vasodilators are started preemptively at this point, since it is easier to wean them in a stable situation than to initiate them during a low cardiac output scenario.

Inotropic and chronotropic pharmacologic stimulation of the graft is also initiated at the end of the reperfusion period. Adrenergic inopressor drugs (adrenaline, noradrenaline) are frequently combined with PDE III-inhibiting inodilator agents (milrinone). Other centers use dobutamine or isoproterenol as first-line inotrope. Escalation of inotropic stimulation is possible with the Ca^{++}-sensitizing inodilator levosimendan.

At a pump flow or cardiac index of 2.4 L/min/m^2, a mean arterial pressure of 60 mmHg at a CVP of 8–10 mmHg or less should be targeted. A radial MAP of less than 50 mmHg under these conditions, despite noradrenaline infusion, should raise the suspicion of a radial to central pressure gradient and vasoplegic syndrome [16]. This constellation occurs quite frequently in patients bridged to transplantation on continuous-flow LVAD, patients under intensified medical therapy for severe heart failure with RAAS inhibition, or after massive blood turnover and long CPB runs. In such situations, radial arterial pressure should be compared to central aortic root pressure, which can be transduced by the surgeon via a needle or vent. Aortic root pressure may exceed radial pressure by up to 30 mmHg (systolic) due to peripheral arterio-venous shunting. For several hours postoperatively, femoral arterial pressure may better reflect central aortic pressures and help to avoid vasopressor overdosing [17].

If central aortic pressure measurement on CPB confirms low systemic vascular resistance at adequate or supranormal pump flow, the addition of vasopressin usually succeeds in restoring pressor response to noradrenaline, without inducing pulmonary vasoconstriction. Vasopressor effect can be further intensified by addition of methylene blue, a guanylate cyclase inhibitor which blocks release of cyclic guanosine monophosphate (cGMP) and thus counteracts vasorelaxation. There is only anecdotal evidence of improvement in outcome with methylene blue rescue [16]. Actions and dosages of inotropes and vasoactives are given in Table 16.1.

Table 16.1 Inotropes and vasoactive drugs used after cardiac transplantation (systematic review in [18])

	Mechanism	Con-tractility	Systemic vasculature		Pulmonary vasculature		Chrono-tropy	Arrhyth-mia risk	Dose range
Inodilators			Con-strictor	Dilator	Con-strictor	Dilator			
Epinephrine	β1, β2, α agonist	++++	+++	+ (low dose)	(+)	0	++	+++	0.05–0.20 mcg/kg/min
Dobutamine	β1 agonist	+++	0	++	0	+	+	+	2–20 mcg/kg/min
Dopamine	DA1, β1, β2, α agonist	+++	++	+ (low dose)	+	–	+	+	2–20 mcg/kg/min (≤5 in RVF)
Isoproterenol	β1, β2 agonist	++++	0	+++	0	++	++++	++++	0.02–0.20 mcg/kg/min
Milrinone	PDE III-Inh. cAMP↑	+++	0	++	0	+	0/+	++	0.5–0.75 mcg/kg/min
Levosimendan	Ca^{++} Sensit. PDE III-inh.	+++	0	++	0	+	+	0	0.05–0.1 mcg/kg/min
Vasopressors									
Norepinephrine	α, β1 agonist	+++	++++	0	+	0	+[a]	+	0.05–0.20 mcg/kg/min
Vasopressin	V1 agonist	0	++++	0	0	(+)	0	0	0.03–0.1 U/min
Pulmonary vasodilators									
Inhaled NO	cGMP↑ offset 1–2 min	0	0	0	0	++	0	0	0.05–40 ppm
Inhaled Iloprost	cAMP↑ offset 1–2 h	0	0	(+)	0	+++	0	0	10–20 mcg q 3 h
Inhaled Epoprostenol (PGI_2 analogue)	cAMP↑ half life 3–5 min	0	0	(+)	0	+++	0	0	10–50 ng/kg/min
Inhaled Milrinone	PDE III-Inh. cAMP↑ half life 1–2 h	(+)	0	(+)	0	++	0	0	50–80 mcg/kg per dose[c]
Systemic & Pulmonary Vasodilators									
Nitroglycerin i.v.	cGMP↑	0[a]	0	++	0	+++	0[a]	0	0.1–7 mcg/kg/min
Nitroprusside i.v.	cGMP↑	0[a]	0	+++	0	+++	0[a]	0	0.1–4 mcg/kg/min
Epoprostenol/Prostacyclin i.v.	cAMP↑ (offset 10 min)	(+)	0	++	0	+++	0	0	1–9 ng/kg/min
Sildenafil po./iv[b]	PDE V inh. cGMP↑	0	0	++	0	+++	(+)	0	20 mg/8 h po 10 mg/8 h iv

[a]Denervated graft/baroreflex disruption in the recipient prevent reflex tachy- or bradycardia
[b][19] [c][20]

Cardiac autonomic innervation is disrupted in the donor heart. It is thus unresponsive to autonomic nervous system stimulation (e.g., baroreceptor reflexes, reflex tachycardia) or indirectly acting chronotropic agents (e.g., ephedrine, atropine). Temporal epicardial atrial and ventricular pacemaker leads are attached. Initially, intrinsic nodal bradycardia may require at least transient pacing. When sinus nodes recover, two P waves may be noted from donor and recipient atria. Atrial or if necessary, A-V sequential pacing is established at a rate of 90–110 bpm in order to provide good preload without distending the RV.

16.3.7.3 Weaning

Venous return is shifted to the patient until CVP reaches a maximum of 10–12 mmHg. Progressive filling and ejection of the heart allows to assess biventricular function visually in the surgical field and by TEE. Right ventricular overload must be strictly avoided. Central aortic pressure is adjusted to a MAP of 65–70 mmHg by reinfusion of CPB circuit volume, further inotropic stimulation and selective pulmonary vasodilation. The retracted PAC is repositioned into the pulmonary artery. It is helpful for monitoring right heart hemodynamics and mixed venous oxygen saturation over the ensuing 24–48 h on ICU, particularly after TEE surveillance ends.

After removal of the venous cannulae, heparin anticoagulation is fully reversed as guided by ACT or Hepcon®.

16.3.8 Transesophageal Echocardiographic (TEE) Assessment

TEE is indispensable during weaning from CPB, during surgical hemostasis, fluid, inotrope and vasoactive treatment, and chest closure. Surgical problems should be identified in the OR, preferably before the chest is closed. Regular TEE, and later TTE-based, re-assessment is continued on ICU.

16.3.8.1 LV Assessment

It focuses on parameters of global systolic function (LVEF), regional wall motion abnormalities, dyssychrony, and parameters of diastolic function. During substantial inotropic stimulation, an underfilled LV (due to hypovolemia, RV dysfunction, pulmonary hypertension) may tend to develop dynamic outflow tract obstruction (e.g., due to systolic anterior motion, SAM, of the anterior mitral leaflet). Early graft dysfunction is suspected if LVEF does not recover to more than 40%.

16.3.8.2 RV Assessment

This includes right atrial (RA) and ventricular (RV) dimensions (RA transverse diameter; RV diastolic dimensions at annulus, mid-portion and from apex to RV annular plane; RV end-diastolic and end-systolic area (RVEDA), as well as RV fractional area change (RVFAC); and tricuspid annular plane systolic excursion (TAPSE). Echo assessment in the OR and on ICU should always be integrated with concurrent invasive hemodynamic measurements.

Features of impending or frank RV dysfunction are, for instance

- RV distension (RV short/long axis ratio > 0.6) and rounding, tricuspid annular dilatation (>40 mm or >2.1 mm per m^2 of BSA)
- impaired global RV function (RV FAC < 35%); depressed tricuspid annular plane systolic excursion (TAPSE) (<16 mm) and peak velocity S' (<10 cm/s);
- impaired or absent RV free wall motion
- inferior/inferoseptal hypo- or akinesis, suggesting regional ischemia from RCA gaseous embolism or occlusion;
- bowing of the IAS towards the left atrium, indicating increased right atrial and/or abnormally low left atrial pressure (RAP/LAP >1),
- leftward shift and paradoxical motion of the IVS;
- progressive tricuspid regurgitation (moderate to severe), hepatic venous systolic flow attenuation or reversal.
- increased RV-RA pressure gradient, indicating increased RV afterload due to pulmonary vasoconstriction or hypertension, or to anastomotic PA stenosis
- loss of RV-RA pressure gradient and equalization of RA and RV pressures during frank RV failure.
- RVOT or RV compression. This may occur during surgical hemostasis or on chest closure, with acute hypotension in response. The chest may need to be left open under sterile dressings for delayed closure.

16.3.8.3 Valve Assessment

It focuses primarily on presence, grade and mechanism of mitral (MR) and tricuspid valve regurgitation (TR). If tricuspid annular dilatation with moderate or severe TR is present, tricuspid annuloplasty is considered (Class II LoE C). Any TR graded intraoperatively as more than mild must be re-evaluated by TTE or TEE within 24 h (Class I LoE C) [21]. MR is frequent early after coming off bypass, but mostly functional by mechanism (e.g., SAM phenomenon) and reversible over time. Significant aortic valve regurgitation is unusual.

16.3.8.4 Surgical Anastomoses

These must be detected in the OR as long as the chest is still open, focusing on caval veins, pulmonary artery, left atrium and pulmonary veins. Narrowing and abnormally increased Doppler flow velocity may indicate obstruction or distortion in SVC, IVC or PA. Stenosis or kinking of the PA anastomosis is suspected from color flow acceleration with increased Doppler gradient; it should be confirmed or ruled out by direct pressure transduction from the surgical field. If necessary, it is addressed surgically.

Caval vein stenosis may occur at the anastomotic level or cannulation sites. Bicaval instead of biatrial anastomosis is nowadays the preferred technique to avoid the risk of sinus node dysfunction and chronic dysrhythmia from right atrial sutures. Typically, an elevated non-pulsatile CVP tracing is transduced from the most cranial CVP lumen, whereas TEE and PA pressures suggest a relatively underfilled, hypovolemic heart. TEE imaging of the SVC in bicaval view will reveal luminal narrowing and abnormally increased flow velocity; any gradient is confirmed by direct needle pressure transduction. Occasionally, surgical revision is required.

Left atrial or biatrial anastomosis may cause typical thickened suture lines in atrial walls and interatrial septum, which, in 2D-TEE imaging, must be discerned from thrombotic mass, or invagination of the atrial wall. Very rarely, obstruction of mitral inflow by excess atrial tissue may cause pulmonary congestion and RV failure.

Pleural and pericardial blood or fluid collection should be monitored regularly by TEE during surgery, prior to chest closure and transfer to ICU, and during any period of hemodynamic instability.

After extubation and later postoperatively, surveillance is continued using transthoracic echocardiography. TTE is useful for early detection of pericardial effusion, for assessment of functional indicators of acute allograft rejection, for stress testing and guidance of EMB [22, 23].

16.4 Postoperative Considerations

16.4.1 Transfer to ICU

Transfer from the OR to ICU, and subsequent admission with transition of care from the anesthesia to the ICU team is a period of significant risk. Preoperative and current patient status, surgical procedures, their results and complications, as well as all current medications and therapies must be communicated in advance to the ICU staff.

During transfer, there must be no interruption of monitoring, mechanical ventilator and temporal pacemaker settings, pharmacological or mechanical organ support, pulmonary vasodilator, fluid or blood component therapy, and chest tube drainage.

On ICU admission, switching of monitors, respirator, syringe pumps etc. should occur sequentially, to allow reassessment after each step. Team handovers should be structured and undisturbed. Transplantation specifics are informations about donor heart ischemia time, and orders by transplant cardiology of immunosuppressant, antibiotics, anticoagulation and laboratory sampling.

16.4.2 Hemodynamic Management

16.4.2.1 Monitoring

Hemodynamic monitoring is continued on ICU as described in the OR after CPB weaning. TEE should be used on indication of any hemodynamic instability. Also, urine and chest tube output should be monitored continuously. During several hours after CPB weaning, biventricular contractility and diastolic function are frequently impaired but usually improve over several hours. Meticulous maintenance of preload and atrioventricular synchrony, preemptive support of biventricular myocardial contractility with inotropes, pulmonary vasodilation and, if necessary, heart rate control by atrial pacing is continued throughout 24–48 postop hours.

16.4.2.2 Rate and Rhythm Control

Cardiac rhythm disturbances are frequent in allografts due to denervation, ischemia-reperfusion injury and surgical suture lines. Bradycardia is overcome with A-V sequential pacing at rates of 90–110 bpm, using the temporary atrial and ventricular pacing wires placed routinely by the surgeon (Class IB). Use of isoproterenol for chronotropy has become infrequent due to its hypotensive side effect. Tachyarrhythmia should be rate-controlled, and if persisting, should alert the care team to rule out rejection. If no adequate chronotropic response has returned three weeks after transplantation, implantation of a permanent pacemaker is recommended [21]. Amiodarone, beta-blockers and non-dihydropyridine calcium channel blockers can be used in heart transplant recipients with few interactions.

16.4.2.3 Inotropic and Vasoactive Drug Support

Compared to routine cardiac surgical patients, transplant recipients require more prolonged inotropic and vasoactive drug support. Regimens for hemodynamic drug support vary institutionally, but most suggest the following agents. Single or combined administration may be indicated in order to balance inotropic action with effects on pulmonary and systemic vascular resistance.

There is consensus that preemptive administration of inotropic agents is useful (Class I C). Systemic vasodilation is most often achieved already with the use of inodilator drugs like dobutamine or milrinone. Due TO their additive vasodilator effect, combination of milrinone with levosimendan should be avoided. Inotropes should be weaned slowly over 3–5 postoperative days (Class I C) [21].

Vasopressor agents are useful to restore mean arterial pressure and RV perfusion from vasodilatory hypotension as long as cardiac output and mixed venous oxygen saturation remain adequate. Noradrenaline, as a pulmonary vasoconstrictor, should rather be combined with low-dose vasopressin, which does not constrict pulmonary vessels, instead of escalating noradrenaline to high doses far beyond 0.2 mcg/kg/min.

Pure vasodilators are used most often to reduce pulmonary vascular resistance, i.e., RV afterload. Non-selective intravenous vasodilators (nitroglycerine, sodium nitroprusside) reduce both pulmonary and systemic vascular resistance. They should be given only in the absence of systemic hypotension. (Class IIa C) [21].

Preference should be given to agents with pulmonary selectivity (inhaled gaseous nitric oxide (NO), aerosolized iloprost or prostacyclin, oral or intravenous sildenafil). These allow to reduce RV afterload with less hypotension than non-selective vasodilators. (Class IIa C) [21].

The vasoactive NO molecule is endogeneously produced primarily by NO synthase in endothelial cells. It can be exogeneously administered as a medical gas or intravenously supplied by NO donator drugs (e.g., nitroprusside). NO (and also nitroglycerine) activates guanylate cyclase in vascular smooth muscle cells and, via the second messenger cGMP, induces local smooth muscle relaxation. When inhaled as a therapeutic gas, NO reduces PVR in ventilated alveolar units and improves ventilation-perfusion mismatch. As a free radical, inhaled NO is rapidly inactivated by contact with intravascular hemoglobin (half-life, 5–10 s). Therefore, iNO provides selective pulmonary vasodilation without systemic vasodilation. A decrease of elevated PVR in patients with RV dysfunction results in reduced pulmonary arterial pressure and RV afterload, or increased cardiac output and LV filling, or both.

iNO inactivation by hemoglobin results in clinically negligible methemoglobin formation. Within a respiratory gas mixture the NO radical is also oxidated to toxic NO_x moieties. Several manufactureres produce NO application devices for use with respirators (INOmax DSIR®, Mallinckrodt; NOxBOX®,UK; SoKinox®, Air Liquide Santé). These provide exact and constant inspiratory NO gas dosing with continuous monitoring of inspired concentration and toxic by products.

Inhaled NO has the specific risk of rebound pulmonary vasoconstriction on sudden withdrawal, and of mild toxicity (NOx, methemoglobin). Therefore patients should be weaned gradually from iNO therapy within 12–24 h, with the smallest reduction steps below concentrations of 5 ppm. If necessary, this can be aided by intermittent inhalation of aerosolized iloprost, which can be continued after extubation using portable nebulizer devices. Also, iNO weaning can be facilitated by oral treatment with sildenafil, an inhibitor of Type V phosphodiesterase, and hence, of cGMP breakdown.

Prostanoids like prostacyclin (PgI_2) and its longer acting analogue iloprost relax vascular smooth muscle cells via adenylate cyclase activation and second-messenging via cAMP. For inhalative use, their aqueous solution is aerosolized and delivered to the alveolar space by using portable ultrasonic or vibrating mesh nebulizers (droplet diameter, 3–5 μm). When inhaled, selectivity of their pulmonary vasodilatory effect is dose-dependent and less than that of iNO [24]. Also, prostanoid inhalation is usually not accompanied by improved oxygenation. High inhalative doses may induce systemic vasodilation (facial flush, hypotension). The extent of PVR reduction is similar or slightly superior to iNO. While prostacycline has a half-life of only about 3 min, iloprost is a stable prostacyclin analogue with a longer half-life of 20–30 min, and hence, with 30–60 min duration of effect. In patients with pulmonary arterial hypertension inhaled iloprost improves pulmonary hemodynamics and exercise capacity [25]. Inhaled iloprost can also be combined with oral sildenafil to enhance and prolong its pulmonary vasodilatory effects [26].

Milrinone is an inhibitor of phosphodiesterase III and is widely used as IV inotrope. By inhibiting the degradation of the second messenger cAMP, milrinone also relaxes vascular smooth muscle cells. In aerosolized form it has been used, off label, as long-acting (>1–2 h) inhaled pulmonary vasodilator. A recent RCT found that compared with placebo, milrinone inhalation improved hemodynamics, but did not reduce incidence of RV failure in high risk cardiac surgical patients [20]. Combination of inhaled aerosolized milrinon with inhaled prostacycline produced additive effects and reduced vasoactive drug requirement in high risk cardiac surgical patients [27, 28].

16.4.2.4 Management of Hemodynamic Complications

Severe postoperative hemodynamic complications are mostly due to early graft dysfunction of RV and/or LV, or due to bleeding, surgical complications, pulmonary hypertension or acute allograft rejection (secondary graft dysfunction).

Primary and Secondary Graft Dysfunction

Graft dysfunction and failure accounts for 31–42% of 30-day mortality and is the leading cause of early death after heart transplantation, followed by multi-organ failure [5, 29]. For categorization of risk, the RADIAL score has been developed (RADIAL: recipient right (R) atrial pressure ≥ 10 mmHg; age (A) ≥ 60 y; diabetes (D), and inotrope (I) dependence; donor age (A) ≥ 30 y, and length (L) of ischemia ≥240 min) [30].

Primary Graft Dysfunction (PGD) is defined as

- left or biventricular (PGD-LV with LV or BV dysfunction), or right ventricular (PGD-RV) dysfunction,
- which occurs within the initial 24 post-transplantation hours,
- which has no identifiable secondary cause,
- which requires prolonged inotropic or mechanical circulatory support, and possibly retransplantation [31].

A incidence of PGD between 2.5 and 32% is reported in the literature, and is associated with an increased 30 day mortality of 37% [29, 30, 32]. Management is reported to require intra-aortic balloon pumping in 50%, mechanical support in 27% and renal replacement therapy in it 61%, and it substantially prolongs ICU stay [32].

PGD may be graded as mild, moderate, or severe, depending on cardiac function and extent of inotrope and mechanical support [29] (Table 16.2).

Etiology and risk of PGD are related to issues of

- the donor (age, female sex, cause of brain death),
- the recipient (age, pulmonary hypertension, dependence on inotropes, respirator, and MCS)
- the procedure (ischemic time, donor-to-recipient weight mismatch) [29].

Table 16.2 Definition of Severity Scale for Primary Graft Dysfunction (PGD)

1. PGD-Left ventricle (PGD-LV):	*Mild PGD-LV: One* of the following criteria must be met:	LVEF ≤40% by echocardiography, *or* Hemodynamics with RAP >15 mm Hg, PCWP >20 mm Hg, CI < 2.0 L/min/m^2 (lasting more than 1 h) requiring Low-dose inotropes
	Moderate PGD-LV: Must meet one criterion from I *and* another criterion from II:	I. *One* criteria from the following: Left ventricular ejection fraction ≤40%, *or* Hemodynamic compromise with RAP >15 mm Hg, PCWP >20 mm Hg, CI < 2.0 L/min/m^2, hypotension with MAP <70 mm Hg (lasting more than 1 h) II. *One* criteria from the following: i. High-dose inotropes—Inotrope score > 10[a] *or* ii. Newly placed IABP (regardless of inotropes)
	Severe PGD-LV	Dependence on Left or biventricular mechanical support including ECMO, LVAD, BiVAD, or percutaneous LVAD. Excludes requirement for IABP
2. PGD-right ventricle (PGD-RV):	Diagnosis requires either both i and ii, or iii alone:	i. Hemodynamics with RAP >15 mm Hg, PCWP <15 mm Hg, CI < 2.0 L/min/m^2 ii. TPG <15 mm Hg and/or pulmonary artery systolic pressure < 50 mm Hg, *or* iii. Need for RVAD

Mod. after [29] (*with permission*)
BiVAD biventricular assist device, *CI* cardiac index, *ECMO* extracorporeal membrane oxygenation, *IABP* intra-aortic balloon pump, *LVAD* Left ventricular assist device, *PCWP* pulmonary capillary wedge pressure, *RAP* right atrial pressure, *RVAD* right ventricular assist device, *TPG* transpulmonary pressure gradient
[a]Inotrope score = dopamine (×1) + dobutamine (×1) + amrinone (×1) + milrinone (×l5) + epinephrine (×100) + norepinephrine (×100) with each drug dosed in μg/kg/min

Technical problems may aggravate ischemia-reperfusion injury and contribute to delayed recovery. For instance, the organ may have suffered in the donor, i.e., during terminal catecholamine surge or prolonged high-dose catecholamine infusion, during severe hypotension, massive transfusion or cardiopulmonary resuscitation prior to organ harvest, or during procurement and transport.

Secondary Graft Dysfunction It is assumed when there is an identifiable secondary cause such as hyperacute rejection, pulmonary hypertension, or an iatrogenic complication.

Right Ventricular Dysfunction and Failure

In most instances of PGF the RV is affected, either alone (45%) or as part of biventricular failure (47%) [30]. RV failure still accounts for approximately 20% of early deaths [30, 33]. RV dysfunction is thus a common hemodynamic problem early after cardiac transplantation. This may be due to more liberal acceptance of recipients with secondary pulmonary hypertension but bridged on VAD; of organs from donors who are less stable or less well matched; and of longer storage and transport times.

The normal RV is preload-compliant but highly afterload-sensitive. Even a perfectly healthy donor RV has undergone significant ischemia-reperfusion injury, and resumes its function in a multimorbid recipient. This massively strains its limited functional reserves. Pathophysiological mechanisms leading to RV failure after cardiac transplantation interact in a vicious circle and are illustrated in Fig. 16.2 [18].

RV contractility critically depends on diastolic and systolic coronary perfusion. Maintenance of mean arterial pressure and LV function are therefore absolutely essential.

In the OR and on ICU, a post-ischemic grafted RV may acutely decompensate and fail for a number of reasons:

- RV ischemia due to coronary hypoperfusion may develop during hemorrhagic hypotension; during massive transfusion with RV volume overload; due to surgical manipulation or ischemia from air embolized to the RCA.
- Increased pulmonary vascular resistance (RV afterload) will pre-exist in the recipient, or may be provoked by a long CPB run, massive transfusion, hypercapnia, acidosis, hypoxemia or protamine-induced vasoconstriction. The volume- or pressure-overloaded RV will dilate and fail; progressive TR and leftward shift of the interventricular septum will impair LV filling and lead to hypotension, low cardiac output and ischemic lactic acidosis.

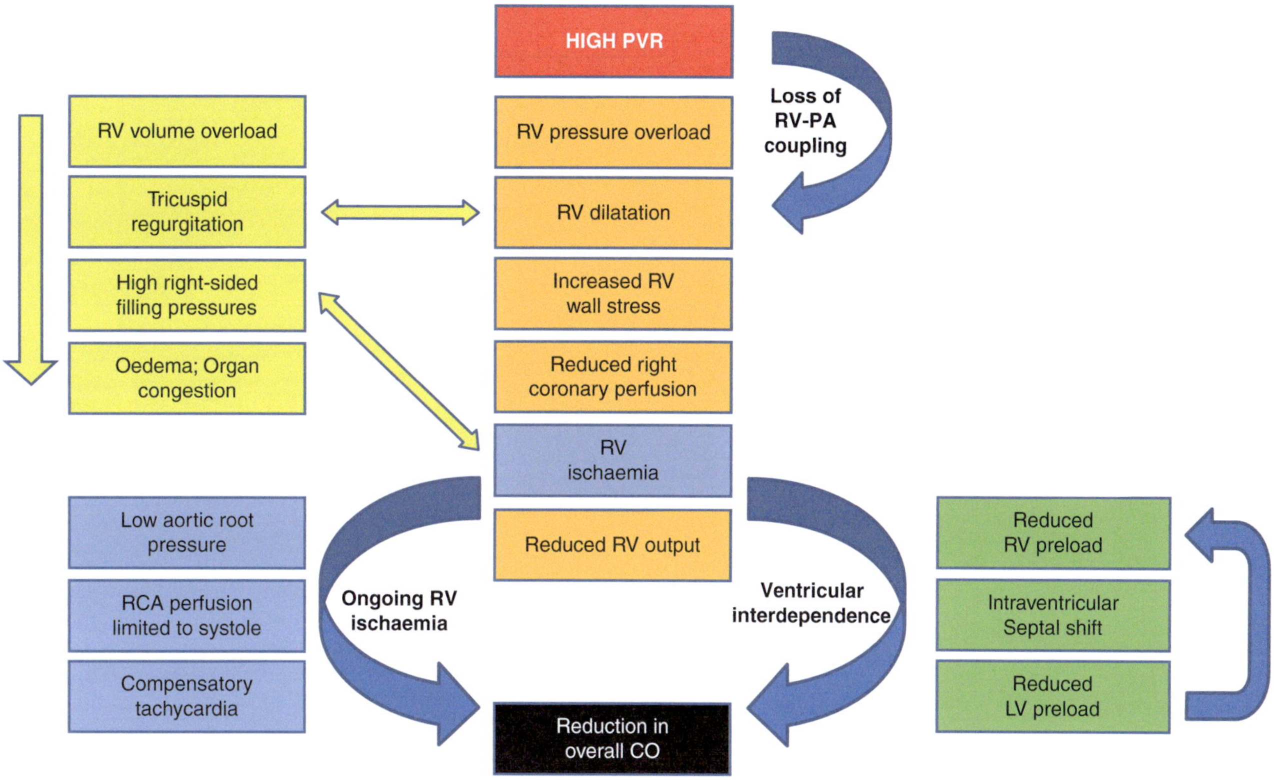

Fig. 16.2 Pathophysiology of right ventricular failure in the setting of high PVR. *CO*, cardiac output; *LV*, left ventricle; *MAPr* mean arterial pressure; *PVR*, pulmonary vascular resistance; *RV*, right ventricle. ([18], with permission)

– Arterial hypotension, low cardiac output and acidosis will worsen ischemia and further increase afterload of the failing RV.

Monitoring and diagnosis of impending RV failure rely on TEE or TTE assessment, and on invasive measurement of RA, RV, PA pressures, cardiac index and mixed venous saturation.

– *Echocardiographic (TEE, TTE) risk indicators* are RV distension and tricuspid annular dilatation; RV free wall and inferior hypo- or akinesis; left-sided shifting and paradoxical motion of the IVS, and bowing of the IAS to the left; depressed TAPSE; progressive tricuspid regurgitation with supranormal RV-RA pressure gradients, indicating increased RV afterload due to PHT or stenosis of the PA anastomosis; low RV-RA pressure gradient and equalization of RA and RV pressures during frank RV failure.
– *Invasive hemodynamic data (PAC)* will provide information about abnormal RV pre- and afterload, PHT, systolic RV failure, pulmonary venous hypertension, transpulmonary pressure gradient and pulmonary vascular resistance (PVR). Low cardiac output (<2.4 L/min/m^2) is confirmed by thermodilution technique and low mixed venous oxygen saturation (<65%).
– In the OR and if the chest remains open, direct observation of RV function may be possible during re-exploration.

Prevention and treatment of RV dysfunction or failure are a continuum starting with reperfusion on CPB [34]. Management is outlined in the following as for primary graft dysfunction. Secondary causes (surgical or other iatrogenic problems, or acute rejection) should be addressed specifically beyond standard supportive measures.

Mainstays in prevention and treatment of early postoperative RV dysfunction are (Fig. 16.3):

– maintenance of arterial normotension (mean arterial pressure MAP should be at least 65–70 mmHg)
– maintenance of sinus/atrial PM rhythm (atrial kick) at mild tachycardia (90–110 bpm)
– baseline inotropic RV and LV stimulation, e.g., with
  • adrenaline (0.05–0.20 mcg/kg/min) and
  • milrinone (loading dose, 25 mcg/kg, maintenance 0.25–0.5 mcg/kg/min)
  • Inotrope dose is adjusted to produce a cardiac index (CI) of ≥2.4 L/min/m^2 and a mixed venous $SO_2 > 65\%$
– RV preload is titrated with fluid, under TEE guidance as feasible, while closely monitoring RV diameters and function, tricuspid regurgitation, interatrial and interven-

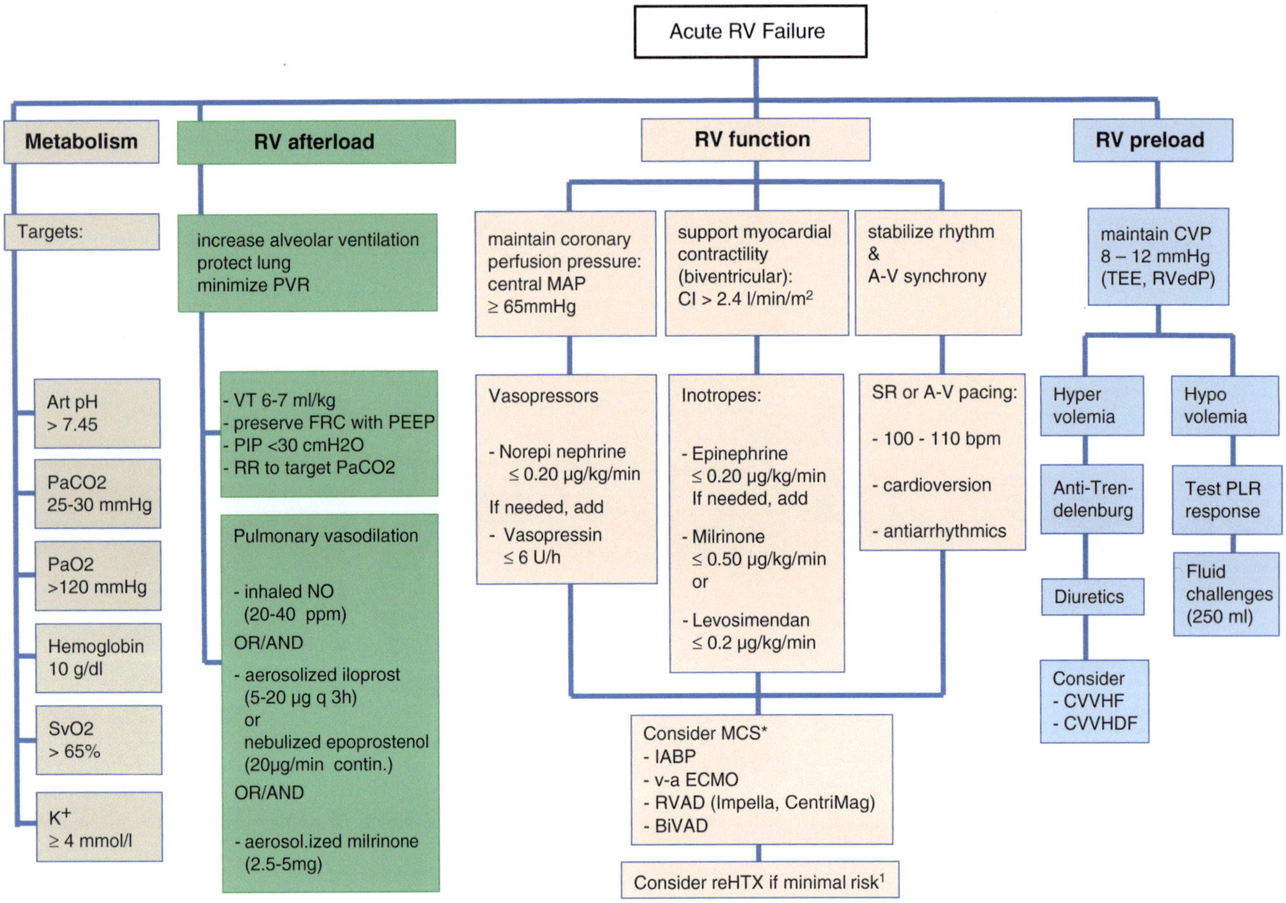

Fig. 16.3 Mainstays in prevention and treatment of early postoperative RV dysfunction

tricular septal motion as well as CVP (maximum, 12 mmHg), PAP and stroke volume response.

- Reduction of PVR/PHT and RV afterload by non-specific measures:
  - mild metabolic alkalosis (bicarbonate) and hyperventilation (hypocapnic $PaCO_2$ of 25–30 mmHg) will vasodilate the lung.
  - high DO_2 providing increased alveolar (>100 mmHg) and mixed venous PO_2 (>40–50 mmHg) will counteract hypoxic pulmonary vasoconstriction
  - non-specific intravenous nitrodilators, e.g., nitroglycerine (0.1–7 mcg/kg/min), sodium nitroprusside (0.1–4 mcg/kg/min), will reduce PVR but also SVR, and should be used with caution. Arterial hypotension is counterproductive for RV contractility at this point.
- Specific pulmonary vasodilator therapy is begun preemptively (in the OR) by many centers, using mostly inhaled nitric oxide (iNO, 20–40 ppm) or inhaled aerosolized iloprost (10–20 mcg q 3 h). If pulmonary hypertension persists at satisfactory LV function (TEE criteria, PCPW <18 mmHg), pulmonary vasodilation may be intensified by combining inhaled NO with inhaled iloprost. Since they work via different signaling pathways, combinations of these agents have been shown to act synergistically [35]. RV afterload reduction goals are to keep PVR < 6 Wood Units and transpulmonary pressure gradient TPG at 5–10 mmHg.
- Systemic afterload (SVR) is adjusted, if necessary, by using noradrenaline (0.05–0.10 mcg/kg/min to maintain central aortic MAP at approximately 70 mmHg and CI and mixed venous SO_2 as above, and lactate <3 mmol/l. In vasoplegic syndrome (e.g., SVR < 800 dyn s cm^{-5} despite high-dose noradrenaline infusion), low-dose vasopressin (0.6–6 U/h) is rather added early to noradrenaline instead of escalating the dosage of the latter. Methylene blue, an inhibitor of guanylate cyclase, may be used as a last-resort attempt to increase SVR, without sufficient evidence as to improvement in outcome [16].

Left or Bi-ventricular Dysfunction

Diagnostic criteria and severity grading are given in table [29]. Inotropic and vasoactive drug selection should take several aspects into account:

- Potential β-1 adrenoceptor downregulation may be circumvened by use of adrenaline (β-1 and β-2 adrenoceptor agonist) and by addition of levosimendan, a combined PDE III inhibitor/calcium sensitizer. Evidence is still inconclusive, however, that levosimendan reduces cardiac surgical mortality in adults with LV dysfunction [36].

- If pulmonary hypertension and RV failure occur secondary to left heart problems, intravenous nitro-vasodilators (nitroglycerine, nitroprusside) reduce afterload and augment output of both ventricles, and should be preferred over selective pulmonary vasodilators (iNO), since the latter may provoke pulmonary edema when pulmonary venous pressure is high.
- Vasodilatory hypotension induced by inodilator drugs (isoproterenol, dobutamine, PDE III inhibitors, levosimendan) may require addition of an inopressor (noradrenaline). The aim is to restore MAP (>65 mmHg) while maintaining a sufficient cardiac index (>2.2–2.4 L/min/m^2), mixed venous SO_2 (>65%), receding lactate levels (<3 mmol/l) and satisfactory urine output (>0.5 ml/kg/h).

Persistent ischemic segmental wall motion abnormalities may indicate causes not amenable to inotropic stimulation. For instance, unappreciated coronary heart disease in a donor, or coronary dissection from coronarography or selective cardioplegia may be present. Additional CABG surgery, reperfusion and extended postoperative inotropic or mechanical cardiac support may be required.

Mechanical Circulatory Support (MCS) for Refractory Graft Failure

If graft failure develops on separation from CPB or postoperatively in ICU, despite exclusion of all correctable causes, and remains unresponsive to treatment with inotropes and vasoactives, MCS should be initiated early. Decisions should be made early in order to avoid ventricular distension, prolonged periods of low cardiac output and multi-organ damage. (Class I B) [21].

Depending on the stage the procedure is in (CPB cannulation in place or removed; chest open or closed) and location (OR or ICU), this is accomplished either after returning first to CPB, or by central or peripheral vascular access. Device selection depends on etiology and prognosis of graft failure, presence of concomitant pulmonary failure, and on institutional preferences.

Use of intraaortic balloon pump (IABP) reduces afterload of the LV and augments diastolic coronary perfusion of both ventricles. Since the normal RV myocardium depends on both diastolic and systolic perfusion, IABP may be more beneficial for LV than for RV recovery. Of note, recent studies in infarct-related cardiogenic shock did not find improved outcome with IABP use [37].

Veno-arterial ECMO affords immediate diastolic decompression and systolic unloading of the RV and the pulmonary circulation. It also reduces volume (but not pressure) workload of the LV. It supports respiratory gas exchange, and is therefore first choice if respiratory failure accompanies cardiac graft failure. ECMO has been used as initial modality of MCS (81%) in large single-center series [38]. Risks of bleeding due to anticoagulation and of infection are significant. If the heart does not eject, overdistension may be prevented by placing an LV vent surgically or via an Impella® pump (Abiomed). Central ECMO cannulation usually requires the chest to remain open, but allows rapid revision of bleeding complications. Cannulation through the chest or upper abdominal wall [29], or peripheral cannulation via femoral or axillary access allow earlier chest closure. This reduces the risk of infection under immunosuppression, but measures must be taken to provide distal limb perfusion. After early graft failure in adults, weaning from ECMO can be achieved in more than 80% [39], with survival at 30 days after transplantation ranging from 50% to 80% [40, 41]. In PGF after pediatric heart transplantation, ECMO is already considered first choice for MCS (Class IIa C) [21].

The RV can be mechanically assisted by insertion of a percutaneous RVAD, e.g., of a continuous-flow pump (Impella® RP Right Ventricular Assist Device, Abiomed), or with external RVAD (e.g., Levitronix CentriMag). Prerequisites are adequate pulmonary gas exchange and preserved LV function.

LVADs or biventricular assist devices require preserved pulmonary gas exchange, too. Some LVADs may be inserted percutaneously (paracorporeal systems like TandemHeart®, Impella® Cardiac Assist Device), with the advantage of relatively simple implantation, management and explantation [21]. Other temporary, continuous-flow VADs (e.g. Levitronix™ Centrimag) require surgical access and can provide temporary uni- or biventricular support [31].

Weaning from MCS is determined by graft recovery. Outcome is poor, for instance, if more than four days of ECMO support is required [42]. If graft function does not recover within 3–5 days, guidelines recommend to rule out hyperacute and antibody-mediated rejection and to consider institution of long-term mechanical circulatory support as a bridge to recovery, re-transplantation or destination [21].

Typical complications of MCS are stroke, infection, and bleeding, with an incidence in a range of 4% to 7% each, which increases with time on MCS [38].

Postoperative Bleeding and Coagulopathy

Cardiac transplantation carries a high risk of bleeding and massive transfusion particularly in the VAD era. Contributors are residual preoperative anticoagulation, hepatic dysfunction due to chronic venous congestion, extensive pre-CPB surgical dissection, and prolonged reperfusion on CPB. Quantitative and functional loss of plasma and platelets occurs regularly owing to shed blood reprocessing with cell saver machines, as well as to hemodilution, hypothermia and foreign surface activation.

If the post-transplant course is uneventful, and chest drain output has decreased adequately, postoperative anticoagulation is started with iv unfractionated heparin and aspirin, usually between 6 and 12 h after ICU admission. Severe postoperative bleeding, e.g., with chest drainage output during the initial 4 postoperative hours of more than 200 ml/h despite normal or improving coagulation parameters, requires surgical re-exploration.

If diffuse microvascular bleeding persists despite adequate surgical hemostasis and heparin reversal, differential diagnosis is made, combining rapid point-of-care thrombelastometry (viscoelastic clot analysis, e.g., ROTEM®, TEM International GmbH, D; TEG®, Haemonetics Corp., USA) with conventional coagulation tests. Efficacy of these tools in reducing transfusion exposure and morbidity in bleeding patients has been shown [43].

The available therapeutic armamentarium consists of packed red cell (PRBC) and platelet concentrates (PLT), FFP and cryoprecipitate, as well as stable factor concentrates like fibrinogen concentrate, 4-factor prothrombin complex concentrate (containing F. II, VII, IX, X, Proteins S,C, Z), F VIII, recombinant activated factor VII (rFVIIa) and factor XIII. Blood products should be leukocyte-depleted and negative for cytomegalovirus (CMV).

Goal-directed treatment is initiated according to evidence-based algorithms for transfusion and postoperative hemostasis. The detrimental triad of hypothermia (core T < 36 °C), acidosis (pH < 7.3) and ionized hypocalcemia (Ca^{++} < 1.1 mmol/l) must be avoided or treated aggressively [44]. Depending on comorbid risk (cerebrovascular, renal, pulmonary) and bleeding activity, hemoglobin levels are to be maintained between 80 and 90 g/l, platelet count at 100 G/l, and fibrinogen levels (Clauss) at 2.0–2.5 g/l (FIBTEM MCF, 12–14 mm [45]). Antifibrinolytics (tranexamic acid) may be re-introduced.

Overtransfusion carries the risk of transfusion-associated circulatory overload (TACO) and acute RV failure, particularly after cardiac transplantation. Only in emergency scenarios of uncontrolled blood loss, massive transfusion packages of PRBC and FFP (fixed ratio, 1:1 or 2:1) should be resorted to. Guidance of hemostatic therapy by viscoelastic point-of-care testing and transfusion algorithms should be resumed as soon as possible. Abrupt restoration of coagulation potential with prothrombin complex concentrate (PCC) and/or recombinant activated factor VII (rFVIIa) may increase the risk of thromboembolic complications. Use of both concentrates is "off label" in this situation, and should be reserved for rescue scenarios only after all evidence-based options have been exhausted.

Pericardial Effusion and Tamponade

Diagnosis and monitoring is by echocardiography (TTE, TEE). Hemodynamically significant effusions (hypotension, compression of cardiac chambers and equalization of filling pressures) should be drained surgically (Class I C). Effusions without hemodynamic compromise require drainage only if there is a strong suspicion of an infectious etiology (Class IIa C) [21]. Reexploration for any bleeding complications increases the risk of infection and sepsis in the immunosuppressed patient.

16.4.3 Respirator Weaning and Pulmonary Care

Respirator settings should use "low" tidal volumes of 6–7 ml/kg ideal body weight and a PEEP (usually about 5 mbar) sufficient to maintain functional residual capacity (FRC) of the lungs. Cautious lung recruitment maneuvers may be necessary to counteract dependent alveolar collapse. Respirator settings should aim to avoid pulmonary barotrauma, volutrauma, and to prevent negative effects of atelectasis, i.e., pulmonary shunting, alveolar trauma, increased PVR and reduced efficacy of inhaled vasodilators. Initially, mild hypocapnia ($PaCO_2$ 32–35 mmHg) should be maintained by adjusting respirator rate rather than tidal volume.

Respirator weaning should be started as soon as both systemic and pulmonary hemodynamics are stable over several hours. Transition to assisted ventilation modes and then to spontaneous respiration, extubation, and if necessary transient support by non-invasive ventilation techniques are managed as after other cardiac surgeries. Pulmonary vasodilator treatment can be changed, after extubation, to aerosolized iloprost inhaler and/or to orally administered sildenafil.

Recurrent atelectasis and pleural effusions are common. They may require intensive chest physiotherapy and diuretics, or even bronchoscopy, endobronchial suctioning, or additional drainage. Aggressive diagnosis and anti-infectious therapy is required if pneumonia is ruled in. Prolonged perioperative requirement of ventilator, dialysis or VAD support is associated with increased risk of early graft failure and infection [4].

16.4.4 Imaging and Laboratory Testing

On ICU admission, and usually daily thereafter during ICU stay, chest radiograms are taken to assess position of catheters, leads and drains, and to monitor for pneumothorax, atelectasis, pleural effusion, interstitial edema, and infiltrates. Also, echocardiography is performed daily to assess biventricular function, valves and volemia, and to monitor for pericardial and pleural effusion.

Laboratory testing includes, initially, measurement of hemoglobin, blood cell count, arterial and mixed venous blood gas analysis, electrolyte, glucose and lactate several times per day. Depending on center routines, cardiac enzymes, liver and kidney function parameters, coagulation profile, as well as trough levels of immunosuppressants, antibiotics and antiarrhythmics are monitored daily in the early postoperative period. T cell counts, microbiology samples (tracheal secretions, urine), fungal serology and lipid profile are taken twice or once a week.

16.4.5 Infection Control and Antimicrobial Therapy

Recommendations for isolation of solid organ graft recipients are largely based on expert opinion. Reverse isolation and other protected environments are not considered necessary for prevention of infection in solid-organ transplant recipients [46]. On ICU, patients should be nursed separately from other patients, using ICU hygiene precautions (cap, mask, gown, non-sterile gloves, hand washing and disinfection before and after patient care). Institutional practice varies, however, with some centers using reverse isolation in single-bed rooms. Recipients should be equipped with special masks when transported through high-risk areas within the hospital [46].

Perioperative antibiotic prophylaxis, usually with a second-generation cephalosporine active against staphylococcus species, is continued from its preoperative initiation until 48 h, with specific antimicrobial therapy thereafter as required. In case of preexisting infections in recipient or donor, perioperative antibiotic prophylaxis should be selected according to results of sensitivity testing.

In the first weeks after transplantation, bacterial are more common than viral respiratory infections. CMV infection occurs mostly after the first month. CMV prophylaxis is adapted to CMV serologic status of donor and recipient, and is started within 24–48 h after transplantation (Class I A). Also, early postoperative initiation of anti-protozoal prophylaxis is recommended against *Pneumocystis jiroveci*, usually with trimethoprim-sulfamethoxazole [21].

Recipients should have fungal colonization diagnosed or excluded prior to transplantation (Class I B) [47]. Antifungal prophylaxis against mucocutaneous candidiasis (e.g., topical nystatin) is initiated after extubation. Also, prophylaxis with aerosolized amphotericin B during the early post-transplant period appears safe and efficacious [47]. More than half of the invasive fungal infections (Candida and Aspergillus species) occur during the first 3 months after transplantation. Aggressive diagnosis and systemic treatment is required in these immunosuppressed patients.

16.4.6 Renal Dysfunction

Heart transplant recipients are at increased risk of acute kidney injury (AKI). Contributing factors are multiple, i.e., preexisting renal impairment, perioperative hypoperfusion, vasoconstrictor drugs, anemia, hemodilution, transfusion, hemolysis, and renal toxicity of immunosuppressants (e.g., calcineurin inhibitors like cyclosporine, tacrolimus).

Preventive measures are adequate hydration with balanced crystalloid solutions (Ringer's solution) and intravascular normovolemia (blood products, if indicated). CVP should be maintained between 5 and 12 mmHg. Cardiac output, hemoglobin concentration, oxygenation and mean arterial pressure should be optimized such as to provide adequate systemic and renal oxygen delivery [48].

Hydroxyethyl starch solutions have been shown to interfere with renal function and hemostasis and should be avoided. Normal saline causes hyperchloremic acidosis with renal vasoconstriction, and should not be used as a rehydration fluid. Radiocontrast dye exposure should be minimized to avoid contrast-induced nephropathy. For instance, DSE or CT coronary angiography might be considered instead of invasive coronary angiography. Evidence of renal protection against postoperative acute kidney injury by agents like dopamine, fenoldopam, dopexamin, mannitol, bicarbonate, or N-acetylcysteine is poor or lacking [48].

Oligo-anuria of less than 0.5 ml/kg/h is an early symptom of renal dysfunction and impending injury, but neither very sensitive nor specific. The subsequent rise in serum creatinine occurs rather late for timely intervention. As a perspective, rapidly responding urinary biomarkers of acute kidney injury, e.g., tissue inhibitor metalloproteinase-2 (TIMP-2) and/or insulin-like growth factor (IGF)-binding protein-7 (IGFBP7), may help in the future to detect impending kidney injury early enough for timely intervention [48].

If there is significant preoperative renal insufficiency or postoperative functional deterioration, dose and dosing intervals of nephrotoxic agents, e.g., antibiotics and immunosuppressants, need to be adjusted according to eGFR. Nephrotoxic calcineurin inhibitors may be replaced with a renal-sparing alternative, e.g., everolimus.

Postoperative volume overload is treated, first, by intermittent or continuous stimulation of urine output with loop diuretics. Thiazide diuretics and aldosterone antagonists may be added. If the recipient remains or becomes oligo-anuric despite consequent hemodynamic resuscitation, hydration and stimulation, consideration should be given to early renal replacement therapy (RRT) (Class I B). Continuous veno-venous hemofiltration (CVVH) allows hemodynamically well controlled volume removal. Both negative fluid balance and renal replacement are achieved with continuous hemodiafiltration (CVVHD) in hemodynamically unstable patients, and with hemodialysis in stable patients. There is growing evidence that early initiation of RRT for cardiac surgical or critically ill patients with AKI is associated with lower perioperative mortality [49, 50]. Nevertheless, need of post-transplant dialysis is a major risk factor for perioperative and long-term mortality.

16.4.7 Glycemic Control and Nutritional Support

Hyperglycemia, e.g. from cardioplegia, perioperative stress, catecholamines and glucocorticoids, and hypoglycemia, e.g. from "tight" glycemic control, are both associated with inferior outcome [51]. Postoperative blood glucose levels should be kept between 100–150 mg/dl with continuous short-acting insulin infusion on ICU, and conventional euglycemic management thereafter. Vitamine and thyroid hormone substitution may be indicated. Gastroenteral tube feeding with a low caloric intake is usually started early, e.g., on the 2nd postoperative day.

16.4.8 Immunosuppression and Rejection

Depending on transplant center policy, azathioprine 5 mg/kg iv is given preoperatively. Methylprednisolone 1000 mg iv is usually administered prior to reperfusion. Antithymocyte globulin therapy may be introduced between 4 and 12 h operatively, especially in patients at high risk of renal dysfunction. For standard maintenance immunosuppression, a triple combination of the calcineurin inhibitor tacrolimus with mycophenolate mofetil and prednisone is used (as of 2014) in more than 90% of the recipients [5]. In case of progressive impairment of renal function, everolimus may replace calcineurin inhibitors [52].

Significant side effects of immunosuppressant agents for this period are listed in Table 16.3.

Table 16.3 Significant side effects of common immunosuppressants

Agent	Mechanism	Major side effects
Corticosteriods	↓cytokine production, ↓leukocyte chemotaxis, ↓T-cell activation	Hyperglycemia, hypertension, adrenal suppression, peptic ulcer, myopathy, osteoporosis
Azathioprine	↓DNA synthesis, ↓lymphocyte proliferation	Leukopenia, thrombopenia, hepatotoxicity, cholestasis
Mycophenolate mofetil	↓DNA synthesis, ↓lymphocyte proliferation	Leukopenia, GI symptoms
Cyclosporine	↓ T-cell proliferation	Nephrotoxicity, hepatotoxicity, neurotoxicity hypertension, hyperkalemia
Tacrolimus	↓ T-cell activation	Nephrotoxicity, hypertension, hyperkalemia, hyperglycemia, anemia
Antilymphocyte globulin	↑T-cell opsonization & lysis	Anaphylaxis, leukopenia, thrombopenia, fever, hypotension, hepatitis
OKT3	↑T-cell opsonization & lysis	Hypotension, bronchospasm, pulmonary edema, fever, aseptic meningitis, seizures
Rapamycin	↑T-cell apoptosis	Joint pain/swelling, tremor, rash, fever, GI symptoms

↓ reduces/inhibits ↑increases/promotes

16.4.8.1 Hyperacute Rejection

Hyperacute rejection is a rare but catastrophic complication in the immediate reperfusion period [53, 54]. It is mediated by preformed cytotoxic antibodies in the recipient against donor human leukocyte antigen (HLA) antigens. Sensitization of the recipient to major histocompatibility complex (MHC) antigens may have had occurred during previous allogeneic transfusion or transplantation, or to fetal paternal antigens during pregnancy. Already on early clinical assessment during reperfusion in the OR, the graft appears livid due to microvascular thrombosis, and never resumes or rapidly loses its function. Inotrope and vasopressor support typically prove futile, and the patient returns to full mechanical circulatory support (MCS). An intraoperative EMB is obtained for diagnosis. Treatment should start immediately in the OR. It includes high-dose corticosteroids, plasmapheresis, intravenous immunoglobulin and a combination of iv immunosuppressants (e.g., tacrolimus, MMF) (Class IC) [21]. The patient usually remains on MCS as a bridge to retransplantation until a new donor organ can be found, or to destination.

16.4.8.2 Acute Allograft Rejection

Acute rejection (AR) is a (mostly T-cell mediated) immune response to donor histocompatibility antigens in graft myocardium, and accounts for less than 0.5% of 30-day mortality [4]. Risk is associated with extent of HLA mismatch and the immunosuppressive regimen, and is increased with younger recipient age and female sex. AR occurs most frequently within the first year after transplantation. Initial symptoms are non-specific (fatigue, dyspnea, palpitation), while TTE reveals deterioration of LV function. Endomyocardial biopsy (EMB) remains the current standard in surveillance for and diagnosis of AR. A weekly EMB schedule starts in the first postoperative week. EMB is an invasive procedure performed under local anesthesia, usually via a right-sided transjugular approach, in the catheterization laboratory. Damage to the tricuspid valve or chordae is a known complication, with an incidence of less than 1% [55].

The management of antibody mediated rejection (AMR) in heart transplantation is so far not fully standardized. It relies on criteria based on pathology, antibody status and deteriorating ejection fraction. Oral steroid dose may be increased or switched to IV. Intravenous immunoglobulin and plasmapheresis may be initiated [56], or other immunosuppressants are added.

Disclosures B. Eberle MD declares no conflict of interest.
H. Kaiser MD declares no conflict of interest.

References

1. Lund LH, Edwards LB, Kucheryavaya AY, et al. The registry of the International Society for Heart and Lung Transplantation: thirty-second official adult Heart Transplantation Report – 2015; Focus theme: early graft failure. J Heart Lung Transplant. 2015;34(10):1244–54.
2. Madan S, Saeed O, Shin J, et al. Donor troponin and survival after cardiac transplantation: an analysis of the United Network of organ sharing registry. Circ Heart Fail. 2016;9(6):e002909.
3. Trivedi JR, Cheng A, Ising M, et al. Heart transplant survival based on recipient and donor risk scoring: a UNOS database analysis. ASAIO J. 2016; https://doi.org/10.1097/MAT.0000000000000337. Publish Ahead of Print
4. Wever-Pinzon O, Edwards LB, Taylor DO, et al. Association of recipient age and causes of heart transplant mortality: implications for personalization of post-transplant management-An analysis of the International Society for Heart and Lung Transplantation Registry. J Heart Lung Transplant. 2016; https://doi.org/10.1016/j.healun.2016.08.008. [Epub ahead of print]
5. Lund LH, Edwards LB, Dipchand AI, et al. The registry of the International Society for Heart and Lung Transplantation: thirty-third Adult Heart Transplantation Report-2016; Focus theme: primary diagnostic indications for transplant. J Heart Lung Transplant. 2016;35(10):1158–69.
6. Linkins LA, Dans AL, Moores LK, et al. Treatment and prevention of heparin-induced thrombocyte-penia: antithrombotic therapy and prevention of thrombosis, 9th ed: American College of Chest Physicians Evidence-Based Clinical Practice Guidelines. Chest. 2012;141(2 Suppl):e495S–530S.
7. Söhle M, et al. Neuromonitoring in der Kardioanästhesie. Eine gemeinsame Stellungnahme der Deutschen Gesellschaft fur Anästhesiologie und Intensivmedizin (DGAI) und der Deutschen Gesellschaft für Thorax-, Herz- und Gefäßchirurgie (DGTHG). Anästh Intensivmed. 2014;55:2–19.
8. Engelman R, Shahian D, Shemin R, et al. The Society of Thoracic Surgeons practice guideline series: antibiotic prophylaxis in cardiac surgery, part II: antibiotic choice. Ann Thorac Surg. 2007;83(4):1569–76.
9. Lador A, Nasir H, Mansur N, et al. Antibiotic prophylaxis in cardiac surgery: systematic review and meta-analysis. J Antimicrob Chemother. 2012;67:541–50.
10. Massad MG, Cook DJ, Schmitt SK, et al. Factors influencing HLA sensitization in implantable LVAD recipients. Ann Thorac Surg. 1997;64:1120–5.
11. Treleaven J, Gennery A, Marsh J, et al. Guidelines on the use of irradiated blood components prepared by the British Committee for Standards in Haematology blood transfusion task force. Br J Haematol. 2011;152:35–51.
12. Pritchard AE, Shaz BH. Survey of irradiation practice for the prevention of transfusion-Associated graft-versus-host disease. Arch Pathol Lab Med. 2016;140(10):1092–7.
13. Ranucci M, Aloisio T, Carboni G, et al. Acute kidney injury and hemodilution during cardiopulmonary bypass: a changing scenario. Ann Thorac Surg. 2015;100(1):95–100.
14. Myles PS, Smith JA, Forbes A, et al. Tranexamic acid in patients undergoing coronary-artery surgery. N Engl J Med. 2016;376(2):136–48. [Epub ahead of print]
15. Grigore AM, Grocott HP, Mathew JP, et al. The rewarming rate and increased peak temperature alter neurocognitive outcome after cardiac surgery. Anesth Analg. 2002;94(1):4–10.
16. Belletti A, Musu M, Silvetti S, et al. Non-Adrenergic vasopressors in patients with or at risk for vasodilatory shock. a systematic review and meta-analysis of randomized trials. PLoS One. 2015;10:e0142605.
17. Manecke GR Jr, Parimucha M, Stratmann G, et al. Deep hypothermic circulatory arrest and the femoral-to-radial arterial pressure gradient. J Cardiothorac Vasc Anesth. 2004;18:175–9.
18. Price LC, Wort SJ, Finney SJ, et al. Pulmonary vascular and right ventricular dysfunction in adult critical care: current and emerging options for management: a systematic literature review. Crit Care. 2010;14(5):R169.
19. Bonet LA, Guillén RV, Lázaro IS, et al. Intravenous sildenafil in right ventricular dysfunction with pulmonary hypertension following a heart transplant. Heart Int. 2014;9:22–5.
20. Denault AY, Bussières JS, Arellano R, et al. A multicentre randomized-controlled trial of inhaled milrinone in high-risk cardiac surgical patients. Can J Anaesth. 2016;63:1140–53.
21. Costanzo MR, et al. The International Society of Heart and Lung Transplantation Guidelines for the care of heart transplant recipients. J Heart Lung Transplant. 2010;29:914–56.
22. Mondillo S, Maccherini M, Galderisi M. Usefulness and limitations of transthoracic echocardiography in heart transplantation recipients. Cardiovasc Ultrasound. 2008;6:2.
23. Stengel S, Allemann Y, Zimmerli M, et al. Doppler tissue imaging for assessing left ventricular diastolic dysfunction in heart transplant rejection. Heart. 2001;86:432–7.
24. Walmrath D, Schneider T, Schermuly R, et al. Direct comparison of inhaled nitric oxide and aerosolized prostacyclin in acute respiratory distress syndrome. Am J Respir Crit Care Med. 1996;153:991–6.
25. Hoeper MM, Schwarze M, Ehlerding S, et al. Long-term treatment of primary pulmonary hypertension with aerosolized iloprost, a prostacyclin analogue. N Engl J Med. 2000;342:1866–70.
26. Ghofrani HA, Rose F, Schermuly RT, et al. Oral sildenafi l as long-term adjunct therapy to inhaled iloprost in severe pulmonary arterial hypertension. J Am Coll Cardiol. 2003;42:158–64.
27. Haraldsson SA, Kieler-Jensen N, Ricksten SE. The additive pulmonary vasodilatory effects of inhaled prostacyclin and inhaled milrinone in postcardiac surgical patients with pulmonary hypertension. Anesth Analg. 2001;93:1439–45.
28. Laflamme M, Perrault LP, Carrier M, et al. Preliminary experience with combined inhaled milrinone and prostacyclin in cardiac surgical patients with pulmonary hypertension. J Cardiothorac Vasc Anesth. 2015;29:38–45.
29. Kobashigawa J, Zuckermann A, Macdonald P, et al. Report from a consensus conference on primary graft dysfunction after cardiac transplantation. J Heart Lung Transplant. 2014;33(4):327–40.
30. Cosío Carmena MD, Gómez Bueno M, Almenar L, et al. Primary graft failure after heart transplantation: characteristics in a contemporary cohort and performance of the RADIAL risk score. J Heart Lung Transplant. 2013;32:1187–95.
31. Thomas HL, Dronavalli VB, Parameshwar J, et al. Steering group of the UK cardiothoracic transplant audit. Incidence and outcome of Levitronix CentriMag support as rescue therapy for early cardiac allograft failure: a United Kingdom national study. Eur J Cardiothorac Surg. 2011;40:1348.
32. Dronavalli VB, Rogers CA, Banner NR. Primary cardiac allograft dysfunction-validation of a clinical definition. Transplantation. 2015;99:1919–25.
33. Hosenpud JD, Bennett LE, Keck BM, et al. The registry of the International Society for Heart and Lung Transplantation:

seventeenth official report-2000. J Heart Lung Transplant. 2000;19:909–31.
34. Stobierska-Dzierzek B, Awad H, Michler RE. The evolving management of acute right-sided heart failure in cardiac transplant recipients. J Am Coll Cardiol. 2001;38:923–31.
35. Antoniou T, Koletsis EN, Prokakis C, et al. Hemodynamic effects of combination therapy with inhaled nitric oxide and iloprost in patients with pulmonary hypertension and right ventricular dysfunction after high-risk cardiac surgery. J Cardiothorac Vasc Anesth. 2013;27:459–66.
36. Wang B, He X, Gong Y, Cheng B. Levosimendan in Patients with Left Ventricular Dysfunction Undergoing Cardiac Surgery: An Update Meta-Analysis and Trial Sequential Analysis. Biomed Res Int. 2018. https://doi.org/10.1155/2018/7563083.
37. Unverzagt S, Buerke M, de Waha A, et al. Intra-aortic balloon pump counterpulsation (IABP) for myocardial infarction complicated by cardiogenic shock. Cochrane Database Syst Rev. 2015;3:CD007398.
38. Mihaljevic T, Jarretta CM, Gonzalez-Stawinskia G, et al. Mechanical circulatory support after heart transplantation. Eur J Cardiothorac Surg. 2012;41:200–6.
39. Lima EB, Cunha CR, Barzilai VS, et al. Experience of ECMO in primary graft dysfunction after orthotopic heart transplantation. Arq Bras Cardiol. 2015;105:285–91.
40. D'Alessandro C, Aubert S, Golmard JL, Praschker BL, et al. Extracorporeal membrane oxygenation temporary support for early graft failure after cardiac transplantation. Eur J Cardiothorac Surg. 2010;37:343–9.
41. Lehmann S, Uhlemann M, Etz CD, et al. Extracorporeal membrane oxygenation: experience in acute graft failure after heart transplantation. Clin Transpl. 2014;28(7):789–96.
42. Chou NK, Chi NH, Wu IW, et al. Extracoporeal membrane oxygenation to rescue cardiopulmonary failure after heart transplantation: a single-center experience. Transplant Proc. 2010;42:943–5.
43. Wikkelsø A, Wetterslev J, Møller AM, Afshari A. Thromboelastography (TEG) or thromboelastometry (ROTEM) to monitor haemostatic treatment versus usual care in adults or children with bleeding. Cochrane Database Syst Rev. 2016;8:CD007871.
44. Rossaint R, Bouillon B, Cerny V, et al. The European guideline on management of major bleeding and coagulopathy following trauma: fourth edition. Crit Care. 2016;20:100. https://doi.org/10.1186/s13054-016-1265-x.
45. Ranucci M, Baryshnikova E. Fibrinogen supplementation after cardiac surgery: insights from the Zero-Plasma trial (ZEPLAST). Br J Anaesth. 2016;116(5):618–23.
46. Soave R. Prophylaxis strategies for solid-organ transplantation. Clin Infect Dis. 2001;33(Suppl 1(s1)):S26–31.
47. Husain S, Sole A, Alexander BD, et al. The 2015 International Society for Heart and Lung Transplantation Guidelines for the management of fungal infections in mechanical circulatory support and cardiothoracic organ transplant recipients: executive summary. J Heart Lung Transplant. 2016;35(3):261–82.
48. Zarbock A, Milles K. Novel therapy for renal protection. Curr Opin Anaesthesiol. 2015;28(4):431–8.
49. Liu Y, Davari-Farid S, Arora P, et al. Early versus late initiation of renal replacement therapy in critically ill patients with acute kidney injury after cardiac surgery: a systematic review and meta-analysis. J Cardiothorac Vasc Anesth. 2014;28:557–63.
50. Zarbock A, Kellum JA, Schmidt C, et al. Effect of early vs delayed initiation of renal replacement therapy on mortality in critically Ill patients with acute kidney injury: the ELAIN randomized clinical trial. JAMA. 2016;315(20):2190–9.
51. Johnston LE, Kirby JL, Downs EA, et al. Postoperative hypoglycemia is associated with worse outcomes after cardiac operations. Ann Thorac Surg. 2016; https://doi.org/10.1016/j.athoracsur.2016.05.121. [Epub ahead of print]
52. Lesche D, Sigurdardottir V, Setoud R, et al. Influence of CYP3A5 genetic variation on everolimus maintenance dosing after cardiac transplantation. Clin Transpl. 2015;29(12):1213–20.
53. Kemnitz J, et al. Hyperacute rejection in heart allografts. Pathol Res Pract. 1991;187:23–9.
54. Michaels PJ, et al. Humoral rejection in cardiac transplantation: risk factors, hemodynamic consequences and relationship to transplant coronary artery disease. J Heart Lung Transplant. 2003;22:58–69.
55. Strecker T, Rösch J, Weyand M, Agaimy A. Endomyocardial biopsy for monitoring heart transplant patients: 11-years-experience at a german heart center. Int J Clin Exp Pathol. 2013;6(1):55–65.
56. Chih S, Tinckam KJ, Ross HJ. A survey of current practice for antibody-mediated rejection in heart transplantation. Am J Transplant. 2013;13:1069–74.

Organ Preservation and Implantation

17

Friedhelm Beyersdorf and Johannes Scheumann

17.1 Introduction

On December 3, 2017 there will be the 50th Anniversary of the first successful human heart transplantation held in Cape Town, South Africa. While it was a revolutionary operation in 1967, it is nowadays a routine treatment with over 2500 heart transplants are performed annually and still the gold standard for patients in terminal heart failure.

Even though there are still many drawbacks after transplantation, e.g. rejection, infection, severe side effects of immunosuppressive drugs, limited very long-term results (mostly due to chronic rejection or chronic transplantation atherosclerosis) [12], it still represents a much better quality of life as compared to the alternative treatment of implantation of left ventricular assist devices (LVAD) [11]. Heart transplantation remains the gold standard therapy for end-stage heart failure patients [34], even though the short and medium-term results (2–4 years follow-up) of most current LVADs are very promising [26, 38] and are improving steadily.

Currently the worldwide major problem with transplantation is donor organ shortage and – at the same time – the increased incidence of terminal heart failure. In certain countries (e.g. Germany) there is an up to 5 year waiting time on the transplant list for the "T" status. Even for High Urgency (HU) patients waiting time over 6 months for certain blood groups (type B) is not unusual.

This shortage of donors has led to an interest in both, usage of marginal donors and organ donation after circulatory death (DCD). DCD hearts were already used in the first human heart transplant in 1967 [4]. Recently Dhital et al. have reported successful transplantation of DCD hearts in 4 patients [8]. Further experimental studies are being carried out in order to improve the current results [24]. In addition reperfusion modifications were applied in these studies (e.g. reperfusion solution that included adenosine, cyclosporine, and an acid pH) showing excellent results in the machine perfusion and controlled reperfusion group [23].

The acceptance of so-called "marginal donors" is also increasingly discussed and more and more used in order to prevent an even higher mortality rate on the HTX waiting list or to avoid implantation of mechanical circulatory assist devices as the last option for deteriorating patients. Many patients on the HU list try to avoid by any means the implantation of an LVAD, because they know that they will loose their HU status after an uneventful LVAD implantation. The prolonged waiting period results in several cases in a very critical hemodynamic status for a long period of time, making any transplantation difficult – if not impossible.

Organ preservation and the implantation technique are therefore of utmost importance and will be described in detail in the next paragraphs.

17.2 Different Definitions of Ischemic Tolerance

The general term "ischemic tolerance" usually describes the duration of complete ischemia after which survival of cells or organs is possible.

However there are at least three completely different situations where the term "ischemic tolerance" can and will be used:

- Normal blood reperfusion is reestablished after a period of ischemia, i.e. "ischemic tolerance with normal blood reperfusion" (ISTO-BLOREP). This is the most often used definition for "ischemic tolerance".
- Duration of cellular integrity during ischemia without any reperfusion; i.e. duration of cell membrane stability, mitochondrial integrity, etc.

F. Beyersdorf (✉) · J. Scheumann
Department of Cardiovascular Surgery, University Heart Center Freiburg, Freiburg, Germany
e-mail: Friedhelm.beyersdorf@universitaets-herzzentrum.de

D. S. Feldman, P. Mohacsi (eds.), *Heart Failure*, Cardiovascular Medicine, https://doi.org/10.1007/978-3-319-98184-0_17

Table 17.1 Time differences of ischemic tolerance of cells without reperfusion, with normal blood reperfusion and controlled reperfusion

	ISTO-BLOREP	ISTO-NOREP	ISTO-COREP
Neurologic tissue (e.g. brain cells) (min)	3–5 Astrup et al. [3]	60 Hossmann et al. [17]	20 Taunyane et al. [31]
Cardiac muscle cells (h)	<2 Allen et al. [1]	6 Sjöstrand et al. [30]	6 Allen et al. [1]
Skeletal muscle cells (h)	<6 Beyersdorf et al. [6]	6 Beyersdorf et al. [6]	>6 Mitrev et al. [22]

ISTO-BLOREP
ISTO-NOREP
ISTO-COREP

- This "ischemic tolerance without reperfusion" (ISTO-NOREP) is always longer than the "ischemic tolerance with normal blood reperfusion" (Table 17.1). In other words the initial reperfusion period with normal blood poses an additional (reperfusion) injury to the damage already imposed by ischemia [10].
- Instead of using normal blood as the initial reperfusate after an ischemic insult, an alternative approach is to treat the damaged cells during the initial reperfusion period (20–30 min) by modifying the conditions of reperfusion (i.e. blood pressure, flow, temperature, etc.) and the composition of the initial reperfusate (i.e. calcium, osmolarity, pH, oxygen content, etc.). This treatment is known as "controlled reperfusion" [5, 7]. Ischemic tolerance after controlled reperfusion (ISTO-COREP) is significantly longer as compared to the ischemic tolerance after normal blood reperfusion (ISTO-BLOREP) (Table 17.1).

Therefore, in order to prolong the viability of organs after an ischemic insult, different strategies can be used:

1. Protecting the heart during explantation, transport and implantation
2. Avoid or at least shorten the ischemic period
3. Treat the ischemically damaged organ by a period of controlled reperfusion

17.3 Organ Preservation During Explantation, Transport and Implantation

Crystalloid cardioplegia is the method of choice for myocardial protection during explantation in most centers. This is almost always followed by cold storage in ice using different bags. During implantation various forms of maintaining a cold environment (ice slush, ice pads, etc.) are being used. This cold ischemic storage has been the method of choice for myocardial preservation since the beginning of HTX in 1967.

17.4 Organ Preservation by Ex-vivo-Perfusion During Transport

The technique of ex-vivo (machine) perfusion was already used in the 60ies and 70ies of the last century in order to achieve optimal conservation of organs for transplantation. With the development of organ-specific storage solutions in the 80ies, the quality of preservation increased significantly and the more cumbersome machine perfusion techniques were abandoned. However with the increased use of marginal donors there is now a revival of the machine perfusion techniques. The optimal perfusion technique should allow:

- Long preservation of marginal organs
- Viability testing of organs before transplantation, and
- Treatment/resuscitation of organs between explantation and implantation

In order to improve the quality of myocardial preservation and decrease ischemia during transport, attempts were made during the last decade to perfuse explanted organs instead of using cold ischemic storage [20]. These perfusion machines are in clinical use for kidney, lung and heart transplantation.

The use of kidney perfusion machines is in routine use in case of a cardiac arrested donor with the aim not only to decrease ischemic time but also to assess the quality of the organ [20].

In lung transplantation, ex vivo perfusion is used to resuscitate marginal lungs [20]. A recent retrospective study from Toronto and Lausanne has shown that the ischemic tolerance with normal blood reperfusion (ISTO-BLOREP) can be doubled by a normothermic perfusion (ex vivo perfusion) and ventilation of the lungs in between cooling phases for ex-and implantation [37]. In addition a significant reduction in severe primary lung-transplant-dysfunction was seen in the prospective, randomized INSPIRE-Trial [36].

The Organ Care System (OCS, Transmedics Co.) (Fig. 17.1) is the only perfusion machine clinically available for HTX. The quality of perfusion of the cardiac allograft is assessed by (a) measuring the mean aortic pressure and the coronary blood flow and by (b) comparing inflow and outflow serum lactate concentrations. When the metabolism of the cardiac allograft remains anaerobic, this is a strong indicator for onging ischemic despite perfusion [16, 20].

Several studies have been published showing improved outcomes after OCS usage as compared to cold storage [13, 14, 19]. A randomized study (PROCEED II trial) showed no

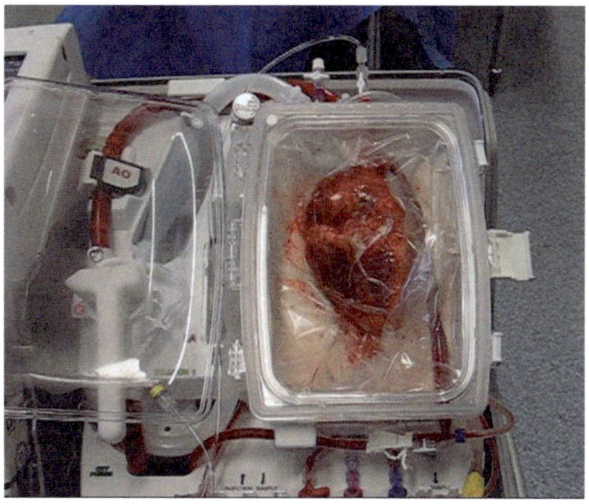

Fig. 17.1 The transport unit of the Organ Care System with ex vivo perfusion of a human heart (University of Freiburg, Germany). (analog Fig. 17.1 aus [20])

significant differences between the OCS and the cold storage groups (and non-inferiority of the OCS group) including only non-marginal donors [2]. However in this study the total preservation time was significantly longer for the OCS group (324 min) compared to the cold ischemic group (195 min), i.e. OCS was able to generate the same good results even after longer ex vivo preservation [2].

In addition, animal studies [15, 18, 32, 33, 35] as well as clinical reports [8, 20] have shown the superiority of the OCS in cases of organ donation after circulatory death.

Nevertheless, prerequisites for the usage of this promising new method of organ preservation is the need for proper experience and a high number cases with OCS usage for the whole team.

17.5 Implantation Techniques

The implantation procedure covers the preparation of the recipient, the implantation of the graft as well as the initial reperfusion period and the phase after the cardiopulmonary bypass (CPB) has been stopped. Heart transplantation should be a well-organized event [28] and attention to every detail of the procedure is of utmost importance.

During heart implantation, the goal is to allow a safe and anatomical correct implantation. Little has been changed from the initial procedure used by Lower and Shumway in dogs in the late 1950s and early 1960s [21]. However in most centers the original standard method is being replaced by the bicaval technique [25, 29], which is characterized by 2 arterial, 1 left atrial and 2 caval anastomoses, preserving the right atrium intact and leaving only a small posterior part of recipient left atrial tissue between both pulmonary veins [27].

17.5.1 Preparation of the Recipient

A majority (> 50%) of the current recipients of heart allografts had undergone one, two or even more cardiac operations before the transplantation (e.g. coronary artery bypass grafting, valve operations, LVAD implantation, etc.). Therefore dissection of the chest and removal of the diseased heart may be a difficult and time-consuming part of the transplantation. The entire timetable of the procurement, transport and arrival in the hospital is an important logistical part in order to avoid unnecessary ischemia for the donated organ. Machine perfusion allows the best timing in terms of shorting the ischemic period in those cases.

In those patients with previous cardiac operations, only the aorta and the right atrium need to be dissected before cannulation. However in order to avoid long perfusion times on cardiopulmonary bypass (CPB) and improve hemostasis before the implantation starts, it is often beneficial – when possible – to dissect the heart as much as possible without CPB and without heparinization. During this maneuver special attention has to be paid to avoid potential embolization of thrombotic material often present in the dilated left ventricle or left atrium. Even if the donor heart is not in the operating room (OR) the extra time can be spend on a meticulous hemostasis of the recipient and the chest can be packed with sponges.

Due to previous cardiac operations and the necessity to have a rather long aortic segment for the anastomosis, aortic cannulation is usually performed with an aortic arch cannula using the Seldinger technique. Venous cannulation is done with separate very distal cannulation of the superior vena cava (26 F in diameter) in order to allow a conveniend anastomosis in the bicaval technique. Cannulation of the inferior vena cava via the right atrium is performed in an area that is not too thin walled (cannula usually 28F in diameter). Both venae cavae are transsected 2/3 of their circumference and a strip of the backwall of the right atrium is left in place to avoid complete retraction of the venae cavae.

17.5.2 Preparation of the Donor Heart

The pulmonary artery and the aorta from the donor heart are being separated (Fig. 17.2). The pulmonary artery is trimmed just proximal to its bifurcation and the aorta is trimmed just proximal to the takeoff of the innominate artery [28]. The pulmonary veins are being identified and connected to create a left atrial cuff. In the bicaval technique the superior vena cava is left as long as possible.

The fossa ovalis is always examined for a patent foramen ovale. If present it is closed with 4–0 monofilament polypropylene running suture in two layers.

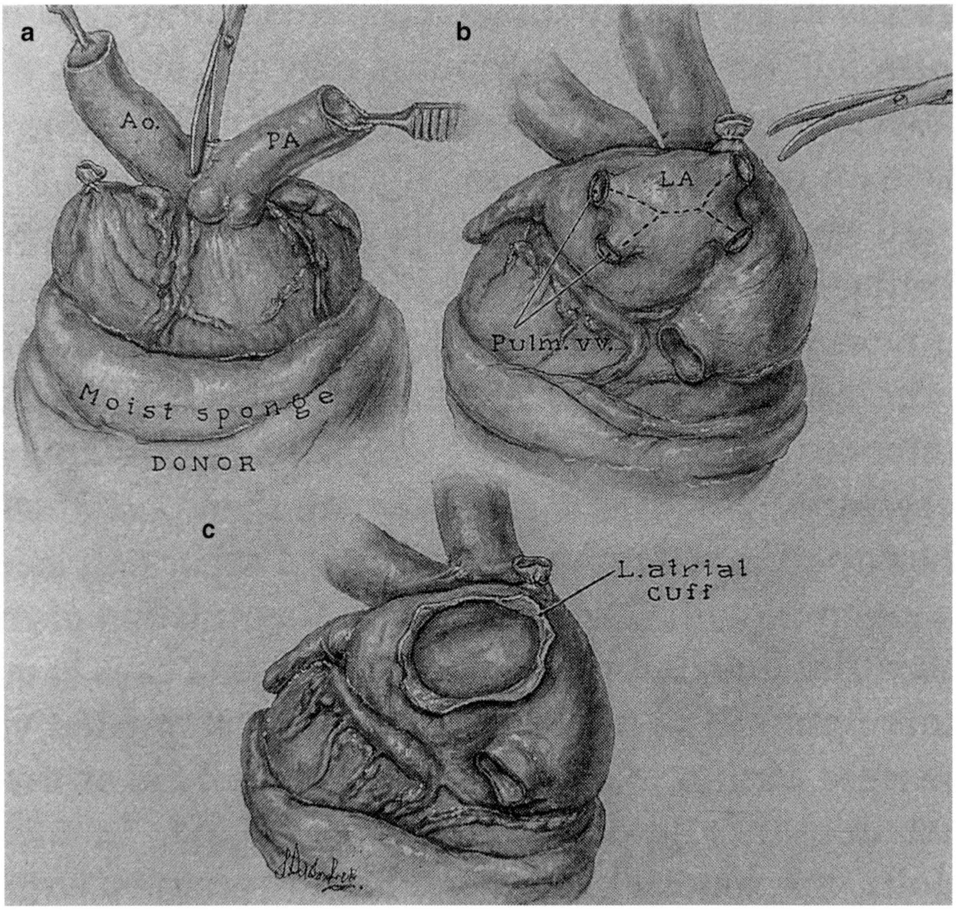

Fig. 17.2 Preparation of the donor heart. (Reproduced from Fig. 15.2 from Shumway and Shumway, p. 164)

17.5.3 Explantation of the Recipient's Heart

Before total cardiopulmonary bypass is established, the operative field is continuously flushed with carbon dioxide (CO2).

After clamping the ascending aorta, the native right atrium is opened anteriorly and a cardiotomy sucker is inserted. Then the left atrium is opened via the foramen oval and the sucker is placed in the left atrium. Thereafter the aorta and the pulmonary artery are divided just above the anulus (Fig. 17.3). This will allow preparation of the aortic and pulmonary valve from the diseased explanted heart and later usage as homografts.

As the next step, the incision in the right atrium is extended inferiorly toward and then into the coronary sinus. Care has to be taken to completely remove the coronary sinus to prevent later bleeding from collaterals connecting with the coronary sinus. For the bicaval technique, the right atrium is trimmed as much as possible, but the backwall of the right atrium is left in place, in order to avoid a retraction of the superior and inferior vena cava, which might occur after complete circumferential dissection of the both cavae.

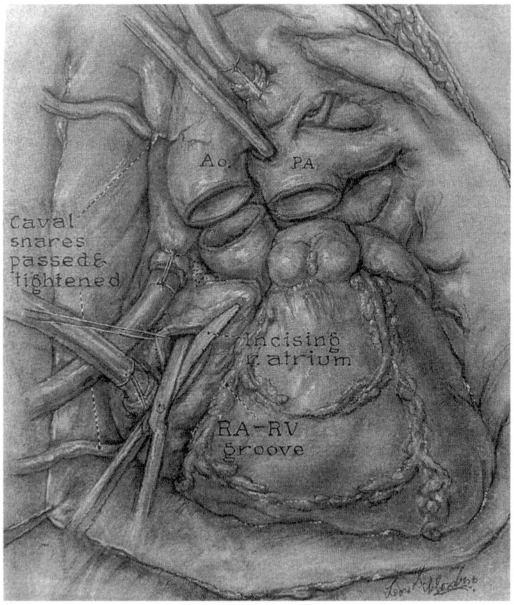

Fig. 17.3 Explantation of the recipient's heart. (Reproduced from Fig. 15.3 from Shumway and Shumway, p. 165)

The explantation of the heart continues by opening the roof of the left atrium and identifying the left pulmonary veins. The left atrial appendage can be left in situ as an anatomical marker, until shortly before the donor heart is being implanted.

Finally the excised heart is being removed from the chest and the pericardial sac is being irrigated with cold saline. The left atrial cuff is being trimmed and any bleeding spots are being taken care of at this stage.

17.5.4 Implantation of the Donor Heart

The left atrium is being anastomosed first with a 120 cm long, 3–0 monofilament polypropylene running suture (Fig. 17.4). During the initial sutures, the donor heart is held above the pericardial sac and it is lowered into the chest cavity thereafter. Epicardial cooling with cold saline or ice can be achieved while it is being implanted. To assure a good suture line with perfect endothelial lining, we prefer suturing of atrial walls outside-in (donor heart) and then inside-out (recipient heart) (Fig. 17.5). After completion of the left atrial anastomosis, this cavity is filled with cold saline solution.

As the next step, the inferior vena cava anastomosis is done next with a 4–0 monofilament polypropylene running suture. Optimal alignment of the recipient's vena cava inferior and the donor's cava is of utmost importance to avoid any kinking or distortion with subsequent stenosis.

The superior vena cava anastomosis is usually done as the last part of the transplantation in order to shorten the ischemic time and to allow a better judgment of the length of the cava while the hart is being beating and filled with blood.

The next step is the anastomosis of the pulmonary artery. It is important to cut the pulmonary artery very short in order to prevent kinking, which was found to be a case of postoperative right heart failure [9]. In general, the pulmonary valve of the donor heart should be anastomosed almost to the pulmonary bifurcation of the recipient, in order to avoid kinking. Kinking might also occur if the aorta and the pulmonary artery are not completely separated from each other. In addition, any rotation of the pulmonary anastomosis has to be avoided. The pulmonary artery wall is a very delicate structure and the stiches have to be made very close together. In certain cases, a pericardial strip should be used to avoid suture holes in the pulmonary wall.

The last step during the period of aortic cross-clamping is the aortic anastomosis. Frequently there is a size discrepancy between the donor and the recipient aorta, which need to be compensated by the 4–0 monofilament polypropylene running suture by using the inlay technique. If the quality of the aortic wall is rather bad (atherosclerotic, thin, calcified), the Blalock technique with or without pericardial strips should be used.

During the last part of the anastomosis, the snare of the inferior vena cava is removed and the heart is being filled with blood from the lungs. A meticulous de-airing procedure is carried out with a needle vent in the ascending aorta.

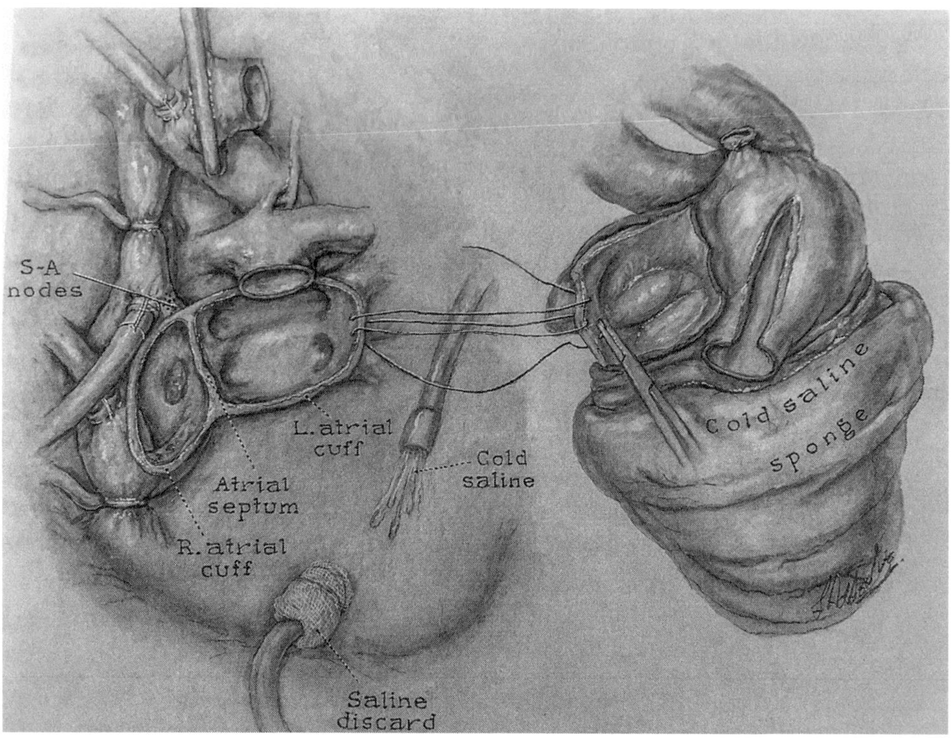

Fig. 17.4 Implantation of the donor heart. (Reproduced from Fig. 15.4 from Shumway and Shumway, p. 166)

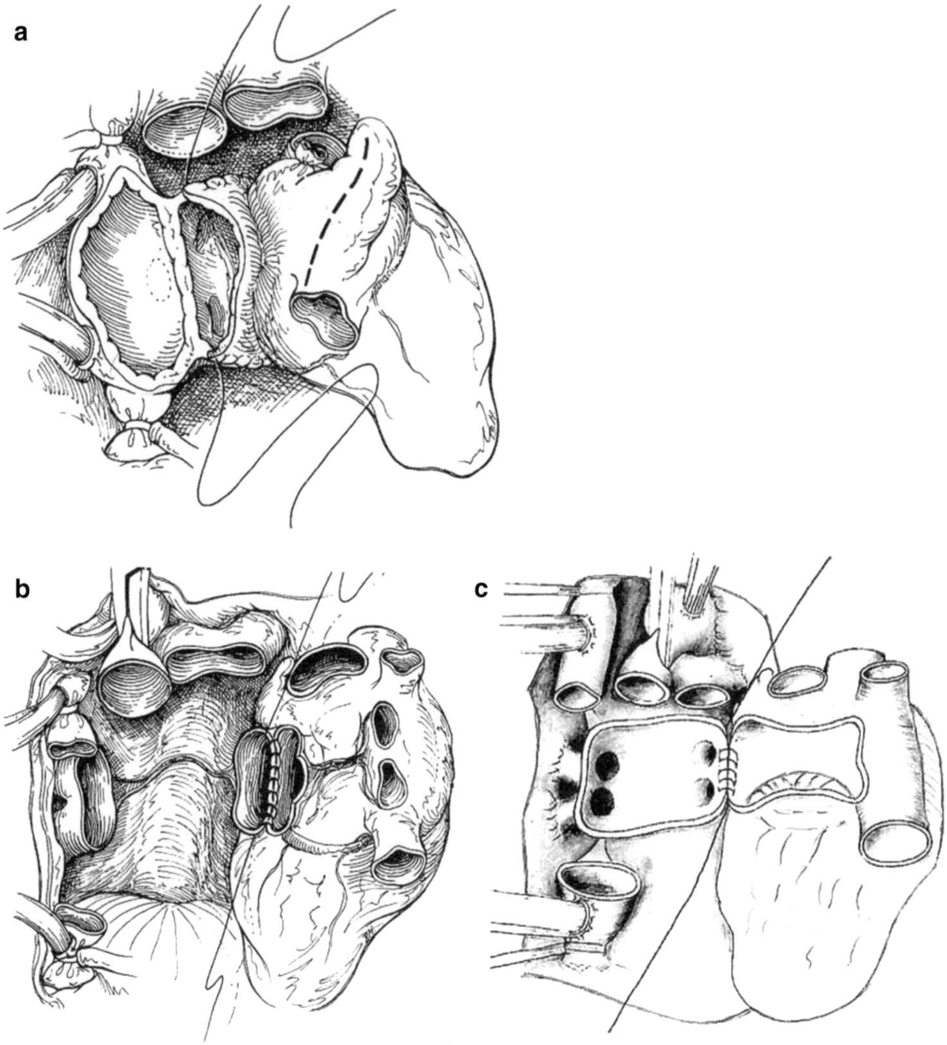

Fig. 17.5 Preferred suturing technique during heart transplantation

17.5.5 Reperfusion Period

Shortly before the aortic clamp is removed, terminal warm blood cardioplegic reperfusion is given into the aorta for 3 min. Some centers do prefer to use leucocyte filters in the CPB circuit during this phase.

Perioperative immunosuppression is an integral part of heart transplantation during this period. At time of skin incision 1 g of methylprednisolone is administered intravenously.

After removal of the cross-clamp, the superior vena cava anastomosis is being performed taking care to avoid any stenosis in this area. A pressure measurement is done directly by needle insertion in the proximal and distal portion of the anastomosis. Care has to be taken to avoid (a) a "purse-string effect" when using a running suture, and (b) a rotation of the superior vena cava (the right atrial appendage can serve as an anatomical landmark).

The reperfusion duration with CPB on the beating empty heart is approx. 1/3 of the total ischemic time. Thereafter CPB is slowly weaned off.

Full hemodynamic and echocardiographic monitoring is used to assess the function of the heart during this period.

In addition the reperfusion period can be used to remove all preexisting devices, such as pacemakers, defibrillators, driveline from LVADs, etc.

Pericardial closure will be done if there is some pericardium left. In cases of second or third re-do, pericardial substitutes, such as Goretex membrane can be used to cover the transplanted heart.

To achieve a perfect hemostasis after transplantation cannot be overstated. Many patients have had previous cardiac operations, are on anticoagulation (antiplatelet therapy, warfarin, etc.), or have impaired renal and liver function to start with. Postoperative bleeding with subsequent tamponade or the necessity to give blood products can result in an increased mortality and morbidity after transplantation. Especially in the high percentage of patients who are already in a borderline condition before the transplant or who are waiting on the high-urgency list, postoperative bleeding can result in immediate cardiogenic shock with subsequent multi-organ failure.

References

1. Allen BS, Okamoto F, Buckberg GD, Bugyi H, Young H, Leaf J, Beyersdorf F, et al. Immediate functional recovery after six hours of regional ischemia by careful control of conditions of reperfusion and composition of reperfusate. J Thorac Cardiovasc Surg. 1986;92(3 Pt 2):621–35.
2. Ardahali A, Esmailian F, Deng M, Soltesz E, Hsich E, Naka Y, et al. Ex vivo perfusion of donor hearts for human heart transplantation (PROCEED II): a prospective, open-label, multicentre, randomized non-inferiority trial. Lancet. 2015;385:2577–84.
3. Astrup J, Siesjö BK, Symon L. Thresholds in cerebral ischemia – the ischemic penumbra. Stroke. 1981;12(6):723–5.
4. Barnard CN. The operation. A human cardiac transplant: an interim report of a successful operation performed at Groote Schuur Hospital, Cape Town. S Afr Med J. 1967;41:1271–4.
5. Beyersdorf F. The use of controlled reperfusion strategies in cardiac surgery to minimize ischaemia/reperfusion damage. Cardiovasc Res. 2009;83:262–8.
6. Beyersdorf F, Unger A, Wildhirt A, Kretzer U, Deutschländer N, Krüger S, Matheis G, Hanselmann A, Zimmer G, Satter P. Studies of reperfusion injury in skeletal muscle: preserved cellular viability after extended periods of warm ischemia. J Cardiovasc Surg. 1991;32(5):664–76.
7. Buckberg GD. Studies of controlled reperfusion after ischemia. J Thorac Cardiovasc Surg. 1986;92:483–7.
8. Dhital KK, Iyer A, Connellan M, Chew HC, Gao L, Doyle A, et al. Adult heart transplantation with distant procurement and ex-vivo preservation of donor hearts after circulatory death: a case series. Lancet. 2015;385:2585–91.
9. Dreyfus G, Jebara VA, Couetil JP, Carpentier A. Kinking of the pulmonary artery: a treatable cause of acute right heart failure after heart transplantation. J Heart Transplant. 1990;9:575–6.
10. Eltzschig H, Eckle T. Ischemia and Reperfusion – from mechanism to translation. Nat Med. 2011;17:1391–401.
11. Emin A, Rogers CA, Banner NR, et al. Quality of life of advanced chronic heart failure: medical care, mechanical circulatory support and transplantation. Eur J Cardiothorac Surg. 2016;50:269–73.
12. Fellström B. Transplantation atherosclerosis. J Intern Med. 1996;240:253–7.
13. Garcia Sáez D, Zych B, Sabashnikov A, Bowles CT, de Robertis F, Mohite PN, et al. Evaluation of the organ care system in heart transplantation with an adverse donor/recipient profile. Ann Thorac Surg. 2014;98:2099–105.
14. Garcia Sáez D, Zych B, Mohite PN, Sabashnikov A, Patil NP, Popov A, et al. LVAD bridging to heart transplantation with an ex-vivo allograft preservation shows significantly improved outcomes: a new standard of care? J Heart Lung Transpl. 2015;34:S95.
15. Garcia Sáez D, Elbetanony A, Lezberg P, Hassanein A, Bowles CT, Popov AF, et al. Ex-vivo heart perfusion after cardiocirculatory death: a porcine model. J Surg Res. 2015;195:311–4.
16. Hamed A, Tsui S, Huber J, Lin R, Poggio RC, Ardehali A. Serum lactate is a highly sensitive and specific predictor of postcardiac transplant outcomes using the Organ Care System. J Heart Lung Transpl. 2009;28:S71.
17. Hossmann KA, Schmidt-Kastner R, Grosse Ophoff B. Recovery of integrative central nervous function after one hour global cerebro-circulatory arrest in normothermic cat. J Neurol Sci. 1987;77(2–3):305–20.
18. Iyer A, Gao L, Doyle A, Rao P, Cropper JR, Soto C, et al. Normothermic ex vivo perfusion provides superior organ preservation and enables viability assessment of hearts from DCD donors. Am J Transplant. 2015;15:371–80.
19. Koerner MM, Ghodsizad A, Schulz U, El Baayosy A, Koerfer R, Tenderich G. Normothermic ex vivo allograft blood perfusion in clinical heart transplantation. Heart Surg Forum. 2014;17:E141–5.
20. Leprince P, Popov AF, Simon AR, Benk C, Siepe M. Ex vivo perfusion of the heart with the use of the Organ Care System. Eur J Cardiothorac Surg. 2016;49:1318–20.
21. Lower RR, Shumway NE. Studies on the orthotopic homotransplantations of the canine heart. Surg Forum. 1960;11:18–23.
22. Mitrev Z, Beyersdorf F, Hallmann R, Poloczek Y, Ihnken K, Herold H, Unkelbach U, Zimmer G, Freisleben HJ, Satter P. Reperfusion injury in skeletal muscle: controlled limb reperfusion reduces local and systemic complications after prolonged ischaemia. Cardiovasc Surg. 1994;2(6):737–48.
23. Ou R, Lim YW, Choong JW, et al. Low-flow hypothermic crystalloid perfusion is superior to cold storage during prolonged heart preservation. Transplant Proc. 2014;46:3309–13.
24. Rosenfeldt F, Ou R, Salamonsen R, Marasco S, Zimmet A, Byrne J, Cosic F, Saxena P, Esmore D. A novel combination technique of cold crystalloid perfusion but not cold storage facilitates transplantation of canine hearts donated after circulatory arrest. J Heart Lung Transplant. 2016;35:1358–64.
25. Sarsam MA, Campbell CS, Yonan NA, Deiraniya AK, Rahman AN. An alternative surgical technique in orthotopic cardiac transplantation. J Card Surg. 1993;8:344–9.
26. Schmitto JD, Zimpfer D, Fiane AE, Larbalestier R, Tsui S, Jansz P, Simon A, Schueler S, Strueber M. Long-term support of patients recieving a left ventricular assist device for advanced heart failure: a follow-up analysis of the Registry to Evaluate the HeartWare Left Ventricular Assist System. Eur J Cardiothorac Surg. 2016;50:834–8.
27. Schnoor M, Schäfer T, Lühmann D, Sievers HH. Bicaval versus standard technique in orthotopic heart transplantation: A systematic review and meta-analysis. J Thorac Cardiovasc Surg. 2007;134:1322–31.
28. Shumway SJ. Operative Techniques in Heart Transplantation. In: Shumway SJ, Shumway NE, editors. Thoracic Transplantation. Cambridge, MA: Blackwell Science; 1995. p. 163–73.
29. Sievers HH, Weyand M, Kraatz EG, Bernhard A. An alternative technique for orthotopic cardiac transplantation, with preservation of the normal anatomy of the right atrium. Thorac Cardiovasc Surg. 1991,39:70–2.
30. Sjostrand F, Allen BS, Buckberg GD, Okamoto F, Young H, Bugyi H, Beyersdorf F, Barnard RJ, Leaf J. Electron microscopic studies: importance of embedding techniques in quantitative evaluation of cardiac mitochondrial structure during regional ischemia and reperfusion. J Thorac Cardiovasc Surg. 1986;92(3 Pt 2):513–24.
31. Taunyane IC, Benk C, Beyersdorf F, et al. Preserved brain morphology after controlled automated reperfusion of the whole body following normothermic circulatory arrest time of up to 20 minutes. Eur J Cardiothorac Surg. 2016;50(6):1025–34.
32. Tolboom H, Makhro A, Rosser BA, Wilhelm MJ, Bogdanova A, Falk V. Recovery of donor hearts after circulatory death with normothermic extracorporeal machine perfusion. Eur J Cardiothorac Surg. 2015;47:173–9.
33. Tolboom H, Olejnickova V, Reser D, Rosser B, Wilhelm MJ, Gassmann M, et al. Moderate hypothermia during ex vivo machine perfusion promotes recovery of hearts donated ater circulatory death. Eur J Cardiothorac Surg. 2016;49:25–31.
34. Trivedi JR, Rajagopal K, Schumer EM, Birks EJ, Lenneman A, Cheng A, Slaughter MS. Differences in status 1A heart transplantation survival in the continuous flow left ventricular assist device era. Ann Thorac Surg. 2016;102:1512–6.
35. Van Caenegem O, Beauloye C, Bertrand L, Horman S, Lepropre S, Sparavier G, et al. Hypothermic continuous machine perfusion enables preservation of energy charge and functional recovery of hearts grafts in an ex vivo model of donation following circulatory death. Eur J Cardiothorac Surg. 2016;49:1348–53.
36. Warnecke G, et al. Organ Care System (OCS) Lung INSPIRE International Trial Results (abstract OLB05). Transplan Int. 2015;28(Suppl):131.3–4.

37. Yeung JC, et al. Outcomes after transplantation of lungs preserved for more than 12 h: retrospective study. Lancet Respiratory Med. 2016;5:119–24. https://doi.org/10.1016/S2213-2600(16)30323-X.
38. Zimpfer D, Netuka I, Schmitto JD, Pya Y, Garbade M, Moshuis M, Beyersdorf F, Marasco S, Rao V, Damme L, Sood P, Krabatsch T. Multicentre clinical trial experience with the HeartMate 3 left ventricular assist device: 30-day outcomes. Eur J Cardiothorac Surg. 2016;50:548–54.

Part IX

Heart Transplantation (II, Medical)

Patient Selection, Pretransplant Management, Donor and Recipient Matching

18

David S. Feldman, Sudha P. Jaganathan, and Parvathi Mudigonda

18.1 Patient Selection

After reversible causes of HF have been addressed and medical and surgical treatments optimized, including cardiac resynchronization therapy (CRT), the next step is to determine whether a patient meets criteria for advanced HF therapy. The process of patient selection and pre-transplant management is comprehensive and multidimensional. Objective risk markers and risk scores such as NT-pro BNP and HF models are routinely used in risk stratification, but they often do not encompass the entire clinical spectrum of an individual [2]. The following are key patient characteristics that may help identify suitable patients for advanced therapies:

18.1.1 Recipient Selection

1. Refractory HF or cardiogenic shock requiring continuous inotrope infusion or mechanical circulatory support or intra aortic balloon pump. Low perfusion state with resultant end-organ failure (most commonly renal or hepatic) warrants urgent referral to prevent irreversible end-organ damage.
2. Cardiopulmonary exercise test (CPET) to measure aerobic capacity: The 2016 ISHLT guidelines suggest a maximal cardiopulmonary exercise test be defined as a respiratory exchange ratio (RER) >1.05 and achievement of anaerobic threshold on optimal pharmacologic therapy. VO_2 max and VE-VCO_2 slope correlate with prognosis. VO_2 max is the maximum rate of oxygen consumption during incremental exercise and is dependent on patient effort. The VE-VCO_2 slope is minute ventilation relative to amount of carbon dioxide production and is effort independent [3]. Presence of a CRT device no longer influences VO_2 max cutoffs. The following are threshold values to prompt referral:
   (a) Patients intolerant of β-blockers: VO_2 max ≤14 mL/kg/min
   (b) Patients on β-blockers: VO_2 max ≤12 mL/kg/min
   (c) With submaximal effort (RER <1.05), use VE-VCO_2 slope > 35
   (d) Patients <50 years and women, reasonable to use alternate standards
   (e) Obese patients, adjusting VO_2 max to lean body mass may be considered (VO_2 max <19 mL/kg/min)
3. HF prognostic models such as the Seattle Heart Failure Model (SHFM) or Heart Failure Survival Score (HFSS) should be used along with CPET to guide listing in ambulatory patients [3–7]. SHFM in particular, risk stratifies patients based on the impact of newer HF therapies on survival, including device therapies [6].
   (a) SHFM: >20% score aids in predicting 1 year mortality
   (b) HFSS in medium-high risk categorization prioritizes the ambulant patient
   (c) Neither should be use as sole criterions for listing
   (d) Convenient and easy to use for the medical practitioner with calculators available on the internet or as an application on hand-held devices
4. Functional Comorbidities
   (a) Age. In the early era of transplant, eligible patients were less than 50–55 years old. Decreased survival correlated with increasing donor and recipient age [3].
      (i) Recommended age threshold is ≤70 years
      (ii) Carefully selected patients >70 years may be considered [3]
   (b) Weight. A body mass index (BMI) of >35 kg/m^2 as pre-transplant body mass index is associated with poor outcomes after transplantation. Weight loss to achieve a BMI ≤ 35 kg/m^2 before listing is recommended [3].

D. S. Feldman (✉)
Division of Cardiology, Department of Medicine, University of Cincinnati, Cincinnati, OH, USA
e-mail: FELDMADS@ucmail.uc.edu

S. P. Jaganathan · P. Mudigonda
University of Cincinnati, Cincinnati, OH, USA

D. S. Feldman, P. Mohacsi (eds.), *Heart Failure*, Cardiovascular Medicine, https://doi.org/10.1007/978-3-319-98184-0_18

(c) Malignancy. Collaboration with oncologists to individualize risk stratification of tumor recurrence is recommended, given the heterogeneous nature of neoplasms. Transplantation can be considered when risk of recurrence is low, treatment responsive and there is no evidence of metastasis.
(d) Frailty. An assessment of frailty with at least 3 out of the following 5 symptoms can augment eligibility assessment: muscle loss, slow walking speed, low levels of physical activity, >10 pound weight loss within 1 year, and fatigue.

5. Medical Comorbidities
   (a) Pulmonary hypertension exists in many patients with advanced heart failure and portends a poor prognosis post-transplant with many who succumb to death from right HF. It is important to identify and risk stratify patients based on their resting pulmonary arterial pressure and pulmonary vascular resistance (PVR) [3, 8].
      (i) In Patients who are listed, a RHC should be performed at a 3–6 month interval especially with worsening symptoms or the presence of a reversible cause of pulmonary hypertension [3].
      (ii) A vasodilatory challenge can be done when the pulmonary artery systolic pressure is greater than 50 mm hg with either a trans pulmonary gradient (TPG) >15 or the PVR >3 Wood Units [3, 8].
      (iii) If the vasodilatory challenge fails to improve hemodynamics, patients can be admitted to the hospital to undergo a trial of medical therapy or if unsuccessful, an unloading trial of mechanical therapies such as left ventricular assist device (LVAD) or an intra-aortic balloon pump (IABP)
      (iv) After such therapies, reevaluation of hemodynamics should be undertaken to ascertain reversibility of pulmonary hypertension. Pulmonary vascular hemodynamics that are refractory to either medical or mechanical therapies is a contraindication to heart transplantation [3].
   (b) Diabetes Mellitus: patients with end organ damage (other than non-proliferative retinopathy) or poor glycemic control (HbA1C > 7.5% or 58 mmol/mol) is a relative contraindication to heart transplantation.
   (c) Renal dysfunction: an eGFR <30 ml/min/1.73 m^2 with irreversible renal injury is a contraindication for heart transplantation alone. However, otherwise eligible patients should be considered for a heart-kidney transplantation.
   (d) Peripheral and cerebrovascular disease: Progression of vascular disease may be accelerated after heart transplantation [3, 8]. As such, severe cerebrovascular disease with clinical manifestations is an absolute contraindication. Peripheral arterial disease is a relative contraindication when it limits exercise capacity and is not amenable to revascularization.
   (e) Active systemic infections: Generally considered an absolute contraindication in the presence of a potentially treatable organism or active viremia [8].
   (f) Tobacco and Substance Dependence. Active tobacco use in the last 6 months is a relative contraindication, as it has been associated with poor outcomes. Formal education for tobacco cessation and providing necessary modalities to aide in quitting is imperative in both the pre and post transplantation period. This includes exposure to second hand smoke. Studies have demonstrated an increased incidence in coronary allograft vasculopathy (CAV) in patients who smoke post-transplant [8]. Patients that actively use substances, including alcohol, are not considered for transplantation. Patients that have completed a structured rehabilitation program within 24 months of exposure may be considered for listing for transplantation.
   (g) Psycho-social Evaluation. A thorough psychosocial assessment, including ability to give informed consent, should be performed prior to listing. In patients with poor social support, noncompliance, severe cognitive-behavioral disability or dementia, the arduous clinical commitments can pose potential harm. A heart transplant cannot be recommended.

Special considerations for a group of potential recipients are mentioned in the 2016 International Society for Heart Lung Transplantation (ISHLT) guidelines. These include patients with restrictive and infiltrative cardiomyopathy and patients with certain infectious diseases. On the other end of the spectrum, a greater proportion of patients surviving into adulthood with congenital heart disease, are adding to the pool for candidacy for heart transplantation [3, 9]. These patients require specific considerations and prognostication prior to listing for heart transplantation.

18.1.2 Donor Selection

The continued mismatch between donor organ supply and demand as well as focus on institutional outcomes in heart transplantation means having a better understanding of not only recipient criteria but of donor risk factors that affect patient and graft survival [1]. Apart from the primary survey of donors which include confirmation of brain death, laboratory tests, identification of co-morbidities, and demographics, a more heart specific assessment is needed such as cardiac biomarkers, electrocardiograms, echocardiogram, assessment of use of inotropic support, and coronary angiogram when indicated.

Age of the donor is a major component in the selection process with an ideal age being <55 years old and might be an independent risk factor for long term mortality [1]. Hearts from donors younger than 45 years old will be able to withstand both the perils of heart transplant surgery and recipient factors like underlying co morbidities and hemodynamic instabilities [10]. Donor hearts between the ages of 45–55 years of age are not as resilient and require to be used in the projected ischemic time of less than 4 h [10]. Based on UNOS data, 50% of heart donors are between 18–34 years of age [1].

Echocardiographic assessment is important in ascertaining cardiac function of the donor heart. Depressed left ventricular function (LV function <40% despite optimization of hemodynamics), valvular disease, and in particular, left ventricular hypertrophy (LVH) all predict recipient survival.

In efforts to expand the donor pool, special considerations and exceptions are made with focus on optimizing, recovering and repairing a potential donor heart to make it suitable for heart transplantation [1].

18.2 Pre-transplantation Management

The United Network of Organ Sharing (UNOS) assigns all transplant candidates a "status" which prioritizes them based on their medical condition. Status 1A defines patients who are seriously ill, on high dose inotropes or on mechanical circulatory support (MCS). Patients with status 1b are on lower dose inotropes and/or with MCS but can be managed at home and status 2 patients are usually ambulatory and not on inotrope therapy [6]. Based on listing status and availability of potential organs, alternatives to transplantation, continual laboratory and hemodynamic assessment will have to be done in a multidisciplinary fashion to optimize survival and quality of life.

Dynamic listing algorithms are in place for listed patients in the outpatient ambulatory setting who are not dependent on inotropic therapy. This requires continual reevaluation at 3–6 month intervals with cardiopulmonary exercise stress testing and HFSS after maximizing pharmacologic and device therapy (implantable cardioverter defibrillator and cardiac resynchronization therapy (CRT)) [3]. Such patients can be assessed for delisting if hemodynamics have improved.

18.2.1 MCS and Inotrope Use

The use of MCS has been favored over the last two decades for patients that are eligible for transplantation and also considered for patients with potentially reversible or treatable comorbidities prior to transplantation [3]. Twenty eight percent of transplant recipients between 2006–2012 had a ventricular assist device per recent data from the ISHLT. Some studies also suggest a mortality benefit in patients with prior LVAD even up to 1 year post transplantation [6] despite the additional risk associated with implantation and complications arising from the device. With better survival conferred on the transplant waiting list, clinicians now prefer using LVAD as a "bridge-to-transplant" therapy versus inotrope or intra-aortic balloon pump use.

Less favored pre-transplantation therapy are usage of inotropes which include medications like intravenous dobutamine and milrinone. Usually, these are reserved as more palliative therapies and can be used as a bridge to either transplantation or LVAD. Mortality is high in these patients with nearly 100% at 1 year [6].

18.2.2 Pre-transplantation Infection Screen and Vaccination

A pre-transplant infectious screen may reveal a lack of immunity to common pathogens that prove to be detrimental post-transplantation [11]. Patients with end stage organ disease are susceptible to a host of diseases that potentially can be life threatening. A pre-transplant screen of active and latent infections should be carried out in all potential candidates for transplantation. This includes a thorough dental evaluation prior to listing. Accordingly, vaccination should be completed prior to transplantation as vaccination afterwards is less likely to be effective [11]. The importance of patient education regarding potential infections a post-transplant candidate might be susceptible to as well as preventative strategies are imperative as part of the pre-transplantation screen [11]. The clinician must also be aware that apart from educating the candidate regarding common pathogens, potential sources such as pets, environmental exposure, and food source for example must also be advised.

18.2.3 Sensitization in the Pre-heart Transplant Patient

An important part of managing pre-transplant candidates is identifying and treating the sensitized patient. Sensitization refers to the development of circulating antibodies against human leukocyte antigen (HLA). A serious consequence of this is increased risk of hyperacute rejection, decreased survival, and development of cardiac allograft vasculopathy post-transplantation. Historically, patients with increased risk of sensitization are ones who have exposure to blood transfusion, multi-parous women, prior organ transplant, and more importantly, placement of an LVAD [12]. Usually patients with a VAD have also had exposure to blood products.

The preferred screening tool to detect the presence of circulating anti-HLA antibodies is the panel-reactive antibody (PRA) test. A higher percentage of PRA positive results are usually associated with worse outcomes. Although lacking specificity, a high pre-transplant PRA result is associated with lower survival and higher rates of rejection after transplant. Non-HLA antibodies have also been implicated in poor graft survival although the ability to test for these are not as refined as it is for the HLA antibodies. These include certain autoantibodies and antibodies against major histocompatibility complex (MHC) Class I and Class II and its avoidance and removal have led to better outcomes. While on the waitlist, patients should be screened for circulating antibodies about every 6 months [10, 12]. In patients with detectable circulating antibodies the frequency of screening is every 3 months and every 2–4 weeks in any transplant candidate that has had a sensitizing event [10].

While increased sensitization does not preclude transplant eligibility, the wait times for transplantation are significantly longer than for those who are not sensitized [12]. In turn, higher wait time translates into increased mortality. According to the 2010 ISHLT guidelines on care of heart transplant recipients, a PRA usually of greater than 10% will require further evaluation regarding the benefits of de-sensitization [10]. De-sensitization therapies include IV immunoglobulin (Ig) infusion, plasmapheresis, and rituximab [10, 12] and after appropriate therapy, PRAs should be checked 1–2 weeks later with the goal to lower risk of hyperacute rejection.

18.3 Donor and Recipient Matching

When transplant centers accept patients onto the wait list, they are registered in a national, centralized database linking all transplant candidates and donors. For every organ that becomes available, the program generates a list of potential recipients based on severity of disease, patient demographics and specific laboratory data inputted earlier. Donor-recipient matching not only involves objective criteria such as blood type, body size, and crossmatching based on allosensitization, but also geographic disparity, severity of illness in the recipient, and the recipient wait time on the transplant list [13]. With these variables, the organ procurement organization works closely with the recipients transplant center to ensure the best possible match between recipient and donor. To allow alternatives for the high risk heart transplant recipient, some institutions have an extended criterion and allow the use of "marginal" donor organs. This alternative list when compared to patients with LVAD as destination therapy, were shown to have similar survival rates [1].

The recommendations for donor-recipient size matching are based on ISHLT 2010 guidelines and recommend use of donor hearts whose body weight is no greater than 30% below that of the recipient [10]. Size matching also encompasses height matching and consideration of chest size especially in those recipients with prior LVAD and/or sternotomies. Gender matching is also considered as gender mismatch is usually observed in male recipients of female hearts and correlates with increased rates of rejection and mortality [1].

Evaluation of allosensitization plays a large role in donor-recipient matching because, as mentioned in the prior section, the increased risk of rejection and mortality in the sensitized recipient. Several crossmatching tools are available to assist in finding an ideal match.

1. Prospective: this involves matching the donor with the recipient by directly acquiring and testing blood. This approach is geographically challenging therefore predominantly involves using organs procured locally. For obvious reasons, this can lead to increased wait times and rate of death while on the wait list [1, 12].
2. Retrospective: involves a direct comparison between the donor and recipient blood with results being available after the organ has been used for transplantation. It's a technique used when prospective crossmatching is not available.
3. Virtual: In 2001, Duke University Medical Center implemented virtual crossmatching to alleviate the geographical disparity that existed with prospective crossmatching [12]. It involves comparing the recipient specific PRAs with the donor HLA antigens and decisions are made based on this. However, this is only as accurate as the last blood sample obtained from the recipient and therefore, any sensitizing events occurring in between can skew the match. With the implementation of virtual crossmatching, the donor pool has largely increased with more sensitized patients being successfully transplanted.

18.3.1 Marginal Donors

With the limited and static donor pool, more institutions are allowing the use of "marginal" donors. This term incorporates donors that do not meet the ideal criteria in terms of age and may have structural heart disease and/or criteria for high risk behavior which include infectious diseases such as HIV, Hepatitis B or C, history of drug abuse or recent incarceration. A marginal donor can also constitute donors with higher than allowed ischemic time. This can be further divided into adequate donors with some features suggestive of high risk and the true marginal donors that meet the above criteria [14].

Of the various risk models that exist in predicting recipient survival after receiving a marginal donor heart, ischemic time posed the highest risk followed by age [14]. Another risk model developed in Europe called the European Transplant Heart Donor Score (HDS) showed that age and presence of LVH were independent predictors of mortality [14]. Despite this, more research into this field is needed to improve donor suitability.

18.4 Conclusion

Various regulations and standardizations are in place to appropriately allocate hearts for transplantation. Patients are meticulously selected based on numerous criteria and then assigned a status based on UNOS criteria. This is a continual process and requires frequent reevaluation at appropriate time intervals by medical practitioners. Although the advancements in medical therapy, MCS, and device therapy have significantly lowered mortality in this specific patient population, heart transplantation remains the gold standard in treatment [14]. With strategies to increase the donor pool, efforts to reduce the waitlist, and increase the effectiveness of treating the sensitized patient, we can maximally utilize a scarce resource.

References

1. Ahmet K, et al. Donor selection in heart transplantation. J Thorac Dis. 2014;6(8):1097–104.
2. Crespo-Leiro MG, et al. Advanced heart failure: a position statement of the Heart Failure Association of the European Society of Cardiology. Eur J Heart Fail. 2018.
3. Mehra MR, et al. The 2016 International Society for Heart Lung Transplantation listing criteria for heart transplantation: A 10 year update. J Heart Lung Transplant. 2016;35(1):1–23.
4. Gardner RS, et al. Who needs a heart transplant? Eur Heart J. 2006;27:770–2.
5. Fanaroff AC, et al. Patient selection for advanced heart failure therapy referral. Crit Pathw Cardiol. 2014;13(1):1–5.
6. Alraies CM, Eckman P. Adult heart transplant: indications and outcomes. J Thorac Dis. 2014;6(8):1120–8.
7. AbouEzzeddine OF, Redfield MM. Who has advanced heart failure? definition and epidemiology. Congest Heart Fail. 2011;17(4):160–8.
8. de Jonge N, Kirkels JH, et al. Guidelines for heart transplantation. Neth Hear J. 2008;16(3):19–87.
9. Tonsho M, et al. Heart transplantation: challenges facing the field. Cold Spring Harb Perspect Med. 2014;4:a015636.
10. Costanzo MR, et al. The International Society of Heart and Lung Transplantation guidelines for the care of heart transplant recipients. J Heart Lung Transplant. 2010;29(8):914–56.
11. Avery RK. Recipient screening prior to solid-organ transplantation. Clin Infect Dis. 2002;35:1513–9.
12. Kobashigawa J, et al. Report from a consensus conference on the sensitized patient awaiting heart transplantation. J Heart Lung Transplant. 2009;28(3):213–25.
13. U.S. Department of Health and Human Services. https://www.organdonor.gov/about/process/matching.html.
14. Hsich EM. Matching the market for heart transplantation. Circ Heart Fail. 2016;9(4):e002679.
15. Khush KK, et al. National decline in donor heart utilization with regional variability: 1995–2010. Am J Transplant. 2015;15(3):642–9.

Part X

Heart Transplantation (III)

Immunosuppression, Including Drug Toxicity, Interactions, New Immunosuppressants in the Pipeline

19

Denise Wang, Bruno Meiser, Howard J. Eisen, and Sandra Eifert

19.1 Basic Immunosuppression for Transplant

The success of organ transplantation depends on the prevention of the allograft rejection with immunosuppression. The three types of rejections are hyperacute, acute, and chronic and are categorized by when the rejection occurs, and the mechanisms of organ injury. The type of tissue, specificity and memory of the lymphocytes, and the type of organ being transplanted are factors that dictate the risk of the type of rejection that may occur.

Hyperacute rejection is a type II hypersensitivity reaction that manifests within minutes to hours after the reperfusion of the organ. Preformed antibodies bind to the endothelial cells of the graft and cause complement activation, recruitment of phagocytic cells, platelet activation, and complement deposition. The response can cause thrombosis, swelling, and hemorrhage that are common to type II hypersensitivity reactions. Individuals with prior transplants and blood transfusions are susceptible to hyperacute rejections. This type of rejection is often prevented with ABO matching, panel reactive antibody (PRA) tests and the virtual cross match [1].

Acute rejection is a T-cell-mediated immune response characterized by the infiltration of lymphocytes and macrophages to the graft. The response occurs by a three-signal model. Antigen-presenting cells (APCs), such as dendritic cells and macrophages, from the graft and surrounding tissues travel to secondary lymphoid organs of the recipient to present foreign antigen on their major histocompatibility complex (MHC) to CD3/T cell receptors (TCRs) on T cells, which constitutes signal 1. Signal 2 is a costimulatory signal that involves CD80 and CD86 on APCs engaging CD28 on T cells (Fig. 19.1). Both signal 1 and 2 are required to activate the calcium-calcineurin pathway, renin-angiotensin system (RAS)-mitogen-activated protein (MAP) kinase pathway, and the nuclear factor-κB (NF-κB) pathway [2]. These pathways activate nuclear factor of activated T cells (NFAT), MAP kinase, and NF-κB to promote the production of cytokines and molecules such as interleukin-2 (IL-2), interleukin-15 (IL-15), CD154, and CD25. Signal 3 is the activation of mammalian target of rapamycin (mTOR), Janus kinase 3 (JAK3), and MAP kinase signaling pathways by the cytokines and molecules for cell proliferation as a response to signals 1 and 2. The proliferation and differentiation following signal 3 leads to an increase in effector T cells and the activation of B cells [3]. The effector T cells initiate an inflammatory response that can result in acute rejection through the loss of organ function. Individuals who are not properly immunosuppressed or sensitized to the transplant can have acute rejections within days of the transplantation. The highest occurrence of acute rejections is within the first 3 months. Thus, immune suppression during these months is crucial to avoid the recipient's immune system from mounting a response against the allograft. Unlike the lack of therapeutic options in hyperacute rejections, immunosuppressive agents are used to treat and to decrease the likelihood of acute rejections. Reversal of damage with immunosuppressants is sometimes possible. Immunophilin ligands, mycophenolic acids, corticosteroids, and immunoglobulin-based agents are types of immunosuppressants that are commonly used. Induction therapy comprised of immunosuppressive agents from various classes that usually starts at the beginning of transplantation may decrease the risk for acute rejection.

The original version of this chapter was revised. A correction to this chapter can be found at https://doi.org/10.1007/978-3-319-98184-0_28

D. Wang · H. J. Eisen (✉)
Drexel University College of Medicine, Philadelphia, PA, USA
e-mail: Howard.Eisen@DrexelMed.edu

B. Meiser · S. Eifert
Ludwig Maximillians University of Munich Medical Center, Munich, Germany

D. S. Feldman, P. Mohacsi (eds.), *Heart Failure*, Cardiovascular Medicine, https://doi.org/10.1007/978-3-319-98184-0_19

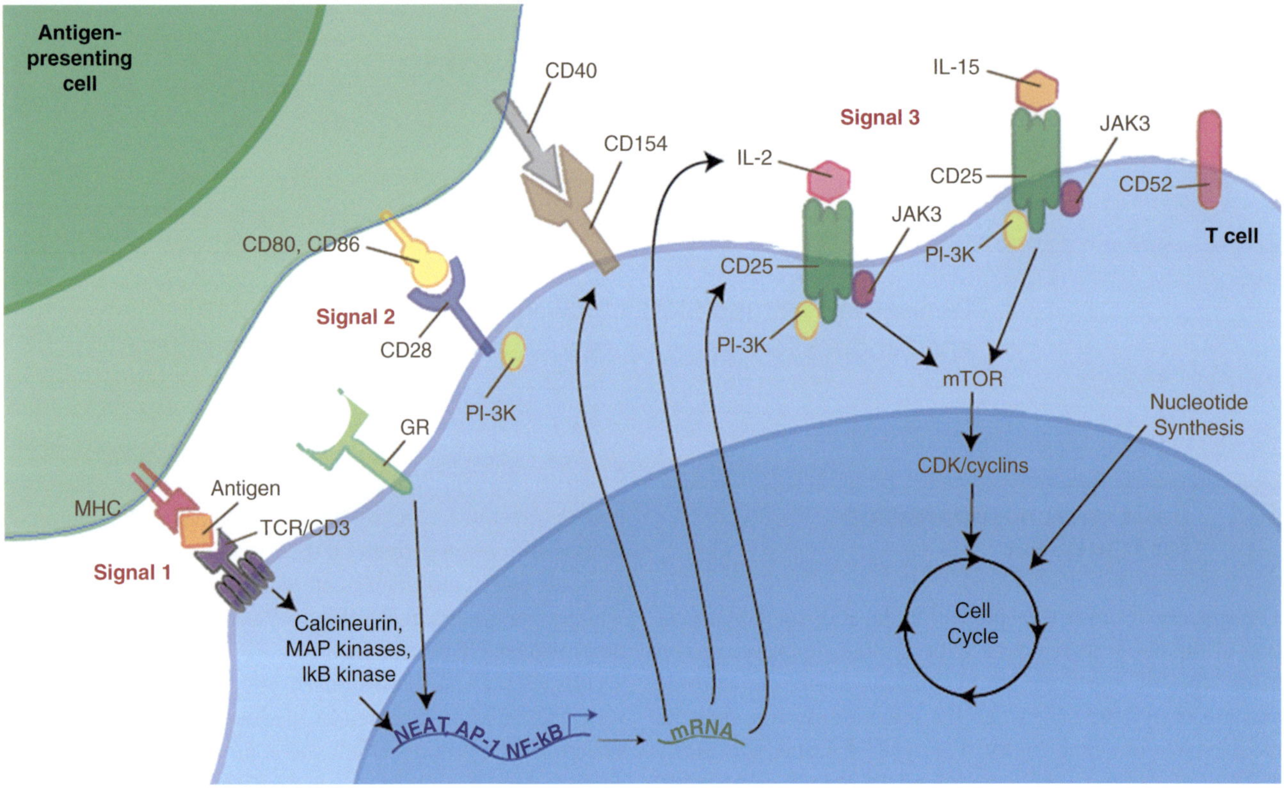

Fig. 19.1 Mechanism of T-cell-mediated rejection. Signal 1 – Antigen-presenting cells (APC) presents antigen on major histocompatibility complex (MHC) to T cell receptor (TCR) on T cells. Signal 2 – CD80 and CD86 on APCs engage CD28 on T cells. Signal 1 and 2 leads to activation of calcium-calcineurin pathway, renin-angiotensin system (RAS)-mitogen-activated protein (MAP) kinase pathway, and nuclear factor-κB (NF-κB) pathway. These three pathways promotes expression of cytokines and molecules to activate signal 3. Signal 3 – Cytokines and molecules induce T cell proliferation

Chronic rejection is a type IV/delayed type hypersensitivity and can occur within months to years that results in the fibrosis and scarring of the allograft. This type of rejection is humoral and T-cell-mediated and causes the proliferation of inflammatory lesions around the graft vasculature. Macrophages activated by T cells respond to growth factors and induce antigen-specific injury that causes increased fibrosis, ischemia, and cell death leading to cardiac allograft vasculopathy (CAV). Chronic rejection may also involve parenchymal transdifferentiation into mesenchymal cells [4] and cell senescence [5]. The damage done to the allograft is irreversible and gradual. It is the primary cause of graft loss, morbidity and mortality beyond the first year post-transplant. Early and consistent immunosuppression with the agents used for acute rejections helps lengthen the time of allograft function and may delay or prevent chronic rejection. At late stages of chronic rejection, re-transplantation is the only definitive treatment. Certain immunosuppressive agents such as mTOR inhibitors may mitigate CAV [6, 7]. Therefore, immunosuppression is an important aspect of transplantation.

19.2 Standard Immunosuppression

For solid organ transplants, immunosuppressants are used to prevent host vs. graft disease, the recipient's immune system attacking the allograft. Immunosuppressive agents include immunophilin ligands, mycophenolic acids, corticosteroids, and immunoglobulin-based agents. Immunophilin ligands commonly used in transplant management are calcineurin inhibitors that include cyclosporine and tacrolimus, and mTOR inhibitors that include sirolimus (rapamycin) and everolimus. Mycophenolic acids are antiproliferative agents derived from penicillium molds that selectively inhibit de novo purine synthesis, targeting

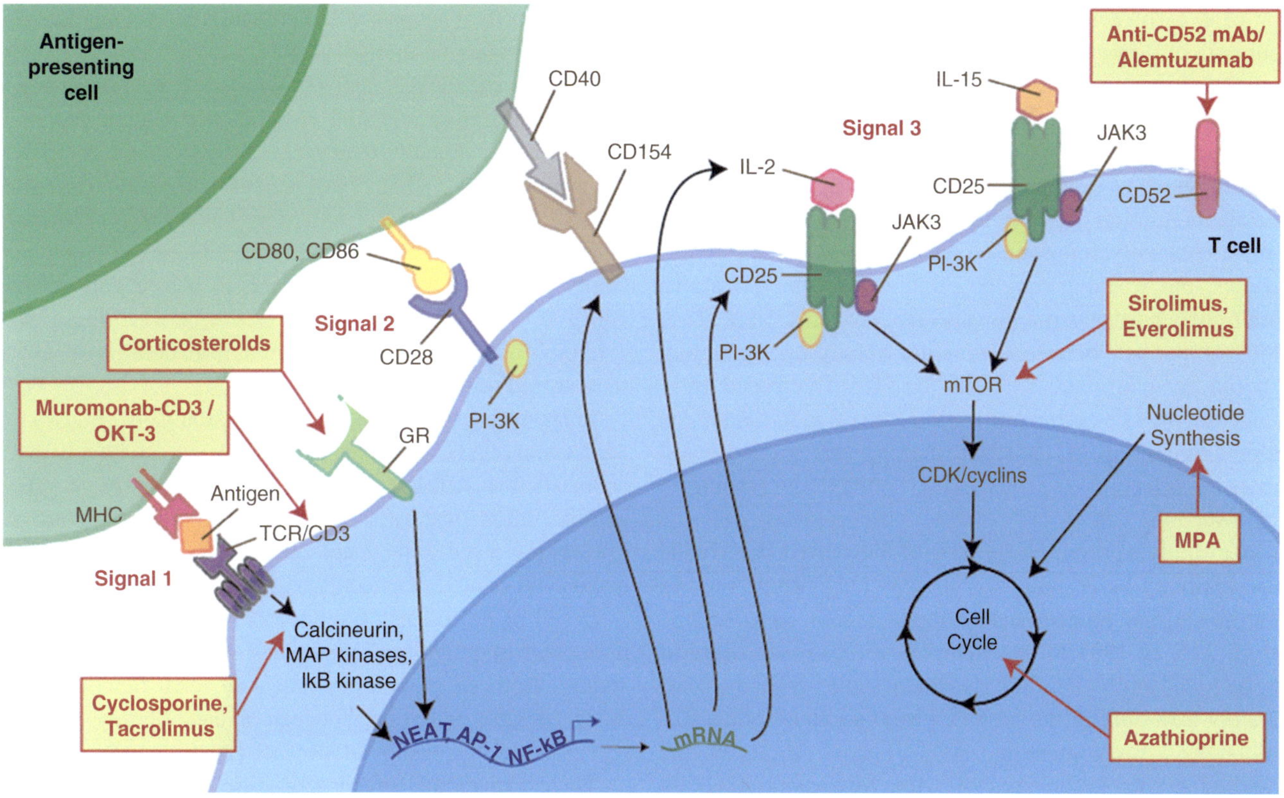

Fig. 19.2 Targets and Pathways of Immunosuppressive Agents. Calcineurin inhibitors – Cyclosporine and tacrolimus inhibit IL-2 transcription to block T cell activation. Mycophenolic acids (MPA) – Mycophenolate mofetil and Myfortic inhibit guanosine monophosphate nucleotide synthesis, preventing de novo purine synthesis within T and B cells. mTOR inhibitors – Sirolimus and everolimus inhibit mTOR to prevent G1 to S progression in cell cycle of T cells. Anti-CD3 – Muromonab-CD3 (OKT3) internalizes the T cell receptor. Anti-CD52 – Alemtuzumab depletes CD52 expressing lymphocytes. Azathioprine (AZA) is a prodrug of mercaptopurine that interferes with purine nucleic acid metabolism

lymphocytes [8]. Mycophenolate mofetil (MMF/CellCept) and mycophenolate sodium (Myfortic) are used frequently. Corticosteroids, like prednisone, decrease cytokine transcription to suppress B and T cell functions and to reduce the body's inflammatory response [9]. They are used for induction therapy, rescue from acute rejection, and immunosuppression maintenance in transplantation. Immunoglobulin-based agents include basiliximab and anti-thymocyte globulin that deplete antibodies. These agents are used perioperatively during induction therapy and postoperatively to prevent acute rejections and to maintain the allograft function. Triple drug therapy of a calcineurin inhibitor, an antiproliferative agent, and a corticosteroid is generally used. The selection of immunosuppressants to use is dependent on the risk of rejection of the recipient. Risk factors include pregnancy, mechanical circulatory assist device usage, surgeries requiring transfusions, and comorbidities (infection, renal failure, diabetes).

Live vaccines should be avoided in patients using immunosuppressive agents because patients on immunosuppression therapy have a higher chance of acquiring infections. Even with the potential risk, immunosuppressive agents are used to attain host-graft adaption to ensure a successful long term transplantation. While on immunsuppression, patients need to be monitored closely to avoid toxicities, drug interactions, and poor immunosuppression that can lead to adverse effects or rejection of the allograft [3] (Fig. 19.2).

19.3 Induction Therapy

19.3.1 Concept of Induction

Induction therapy was established after the empirical observation that in the perioperative period after transplantation a more intense immunosuppression is required to prevent early acute rejection. Induction therapy mainly consists of poly- or monoclonal antibodies that target specific epitopes on the surface of both B and T cells. Prophylactic mono- or polyclonal antibodies may result in lower rejection and mortality rates, or may even facilitate development of tolerance to the allograft. Furthermore, delayed initiation of nephrotoxic immunosuppressive drugs in patients with compromised renal function and early glucocorticoid weaning may be possible. Recommendations are mostly derived from retrospective analyses. Data about the comparison between induction versus non-induction should be interpreted with caution [10]. Decreased early rejection may be exchanged for an increase in late rejection after completion of induction therapy and for increased rates of infection and malignancy potentially associated with such therapy.

Currently, approximately 50% of the centers worldwide use antibody-based induction therapy [11]. While the use of the murine monoclonal antibody OKT3 has declined from 22% in 1995 to less than 1% in 2015, the share of polyclonal antibodies has remained stable with approximately 20% during the past 12 years. Although, new formulations (thymoglobulin, ATG-F) have replaced the antibodies used in the past (ATGAM, Minnesota-ATG). At present, anti-IL-2 receptor antibodies are the agents (30%) most frequently used for induction therapy after heart transplantation.

19.3.2 Polyclonal Antibodies

Heterologous antibody preparations derived from immunized animals have been used in transplantation since the 1960s, both as induction and rescue therapies. Polyclonal antibodies induce dose-dependent T cell depletion in blood and peripheral lymphoid tissues, most likely through complement-dependent cell lysis and activation-associated apoptosis mechanisms. Given their broad spectrum of activities, their anti-rejection properties are believed to be mediated by mechanisms other than T cell depletion, including costimulation blockade, adhesion molecule modulation, and B cell depletion [12–14]. This broad spectrum of activity is also responsible for the antibodies' toxicities, including thrombocytopenia and leukopenia.

Polyclonal antibodies are derived by immunization of rabbits (thymoglobulin, ATG) or horses (ATGAM) with human thymocytes. Induction with polyclonal antibodies has been linked in some studies to higher rates of post-transplant lymphoproliferative disorder (PTLD). In contrast, data from a registry that included 25,000 transplant patients failed to reveal such an association. Moreover, ATG may have a protective effect against PTLD if antiviral prophylaxis is used after induction therapy [15].

One retrospective analysis showed that ATG-treated patients had fewer rejection episodes and a trend towards less graft vasculopathy than recipients who were not given induction therapy [16]. Two studies comparing different polyclonal antibodies formulations have shown different results. One study showed less rejection in 342 patients treated with thymoglobulin compared to 142 patients treated with ATG [17]. However, no difference between these two antibody formulations was seen in a 50-patient prospective randomized trial [18].

In recent years, shorter ATG application (5 vs. 7 days) or adjustment of ATG dose have shown to lower the lymphocyte count (below <100/μL). While shorter duration of ATG administration was associated with increased rates of rejection, dosage adjustment of ATG according to T cell counts was related to a decrease of rejection rates [19].

Delay of calcineurin inhibitor (CNI) therapy under the protection of polyclonal antibodies was examined in two studies. Both showed improvement of renal function with delay of CNI initiation between 5 and 12 days. Acute rejection incidences did not increase [20, 21].

Three polyclonal preparations are currently used for induction: two rabbit-derived antibody preparations, Fresenius-ATG (Fresenius) and Thymoglobuline (Genzyme), and 1 horse derived product ATGAM (Upjohn).

19.3.3 IL-2 Receptor Antagonists

Use of Interleukin-2 receptor (IL-2R) antagonists for induction therapy has increased in the past few years, with 20–30% of patients undergoing heart transplantation are currently treated with IL-2R antagonists [11]. Initially, two specific monoclonal antibodies binding to CD25 (IL-2R), daclizumab and basiliximab, were developed. They were designed to reduce the limitations of former nonhuman antibody specimens by creating a chimeric human/murine (basiliximab) or humanized (daclizumab) monoclonal antibody that specifically binds to the IL-2R on activated T lymphocytes. This action prevents their T lymphocyte expansion without the associated development of serum sickness caused by mouse, rabbit, or horse derived proteins [22]. Daclizumab (Zenapax) was discontinued by the manufacturer in 2009 due to diminishing market demand.

Basiliximab was first used in renal transplantation. Later, it was increasingly used in heart transplantation recipients as induction therapy or in the case of graft rejection. The antibody should be administrated intravenously within

2–24 h after transplantation. Repeated administration should be undertaken within 4 days (half-life: 7.2 days). When a dosage of 2.5–25 mg is given twice (day 0 and day 4), approximately 90% of available IL-2 receptors on T lymphocytes are described to be blocked. This dosage should be maintained for 4–6 weeks [23, 24].

Trials comparing IL-2 receptor antagonists without induction have led to contradictory results. Beniaminovitz reported the results of daclizumab induction in a prospective, randomized, open-label pilot trial. Although rejection decreased during the first 3 months after transplantation, there was no difference in rejection and survival at 1 year [23]. This small trial of 55 patients was followed by a 434 patient involving prospective, randomized, double-blinded, multi-centered trial that showed significantly fewer acute rejection episodes at 12 months post-transplantation (35.6% vs. 47.7%) with daclizumab [25]. The use of daclizumab to treat rejection was associated with a higher risk of death from infection in the daclizumab group.

A prospective, randomized trial of basiliximab induction versus placebo in 56 patients was unable to show significant differences between these treatment groups in regard to adverse events, but it did demonstrate a lower incidence of (first biopsy-proven) acute rejections [26]. A retrospective comparison of 25 patients with renal insufficiency treated with basiliximab and a CNI delay of 4 days versus 33 patients without induction demonstrated similar survival and rejection rates [27]. Two retrospective studies compared the use of an IL-2 receptor antagonist with OKT3 and reported conflicting results. One study showed less allograft rejection in the IL-2 receptor blocker group, while the other revealed no differences in rejection between groups [28, 29].

A total of five trials compared thymoglobulin with basiliximab. All studies showed fewer rejection episodes in thymoglobulin groups [16, 22, 30]. However, infection rates were lower in the basiliximab groups, while survival rates were similar. A prospective comparison of thymoglobulin with daclizumab failed to detect differences in survival, rejection, or infection rates [31].

19.3.4 Alemtuzumab

Alemtuzumab (Campath-1H) is a humanized rat anti-CD52 monoclonal antibody that rapidly depletes CD52 expressing lymphocytes in central and peripheral lymphoid tissues and results in a long-lasting lymphopenia. It might combine the potent depleting capabilities of polyclonal antibodies with the benefits of humanized monoclonal antibodies, including ease of administration, consistent activity, and safety. While the agent has been used as induction therapy in in kidney transplant recipients [32], the use of Campath for heart transplantation is under investigation. First results indicate that it decreases the incidence of early acute cellular rejection and maintains immunosuppression at lower dosages [33].

19.3.5 Muromonab-CD3 (OKT3)

Muromonab-CD3 (OKT3) is a murine monoclonal antibody that binds to the CD3 molecule, causing internalization of the T cell receptor and simultaneous T cell activation and depletion. OKT-3 was the first monoclonal antibody approved for clinical use in humans.

The use of OKT3 as an inductive therapeutic has dramatically decreased during the last decade, making its availability in the future uncertain. Comparison of OKT3 versus no induction was described mostly in the 1990s and showed no influence on rejection or survival. A 9-year experience with 85 patients treated with OKT3 compared to 29 patients who did not undergo induction therapy found no differences between the two groups [34]. A review of the literature up until 1992 by Carrier et al. concluded that the use of OKT3 was not associated with any mortality benefit in heart transplantation [35]. Furthermore, OKT3 administration proved to be associated with a number of important acute and long-term side effects. The first drug doses can typically cause a cytokine release syndrome; long-term adverse reactions include an increased risk of life-threatening opportunistic infections. In addition, anti mouse antibodies may develop, which could be associated with anaphylactic reactions or therapeutic failure. While in one study, the prolonged use of OKT3 for prophylaxis of acute rejection after heart transplantation has been associated with a higher risk for PTLD [36], newer reports have shown a reduction in lymphoma incidence [10, 37].

19.4 Calcineurin Inhibitors

Calcineurin (CN) is an enzyme that dephosphorylates the nuclear factor of activated T cell complex (NF-ATC), which regulates the transcription promotor of Interleukin 2 (IL-2) production. CN is activated when an antigen-presenting cell interacts with a T cell receptor, leading to an upregulation of IL-2 followed by the production of cytokines mediated by activated and stimulated T lymphocytes [38]. It is discussed that the absolute amount of produced IL-2 influences the extent of the immune system response.

Drugs blocking CN are named calcineurin inhibitors (CNIs); cyclosporine A (CYA) and tacrolimus (TAC) are the most prominent agents. CYA and TAC bind a specific immunophilin to form a complex that interacts with intracellular CN to inhibit the expression of genes of proinflammatory cytokines. Reduced cytokine production prevents T cell activation and proliferation, upregulates adhesion molecules, and decreases the inflammatory response [10].

Besides the generalized adverse effects of all immunosuppressive compounds caused by their interaction with the immune system, CNIs are particularly associated with nephrotoxic and neurologic side effects. Dose reduction or even avoidance of CNIs in heart transplantation protocols have been studied extensively [39]. CNIs are still considered to be the most important part of immunosuppression after heart transplantation [11].

19.4.1 Cyclosporine

CYA is a lipophil, cyclic polypeptide consisting of 11 amino acids. It binds to cyclophylin (CpN) to form a complex that inhibits CpN, resulting in a suppression of activated T cells and B-cell function. CYA was isolated from the fungus, *Tolypocladium inflatum*, found at the Hardanger Vidda in Norway in 1971. It was initially investigated as an antifungal antibiotic. Its immunosuppressive activity was first reported by Borel in 1976 [40]. Thereafter, the effectiveness in animal and human studies was investigated by Calne and coworkers in Cambridge [41]. They discovered that CYA improved heterogenic heart allografts in rats [42]. The effectiveness of CYA was confirmed in renal transplant recipients [43]. These early studies also recognized potential disadvantages of CYA, such as high rates of lymphoma [43] and its nephrotoxic side effects [44, 45].

The Stanford group introduced CYA into clinical practice for heart transplantation [46]. After evaluating CYA after heterotopic and orthotopic heart transplantation in monkeys, they administered CYA in 66 patients and revealed a unique survival of 80% after 1 year. In the initial clinical phase, the fixed CYA dose was 18 mg/kg per day in combination with azathioprine and corticosteroids [47, 48]. The application method was later modified to an administration adapted to measurements of CYA blood trough levels using a target range of 100–300 ng/ml, followed by a decrease to 100–300 ng/ml for the first month and thereafter lowered to 50–150 ng/ml, given in combination with AzA and ATG (for the first 7 days after heart transplantation).

Compared to the initially available oil-based compound, the later introduced microemulsion revealed better gastrointestinal (GI) absorption and a more reliable pharmacokinetic profile [49], leading to significant reductions of rejection episodes requiring antilymphocyte antibody therapy (6.9 vs. 17.7%, $p = 0.002$), CS dose (0.37 vs. 0.48 mg/kg/day, $p = 0.034$) and treatment failures (3.7 vs. 9.4%, $p = 0.037$) at 24 months [50] as demonstrated in a randomized trial. The renal CYA excretion was proven to be only 6%. Metabolism of CYA occurs via the cytochrome P-450 (CYP450) enzyme system to at least 30 metabolites, and multiple drugs as well as certain foods interacting with the CYP-450 may alter CYA concentrations. Vice versa, CYA inhibits CYP3A4 enzymes and alters the metabolism of other drugs [10].

Monitoring of CYA levels and renal function with appropriate dose adjustments at the time of initiation and discontinuation is essential. Measurement of 12-h trough CYA concentrations remains the standard approach for monitoring CYA therapy despite evidence that it may underestimate the total CYA exposure. Evaluation of 2-h post-dose concentrations (C2) in de novo and stable heart transplant recipients has revealed variable results. In some studies, C2 levels identified patients at risk of receiving inappropriately high CYA doses with a certain susceptibility to experience drug toxicity [20]. Maintenance of a low C2 level in heart transplant recipients given antibody therapy was associated with preserved renal function without increased risk of acute rejection or compromise of heart transplant survival [51]. Compared to 28 historical controls monitored only with CYA trough levels, 28 heart transplant recipients monitored with both C2 and trough levels had a slight reduction of EMB proven rejection (21 vs. 39% $p =$ ns), a significant reduction in 3A rejection (5 vs. 11% $p < 0.002$) and a lower glomerular filtration rate (GFR) [52]. Nevertheless, determination of CYA C0 trough levels (measurement before next dose) is clinically much more practical. The fact that maintaining therapeutic C0 drug levels has been related to good allograft and patient outcomes makes CYA still commonly used [10, 50, 53].

Nowadays recommended CYA dosages for initial intravenous application are either 2–4 mg/kg once a day continuously over 24 h or alternatively, 1–2 mg/kg twice a day over 4–6 h. Subsequent oral application using a dose of 8–12 mg/kg/day in 2 divided doses is popular. Afterwards, dosage is adjusted to target trough levels and dosage reduction is aimed to as low as 3–5 mg/kg/day in the long term follow up of patients without rejection episodes. CYA levels are usually kept highest in the first year post-transplantation (200–350 ng/mL) and then lowered (100–200 ng/mL). Target drug levels should be individualized with regard to CYA related toxicities, specifically renal dysfunction, infections, and malignancies.

19.4.2 Tacrolimus

TAC inhibits CN by forming a complex with the FK506 binding protein, resulting in suppressed T lymphocyte activation and cytokine production. The structure of the macrolide antibiotic isolated from *Streptomyces tsukubaensis* is more similar to rapamycin than to CYA. TAC was described 7 years after the introduction of CYA [54] and evaluated to be much more potent [55].

Armitage reported on its first clinical use in 10 heart transplant recipients in combination with steroids at the University of Pittsburgh [56, 57]. When orally administered, the absorption half-life is 5–6 h and the bioavailability is about 20%, depending on diet of the patient (grapefruit juice increases the bioavailability of TAC and fatty foods reduce the bioavailability); it is mainly absorbed in the duodenum and jejunum. About 75–99% is bound to proteins, and the elimination half-life is 11.7 h. Impaired liver function amplifies the bioavailability. TAC has large inter-individual and intra-individual variations in pharmacokinetics. It is excreted intestinally [58].

The rate and extent of TAC absorption is variable. In certain ethnic groups, such as African Americans, bioavailability may be highly diminished. The compound also undergoes extensive metabolism via the CYP3A system and several drugs may alter its action. Some studies in heart transplant recipients have shown an acceptable correlation between trough concentrations and 12-h AUC [39, 59]. Although some small studies have indicated that 2–4 h post-dose levels might be more representative of TAC exposure than measurement of trough levels, data correlating this TAC monitoring method with heart allograft outcomes are lacking [60].

Multiple single-center and multi-center randomized comparisons between de novo use of TAC and CYA after heart transplantation are available [61–65]. While in most investigations patient survival was similar, TAC treated patients showed less side effects of hypertension, hyperlipidemia, and renal dysfunction [66]. There might, however, be a higher incidence of post-transplant diabetes under tacrolimus [61]. Furthermore, the incidence of acute rejection episodes in TAC treated patients seems to be lower than CYA treated patients. In the largest comparison study, 314 de novo heart transplant recipients were randomized to either TAC or CYA in combination with azathioprine and glucocorticoids [61]. While patient's survival after 18 months was similar among both groups, TAC treated patients had a lower incidence of biopsy-proven moderate or severe acute cellular rejection at 6 months (28% vs 42%, $p = 0.013$). Also, TAC is increasingly used in children [67].

TAC is normally given orally. Drug dosing starts with 0.1–0.3 mg/kg/day and is titrated to achieve therapeutic 12-h trough levels in the first 6 months after transplantation of 10–15 ng/mL, and in stable patients thereafter of 5–10 ng/mL. If intravenous administration is used, one-third to one-tenth of the oral daily dose should be given as a continuous infusion over 24 h.

In the meantime, TAC is available as an extended release once-daily product. This TAC formula is best taken in the morning [68]. In renal and liver transplant recipients, conversion from the original twice-daily TAC to the once-daily preparation was associated with unchanged drug pharmacokinetic profile, safety, and allograft outcomes at 2 years after conversion [10, 69, 70].

19.5 Cytotoxic Agents

19.5.1 Mycophenolate Mofetil (MMF/CellCept)

Mycophenolate mofetil is a prodrug of mycophenolic acid that reversibly inhibits inosine-5′-monophosphate dehydrogenase (IMPDH) to prevent the synthesis of guanosine monophosphate nucleotides [71]. Mycophenolate mofetil selectively inhibits de novo purine synthesis and not the purine salvage pathway. This discriminatory inhibition is important because MMF can specifically target lymphocytes without injuring other organs [72, 73], especially since lymphocytes completely depend on the de novo purine synthesis. Additionally, MMF reduces the expression of adhesion molecules, such as VCAM-1, E-selectin, and P-selectin to decrease the recruitment of inflammatory cells to the allograft [76]. Mycophenolate mofetil also prevents fibrosis by inhibiting fibroblast functions [75]. With these actions, MMF can help reverse ongoing acute rejection and prevent rejection. Furthermore, MMF is used with other drugs to increase immunosuppression. Using MMF with calcineurin inhibitors has demonstrated better patient and graft survival and reduced allograft rejection [76, 77]. However, absorption of MMF is reduced by cyclosporine, so dosage of MMF may need to be adjusted for MMF to be within therapeutic range.

Mycophenolate mofetil does not require monitoring, lacks organ toxicity, and has low cardiovascular risk [3]. It is often the drug used in steroid-free treatment. Most of the adverse effects of MMF are gastrointestinal and hematologic. This includes nausea, vomiting, diarrhea, joint pain, pancytopenia, hypertension, and hyperglycemia. However, these side effects are less severe than those associated with azathioprine, so MMF has been used over azathioprine. Mycophenolate mofetil should not be used in patients with severe renal impairment, patients contemplating pregnancy or are pregnant, and patients with severe gastrointestinal disordered. Mycophenolate mofetil has embryofetal toxicity, gastrointestinal side effects, and nephrotoxicity. Since MMF has similar functions as Myfortic or azathioprine, it should not be used concomitantly with these agents. Myphenolate mofetil should not be used with antacids with magnesium and aluminum hydroxides, proton pump inhibitors, cholestyramine, sevelamer, and certain antibiotics [78]. If MMF were to be used with these drugs, its dosage needs to be adjusted to be within therapeutic range. Antacids with magnesium and aluminum hydroxides and proton pump inhibitors cause decreased therapeutic effect by decreasing MMF solubility due to the increase in pH. Sevelamer also decrease the therapeutic effect of MMF. If needed, MMF can be administered 2 h after sevelamer [78]. Mycophenolate mofetil depends on enterohepatic recirculation to convert to its active form in the liver, so it should not be used with drugs, like cholestyramine or bile acid sequestrants, that hinder enterohepatic recirculation. Antibiotics, such as rifampin or ciprofloxacin, cause reduced MMF concentration [78]. Thus, dosage of MMF would need to be adjusted to improve efficacy.

19.5.2 Myfortic (Mycophenolate Sodium)

Myfortic (mycophenolate sodium) is the enteric-coated version of MMF. Its slow-releasing formulation of mycophenolic acid decreases the gastrointestinal side effects that are seen with MMF usage. Myfortic should not be used with drugs similar to MMF or are contraindicated with MMF, such as azathioprine, antacids with magnesium and aluminum hydroxides, choestyramine, bile acid sequestrants, sevelamer, and certain antibiotics [79].

19.6 Corticosteroids

Corticosteroids inhibit NF-κB to decrease cytokine transcription and to synthesize lipocortins to prevent arachidonic acid release [9]. This action suppresses B and T cell function and induces T cell apoptosis. Corticosteroids also inhibit IL-1, IL-6, IL-2, INF-γ, and TNF-α to decrease the number of lymphocytes in circulation and reduce chemotaxis activity [9]. It is widely used, specifically for transplantation and autoimmune and inflammatory disorders, to depress unwanted inflammatory responses. Anticoagulants, anticonvulsants, non-steroidal anti-inflammatory drugs (NSAIDs) are generally avoided when using corticosteroids or require dosage adjustments to be within therapeutic range [80]. Long-term use of corticosteroids can cause glucose intolerance leading to hyperglycemia, osteoporosis with avascular necrosis of bone, acne, hypertension, cataracts, diabetes, dyslipidemia, peptic ulcer formation, gastrointestinal bleeding, pancreatitis, personality changes, and iatrogenic cushingoid syndrome [80]. To avoid adverse effects from long-term use of corticosteroids but retain the immunosuppressive benefits, corticosteroids are given at a high dose intravenously before and after transplant surgery. Patients are switched to oral corticosteroids and start tapering the dose around 6 months after transplantation. The goal is to withdraw steroid therapy within the first year of transplantation if the patient is adequately immunosuppressed. Corticosteroids is the first line of therapy when signs of acute rejection appear [81, 82].

Prednisone, a prodrug of prednisolone, is the most widely used corticosteroids for transplantation. Like the mechanism of action of other corticosteroids, its mechanism of action mimics cortisol. The targeted glucocorticoid receptor is bound to stabilizing proteins, such as heat shock protein 90 (Hsp90) [83]. Once the corticosteroid binds the receptor, the associated molecules and Hsp90 is released. The steroid-receptor complex dimerizes and enters the nucleus to control gene transcription. This results in a reduction in the inflammatory and immune responses through increased synthesis of an inhibitor of phospholipase A_2 (PLA_2) and a decreased synthesis of cyclooxygenase-2 (COX-2), prostaglandins, leukotrienes, cytokines, and other signaling molecules. It specifically increases the catabolic rate of IgG and lowers IgG circulation. Side effects may include adrenal insufficiency, growth inhibition, salt retention, and the previously mentioned long-term adverse effects of using corticosteroids [80].

19.7 mTOR Inhibitors

19.7.1 Sirolimus (Rapamycin)

Sirolimus (rapamycin) is a macrolide antibiotic from *Streptomyces hygroscopius* that inhibits mTOR and has no discrimination between inhibiting mTORC1 and mTORC2 [84]. It binds FKBP12 and signals through PI_3K/AKT/mTOR pathway to block T cell progression from G1 to S phase and inhibits IL-2, IL-4, and IL-15 [3]. The consequent reduction of cytokines blocks T cell activation and B cell differentiation. Common adverse effects include peripheral edema, hypertension, abdominal pain, nausea, diarrhea, headache, fever, thrombocytopenia, insulin resistance, delayed wound healing, and hyperlipidemia [85]. Since sirolimus is metabolized by CYP3A4, it should not be used with drugs that induce or inhibit CYP3A4 to maintain therapeutic efficacy. Common drugs that would increase sirolimus blood concentrations are bromocriptione, cimetidine, cisapride, clotrimazole, danazol, diltiazem, fluconazole, protease inhibitors, metoclopramide, nicardipine, troleandomycin, and verapamil [85]. Carbamazepine, phenobarbital, phenytoin, rifapentine, and St. John's Wort can decrease its concentration [85]. This includes avoiding grapefruit juice while taking sirolimus [85]. Therefore, if the agents are to be used with sirolimus, they should not be used simultaneously and need sirolimus concentration needs to be monitored to prevent toxicity and to ensure therapeutic effect. Patients with hepatic impairment require lower doses of sirolimus to reduce the risk of toxicity. The drug is not used with cyclosporine due to increased nephrotoxicity, thrombocytopenia, and hypertension from cyclosporine being a substrate and inhibitor of CYP3A4 [86].

19.7.2 Everolimus

Everolimus is a derivative of sirolimus and has a similar mechanism of action. It is also a substrate of CYP3A4 and has the same drug interactions as sirolimus. Unlike sirolimus, it preferentially inhibits mTORC1 with no mTORC2 inhibition, which results in blocking the negative feedback and not the positive feedback to AKT [87]. This lowers the insulin resistance and diabetes risk that are associated with sirolimus, and everolimus has been shown to reduce CAV through reduced lipoprotein-associated phospholipase A_2 ($Lp-PLA_2$) activity and oxidative stress in heart transplant recipients [88]. However, everolimus retains many of the other adverse effects of sirolimus, such as diarrhea, headache, abdominal pain, fatigue, peripheral edema, hyperlipidemia, and thrombocytopenia [87]. It should not be used with angiotensin-converting enzyme (ACE) inhibitors because concomitantly they increase the risk for angioedema [87]. Everolimus helps prevent endomyocardial remodeling after heart transplantation [89]. When compared to sirolimus, everolimus has been shown to have fewer major adverse cardiac events [90]. Everolimus compared to azathioprine has been shown to reduce the frequency of rejection and CMV infections but also reduces the incidence and severity of CAV as defined by intravascular ultrasound (IVUS) [91]. Everolimus was associated with increased creatinine and decreased GFR when compared to azathioprine and regardless of cyclosporine levels [91]. Two doses of everolimus with reduced dose cyclosporine were also compared to MMF with standard dose cyclosprine in the largest clinical trial in cardiac transplantation [92]. Higher dose everolimus (3.0 mg daily) was associated with increased mortality and this arm of the study was terminated by the DSMB early. There was increased mortality at 12 months but not at 24 months in the everolimus 1.5 mg daily group compared to MMF but this was due to deaths from infections in patients also receiving induction therapy [92]. Patients treated with low dose cyclosporine did not have decreased renal function as compared to MMF patients while those who were treated with everolimus and standard dose cyclopsporine had decreased renal function [92]. Everolimus reduced the incidence and severity of CAV as defined by IVUS and even in patients at higher risk of CAV such as diabetics [92, 93].

An alternative strategy was proposed in the SCHEDULE study from Scandinavia which employed a protocol of initiating everolimus and weaning off cyclosporine by 7–11 weeks [94]. These patients had improved renal function compared to the cyclosporine control groupand had a lower incidence and less severity of CAV compared to the cyclopsorine controls. There was no difference in survival but there was a small number of everolimus patients who needed to be placed back on cyclosporine because there were several ISHLT 2R rejection episodes [95] (Fig. 19.3).

19.8 Experimental Immunosuppressants in Pipeline

Rituximab, an anti-CD20 monoclonal antibody has been used to treat lymphomas and antibody-mediated rejection and to mitigate antibody sensitization in cardiac transplant recipients. Rituximab was studied in a randomized clinical trial as part of the NIH Clinical Trials in Organ Transplantation (CTOT-11) to reduce the severity of CAV. 163 heart transplant recipients either received Rituximab or placebo beginning 0–12 days post-transplant. The primary endpoint, percent atheroma volume defined by IVUS and a measure of CAV was surprisingly increased in the Rituximab group compared to controls [95].

There is interest in targeting other mediators of inflammation to prevent rejection. One such target is IL-6 against which the monocloncal antibody tocilizamab is directed and has been approved as a treatment for rheumatoid arthritis. It is now being considered in clinical trials in cardiac transplantation.

Class	Immunosuppressant	Mechanism of Action	Toxicities	Interactions
calcineurin inhibitor	cyclosporine	binds cyclophilin to form a complex that inhibits calcineurin and T cell activation	nephrotoxicity, hypertension, hyperlipidemia, neurotoxicity, gingival hyperplasia, hirsutism, osteoporosis, tremor	
calcineurin inhibitor	tacrolimus	binds FKBP12 to prevent T cell activation	similar to cyclosporine; increased risk of diabetes and neurotoxicity; lower incidence of hypertension, hyperlipidemia, hirsuitism, gingival hyperplasia	
corticosteroid	prednisone	suppress B and T cell function; induce T cell apoptosis	adrenal suppression, growth inhibition, salt retention	anticoagulants, anticonvulsants, NSAIDs
immunoglobulin-based	basiliximab	humanized or chimeric monoclonal anti-CD25 antibody	hypersensitivity reactions (uncommon)	
immunoglobulin-based	anti-thymocyte globulin	animal-derived polyclonal antibodies against human T cells	cytokine-release syndrome, thrombocytopenia, leukopenia, serium sickness	
mTOR inhibitor	sirolimus (rapamycin)	bind FKBP12 to prevent T cell proliferation; inhibits mTORC1 and mTORC2	thrombocytopenia, insulin resistance, hyperlipidemia, impaired wound healing	CYP3A4 substrates and inhibitors
mTOR inhibitor	everolimus	bind FKBP12 to prevent T cell proliferation; preferentially inhibits mTORC1	similar to sirolimus; lower insulin resistance and diabetes than sirolimus	CYP3A4 substrates and inhibitors, ACE inhibitors
mycophenolic acid	mycophenolate mofetil	block de novo purine synthesis to prevent T and B cell proliferation	diarrhea, thrombocytopenia, hypertension, hyperglycemia	enterohepatic recirculation inhibitors, sevelamer, rifampin, ciprofloxacin
mycophenolic acid	Myfortic (mycophenolate sodium)	block de novo purine synthesis to prevent T and B cell proliferation	similar to mycophenolate with lessened gastrointestinal symptoms	enterohepatic recirculation inhibitors, sevelamer, rifampin, ciprofloxacin

Fig. 19.3 Table of immunosuppressants with mechanism of action, toxicities, and interactions

References

1. Eng HS, Leffell MS. Histocompatibility testing after fifty years of transplantation. J Immunol Methods. 2011;369(1–2):1–21.
2. Wang D, Matsumoto R, You Y, et al. CD3/CD28 costimulation-induced NF-kappaB activation is mediated by recruitment of protein kinase C-theta, Bcl10, and IkappaB kinase beta to the immunological synapse through CARMA1. Mol Cell Biol. 2004;24:164–71.
3. Halloran PF. Immunosuppressive drugs for kidney transplantation. N Engl J Med. 2004;351:2715–29.
4. Robertson H, Ali S, McDonnell BJ, Burt AD, Kirby JA. Chronic renal allograft dysfunction: the role of T cell-mediated tubular epithelial to mesenchymal cell transition. J Am Soc Nephrol. 2004;15:390–7.
5. Halloran PF, Melk A, Barth C. Rethinking chronic allograft nephropathy: the concept of accelerated senescence. J Am Soc Nephrol. 1999;10:167–81.
6. Raichlin E, Bae JH, Khalpey Z, et al. Conversion to sirolimus as primary immunosuppression attenuates the progression of allograft vasculopathy after cardiac transplantation. Circulation. 2007;116:2726–33.
7. Sanchez-Fructuoso AI, Sanchez-Fructuoso AI. Everolimus: an update on the mechanism of action, pharmacokinetics and recent clinical trials. Expert Opin Drug Metab Toxicol. 2008;4:807–19.
8. Carr SF, Papp E, Wu JC, et al. Characterization of human type I and type II IMP dehydrogenases. J Biol Chem. 1993;268:27286–90.
9. Coutinho AE, Chapman KE. The anti-inflammatory and immunosuppressive effects of glucocorticoids, recent developments and mechanistic insights. Mol Cell Endocrinol. 2011;335:2.
10. Taylor D, Meiser B, Webber S. The international society of heart and lung transplantation guidelines for the care of heart transplant recipients task force 2: immunosuppression and rejection (Nov. 8, 2010).
11. Lund LH, Edwards LB, Kucheryavaya AY, et al. The registry of the International Society for Heart and Lung Transplantation: thirty-second official adult heart transplantation report–2015; focus theme: early graft failure. J Heart Lung Transplant. 2015; 34:1244.
12. Bourdage JS, Hamlin DM. Comparative polyclonal antithymocyte globulin and antilymphocyte/antilymphoblast globulin anti-CD antigen analysis by flow cytometry. Transplantation. 1995;59(8):1194–200.
13. Rebellato LM, Gross U, Verbanac KM, Thomas JM. A comprehensive definition of the major antibody specificities in polyclonal rabbit antithymocyte globulin. Transplantation. 1994;57(5):685–94.
14. Genestier L, Fournel S, Flacher M, Assossou O, Revillard JP, Bonnefoy-Berard N. Induction of Fas (Apo-1, CD95) mediated apoptosis of activated lymphocytes by polyclonal antithymocyte globulins. Blood. 1998;91(7):2360–8.
15. Crespo-Leiro MG, Alonso-Pulpon L, Arizon JM, et al. Influence of induction therapy, immunosuppressive regimen and anti-viral prophylaxis on development of lymphomas after heart transplantation: data from the Spanish post-heart transplant tumour registry. J Heart Lung Transplant. 2007;26(11):1105–9.
16. Carrier M, White M, Perrault LP, et al. A 10-year experience with intravenous thymoglobuline in induction of immunosuppression following heart transplantation. J Heart Lung Transplant. 1999;18(12):1218–23.
17. Zuckermann AO, Grimm M, Czerny M, et al. Improved long-term results with thymoglobuline induction therapy after cardiac transplantation: a comparison of two different rabbit-antithymocyte globulines. Transplantation. 2000;69(9):1890–8.
18. Schnetzler B, Leger P, Volp A, Dorent R, Pavie A, Gandjbakhch I. A prospective randomized controlled study on the efficacy and tolerance of two antilymphocytic globulins in the prevention of rejection in first-heart transplant recipients. Transpl Int. 2002;15(6): 317–25.
19. Koch A, Daniel V, Dengler TJ, Schnabel PA, Hagl S, Sack FU. Effectivity of a T-cell-adapted induction therapy with anti-thymocyte globulin (Sangstat). J Heart Lung Transplant. 2005;24(6):708–13.
20. Delgado DH, Rao V, Hamel J, Miriuka S, Cusimano RJ, Ross HJ. Monitoring of cyclosporine 2-hour post-dose levels in heart transplantation: improvement in clinical outcomes. J Heart Lung Transplant. 2005;24(9):1343–6.
21. Cantarovich M, Giannetti N, Barkun J, Cecere R. Antithymocyte globulin induction allows a prolonged delay in the initiation of cyclosporine in heart transplant patients with postoperative renal dysfunction. Transplantation. 2004;78(5):779–81.
22. Mattei MF, Redonnet M, Gandjbakhch I, et al. Lower risk of infectious deaths in cardiac transplant patients receiving basiliximab versus anti-thymocyte globulin as induction therapy. J Heart Lung Transplant. 2007;26(7):693–9.
23. Beniaminovitz A, Itescu S, Lietz K, Donovan M, Burke EM, Groff BD, et al. Prevention of rejection in cardiac transplantation by blockade of the interleukin-2 receptor with a monoclonal antibody. N Engl J Med. 2000;342(9):613–9.
24. Nashan B, Moore R, Amlot P, Schmidt AG, Abeywickrama K, Soulillou JP. Randomised trial of basiliximab versus placebo for control of acute cellular rejection in renal allograft recipients. CHIB 201 international study group. Lancet. 1997;350(9086): 1193–8.
25. Hershberger RE, Starling RC, Eisen HJ, et al. Daclizumab to prevent rejection after cardiac transplantation. N Engl J Med. 2005;352(26):2705–13.
26. Mehra MR, Zucker MJ, Wagoner L, et al. A multicenter, prospective, randomized, double-blind trial of basiliximab in heart transplantation. J Heart Lung Transplant. 2005;24(9):1297–304.
27. Rosenberg PB, Vriesendorp AE, Drazner MH, et al. Induction therapy with basiliximab allows delayed initiation of cyclosporine and preserves renal function after cardiac transplantation. J Heart Lung Transplant. 2005;24(9):1327–31.
28. Almenar L, Garcia-Palomar C, Martinez-Dolz L, et al. Influence of induction therapy on rejection and survival in heart transplantation. Transplant Proc. 2005;37(9):4024–7.
29. Cuppoletti A, Perez-Villa F, Vallejos I, Roig E. Experience with single-dose daclizumab in the prevention of acute rejection in heart transplantation. Transplant Proc. 2005;37(9):4036–8.
30. Carlsen J, Johansen M, Boesgaard S, et al. Induction therapy after cardiac transplantation: a comparison of antithymocyte globulin and daclizumab in the prevention of acute rejection. J Heart Lung Transplant. 2005;24(3):296–302.
31. Chou NK, Wang SS, Chen YS, et al. Induction immunosuppression with basiliximab in heart transplantation. Transplant Proc. 2008;40(8):2623–5.
32. Morris PJ, Russell NK. Alemtuzumab (Campath-1H): a systematic review in organ transplantation. Transplantation. 2006;81:1361.
33. Teuteberg J, Shullo M, Zomak R, et al. Alemtuzumab induction facilitates corticosteroid-free maintenance immunosuppression inhuman cardiac transplantation. J Heart Lung Transplant. 2008;27(2):S201–2.
34. Adamson R, Obispo E, Dychter S, et al. Long-term outcome with the use of OKT3 induction therapy in heart transplant patients: a single-center experience. Transplant Proc. 1998;30(u):1107–9.
35. Carrier M, Jenicek M, Pelletier LC. Value of monoclonal antibody OKT3 in solid organ transplantation: a metaanalysis. Transplant Proc. 1992;24(6):2586–91.
36. Swinnen LJ, Costanzo-Nordin MR, Fisher SG, et al. Increased incidence of lymphoproliferative disorder after immunosuppression with the monoclonal antibody OKT3 in cardiac-transplant recipients. N Engl J Med. 1990;323(25):1723–8.
37. Opelz G, Dohler B. Lymphomas after solid organ transplantation: a collaborative transplant study report. Am J Transplant. 2004;4(2):222–30.

38. Yamashita M, Katsumata M, Iwashima M, Kimura M, Shimizu C, Kamata T, et al. T cell receptor-induced calcineurin activation regulates T helper type 2 cell development by modifying the interleukin 4 receptor signaling complex. J Exp Med. 2000;191(11):1869–79.
39. Meiser BM. The best dosing for initial tacrolimus application is trough level adapted! Transplantation. 2005;79(1):10–1.
40. Borel JF, Feurer C, Gubler HU, Stahelin H. Biological effects of cyclosporin A: a new antilymphocytic agent. Agents Actions. 1976;6(4):468–75.
41. Nagao T, White DJ, Calne RY. Kinetics of unresponsiveness induced by a short course of cyclosporin a. Transplantation. 1982;33(1):31–5.
42. Kostakis A. Early experience with cyclosporine: a historic perspective. Transplant Proc. 2004;36(2 Suppl):22S–4S.
43. Merrill JP. Publications of John P. Merrill. Nephron. 1978;22(1–3):265–80.
44. Kahan BD. Cyclosporine: nursing and paraprofessional aspects. Transplant Proc. 1983;15(4 Suppl 1–2):3109–83.
45. Kahan BD. Cyclosporine: a revolution in transplantation. Transplant Procs. 1999;31(1-2A):14S–5S.
46. Oyer PE. Heart transplantation in the cyclosporine era. Ann Thorac Surg. 1988;46(5):489–90.
47. Wallwork J, McGregor CG, Wells FC, Cory-Pearce R, English TA. Cyclosporin and intravenous sulphadimidine and trimethoprim therapy. Lancet. 1983;1(8320):366–7.
48. Cabrol C, Gandjbakhch I, Guiraudon G, Pavie A, Villemot JP, Viars P, et al. Heart transplantation. Our experience at the Pitie Hospital in Paris. Bull Acad Natl Med. 1982;166(2):235–50.
49. Cooney GF, Jeevanandam V, Choudhury S, Feutren G, Mueller EA, Eisen HJ. Comparative bioavailability of Neoral and Sandimmune in cardiac transplant recipients over 1 year. Transplant Proc. 1998;30(5):1892–4.
50. Eisen HJ, Hobbs RE, Davis SF, et al. Safety, tolerability, and efficacy of cyclosporine microemulsion in heart transplant recipients: a randomized, multicenter, doubleblind comparison with the oil-based formulation of cyclosporine–results at 24 months after transplantation. Transplantation. 2001;71(1):70–8.
51. Cantarovich M, Ross H, Arizon JM, et al. Benefit of Neoral C2 monitoring in de novo cardiac transplant recipients receiving basiliximab induction. Transplantation. 2008;85(7):992–9.
52. Barnard JB, Thekkudan J, Richardson S, et al. Cyclosporine profiling with C2 and C0 monitoring improves outcomes after heart transplantation. J Heart Lung Transplant. 2006;25(5):564–8.
53. Oyer P, Stinson E, Jamieson S, et al. CYA in cardiac transplantation: a 2 1/2 year follow-up. Transplant Proc. 1983;15:2546.
54. Kino T, Hatanaka H, Miyata S, Inamura N, Nishiyama M, Yajima T, et al. FK-506, a novel immunosuppressant isolated from a streptomyces. II. Immunosuppressive effect of FK-506 in vitro. J Antibiot. 1987;40(9):1256–65.
55. Ochiai T, Nakajima K, Nagata M, Suzuki T, Asano T, Uematsu T, et al. Effect of a new immunosuppressive agent, FK 506, on heterotopic cardiac allotransplantation in the rat. Transplant Proc. 1987;19(1 Pt 2):1284–6.
56. Armitage JM, Kormos RL, Morita S, Fung J, Marrone GC, Hardesty RL, et al. Clinical trial of FK 506 immunosuppression in adult cardiac transplantation. Ann Thorac Surg. 1992;54(2):205–10. discussion 10–1
57. Armitage JM, Kormos RL, Fung J, Starzl TE. The clinical trial of FK 506 as primary and rescue immunosuppression in adult cardiac transplantation. Transplant Proc. 1991;23(6):3054–7.
58. Taylor DO, Barr ML, Meiser BM, Pham SM, Mentzer RM, Gass AL. Suggested guidelines for the use of tacrolimus in cardiac transplant recipients. J Heart Lung Transplant. 2001;20(7):734–8.
59. Park SI, Felipe CR, Pinheiro-Machado PG, Garcia R, Tedesco-Silva H Jr, Medina-Pestana JO. Circadian and time-dependent variability in tacrolimus pharmacokinetics. Fundam Clin Pharmacol. 2007;21(2):191–7.
60. Langers P, Press RR, den Hartigh J, et al. Flexible limited sampling model for monitoring tacrolimus in stable patients having undergone liver transplantation with samples 4 to 6 hours after dosing is superior to trough concentration. Ther Drug Monit. 2008;30(4):456–61.
61. Grimm M, Rinaldi M, Yonan NA, et al. Superior prevention of acute rejection by tacrolimus vs. cyclosporine in heart transplant recipients–a large European trial. Am J Transplant. 2006;6:1387.
62. Groetzner J, Meiser BM, Schirmer J, et al. Tacrolimus or cyclosporine for immunosuppression after cardiac transplantation: which treatment reveals more side effects during long-term follow-up? Transplant Proc. 2001;33:1461.
63. Meiser BM, Uberfuhr P, Fuchs A, et al. Single-center randomized trial comparing tacrolimus (FK506) and cyclosporine in the prevention of acute myocardial rejection. J Heart Lung Transplant. 1998;17:782.
64. Reichart B, Meiser B, Viganò M, et al. European multicenter Tacrolimus (FK506) heart pilot study: one-year results–European Tacrolimus multicenter heart study group. J Heart Lung Transplant. 1998;17:775.
65. Taylor DO, Barr ML, Radovancevic B, et al. A randomized, multicenter comparison of tacrolimus and cyclosporine immunosuppressive regimens in cardiac transplantation: decreased hyperlipidemia and hypertension with tacrolimus. J Heart Lung Transplant. 1999;18:336.
66. Kobashigawa JA, Stevenson LW, Brownfield ED, Gleeson MP, Moriguchi JD, Kawata N, et al. Corticosteroid weaning late after heart transplantation: relation to HLA-DR mismatching and long-term metabolic benefits. J Heart Lung Transplant. 1995;14(5):963–7.
67. Dipchand AI, Rossano JW, Edwards LB, et al. The registry of the International Society for Heart and Lung Transplantation: eighteenth official pediatric heart transplantation report—2015; focus theme: early graft failure. J Heart Lung Transplant. 2015;34:1233–43.
68. Cross SA, Perry CM. Tacrolimus once-daily formulation: in the prophylaxis of transplant rejection in renal or liver allograft recipients. Drugs. 2007;67(13):1931–43.
69. Alloway R, Steinberg S, Khalil K, et al. Two years postconversion from a prograf-based regimen to a oncedaily tacrolimus extended-release formulation in stable kidney transplant recipients. Transplantation. 2007;83(12):1648–51.
70. Florman S, Alloway R, Kalayoglu M, et al. Once-daily tacrolimus extended release formulation: experience at 2 years postconversion from a Prograf-based regimen in stable liver transplant recipients. Transplantation. 2007;83(12):1639–42.
71. Allison AC, Eugui EM. Purine metabolism and immunosuppressive effects of mycophenolate mofetil (MMF). Clin Transpl. 1996;10:77–84.
72. Giblett ER, Anderson JE, Cohen F, Pollara B, Meuwissen HJ. Adenosine-deaminase deficiency in two patients with severely impaired cellular immunity. Lancet. 1972;2:1067–9.
73. Allison AC, Hovi T, Watts RWE, Webster ADB. Immunological observations on patients with the Lesch-Nyhan syndrome, and on the role of de-novo purine synthesis in lymphocyte transformation. Lancet. 1975;2:1179–83.
74. Blaheta RA, Leckel K, Wittig B, et al. Mycophenolate mofetil impairs transendothelial migration of allogeneic CD4 and CD8 T-cells. Transplant Proc. 1999;31:1250–2.
75. Morath C, Schwenger V, Beimler J, et al. Antifibrotic actions of mycophenolic acid. Clin Transpl. 2006;20:25–9.
76. Meier-Kriesche HU, Steffen BJ, Hochberg AM, et al. Long-term use of mycophenolate mofetil is associated with a reduction in the incidence and risk of late rejection. Am J Transplant. 2003;3:68–73.

77. Gourishankar S, Hunsicker LG, Jhangri GS, Cockfield SM, Halloran PF. The stability of the glomerular filtration rate after renal transplantation is improving. J Am Soc Nephrol. 2003;14:2387–94.
78. CellCept [package insert]. South San Francisco: Genentech USA, Inc.; 2015.
79. Myfortic [package insert]. East Hanover: Novartis Pharmaceutical Corporation; 2016.
80. Prednisone [package insert]. Columbus: Roxane Laboratories; 2012.
81. Lindenfeld J, Miller GG, Shakar SF, et al. Drug therapy in the heart transplant recipient: part I: cardiac rejection and immunosuppressive drugs. Circulation. 2004;110:3734–40.
82. Lindenfeld J, Miller GG, Shakar SF, et al. Drug therapy in the heart transplant recipient: part II: immunosuppressive drugs. Circulation. 2004;110:3858–65.
83. Grad I, Picard D. The glucocorticoid responses are shaped by molecular chaperones. Mol Cell Endocrinol. 2007;275(1–2):2–12.
84. Lamming DW, Ye L, Katajisto P, Katajisto P, Goncalves MD, Saitoh M, Stevens DM, Davis JG, Salmon AB, Richardson A, Ahima RS, Guertin DA, Sabatini DM, Baur JA, et al. Rapamycin-induced insulin resistance is mediated by mTORC2 loss and uncoupled from longevity. Science. 2012;335(6076):1638–43.
85. Rapamune [package insert]. Philadelphia: Wyeth Pharmaceuticals Inc.; 2015.
86. MacDonald AS. A worldwide, phase III, randomized, controlled, safety and efficacy study of a sirolimus/cyclosporine regimen for prevention of acute rejection in recipients of primary mismatched renal allografts. Transplantation. 2001;71:271–80.
87. Afinitor [package insert]. East Hanover: Novartis Pharmaceuticals Corp.; 2016.
88. Rosing K, Fobker M, Kannenberg F, Gunia S, Dell'aquila AM, Kwiecien R, Nofer J. Everolimus therapy is associated with reduced lipoprotein-associated phospholipase A2 (Lp-Pla2) activity and oxidative stress in heart transplant recipients. Atherosclerosis. 2013;230(1):164–70.
89. Hiemann NE, Wellnhofer E, Lehmkuhl HB, Knosalla C, Hetzer R, Meyer R. Everolimus prevents endomyocardial remodeling after heart transplantation. Transplantation. 2011;92:1165e72.
90. Jensen L, Thayssen P, Christiansen E, et al. Safety and efficacy of Everolimus- versus Sirolimus-eluting stents: 5-year results from SORT OUT IV. J Am Coll Cardiol. 2016;67(7):751–62.
91. Eisen HJ, Tuzcu EM, Dorent R, Kobashigawa J, Mancini D, Valantine-Von Kaeppler HA, Starling RC, Sorensen K, Hummel M, Lind JM, Abeywickrama KH, Bernhardt P. Everolimus for the prevention of allograft rejection and vasculopathy in cardiac transplant recipients. N Engl J Med. 2003;349:847–58.
92. Eisen HJ, Kobashigawa J, Starling RC, Pauly DF, Kfoury A, Ross H, Wang SS, Cantin B, Van Bakel A, Ewald G, Hirt S, Lehmkuhl H, Keogh A, Rinaldi M, Potena L, Zuckermann A, Dong G, Cornu-Artis C, Lopez P. Everolimus versus mycophenolate mofetil in heart transplantation: a randomized, multicenter trial. Am J Transplant. 2013;13:1203–16.
93. Kobashigawa JA, Pauly DF, Starling RC, Eisen H, Ross H, Wang SS, Cantin B, Hill JA, Lopez P, Dong G, Nicholls SJ. A2310 IVUS substudy investigators. Cardiac allograft vasculopathy by intravascular ultrasound in heart transplant patients: substudy from the everolimus versus mycophenolate mofetil randomized, multicenter trial. JACC Heart Fail. 2013;5:389–99.
94. Andreassen AK, Andersson B, Gustafsson F, Eiskjaer H, Rådegran G, Gude E, Jansson K, Solbu D, Karason K, Arora S, Dellgren G, Gullestad L, SCHEDULE investigators. Everolimus initiation with early Calcineurin inhibitor withdrawal in De novo heart transplant recipients: three-year results from the randomized SCHEDULE study. Am J Transplant. 2016;4:1238–47.
95. Chandraker A, Kobashigawa J, Stehlik J, Givertz M, Pierson R, Pinney S, Joren M, Nissen S, Guleria I, Morrison Y, Armstrong B, Bridges N, Sayegh M, Starling R. Rituximab induction in cardiac transplantation is associated with accelerated coronary artery vasculopathy: CTOT11. [abstract]. Am J Transplant. 2016; 16 (suppl 3).

Acute Rejection

20

Michelle M. Kittleson and Jon A. Kobashigawa

20.1 Immunosuppression

20.1.1 General Principles

Most immunosuppressive regimens used in heart transplantation consist of a combination of several agents used concurrently and use several general principles. The first general principle is that immune reactivity and tendency toward graft rejection are highest early (within the first 3–6 months) after graft implantation and decrease over time. Thus, most regimens use the highest levels of immunosuppression immediately after surgery and decrease levels over the first year. The second general principle is to use low doses of several drugs without overlapping toxicities in preference of higher (and more toxic) doses of fewer drugs whenever feasible. The third principle is that excessive immunosuppression is undesirable because it places patients at risk for infection in the short-term and malignancy in the long-term.

20.2 Recognition and Treatment of Acute Rejection

20.2.1 Diagnosis

Transplant rejection remains one of the major causes of death after heart transplantation [1] and is classified as hyperacute rejection, acute cellular rejection, or antibody mediated rejection. Hyperacute rejection is rare but may occur in the setting of circulating preformed antibodies to major histocompatability antigens (HLA) in the donor. Possible risk factors include presensitization after blood transfusions, multiparity, and previous organ grafts [2]. Hyperacute rejection manifests as severe graft failure within the first few minutes to hours after transplantation. Without inotropic and mechanical circulatory support, plasmapheresis and intense immunosuppression, the recipient usually does not survive.

While the presentation of hyperacute rejection is dramatic, the signs and symptoms of acute rejection are generally nonspecific and may only manifest in the late stages. Patients may present with fatigue, low-grade fevers, heart failure (HF) symptoms, or hypotension. Occasionally, rejection will manifest as atrial arrhythmias or a new pericardial effusion. On examination, patients may have an elevated jugular venous pressure or a new S3 gallop. However, the majority of patients with acute cellular or antibody-mediated rejection are asymptomatic without signs of allograft dysfunction.

Because symptoms are often vague, routine testing for rejection is standard practice. Unlike renal or liver transplantation, there are no laboratory markers for rejection in heart transplantation and the endomyocardial biopsy remains the cornerstone of rejection surveillance. Despite its limitations (sampling error and interobserver variability of interpretation among pathologists), biopsies have remained the gold standard for the diagnosis of acute allograft rejection. They are performed most often via the right internal jugular vein or femoral vein by introducing a bioptome into the right ventricle (RV) and obtaining three to five pieces of endomyocardium, typically from the RV septum (Fig. 20.1).

While the timing of biopsies will vary from center to center, in general biopsies are performed frequently early after transplantation and less frequently over time. Most programs perform surveillance biopsies on a weekly basis for the first 4–6 postoperative weeks and then with diminishing frequency in a stable patient but at a minimum of every 3 months for the first postoperative year. The need for continued surveillance biopsies after the first year in clinically stable patients has been questioned [3, 4], but many centers con-

M. M. Kittleson · J. A. Kobashigawa (✉)
Cedars-Sinai Smidt Heart Institute, Los Angeles, CA, USA
e-mail: michelle.kittleson@cshs.org; Jon.kobashigawa@cshs.org

D. S. Feldman, P. Mohacsi (eds.), *Heart Failure*, Cardiovascular Medicine, https://doi.org/10.1007/978-3-319-98184-0_20

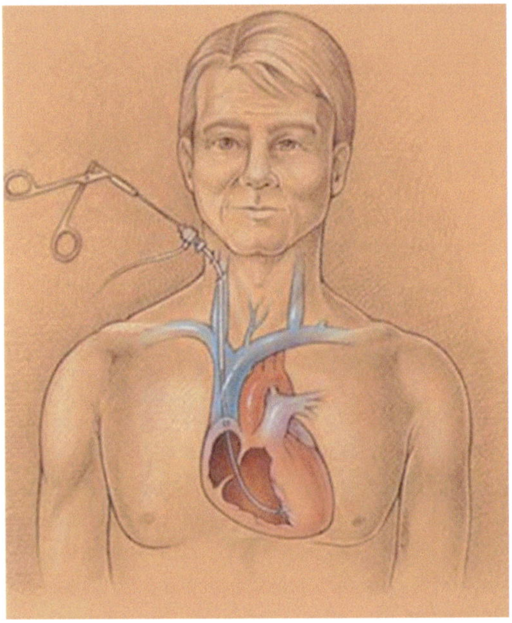

Fig. 20.1 Endomyocardial biopsy via the right internal jugular vein

tinue to perform them on every 4–6 months during the first 5 years after transplantation [5].

The purpose of the endomyocardial biopsy is to assess for myocardial damage in the form of acute cellular rejection (ACR; Fig. 20.2) or antibody-mediated rejection (AMR; Fig. 20.3). The diagnosis of ACR is made in accordance with the revised ISHLT grading scale shown in Table 20.1 [6, 7]. The diagnosis of AMR has achieved standardization after a consensus conference in 2010, shown in Fig. 20.4 [8, 9].

While not required for the diagnosis of AMR, many centers also perform screening for antibodies against human HLA post-transplantation. Strong-, and especially complement-binding, donor-specific anti-HLA antibodies (DSA) are considered potentially cytotoxic [10, 11]. Their presence may merit a change in treatment, depending on the clinical situation, as discussed below.

Although performing an endomyocardial biopsy is straightforward, the morbidity associated with this invasive procedure has led to attempts to identify other means of diagnosing rejection and the gene expression profile (GEP)

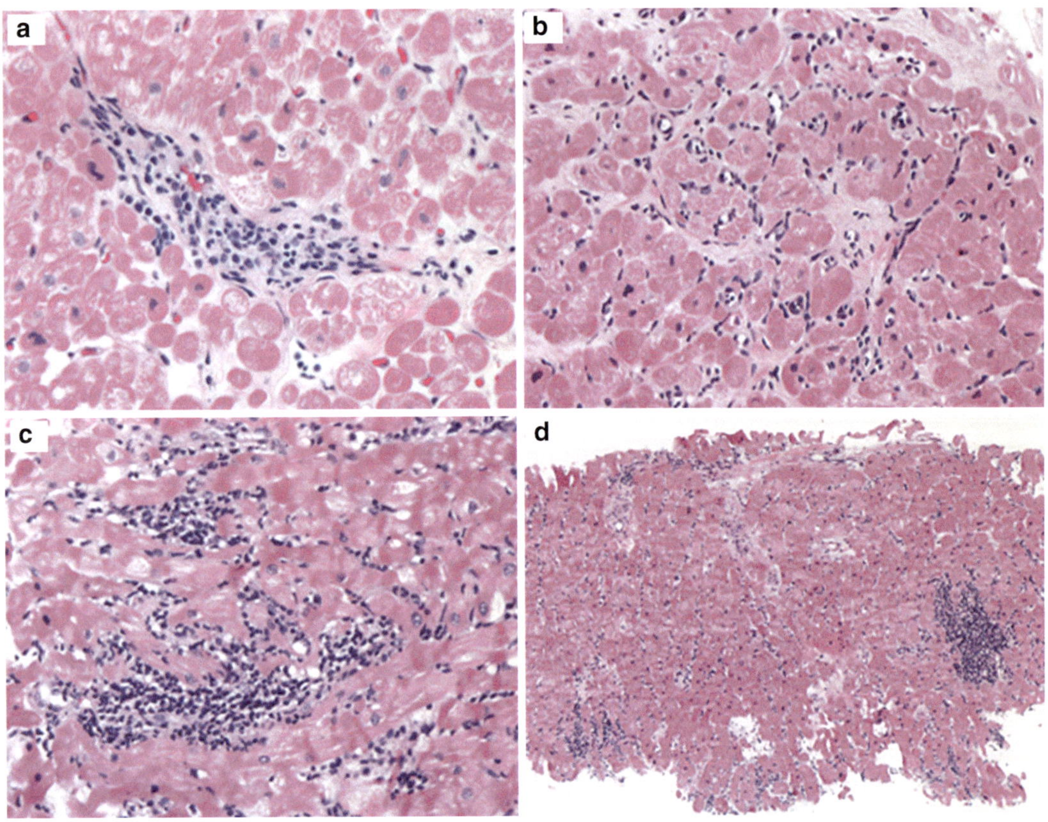

Fig. 20.2 2004 International Society for Heart and Lung Transplantation (ISHLT) acute cellular rejection grading scheme. (**a**) Mild acute rejection characterized by a perivascular cuff of mononuclear inflammatory cells without myocyte damage. This corresponds to focal mild grade 1R. (**b**) Mild acute rejection characterized by a diffuse interstitial pattern. This corresponds to diffuse mild grade 1R. (**c**) Mild acute rejection characterized by a solitary focus of mononuclear cells with rare myocyte damage. This corresponds to focal moderate 1R. (**d**) Moderate acute rejection characterized by multiple foci of inflammation and myocyte damage. This corresponds to multifocal moderate 2R. (**e**) Severe acute rejection showing dense interstitial infiltrates and myocyte damage. This corresponds to diffuse moderate, borderline severe grade 3R. (**f**) Severe acute rejection corresponding to grade 3R

Fig. 20.2 (continued)

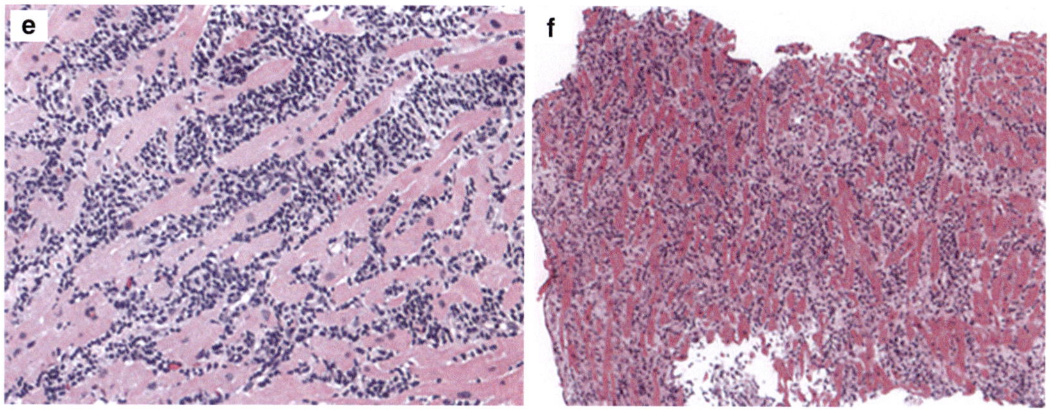

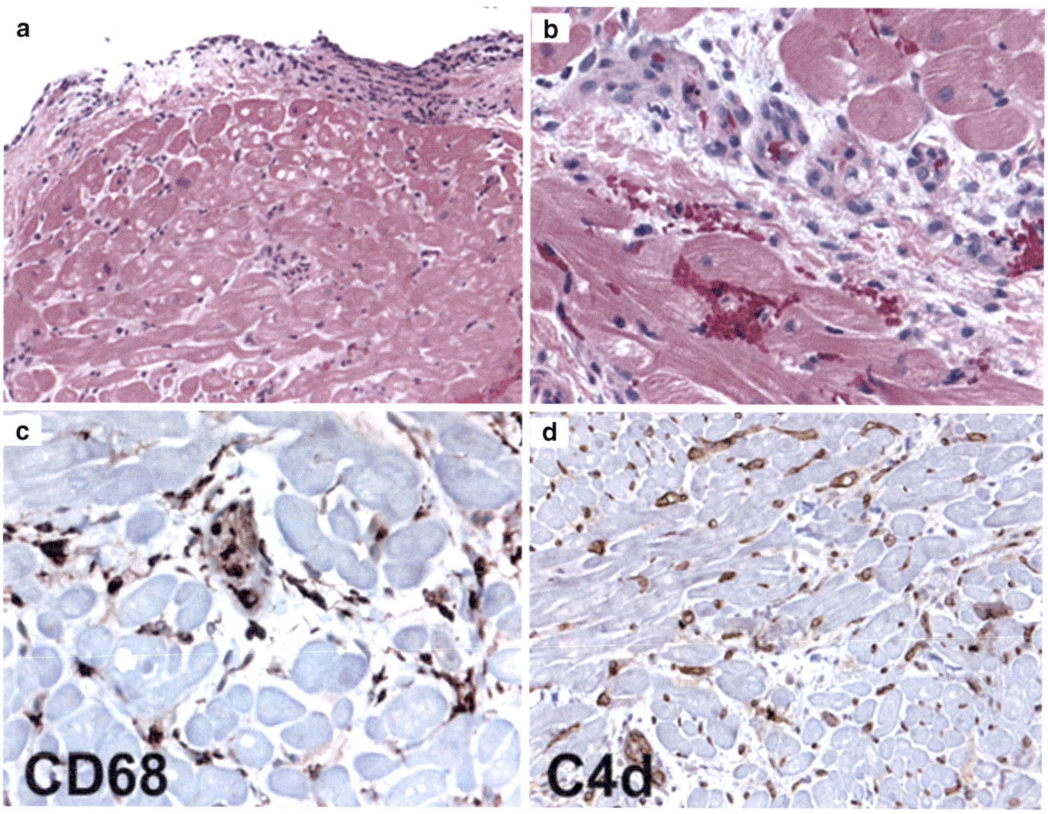

Fig. 20.3 Acute antibody-mediated (humoral) rejection. (**a**) Scanning magnification of endomyocardial biopsy specimen showing a mononuclear cell infiltrate within the endocardium. In the central part of the figure, the small vessel displays prominent endothelial cells. (**b**) High-power magnification showing endothelial cell hyperplasia and perivascular edema. (**c**) CD68 staining of interstitial and intravascular histiocytes. (**d**) Strong, uniform staining of the microvascular for C4d, a marker of complement activation and deposition

Table 20.1 International society for heart and lung transplant standardized cardiac biopsy grading: acute cellular rejection

Grade	Description	Prior classification
0R	No rejection	0
1R, mild	Interstitial and/or perivascular infiltrate with up to one focus of myocyte damage	1A, 1B, 2
2R, moderate	Two or more foci of infiltrate with associated myocyte damage	3A
3R, severe	Diffuse infiltrate with multifocal myocyte damage ± edema ± hemorrhage ± vasculitis	3B, 4

test (AlloMap®, CareDx Inc., San Francisco, CA), an 11-gene expression signature derived from peripheral blood mononuclear cells, has emerged as a noninvasive test with a high negative predictive value for the presence of ACR [12]. In a randomized trial, GEP was shown noninferior to the biopsy in the diagnosis of ACR [13] and also useful early post-transplant [14]. One role of the GEP is to screen low-risk patients at pre-determined intervals with biopsies performed only if the GEP score is abnormal. However, it must be emphasized that patients with a history of, or risk factors for AMR are not candidates for GEP screening, as the test has only been validated for ACR.

20.2.2 Treatment

The management of rejection proceeds in a stepwise fashion based on the severity of rejection detected on biopsy and the patient's presentation (Table 20.2). Biopsies with grade 1R

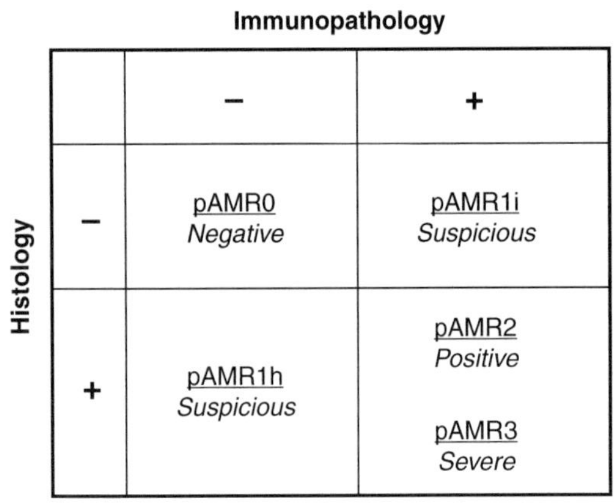

Fig. 20.4 Diagnosis of Antibody-Mediated Rejection. Histologic findings include endothelial activation with intravascular macrophages and capillary destruction. Immunologic findings encompass complement and HLA deposition. The grading scheme stratifies biopsies based on: no histologic or immunologic evidence of antibody-mediated rejection (negative, pAMR0); either histologic or immunologic evidence of antibody-mediated rejection (suspicious, pAMR1h or pARMi, respectively), both histologic and immunologic evidence of antibody-mediated rejection (positive, pAMR2), and a final category for severe findings of myocardial destruction, pAMR3. (Source: Kittleson and Kobashigawa [28]. Permission obtained)

or AMR1, in the absence of clinical or hemodynamic compromise generally merit no intervention.

More serious findings on the biopsy, including Grade 2R or higher and AMR2 or higher warrant treatment. As shown in Table 20.2, the intensity of treatment depends on the patient's presentation. If the patient is asymptomatic (no HF symptoms and normal left ventricular ejection fraction), treatment options include oral pulse steroids, targeting higher levels of immunosuppressive medications, switching from cyclosporine to tacrolimus [15], or switching from MMF to a PSI [16, 17]. Given the equivalent success of intravenous and oral corticosteroid therapy for the treatment of asymptomatic ACR [18], an outpatient course of oral corticosteroids is often the first-line treatment.

Asymptomatic AMR is more challenging. It may be associated with poor outcomes [19–21], but it is unclear whether treatment affects outcomes. At some centers, such patients will receive an oral corticosteroid bolus, consideration of intravenous immune globulin (IV Ig), and monitoring of DSA [8].

For patients with HF symptoms or reduced ejection fraction, treatment is more aggressive, with intravenous corticosteroids and cytolytic therapy with antithymocyte globulin. If there is evidence of AMR2 or higher, patients will also often receive IV Ig. If donor-specific anti-HLA antibodies are present in the setting of AMR, patients may receive more intensive therapy with rituximab or bortezomib. Plasmapheresis may also be used in this setting.

Finally, in patients presenting with cardiogenic shock, empiric aggressive treatment includes intravenous corticosteroids, cytolytic therapy, plasmapheresis, IV Ig, heparin (as patients often have thrombotic occlusion of the cardiac microvasculature on post-mortem examination [22, 23]), and hemodynamic support with intra-aortic balloon counterpulsation or even extracorporeal membrane oxygenation [24].

Any rejection episode should prompt an investigation for precipitating causes such as infection, noncompliance, or drug interactions resulting in subtherapeutic immunosuppressive drug levels. A biopsy should be repeated 2 weeks after completion of treatment to document improvement or resolution of the rejection episode.

Table 20.2 Treatment of acute cellular and antibody-mediated rejection

	Asymptomatic	Reduced EF	Heart failure/Shock
Cellular rejection	Target higher CNI levels Oral steroid bolus + taper MMF → PSI	Oral steroid bolus/taper *or* IV pulse steroids	*Treat based on clinical presentation; do not await biopsy findings* IV pulse steroids Cytolytic therapy (ATG) Plasmapheresis (before ATG dose) IV immune globulin Inotropic therapy IV heparin IABP or ECMO support
Antibody-mediated rejection with no/↓ DSA	Target higher CNI levels MMF → PSI	IV pulse steroids Consider IV immune globulin	
Antibody-mediated rejection with ↑DSA	Oral steroid bolus + taper MMF → PSI Consider IV immune globulin and rituximab	IV pulse steroids IV immune globulin Consider ATG, rituximab or bortezomib	

Adapted from: Kittleson and Kobashigawa [28]

20.3 Long-Term Management

While ACR is often successfully treated with corticosteroids and cytolytic therapy, resulting in a resolution of HF and normalization of the ejection fraction [25], management of AMR is often more complicated. Patients may have a persistent reduction in ejection fraction, restrictive physiology with recurrent HF, and accelerated progression of transplant coronary artery disease [19].

The management of such patients with a persistent drop in ejection fraction after treatment of symptomatic rejection is not well established. Some centers rely on therapies to reduce the levels of DSA, including rituximab and bortezomib, as well as photopheresis to alter the function of T cells [8]. In small case series, such therapies have shown benefit [26, 27], although often such patients go on to require redo heart transplantation.

References

1. Lund LH, Edwards LB, Kucheryavaya AY, et al. The registry of the international society for heart and lung transplantation: thirty-second official adult heart transplantation report-2015; focus theme: early graft failure. J Heart Lung Transplant. 2015;34:1244–54.
2. Kemnitz J, Cremer J, Restrepo-Specht I, et al. Hyperacute rejection in heart allografts. Case studies. Pathol Res Pract. 1991;187:23.
3. Sethi GK, Kosaraju S, Arabia FA, et al. Is it necessary to perform surveillance endomyocardial biopsies in heart transplant recipients? J Heart Lung Transplant. 1995;14:1047.
4. Bestetti R, Theodoropoulos TA, Burdmann EA, et al. Switch from calcineurin inhibitors to sirolimus-induced renal recovery in heart transplant recipients in the midterm follow-up. Transplantation. 2006;81:692–6.
5. Stehlik J, Starling RC, Movsesian MA, et al. Utility of long-term surveillance endomyocardial biopsy: a multi-institutional analysis. J Heart Lung Transplant. 2006;25:1402–9.
6. Billingham ME, Cary NR, Hammond ME, et al. A working formulation for the standardization of nomenclature in the diagnosis of heart and lung rejection: heart rejection study group. The international society for heart transplantation. J Heart Transplant. 1990;9:587.
7. Stewart S, Winters GL, Fishbein MC, et al. Revision of the 1990 working formulation for the standardization of nomenclature in the diagnosis of heart rejection. J Heart Lung Transplant. 2005;24:1710–20.
8. Kobashigawa J, Crespo-Leiro MG, Ensminger SM, et al. Report from a consensus conference on antibody-mediated rejection in heart transplantation. J Heart Lung Transplant. 2011;30:252–69.
9. Berry GJ, Angelini A, Burke MM, et al. The ishlt working formulation for pathologic diagnosis of antibody-mediated rejection in heart transplantation: evolution and current status (2005–2011). J Heart Lung Transplant. 2011;30:601–11.
10. Zeevi A, Lunz J, Feingold B, et al. Persistent strong anti-hla antibody at high titer is complement binding and associated with increased risk of antibody-mediated rejection in heart transplant recipients. J Heart Lung Transplant. 2013;32:98–105.
11. Loupy A, Lefaucheur C, Vernerey D, et al. Complement-binding anti-hla antibodies and kidney-allograft survival. N Engl J Med. 2013;369:1215–26.
12. Deng MC, Eisen HJ, Mehra MR, et al. Noninvasive discrimination of rejection in cardiac allograft recipients using gene expression profiling. Am J Transplant. 2006;6:150–60.
13. Pham MX, Teuteberg JJ, Kfoury AG, et al. Gene-expression profiling for rejection surveillance after cardiac transplantation. N Engl J Med. 2010;362:1890–900.
14. Kobashigawa J, Patel J, Azarbal B, et al. Randomized pilot trial of gene expression profiling versus heart biopsy in the first year after heart transplant: early invasive monitoring attenuation through gene expression trial. Circ Heart Fail. 2015;8:557–64.
15. Kobashigawa JA, Patel J, Furukawa H, et al. Five-year results of a randomized, single-center study of tacrolimus vs microemulsion cyclosporine in heart transplant patients. J Heart Lung Transplant. 2006;25:434–9.
16. Eisen HJ, Kobashigawa J, Starling RC, et al. Everolimus versus mycophenolate mofetil in heart transplantation: a randomized, multicenter trial. Am J Transplant. 2013;13:1203–16.
17. Keogh A, Richardson M, Ruygrok P, et al. Sirolimus in de novo heart transplant recipients reduces acute rejection and prevents coronary artery disease at 2 years: a randomized clinical trial. Circulation. 2004;110:2694–700.
18. Kobashigawa JA, Stevenson LW, Moriguchi JD, et al. Is intravenous glucocorticoid therapy better than an oral regimen for asymptomatic cardiac rejection? A randomized trial. J Am Coll Cardiol. 1993;21:1142–4.
19. Wu GW, Kobashigawa JA, Fishbein MC, et al. Asymptomatic antibody-mediated rejection after heart transplantation predicts poor outcomes. J Heart Lung Transplant. 2009;28:417.
20. Kfoury AG, Hammond ME, Snow GL, et al. Cardiovascular mortality among heart transplant recipients with asymptomatic antibody-mediated or stable mixed cellular and antibody-mediated rejection. J Heart Lung Transplant. 2009;28:781–4.
21. Kfoury AG, Stehlik J, Renlund DG, et al. Impact of repetitive episodes of antibody-mediated or cellular rejection on cardiovascular mortality in cardiac transplant recipients: defining rejection patterns. J Heart Lung Transplant. 2006;25:1277–82.
22. Arbustini E, Roberts WC. Morphological observations in the epicardial coronary arteries and their surroundings late after cardiac transplantation (allograft vascular disease). Am J Cardiol. 1996;78:814–20.
23. Fishbein MC, Kobashigawa J. Biopsy-negative cardiac transplant rejection: etiology, diagnosis, and therapy. Curr Opin Cardiol. 2004;19:166–9.
24. Kittleson MM, Patel JK, Moriguchi JD, et al. Heart transplant recipients supported with extracorporeal membrane oxygenation: outcomes from a single-center experience. J Heart Lung Transplant. 2011;30:1250–6.
25. Michaels PJ, Espejo ML, Kobashigawa J, et al. Humoral rejection in cardiac transplantation: risk factors, hemodynamic consequences and relationship to transplant coronary artery disease. J Heart Lung Transplant. 2003;22:58–69.
26. Patel J, Everly M, Chang D, et al. Reduction of alloantibodies via proteosome inhibition in cardiac transplantation. J Heart Lung Transplant. 2011;30:1320–6.
27. Kirklin JK, Brown RN, Huang ST, et al. Rejection with hemodynamic compromise: objective evidence for efficacy of photopheresis. J Heart Lung Transplant. 2006;25:283–8.
28. Kittleson MM, Kobashigawa JA. Long-term care of the heart transplant recipient. Curr Opin Organ Transplant. 2014;19:515–24.

21 Cardiac Allograft Vasculopathy

Finn Gustafsson

21.1 Definition

Cardiac allograft vasculopathy (CAV) – formerly termed chronic rejection – was described already in 1969, 2 years after the first heart transplant [1]. Soon after the phenomenon was described in details on cadaveric hearts as an obliterative intimal proliferation of the coronary arteries [2]. It became clear that CAV is a disease of the coronary circulation of transplanted hearts distinct from conventional arteriosclerosis. It is a very important complication after heart transplantation as it affects 30–40% of recipients after 5 years and since it is the dominating cause of graft failure and a common cause of death late after transplant [3]. CAV involves not only epicardial arteries but also intramyocardial small arteries and arterioles as well as the cardiac venous vessels (Fig. 21.1). Rapidly, the diagnosis moved from being pathologic-anatomic to become radiologic as coronary angiography was introduced as a routine examination in heart transplant recipients. Typically CAV presents on angiography as diffuse coronary disease with distal arterial obliteration and often also significant proximal stenosis (Fig. 21.2). Further insight to the natural history of CAV was obtained from intravascular ultrasound (IVUS) studies, which have been used primarily for research. Recent developments include use of optical coherence tomography, MRI and CT angiography.

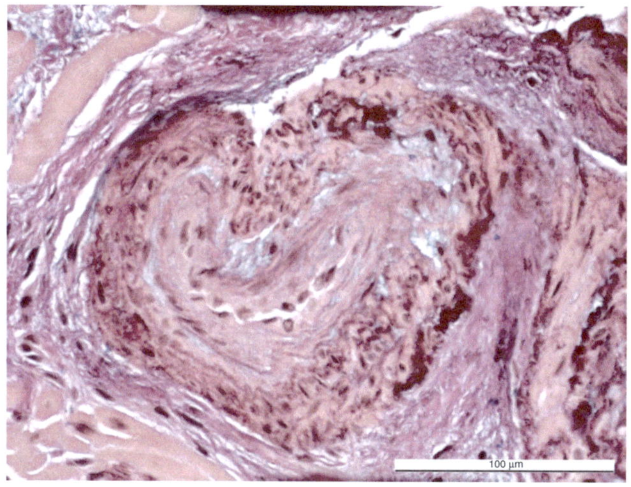

Fig. 21.1 Intramyocardial remodeled small artery with significant initmal proliferation as a result of CAV

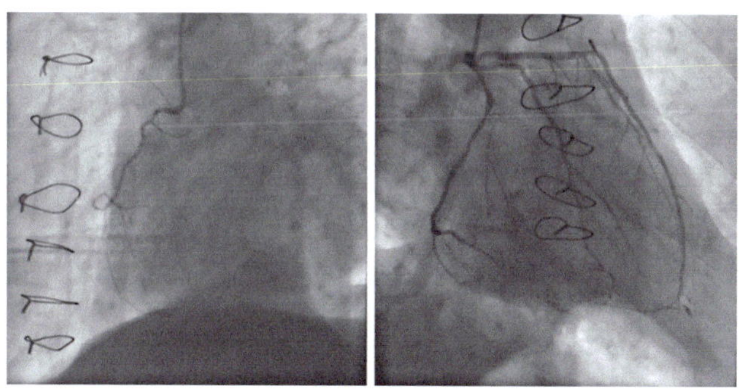

Fig. 21.2 Coronary angiogram of patient 6 years post transplantation showing diffuse narrowing of the branches of the left coronary artery and occlusion of the right coronary artery (ISHLT CAV 2)

21.2 Incidence and Prognostic Importance

CAV can be very aggressive and be present already 1 year after transplantation. In the ISHLT registry the overall prevalence of CAV diagnosed by angiography in survivors at 1, 5, and 10 years after transplantation was 8%, 30%, and 50%, respectively. Higher prevalence is found if the diagnosis is made by IVUS. Prognosis in patients with CAV appears to be improved slightly over time, however, almost one third of the patients dying more than 5 years

F. Gustafsson (✉)
Rigshospitalet, Copenhagen, Denmark
e-mail: finng@dadlnet.dk

D. S. Feldman, P. Mohacsi (eds.), *Heart Failure*, Cardiovascular Medicine, https://doi.org/10.1007/978-3-319-98184-0_21

post transplantation die from CAV [3]. The prognosis clearly also depends on the severity of CAV. Indeed, 5 year mortality in patients with severe CAV occurred has been reported to be >50% [4].

21.3 Risk Factors

Several risk factors for CAV, both relating to the donor and the recipient, have been identified [5] (Table 21.1). Recipient factors may be immunological or non-immunological. Recurrent rejection, especially humoral rejection and the development of donor specific HLA antibodies, appears to accelerate CAV [6]. Rejection, however, is not sufficient to induce CAV, as it is well described that a calcineurin inhibitor free, proliferation signal inhibitor based immunosuppressive regimen, which is associated with increased rates of acute rejection episodes, results in a slower progression of CAV early after transplantation [7]. Infection has been proposed to play a role in development of CAV, in particular CMV [8]. Indeed, CMV D+/R- recipients have an increased risk of CAV and CMV infection has been shown to predispose to CAV. In observational studies, aggressive CMV prophylaxis, resulting in lower rates of CMV infection was associated with lower rates of CAV [9].

Classical risk factors for development of arteriosclerosis such as diabetes, hyperlipidemia and hypertension are very common among heart transplant recipients [10]. It has been clearly shown that these factors significantly accelerate CAV development and that intervention against hyperlipidemia (statins) lower the risk of development of vascular disease [11]. Smoking, although a contraindication to transplantation, is resumed in some patients and is a potent risk factor for CAV [12].

Table 21.1 Risk factors for development of cardiac allograft vasculopathy (CAV)

Donor factors
Age
Male sex
Smoking
Hypertension
Recipient factors
Acute rejection (cellular or humoral)
CMV infection
Hyperlipidemia
Obesity
Smoking
Diabetes

21.4 Pathophysiology

CAV is characterized by concentric intimal hyperplasia of the coronary arteries and severe medial hypertrophy of coronary resistance vessels [2]. The processes are confined to the vessels of the transplanted heart and not part of a generalized vascular disease. The endothelial cells of the coronary circulation appear to play a significant role in initiating the process and several circulating and locally derived factors appear to be implicated, such as platelet derived growth factor, vascular endothelial growth factor, TGF-beta and endothelin-1. T-cell derived cytokines upregulate endothelial factors promoting growth and microthrombosis such ICAM-1 and VCAM −1 as well a P-selectin. As CAV progresses it leads to myocardial ischemia or infarction, arrhythmia and graft failure.

21.5 Diagnosis and Surveillance

Unlike conventional coronary arteriosclerosis, CAV may cause uniform remodeling of the coronary vessels which may be difficult to detect by routine angiography (Fig. 21.3). In patients with angiographically normal corornary arteries, IVUS may uncover severe CAV by demonstrating significant intima thickening. Despite this shortcoming of angiography, the current definition of CAV is predominantly based on this technique. An angiographic definition has now been published by ISHLT (Table 21.2) and constitutes the nomenclature to be used for CAV [13].

Due to cardiac denervation, even patients with severe CAV rarely develop classical angina pectoris, but more often present with more unspecific symptoms of dyspnea, fluid retention, palpitations or syncope. Given the lack of specificity of these symptoms and the high prevalence of CAV, surveillance is recommended. ISHLT guidelines recommend annual or biannual angiography to screen for CAV. In patients without early aggressive CAV (i.e. no angiographic evidence for vasculopathy after 3–5 years), non-invasive screening using dobutamine stress echocardiography or myocardial perfusion scintigraphy may be used in asymptomatic patients. These diagnostic modalities may also be preferred as screening tool in patients with significant renal dysfunction in whom contrast use should be minimized [14].

21.6 Prevention and Treatment

At the current time preventive strategies based on statin therapy and immunosuppression based on an mTOR inhibitor (sirolimus, everolimus) have proven effective. Treatment

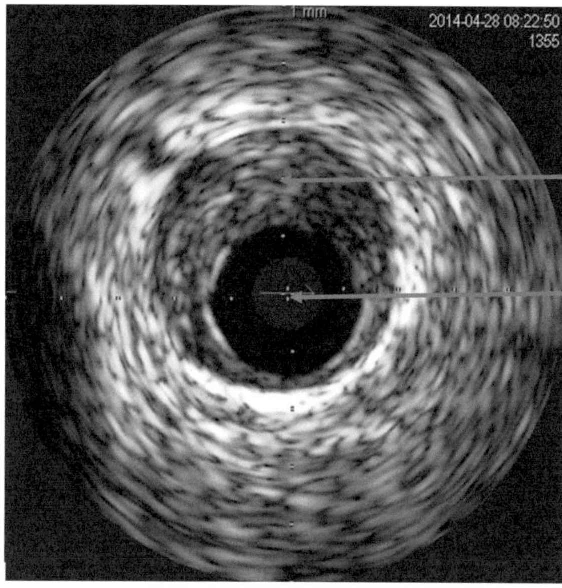

Fig. 21.3 Intravascular ultrasound (IVUS) of anterior descending branch of the left coronary artery from a transplant recipient 1 year after transplantation with angiographically normal arteries

Table 21.2 ISHLT nomenclature for allograft vasculopathy

ISHLT CAV0	No detectable angiographic lesion
ISHLT CAV1 (Mild)	Angiographic left main (LM) >50%, or primary vessel with maximum lesion of >70%, or any branch stenosis >70% (including diffuse narrowing) without allograft dysfunction
ISHLT CAV2 (Moderate)	Angiographic LM >50%; a single primary vessel >70%, or isolated branch stenosis >70% in branches of 2 systems, without allograft dysfunction
ISHLT CAV3 (Severe)	Angiographic LM >50%, or two or more primary vessels >70% stenosis, or isolated branch stenosis >70% in all 3 systems; or ISHLT CAV1 or CAV2 with allograft dysfunction (defined as LVEF <45% or evidence of significant restrictive physiology)

with pravastatin within 2 weeks from transplantation has been demonstrated to significantly lower the rate of CAV, documented both on angiography and IVUS [11]. A similar effect has been documented with simvastatin and both trials of pravastatin and simvastatin showed effect on survival despite the fact that they were moderately sized [15]. Caution must be paid to interaction between statins and immunosuppressants, but statins are recommended for all heart transplant recipients (including children), irrespective of cholesterol levels based on these trials.

Use of sirolimus and everolimus in de novo heart transplant recipients has been associated with lower rates of CAV. Together with a calcineurin inhibitor, both sirolimus and everolimus, have in randomized trials been proven superior to azathioprine [16] and everolimus has also been associated with smaller increase in intimal thickness on IVUS compared with mycophenolate mofetil [17]. Finally, everolimus together with mycophenolate has recently been shown to result in less intima thickness 1 year after transplantation compared with a conventional regimen containing a calcineurin inhibitor and mycophenolate, indicating that the presence of the mTOR inhibitor rather than the absence of another immunosuppressant is the deciding factor for slowing CAV early after transplantation [18].

Later after transplantation switch to an mTOR inhibitor based regimen may slow progression of CAV but the effect is much less pronounced and has not been documented in all studies [19, 20]. When CAV has developed, therapy concentrates on prevention of complications including aspirin for prophylaxis against coronary thrombosis and heart failure therapy if graft dysfunction occurs. Localized coronary stenosis in proximal vessels without obliterated periphery may be treated with percutaneous coronary intervention (PCI) and stenting or very occasionally by coronary artery bypass surgery. The use of prophylactic defibrillators is highly controversial in this setting, since overall prognosis in terms of non-arrhythmic death is difficult to predict in this population.

When advanced CAV develops, and especially when complicated by graft failure, re-transplantation should be considered. CAV is the most common indication for re-transplantation which may yield acceptable results in selected patients [21, 22].

References

1. Thompson JG. Atheroma in a transplanted heart. Lancet. 1969;2(7633):1297.
2. Bieber CP, Stinson EB, Shumway NE, Payne R, Kosek J. Cardiac transplantation in man. VII. Cardiac allograft pathology. Circulation. 1970;41(5):753–72.

3. Lund LH, Edwards LB, Kucheryavaya AY, Benden C, Dipchand AI, Goldfarb S, et al. The registry of the International Society for Heart and Lung Transplantation: thirty-second official adult heart transplantation report—2015; focus theme: early graft failure. J Heart Lung Transplant. 2015;34(10):1244–54.
4. Costanzo MR, Naftel DC, Pritzker MR, Heilman JK III, Boehmer JP, Brozena SC, et al. Heart transplant coronary artery disease detected by coronary angiography: a multiinstitutional study of preoperative donor and recipient risk factors. Cardiac transplant research database. J Heart Lung Transplant. 1998;17(8): 744–53.
5. Stehlik J, Edwards LB, Kucheryavaya AY, Benden C, Christie JD, Dipchand AI, et al. The registry of the International Society for Heart and Lung Transplantation: 29th official adult heart transplant report—2012. J Heart Lung Transplant. 2012;31(10):1052–64.
6. Nath DS, Angaswamy N, Basha HI, Phelan D, Moazami N, Ewald GA, et al. Donor-specific antibodies to human leukocyte antigens are associated with and precede antibodies to major histocompatibility complex class I-related chain a in antibody-mediated rejection and cardiac allograft vasculopathy after human cardiac transplantation. Hum Immunol. 2010;71(12):1191–6.
7. Andreassen AK, Andersson B, Gustafsson F, Eiskjaer H, Radegran G, Gude E, et al. Everolimus initiation and early calcineurin inhibitor withdrawal in heart transplant recipients: a randomized trial. Am J Transplant. 2014 Aug;14(8):1828–38.
8. Delgado JF, Reyne AG, de Dios S, Lopez-Medrano F, Jurado A, Juan RS, et al. Influence of cytomegalovirus infection in the development of cardiac allograft vasculopathy after heart transplantation. J Heart Lung Transplant. 2015;34(8):1112–9.
9. Potena L, Grigioni F, Magnani G, Lazzarotto T, Musuraca AC, Ortolani P, et al. Prophylaxis versus preemptive anti-cytomegalovirus approach for prevention of allograft vasculopathy in heart transplant recipients. J Heart Lung Transplant. 2009;28(5):461–7.
10. Valantine H, Rickenbacker P, Kemna M, Hunt S, Chen YD, Reaven G, et al. Metabolic abnormalities characteristic of dysmetabolic syndrome predict the development of transplant coronary artery disease: a prospective study. Circulation. 2001;103(17):2144–52.
11. Kobashigawa JA, Katznelson S, Laks H, Johnson JA, Yeatman L, Wang XM, et al. Effect of pravastatin on outcomes after cardiac transplantation. N Engl J Med. 1995;333(10):621–7.
12. Arora S, Aukrust P, Andreassen A, Simonsen S, Gude E, Grov I, et al. The prognostic importance of modifiable risk factors after heart transplantation. Am Heart J. 2009;158(3):431–6.
13. Mehra MR, Crespo-Leiro MG, Dipchand A, Ensminger SM, Hiemann NE, Kobashigawa JA, et al. International Society for Heart and Lung Transplantation working formulation of a standardized nomenclature for cardiac allograft vasculopathy-2010. J Heart Lung Transplant. 2010;29(7):717–27.
14. Costanzo MR, Dipchand A, Starling R, Anderson A, Chan M, Desai S, et al. The International Society of Heart and Lung Transplantation Guidelines for the care of heart transplant recipients. J Heart Lung Transplant. 2010;29(8):914–56.
15. Wenke K, Meiser B, Thiery J, Nagel D, von Scheidt W, Steinbeck G, et al. Simvastatin reduces graft vessel disease and mortality after heart transplantation: a four-year randomized trial. Circulation. 1997;96(5):1398–402.
16. Eisen HJ, Tuzcu EM, Dorent R, Kobashigawa J, Mancini D, Valantine-Von Kaeppler HA, et al. Everolimus for the prevention of allograft rejection and vasculopathy in cardiac-transplant recipients. N Engl J Med. 2003;349(9):847–58.
17. Eisen HJ, Kobashigawa J, Starling RC, Pauly DF, Kfoury A, Ross H, et al. Everolimus versus mycophenolate mofetil in heart transplantation: a randomized, multicenter trial. Am J Transplant. 2013;13(5):1203–16.
18. Arora S, Andreassen AK, Andersson B, Gustafsson F, Eiskjaer H, Botker HE, et al. The effect of Everolimus initiation and Calcineurin inhibitor elimination on cardiac allograft vasculopathy in De novo recipients: one-year results of a Scandinavian randomized trial. Am J Transplant. 2015;15(7):1967–75.
19. Ruygrok PN, Webber B, Faddy S, Muller DW, Keogh A. Angiographic regression of cardiac allograft vasculopathy after introducing sirolimus immunosuppression. J Heart Lung Transplant. 2003;22(11):1276–9.
20. Masetti M, Potena L, Nardozza M, Prestinenzi P, Taglieri N, Saia F, et al. Differential effect of everolimus on progression of early and late cardiac allograft vasculopathy in current clinical practice. Am J Transplant. 2013;13(5):1217–26.
21. Goldraich LA, Stehlik J, Kucheryavaya AY, Edwards LB, Ross HJ. Retransplant and medical therapy for cardiac allograft vasculopathy: International Society for Heart and Lung Transplantation registry analysis. Am J Transplant. 2016;16(1):301–9.
22. Lund LH, Edwards LB, Kucheryavaya AY, Benden C, Christie JD, Dipchand AI, et al. The registry of the International Society for Heart and Lung Transplantation: thirty-first official adult heart transplant report--2014; focus theme: retransplantation. J Heart Lung Transplant. 2014;33(10):996–1008.

Part XI

Pulmonary Hypertension

22 Pulmonary Hypertension

Christoph B. Wiedenroth and Eckhard Mayer

22.1 Chronic Thromboembolic Pulmonary Hypertension (CTEPH)

22.1.1 Introduction

Chronic thromboembolic pulmonary hypertension (CTEPH), representing group 4 of the classification of pulmonary hypertension (PH), is defined as a symptomatic PH with a mean pulmonary arterial pressure (PAm) of at least 25 mmHg and normal pulmonary arterial occlusion pressure (PAOP ≤15 mmHg) with pulmonary perfusion defects persisting after a 3 months episode of adequate anticoagulation [5]. Furthermore, there is a mechanical obstructive component, potentially amenable by surgery and a variable degree of secondary vasculopathy [10].

The gold standard treatment is surgical pulmonary endarterectomy (PEA). This complex, but standardized surgical procedure usually leads to normalization of pulmonary hemodynamics. In experienced centers, perioperative risk is low [15, 25]. Unfortunately, up to 1/3 of all CTEPH-patients are inoperable [20]. For inoperable patients, targeted medical treatment with riociguat is available in many countries [6]. Besides medication, balloon pulmonary angioplasty (BPA) is an emerging interventional treatment option for inoperable CTEPH patients [17].

Chronic thromboembolic disease of the pulmonary arteries (CTED) is defined by the same criteria like CTEPH without the finding of PH at rest. Symptomatic patients may be treated surgically [23]. CTED patients with inoperable findings have also been treated successfully by BPA [28].

It is strongly recommended that evaluation and treatment of CTEPH patients is performed in expert centers with an experienced multidisciplinary team [8, 11, 15, 16, 20, 25].

C. B. Wiedenroth (✉) · E. Mayer
Department of Thoracic Surgery, Kerckhoff Heart and Thorax Center, Bad Nauheim, Germany
e-mail: c.wiedenroth@kerckhoff-klinik.de

22.2 Pathophysiology

CTEPH results as a late complication in up to 4% of patients with acute pulmonary embolism [7, 19]. Unresolved thrombi lead to the development of scar tissue, occluding pulmonary artery branches with development of PH with consecutive deterioration of right ventricular function and right heart failure. The high-pressure hyperperfusion of non-obstructed, patent vessels may cause a secondary vasculopathy, leading to further clinical deterioration [12]. This vicious circle compromises the pulmonary and systemic circulation and is associated with a poor prognosis.

22.3 Diagnostic Pathway

Since clinical symptoms are quite unspecific, mean time from first symptoms to diagnosis is 21 months and another 8 months to surgical treatment (PEA) in operable cases [20], underlining the need of a rapid and adaequate diagnostical workup. Usually, first symptom of CTEPH patients is dyspnea under exertion [12].

Regarding the 2015 guidelines of the european society of cardiology and european respiratory society, the following pathway should be used [5]:

History of pulmonary embolism leads to suspicion of CTEPH. Echocardiography is the first diagnostical tool. If signs for pulmonary hypertension are found, VQ-scan (recommended as V/P-SPECT) should be performed, whether to rule out CTEPH or to give another important hint. Regarding CTED patients, cardiopulmonary exercise testing may indicate dead space ventilation.

With suspected CTEPH, patients should be referred to specialized CTEPH centers for further evaluation: WHO functional class, 6 min walk test, pulmonary function testing including lung diffusion capacity for carbon monoxide and blood gas analysis, serum level N-terminal fragment of pro-brain natriuretic peptide (NT-proBNP), and right heart catheterization to

D. S. Feldman, P. Mohacsi (eds.), *Heart Failure*, Cardiovascular Medicine, https://doi.org/10.1007/978-3-319-98184-0_22

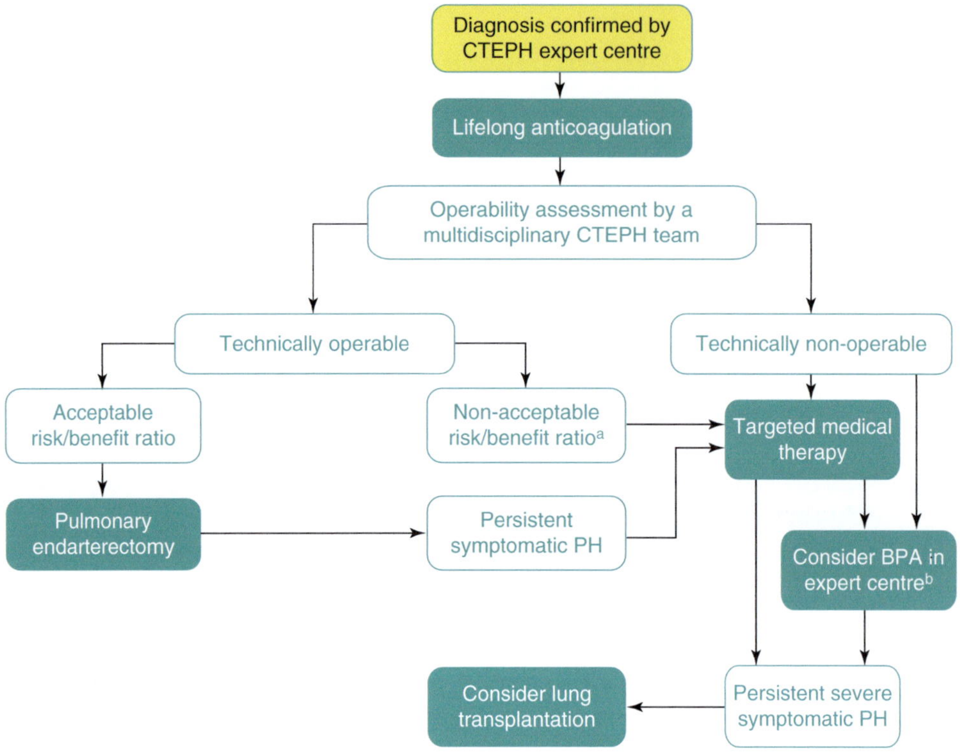

Fig. 22.1 CTEPH treatment algorithm according to ESC/ERS guidelines [5]

determine pulmonary arterial pressures, PAOP, cardiac output and pulmonary vascular resistance (PVR). Computed tomography scans as well as magnetic resonance imaging are used. At last, the gold standard imaging tool for evaluation of operability (and in inoperable cases of target lesions for BPA) is contrast-enhanced digital subtraction angiography.

All patients with CTEPH are discussed in a multidisciplinary conference consisting of experienced PEA-surgeons, interventional radiologists and cardiologists, pulmonologists and anaesthesiologists for further treatment decisions (Fig. 22.1).

22.4 Treatment

22.4.1 Pulmonary Endarterectomy (PEA)

Surgical PEA is the goldstandard treatment of CTEPH and potentially curative [14, 16]. The more PEAs are performed in a center, the lower the mortality rate is, varying between 3.5% and 7.4% [20]. High-volume expert centers are meanwhile reaching mortality-rates of around 2% [13].

However, only 2/3 of all CTEPH-patients are operable. Main reasons for inoperability are peripheral localisation of pulmonary vascular obstructions and in rare cases co-morbidities including severe left heart disease and interstitial lung disease [20].

In specialized centers, PEA surgery is a standardized procedure [3]: using a median sternotomy, patients are connected to the heart-lung-machine for extracorporeal circulation and cooled to 20 °C. PEA is performed in several periods of deep hypothermic circulatory arrest to optimize visualisation and to avoid blood backflow from bronchial arteries. Using a real endarterectomy plane, the scar tissue within the pulmonary vasculature is removed completely (Fig. 22.2), leading to a normalization of parenchymal perfusion.

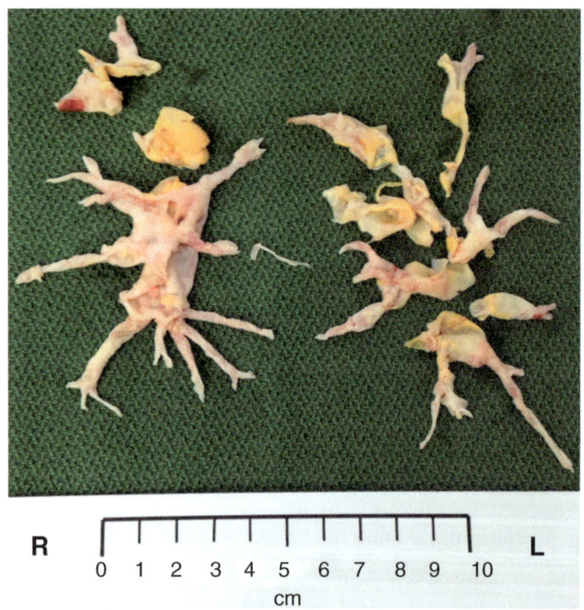

Fig. 22.2 PEA specimen of both pulmonary arteries. Fibrotic material has been removed using a real endarterectomy beginning in the main right and left pulmonary artery to the subsegmental branches

Postoperatively, most of the patients show a significant improvement of physical capacity and an almost complete normalization of pulmonary hemodynamics [14, 16]. Especially in patients with preoperatively very high PVR, a larger proportion of secondary vasculopathy has to be assumed. Therefore, recent data showed usually mild residual PH in up to 50% of operated patients. Patients with moderate to severe PH require additional treatment [2].

For highly selected cases, hybrid procedures combining PEA and BPA have been described [27].

22.4.2 Targeted Medical Treatment

In all CTEPH patients lifelong anticoagulation is recommended. In addition to diuretics and long-term oxygen therapy (in cases with hypoxaemia), in inoperable patients and patients with residual PH following PEA targeted medical treatment with riociguat is recommended. Therefore, operated patients should be reevaluated 6–12 months after PEA with right heart catheterization [5].

Riociguat, a stimulator of the soluble guanylate cyclase (sCG), was the first substance showing an improvement in pulmonary hemodynamics and exercise capacity in a controlled randomized trial [6].

Actually, further substances and combination therapy of targeted medication are under investigation.

22.4.3 Balloon Pulmonary Angioplasty (BPA)

BPA was firstly described by Voorburg et al. in 1988 [26]. The first series of 18 patients was presented in 2001 [4]. In the following years, several centers, especially in Japan, refined the procedure and showed promising improvements of pulmonary hemodynamics and physical capacity with low complication and mortality rates in inoperable CTEPH patients (from initially 3–10% to 0–1.5%) [1, 9, 17, 21, 22, 24]. However, since there is a lack of long term, multicenter data [18], BPA can currently not be recommended as a first line treatment. The benefits of guideline recommended treatment of inoperable CTEPH patients with riociguat and BPA on top have recently been shown [29].

Target lesions for BPA are subsegmental branches of the pulmonary arteries with obstructing scar tissue presenting as webs and bands ("slits") leading to endoluminal stenoses with reduction of parenchymal perfusion.

BPA is performed as a staged procedure using a femoral or jugular access in awake patients. After insertion of a guiding catheter into the target pulmonary arterial branch, a guide wire is placed and the diseased subsegmental branches are dilated by multiple balloon inflations. Hereby, the scar tissue is ruptured, leading to an improvement of the perfusion of the downstream lung parenchyma (Fig. 22.3).

22.5 Summary

CTEPH is a rare, progressive disease with poor prognosis if left untreated. Gold standard therapy is PEA surgery in operable patients, offering a potentially curative treatment option. Targeted medical treatment is recommended in inoperable patients or patients with persisting PH after PEA. Furthermore, BPA can be a therapeutic option for selected inoperable patients.

For an optimal diagnostic and therapeutic management of patients suffering from CTEPH, referral to an expert center is mandatory.

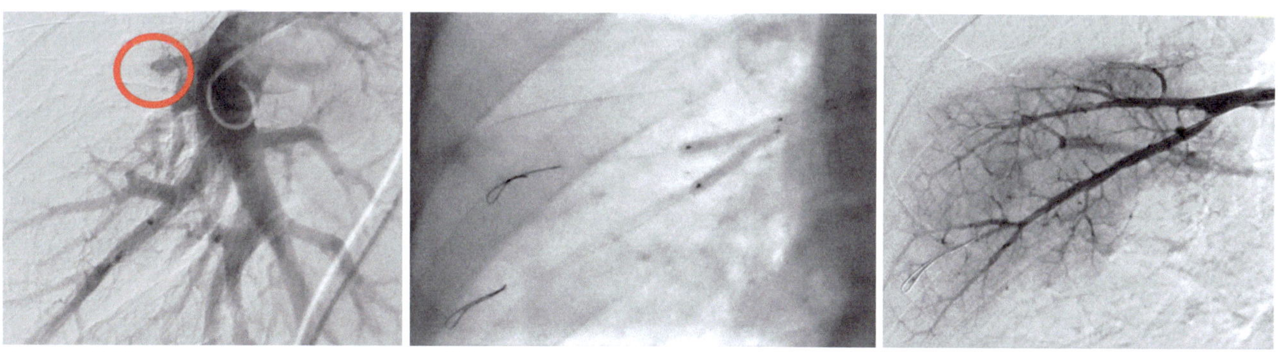

Fig. 22.3 BPA of segment 4 of the right lung in a 79 year old male patient with a PAm of 38 mmHg and a PVR of 6.7 WU

Disclosures CB Wiedenroth has received speaker fees and/or consultant honoraria from Actelion, Bayer AG, BTG, MSD, and Pfizer.

E Mayer has received speaker fees and/or honoraria for consultations from Actelion, Bayer AG, GSK, MSD, and Pfizer.

References

1. Andreassen AK, Ragnarsson A, Gude E, Geiran O, Andersen R. Balloon pulmonary angioplasty in patients with inoperable chronic thromboembolic pulmonary hypertension. Heart. 2013;99(19):1415–20.
2. Cannon JE, Su L, Kiely DG, et al. dynamic risk stratification of patient long-term outcome after pulmonary endarterectomy: results from the United Kingdom National Cohort. Circulation. 2016;133(18):1761–71.
3. Daily PO, Dembitsky WP, Iversen S. Technique of pulmonary thromboendarterectomy for chronic pulmonary embolism. J Card Surg. 1989;4(1):10–24.
4. Feinstein JA, Goldhaber SZ, Lock JE. Balloon pulmonary angioplasty for treatment of chronic thromboembolic pulmonary hypertension. Circulation. 2001;103(1):10–3.
5. Galié N, Humbert M, Vachiery JL, et al. 2015 ESC/ERS Guidelines for the diagnosis and treatment of pulmonary hypertension: The Joint Task Force for the Diagnosis and Treatment of Pulmonary Hypertension of the European Society of Cardiology (ESC) and the European Respiratory Society (ERS): Endorsed by: Association for European Paediatric and Congenital Cardiology (AEPC), International Society for Heart and Lung Transplantation (ISHLT). Eur Respir J. 2015;46(4):903–75.
6. Ghofrani HA, D'Armini AM, Grimminger F, et al. Riociguat for the treatment of chronic thromboembolic pulmonary hypertension. N Engl J Med. 2013;369(4):319–29.
7. Guérin L, Couturaud F, Parent F, et al. Prevalence of chronic thromboembolic pulmonary hypertension after acute pulmonary embolism. Thromb Haemost. 2014;112(3):598–605.
8. Jamieson SW, Kapelanski DP, Sakakibara N, et al. Pulmonary endarterectomy: experience and lessons learned in 1,500 cases. Ann Thorac Surg. 2003;76(5):1457–62.
9. Kataoka M, Inami T, Hayashida K, et al. Percutaneous transluminal pulmonary angioplasty for the treatment of chronic thromboembolic pulmonary hypertension. Circ Cardiovasc Interv. 2012;5(6):756–62.
10. Keogh AM, Mayer E, Benza RL, et al. Interventional and surgical modalities of treatment in pulmonary hypertension. J Am Coll Cardiol. 2009;54(1):67–77.
11. Kim NH, Delcroix M, Jenkins DP, et al. Chronic thromboembolic pulmonary hypertension. J Am Coll Cardiol. 2013;62(25):D92–9.
12. Lang IM, Pesavento R, Bonderman D, et al. Risk factors and basic mechanisms of chronic thromboembolic pulmonary hypertension: a current understanding. Eur Respir J. 2013;41(2):462–8.
13. Lankeit M, Krieg V, Hobohm L, et al. Pulmonary endarterectomy in chronic thromboembolic pulmonary hypertension. J Heart Lung Transplant. 2017;37:250–8. https://doi.org/10.1016/j.healun.2017.06.011.
14. Madani MM, Auger WR, Pretorius V, et al. Pulmonary endarterectomy: recent changes in a single institution's experience of more than 2,700 patients. Ann Thorac Surg. 2012;94(1):97–103.
15. Mayer E. Surgical and post-operative treatment of chronic thromboembolic pulmonary hypertension. Eur Respir Rev. 2010;19(115):64–7.
16. Mayer E, Jenkins D, Lindner J, et al. Surgical management and outcome of patients with chronic thromboembolic pulmonary hypertension: results from an international prospective registry. J Thorac Cardiovasc Surg. 2011;141(3):702–10.
17. Mizoguchi H, Ogawa A, Munemasa M, Mikouchi H, Ito H, Matsubara H. Refined balloon pulmonary angioplasty for inoperable patients with chronic thromboembolic pulmonary hypertension. Minerva Anestesiol. 2012;5(6):748–55.
18. Ogo T. Balloon pulmonary angioplasty for inoperable chronic thromboembolic pulmonary hypertension. Curr Opin Pulm Med. 2015;21:425–31.
19. Pengo V, Lensing A, Prins M, et al. Incidence of chronic thromboembolic pulmonary hypertension after a first episode of pulmonary embolism. N Engl J Med. 2004;350:2257–64.
20. Pepke-Zaba J, Delcroix M, Lang I, et al. Chronic thromboembolic pulmonary hypertension (CTEPH): results from an international prospective registry. Circulation. 2011;124(18):1973–81.
21. Sato H, Ota H, Sugimura K, et al. Balloon pulmonary angioplasty improves biventricular functions and pulmonary flow in chronic thromboembolic pulmonary hypertension. Circ J. 2016;80(6):1470–7.
22. Sugimura K, Fukumoto Y, Satoh K, et al. Percutaneous transluminal pulmonary angioplasty markedly improves pulmonary hemodynamics and long-term prognosis in patients with chronic thromboembolic pulmonary hypertension. Circ J. 2012;76(2):485–8.
23. Taboada D, Pepke-Zaba J, Jenkins DP, et al. Outcome of pulmonary endarterectomy in symptomatic chronic thromboembolic disease. Eur Respir J. 2014;44:1635–45.
24. Taniguchi Y, Miyagawa K, Nakayama K, et al. Balloon pulmonary angioplasty: an additional treatment option to improve the prognosis of patients with chronic thromboembolic pulmonary hypertension. EuroIntervention. 2014;10(4):518–25.
25. Thistlethwaite PA, Madani M, Jamieson SW. Outcomes of pulmonary endarterectomy surgery. Semin Thorac Cardiovasc Surg. 2006;18(3):257–64.
26. Voorburg JA, Cats VM, Buis B, Bruschke AV. Balloon angioplasty in the treatment of pulmonary hypertension caused by pulmonary embolism. Chest. 1988;94:1249–53.
27. Wiedenroth CB, Liebetrau C, Breithecker A, et al. Combined pulmonary endarterectomy and balloon pulmonary angioplasty in patients with chronic thromboembolic pulmonary hypertension. J Heart Lung Transplant. 2016;35(5):591–6.
28. Wiedenroth CB, Olsson KM, Guth S, et al. Balloon pulmonary angioplasty for inoperable patients with chronic thromboembolic disease. Pulm Circ. 2018; https://doi.org/10.1177/204589321775312.
29. Wiedenroth CB, Ghofrani HA, Adameit MSD. Sequential treatment with riociguat and balloon pulmonary angioplasty for patients with inoperable chronic thromboembolic pulmonary hypertension. Pulm Circ. 2018; in press.

Part XII

Mechanical Circulatory Support

23 MCS: Patient Selection

Paul Mohacsi and Pascal A. Berdat

The clinical course of chronic heart failure is usually progressive and characterized by recurrent acute decompensations, if not stabilized by evidence based medical and device therapy, as well as adaptation of life style. Patients with advanced chronic heart failure are moderately to severely symptomatic (class III and IV) and according to the ACC/AHA classification in stage C or D. Progression finally leads to end stage heart failure (refractory symptoms as defined by ACC/AHA as stadium D). Chronic heart failure patients may also deteriorate to cardiogenic shock due to an acute de novo event, such as acute myocardial infarction. Acute heart failure due to such an unexpected event or due to progression of chronic heart failure (leading to a catecholamine dependent and unstable situation) usually triggers the discussion about, whether cardiac transplantation and/or ventricular assist therapy should be considered. However, implantation of a long-term (durable) mechanical circulatory support device (i.e. left ventricular assist device, LVAD) or heart transplantation should not/cannot be done under urgent conditions. It is of utmost importance to first stabilize the patient by using short-term (temporary) mechanical circulatory support (MCS) devices (ECMO, DeltaStream, Levitronix/CentriMag, Impella 2.5, CP or 5.0) as a so-called bridge-to-transplantation strategy.

P. Mohacsi (✉)
CardiovascularCenter Zürich, Hirslanden Clinics Zürich, Zürich, Switzerland

Department of Cardiac Surgery, University Hospital Basel, Basel, Switzerland

Department of Cardiovascular Surgery, University Hospital Bern, Bern, Switzerland

P. A. Berdat
CardiovascularCenter Zürich, Hirslanden Clinics Zürich, Zürich, Switzerland

23.1 Bridge-To-Decision Strategy

Acute heart failure due to a de novo event or decompensation of chronic heart failure must first be investigated and evaluated in a appropriated way. Of course, reversal of the cardiogenic shock and stabilization of the patient must result in sufficient hemodynamics, avoiding multi-organ failure. In the context of cardiogenic shock with or without resuscitation, one of the most important issues is to rule out concomitant ischemic brain damage, which usually needs assistance by experienced neurologists. Gaining time with stabilization finally allows to asses patients' expectations and goals, information, which sometimes has to be collected with the family physician or even more important with the beloved relatives.

Both, because of shortage of cardiac allografts and the bad outcome of implantable MCS devices in INTERMACS level 0–2, patients have to be stabilized first. This can be done by using short-term (temporary) MCS devices. The next section by J. Rogers gives detailed information about the current types of MCS devices for this indication.

23.2 Patient Evaluation

Patient evaluation for MCS is usually very similar to the evaluation of cardiac transplant candidates. Besides body size and weight, analysis of blood group and investigations to rule out infections or tumor diseases, the final issue is to estimate, whether the patient's health conditions allow him to survive at least 5 years on MCS. The determination of a minimum of 5 years of remaining life expectancy has arbitrarily been defined by the experience of experts in the field, balancing costs and effectiveness of MCS. In younger patients (<65 years) implantation of long-term MCS devices inadvertingly raises the question of bridge-to-candidacy, namely bridge-to-transplantation. At present, patients' compliance to accept immunosuppression after a potential transplantation must be guaranteed.

D. S. Feldman, P. Mohacsi (eds.), *Heart Failure*, Cardiovascular Medicine, https://doi.org/10.1007/978-3-319-98184-0_23

Table 23.1 Conditions for evaluation of MCS

Which strategy is the goal?
Bridge to what?
What are the valves and the right coronary artery doing?
Mitral and aortic valves? RCA-supply of the RV?
RV function?
Pulmonary hypertension?
Co-morbidities, especially renal function?
Frailty?[a]
Risk of bleeding on MCS?

[a]*Frailty* is a biologic syndrome of impaired physiologic and homeostatic reserve and increased vulnerability to stressors, resulting from multiple morbidities, aging, and disability [1], with a prevalence of 6.4% in the INTERMACS registry [2]. Frailty contains ≥1 phenotype symptoms: cachexia (loss of muscle mass), weakness, exhaustion, slowness and inactivity. No specific definition has been validated, with exception of the Fried scale [3]. Frailty regression on MCS may occur [4]. *Cardiac cachexia (CC)* is the unintentional non-edematous weight loss of >5% over at least 6 months. CC is linked with older age, longer length of hospital stay and higher costs. CC (19%) ranks among the top three comorbidities of HF, beside malignancies (34%) and COPD (29%). Pathophysiological mechanisms of CC include metabolic and neurohormonal abnormalities [5]. MCS-independent frailty conditions are aging, COPD, cancer, diabetes, osteoporosis, PAVD, cirrhosis and neurologic disease [6]. Preoperative health status (KCCQ) has limited association with outcomes on MCS [7]. For assessment of the *nutritional status*, the prognostic nutritional index (PNI), serum (pre-) albumin and total lymphocyte count might be used as indicators for impaired outcome [8]. Frailty results in significantly longer time to extubation, length of stay, and increased long-term mortality in LVAD patients [9–11].

In case of evaluation for MCS, there are specific conditions, which have to be fulfilled as *conditio sine qua non*, otherwise implantation of a long-term MCS device might be too harmful or even contraindicated. Table 23.1 depicts these specific conditions for MCS. Since patients may stay on MCS for a very long period of time (bridge-to-destination), conditions for usage of long-term LVADs have to be met, as well. "Bridge-to-what?"– or with other words, the treatment strategy of MCS, has repeatedly to be reviewed during follow-up taking into consideration changes in valve function, coronary blood supply, RV-function etc. Especially the function of the RV is crucial in order to define pre-operatively, whether LVAD support will be sufficient. Furthermore, co-morbidities and frailty have to be assessed as well as the risk of anticoagulation-related bleeding after VAD implantation. In order to carefully address all these issues and to reach an optimal pre- and postoperative outcome, timely referral of the patient to heart failure specialists remains a crucial prerequisite.

23.3 Indications for LVAD Therapy 2012 and Before

ESC guidelines 2012 [12] summarized the criteria for "patients potentially eligible for implantation of a ventricular assist device (VAD)" as patients with >2 months of severe symptoms despite optimal medical and device therapy and more than one of the following conditions:

- LVEF <25% and, if measured, peak VO_2 < 12 ml/kg/min
- ≥3 HF hospitalisations in previous 12 months without an obvious precipitating cause
- Dependence on i.v. inotropic therapy
- Progressive end-organ dysfunction (worsening renal and/or hepatic function) due to reduced perfusion and not to inadequate ventricular filling pressure (PCWP ≥20 mm Hg and SBP 80–90 mmHg or CI < 2 L/min/m^2)
- Deteriorating right ventricular (RV) function.

This criteria led to intense discussions, since referring doctors may have thought that potential candidates could wait until the RV deteriorates.

23.4 LVAD Therapy: We Are Living in a New Era!

So far, long term MCS therapy is not only a question of correct indication, but much more also an issue of the right timing. A lot of referring colleagues still believe, that VADs are "artificial hearts" and therefore experimental and should be only considered as "last resort". Interestingly, some colleagues also believe, that VADs are too expensive, ignoring the costs of "conventional" therapeutical alternatives, i.e. implantable cardioverter defibrillators (ICDs), MitraClips, transcatheter aortic heart valve implantations (TAVIs) or sometimes even more expensive chemotherapies for oncological patients. – The impression, that the implantation of a VAD is coming just before patients' demise may come from an illustration of a famous and very good review article of Mariell Jessup [13], which depicts the stages of heart failure and treatment options for systolic heart failure, showing VAD and transplantation just before the final stage of "Hospices". Jessup's article was published just 2 years after the REMATCH trial [14]. However, two- years survival of patients with long-term LVAD therapy for advanced heart failure improved from 38% (REMATCH trial) to 70% [15].

23.5 Indications for LVAD Therapy 2016

Large MCS registries provides us with data, showing the superiority in mortality and morbidity of LVAD support compared to biventricular assist devices (BVAD) [2, 16, 17]. Therefore, it is of utmost importance to preserve RV function, which is a precondition for LVAD implantation.

Guidelines 2012

Table 25 Patients potentially eligible for implantation of a ventricular assist device

Patients with >2 months of severe symptoms despite optimal medical and device therapy and more than one of the following:
• LVEF <25% and, if measured, peak VO_2 < 12 mL/kg/min
• ≥3 HF hospitalizations in previous 12 months without an obvious precipitating cause
• Dependence on i.v. inotropic therapy
• Progressive end-organ dysfunction (worsening renal and/or hepatic function) due to reduced perfusion and not to inadequate ventricular filling pressure (PCWP ≥ 20 mm Hg and SBP ≤80–90 mmHg or CI ≤2 L/min/m²)
• Deteriorating right ventricular function

CI = cardiac index; HF = heart failure; i.v. = intravenous; LVEF = left ventricular ejection fraction; PCWP = pulmonary capillary wedge pressure; SBP = systolic blood pressure.

Guidelines 2016

Table 13.3 Patients potentially eligible for implantation of a left ventricular assist device

Patients with >2 months of severe symptoms despite optimal medical and device therapy and more than one of the following:
LVEF <25% and, if measured, peak VO_2 <12 mL/kg/min.
≥3 HF hospitalizations in previous 12 months without an obvious precipitating cause.
Dependence on i.v. inotropic therapy.
Progressive end-organ dysfunction (worsening renal and/or hepatic function) due to reduced perfusion and not to inadequate ventricular filling pressure (PCWP ≥20 mmHg and SBP ≤80–90 mmHg or CI ≤2 L/min/m²).
Absence of severe right ventricular dysfunction together with severe tricuspid regurgitation.

CI = cardiac index; HF = heart failure; i.v. = intravenous; LVEF = left ventricular ejection fraction; PCWP = pulmonary capillary wedge pressure; SBP = systolic blood pressure; VO_2 = oxygen consumption.

Fig. 23.1 Indications for LVAD implantation

Several guidelines and consensus manuscripts are leading us, when MCS is indicated. The HFA/ESC guidelines were changed in 2016, in that patients get referred earlier to avoid RV failure [18]:

From 2012 [12] to 2016 the timing for LVAD implantation was corrected with respect to the RV function, indicating, that severe RV dysfunction has to be avoided. The ESC/Heart Failure Guidelines 2016 [18] changed the level of recommendations for LVAD implantation in patients with systolic heart failure as bridge-to-transplantation from the recommendation level IB to IIa/C. The level of recommendation for destination therapy remain the same (IIa/B). Figure 23.1 depicts the indications for LVAD implantations according to the ESC/HFA guidelines 2012 and 2016.

The authors of this section believe, that this guideline is recommending LVAD implantation still "too late". They believe, that INTERMACS level 5 ("housebound") should be the very latest for referring patients to a specialized center with repetitive assessment by specialized advanced heart failure cardiologists in order to avoid delayed LVAD implantation.

Several studies were published [19] or are in preparation to answer the right timing with respect to RV function. Currently, most of the dedicated advanced heart failure units are using the INTERMACS profiles for appropriate timing of LVAD implantation [20]. The INTERMACS profiles for right timing of LVAD implantation were included also in the last ESC guidelines for the diagnosis and treatment of acute and chronic heart failure [18].

23.6 Timing for Heart Replacement Therapies

Even if the INTERMACS levels provide us with very helpful pathways as to when to proceed with patient evaluation, the authors believe, that the following issues for an appropriate timing of VAD implantation remain crucial: (1) *Impaired kidney function*. (2) *Pulmonary hypertension*, with temporary contra-indication for heart transplantation, resulting in a bridge-to-candidacy strategy. (3) *Reduced clinical status according to INTERMACS levels*. (4) *Cardiac cachexia* (see above) and (5) *Impaired RV function*, increasing the propensity of Bi-VAD instead of LVAD implantation resulting in the necessity to adhere to a bridge-to-transplantation strategy and impaired outcome.

23.7 Scoring of Life Expectancy in Patients with Advanced Heart Failure

The heart failure survival score (HFSS, Aaronson-Mancini) [Circulation 1997;95:2660–7] is very helpful to assess the risk profile of a patient with advanced heart failure. The HFSS was introduced before betablockers were recommended as evidence-based heart failure therapy and without taking into account, whether the patient had an implanted ICD/CRTD. The HFSS requests the measurement of VO2 max. If the patient is unable to perform cardiopulmonary exercise testing, the Seattle heart failure model (SHFM) might be used as another score (https://depts.washington.edu/shfm/?width=1440&height=900). BNP showed better sensitivity and specificity compared to the HFSS [21].

23.8 Take-Home Messages

It is of utmost importance to refer patients with advanced heart failure to the specialized heart failure cardiologist [22, 23] in time. In contrast to oncological patients, for which the oncologist are usually involved immediately, referring doctors still believe, they can handle heart failure alone [24].The so-called UK NICE-guidelines even recommend to refer patients after myocardial infarction to a heart failure specialist within 2 weeks in order to allow optimal medical management and regular review of the progression of heart failure [25].

23.9 General Remarks

Upcoming European MCS expert consensus manuscript of the European Association of Cardiothoracic Surgery about indications and patient selection will be published in 2018.

The currently available ISHLT guidelines are the last publication on this subject [26]. The next section by Joseph Rogers will give you a summary of the possible VAD systems currently on the market.

References

1. Joyce E. Frailty in advanced heart failure. Heart Fail Clin. 2016;12:363–74.
2. Kirklin JK, Pagani FD, Kormos RL, Stevenson LW, Blume ED, Myers SL, Miller MA, Baldwin JT, Young JB, Naftel DC. Eighth annual INTERMACS report: special focus on framing the impact of adverse events. J Heart Lung Transplant. 2017;36(10):1080–6. https://doi.org/10.1016/j.healun.2017.07.005. Epub 2017 Jul 15.
3. Joseph S, et al. Prospective assessment of frailty using the fried criteria in patients undergoing left ventricular assist device therapy. Am J Cardiol. 2017;120:1349–54.
4. Maurer M, Horn E, Reyentovich A. Can a left ventricular assist device in individuals with advanced systolic heart failure improve or reverse frailty? J Am Geriatr Soc. 2017;65:2383–90.
5. Loncar G, Springer J, Anker M. Cardiac cachexia: hic et nunc. J Cachexia Sarcopenia Muscle. 2016;7:246–60.
6. Flint K, et al. Frailty and the selection of patients for destination therapy left ventricular assist device. Circ Heart Fail. 2012;5:286–93.
7. Flint K, Matlock D, Sundareswaran K. Pre-operative health status and outcomes after continuous-flow left ventricular assist device implantation. J Heart Lung Transplant. 2013;32:1249–54.
8. Yost G, Tatooles A, Bhat G. Preoperative nutritional assessment with the prognostic nutrition index in patients undergoing left ventricular assist device implantation. ASAIO J. 2018;64:52–5.
9. Tse G, et al. Frailty and clinical outcomes in advanced heart failure patients undergoing left ventricular assist device implantation: a systematic review and meta-analysis. JAMDA. 2017;18:255–61.
10. Cooper L, et al. Assessing frailty in patients undergoing destination therapy left ventricular assist device: observations from interagency registry for mechanically assisted circulatory support. ASAIO J. 2017;64:16–23.
11. Dunlay S, et al. Frailty and outcomes after implantation of left ventricular assist device as destination therapy. J Heart Lung Transplant. 2014;33:359–65.
12. McMurray JJV, Adamopoulos S, Anker SD, Auricchio A, Böhm M, Dickstein K, Falk V, Filippatos GS, Fonseca C, Gomez Sanchez MA, Jaarsma T, Køber L, Lip GYH, Maggioni AP, Parkhomenko A, Pieske BM, Popescu BA, Rønnevik PK, Rutten FH, Schwitter J, Seferovic P, Stepinska J, Pedro T, Trindade PT, Voors AA, Zannad F, Zeiher A. ESC guidelines for the diagnosis and treatment of acute and chronic heart failure 2012. Eur J Heart Fail. 2012;14:803–69.
13. Jessup M, Brozena S. Heart failure (review article). N Engl J Med. 2003;348:2007–18.
14. Rose EA, Gelijns AC, Moskowitz AJ, Heitjan DF, Stevenson LW, Dembitsky W, et al. Long-term use of a left ventricular assist device for end-stage heart failure. Randomized Evaluation of Mechanical Assistance for the Treatment of Congestive Heart Failure (REMATCH) Study Group. N Engl J Med. 2001;345:1435–43.
15. Miller LW, Rogers JG. Evolution of left ventricular assist device therapy for advanced heart failure. JAMA. 2018. Published online April 18, 2018. https://doi.org/10.1001/jamacardio.2018.0522.
16. Kirklin JK, Xie R, Cowger J, de By TMMH, Nakatani T, Schueler S, Taylor R, Lannon J, Mohacsi P, Gummert J, Goldstein D, Caliskan K, Hannan MM. Second annual report from the ISHLT Mechanically Assisted Circulatory Support Registry. J Heart Lung Transplant 2018 Jan 31. pii: S1053-2498(18)31295-6. https://doi.org/10.1016/j.healun.2018.01.1294. [Epub ahead of print].
17. De By TMMH, Mohacsi P, Gahl B, Zittermann A, Krabatsch T, Gustafsson F, Leprince P, Meyns B, Netuka I, Caliskan K, Castedo E, Musumeci F, Vincentelli A, Hetzer R, Gummert J; EUROMACS members. The European Registry for Patients with Mechanical Circulatory Support (EUROMACS) of the European Association for Cardio-Thoracic Surgery (EACTS): second report. Eur J Cardiothorac Surg. 2017. https://doi.org/10.1093/ejcts/ezx320.
18. Ponikowski P, Voors, AA, Anker SD, Bueno H, Cleland JGF, Coats AJS, Falk V, Gonzalez-Juanatey JR, Harjola V-P, Jankowska EA, Jessup M, Linde C, Nihoyannopoulos P, Parissis JT (Greece), Pieske B, Riley JP, Rosano GMC, Ruilope LM, Ruschitzka F, Rutten FH, van der Meer P. 2016 ESC guidelines for the diagnosis and treatment of acute and chronic heart failure. Eur Heart J. 2016;37:2129–200.
19. Soliman OI, Akin S, Muslem R, Boersma E, Manintveld OC, Krabatsch T, Gummert JF, de By TMMH, Bogers AJJC, Zijlstra F, Mohacsi P, Caliskan K; EUROMACS Investigators. Derivation and Validation of a Novel Right-Sided Heart Failure Model After Implantation of Continuous Flow Left Ventricular Assist Devices: The EUROMACS (European Registry for Patients with Mechanical Circulatory Support) Right-Sided Heart Failure Risk Score. Circulation. 2017. pii: CIRCULATIONAHA.117.030543. https://doi.org/10.1161/CIRCULATIONAHA.117.030543.
20. Stevenson LW, Pagani FD, Young JB, Jessup M, Miller L, Kormos RL, Naftel DC, Ulisney K, Desvigne-Nickens P, Kirklin JK. INTERMACS profiles of advanced heart failure: the current picture. J Heart Lung Transplant. 2009;28(6):535–41. https://doi.org/10.1016/j.healun.2009.02.015.
21. Rothenburger M, Wichter T, Schmid C, Stypmann J, Tjan TD, Berendes E, Etz C, Pioux A, Löher A, Wenzelburger F, Drees G, Hoffmeier A, Breithardt G, Scheld HH. Aminoterminal pro type B natriuretic peptide as a predictive and prognostic marker in patients with chronic heart failure. J Heart Lung Transplant. 2004;23:1189–97.

22. McDonagh TA, Gardner RS, Lainscak M, Nielson OW, Parissis J, Filippatos G, Anker SD. Heart Failure Association of the European society of cardiology specialist heart failure curriculum. Eur J Heart Fail. 2014;16:151–62.
23. Konstam MA, Jessup M, Francis GS, Mann DL, Greenberg B. Advanced heart failure and transplant cardiology: a Subspeciality is born. J Am Coll Cardiol. 2009;53:834–6.
24. Stewart S, MacIntyre K, Hole DJ, Capewell S, McMurray JJ. More 'malignant' than cancer ? Five-year survival following first admission for heart failure. Europ J Heart Fail. 2001;3:315–22.
25. NICE clinical guideline no 108: chronic heart failure (National clinical guidelines for diagnosis and management in primary and secondary care) August 2010. Royal College of physicians. https://www.ncbi.nlm.nih.gov/pubmedhealth/PMH0046956/pdf/PubMedHealth_PMH0046956.pdf and Cardiology SAC Curriculum for Cardiovascular Medicine. BCS Website, 2010.
26. Feldman D, Pamboukian SV, Teuteberg JJ, Birks E, Lietz K, Moore SA, Morgan JA, Arabia F, Bauman ME, Buchholz HW, Deng M, Dickstein ML, El-Banayosy A, Elliot T, Goldstein DJ, Grady KL, Jones K, Hryniewicz K, John R, Kaan A, Kusne S, Loebe M, Massicotte MP, Moazami N, Mohacsi P, Mooney M, Nelson T, Pagani F, Perry W, Potapov EV, Eduardo Rame J, Russell SD, Sorensen EN, Sun B, Strueber M, Mangi AA, Petty MG, Rogers J. The 2013 International Society for Heart and Lung Transplantation guidelines for mechanical circulatory support: executive summary. J Heart Lung Transplant. 2013;32(2):157–87.

Types of Circulatory Support Devices 24

Joseph G. Rogers

There are many conceptual ways to consider the devices intended to support the circulation: the indication for implantation, type of device, the ventricles supported, the anticipated duration of support and the acuity of patient need. For example, devices used to support a patient in cardiogenic shock following an acute myocardial infarction are different from those used to treat a patient in chronic advanced heart failure who will live permanently on a device. In the remainder of this chapter, mechanical circulatory support devices will be presented as those intended for either short- or long-term support.

24.1 Acute Support Devices

There are several approaches to mechanically supporting the circulation of patients with acute, decompensated heart failure. Device choice depends upon the severity of hemodynamic compromise, device availability, expertise at an individual institution, and the need to support one or both ventricles.

IABP The intra-aortic balloon pump has been the most widely used mechanical circulatory support device in the world over the past 50 years. The device is intuitive to most cardiovascular specialists and can be inserted in a variety of clinical settings including the catheterization laboratory and cardiac care unit. The IABP consists of a 7.5–9.5 Fr catheter inserted in the femoral artery. The device consists of a variably sized balloon that inflates during ventricular diastole and deflates during ventricular systole. The balloon is positioned distal to the left subclavian artery and above the renal arteries. The physiological effect of IABP counterpulsation is augmentation of coronary blood flow, reduced afterload

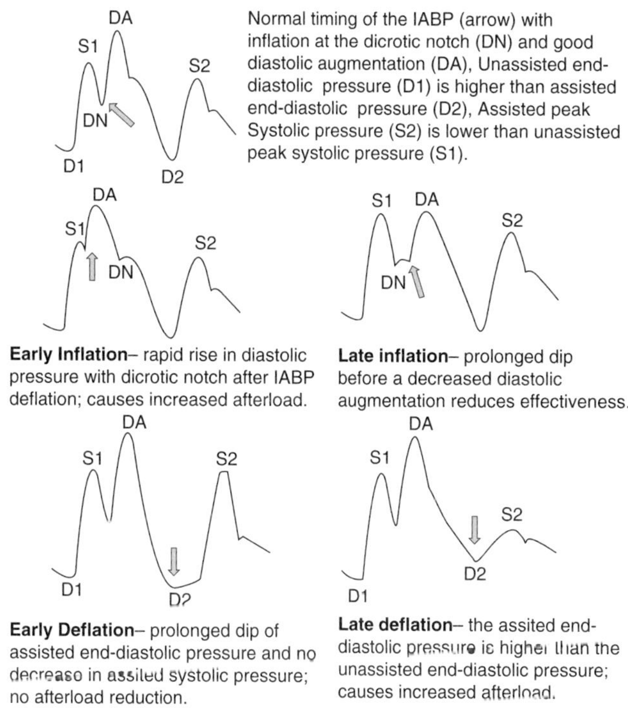

Fig. 24.1 Impact of timing on IABP physiology

in the systemic circulation, and reduced myocardial oxygen consumption [1]. Timing of IABP in the cardiac cycle is critical to maximize the benefit of the device (Fig. 24.1). When appropriately timed, the balloon inflates just after the dicrotic notch in the aortic pressure tracing and deflates prior to the subsequent systole. Early inflation or late deflation results ejection of blood against the partially inflated balloon and increase in left ventricular (LV) afterload and myocardial oxygen consumption. Late inflation or early deflation reduces the hemodynamic benefits of IABP [2].

The IABP has been used in a variety of clinical settings including hemodynamic support in the setting of acute myocardial infarction, high risk percutaneous intervention, and

J. G. Rogers (✉)
Division of Cardiology, Duke University, Durham, NC, USA
e-mail: joseph.rogers@duke.edu

D. S. Feldman, P. Mohacsi (eds.), *Heart Failure*, Cardiovascular Medicine, https://doi.org/10.1007/978-3-319-98184-0_24

cardiogenic shock. The most consistent value of IABP is as an adjuvant to the treatment of myocardial infarction with thrombolytic therapy [3]. The same benefits have not been seen in AMI patients treated with PCI [4]. Data for the treatment of acute cardiogenic shock is less compelling. The recent IABP-Shock II trial randomized 600 patients with cardiogenic shock following myocardial infarction to standard medical therapy or medical therapy in addition to IABP. The 30-day mortality rate approached 40% in both groups and there was no difference in outcomes between the treatment assignments [5].

The majority of complications related to IABP support are related to arterial access. Vascular complications including bleeding or lower extremity ischemia are most frequently reported. Some investigators have been interested in long-term IABP support in patients awaiting heart transplantation and have utilized the device in the axillary position to allow ambulation [6].

Impella The Impella series of devices is capable of providing partial or full support of both left and right ventricular function (Fig. 24.2). The 9 Fr catheter-based system can be inserted peripherally using an over the wire technique or centrally into the aorta. The left ventricular devices are shaped like a pigtail catheter with an incorporated microaxial pump that draws blood from the ventricle and ejects it in to the aorta. The smallest version of the device provide up to 2.5 l/min of output while the larger devices can deliver up to 5 l/min. The right-sided Impella (Impella RP) is inserted via the femoral vein and positioned such that the inflow sits at the inferior vena cava-right atrial junction and the outflow is in the pulmonary artery just above the pulmonic valve.

The Impella products were designed for short-term support and have approval for use up to 6 h. In practice, many centers extend the support duration and tailor it to patient need and effective circulatory support [7].

The Impella 2.5 was tested against IABP in a randomized, clinical trial of 452 patients undergoing high-risk PCI. While the Impella provided superior hemodynamic support, the trial was stopped prematurely for futility of the primary endpoint, 30-day event rate for major adverse events [8]. The IMPRESS trial randomized 48 patients with cardiogenic shock to treatment with either an Impella CP or IABP. The primary endpoint, 30-day and 6-month mortality, was similar in both treatment arms [9]. A recent meta-analysis compared Impella 2.5 and Impella CP to IABP support in patients with cardiogenic shock and was unable to demonstrate improvements in 30-day mortality or left ventricular ejection fraction with Impella [10]. The Impella 5.0 was studied in 16 post-surgical patients who failed to wean from cardiopulmonary bypass. In this experience there was one stroke and one death. The 30-day survival rate was 94% [11]. The Impella RP was evaluated in a non-randomized study of patients with recent right ventricular infarction, or right ventricular failure following LVAD or cardiac surgery. Impella RP support resulted in an increase in cardiac index from 1.8 to 3.3 l/min/m^2 and a reduction in the central venous pressure from 19 to 12 mm Hg. The 30-day survival was 73% [12]. The major complications of the Impella devices relate to access site bleeding. The Impella requires systemic anticoagulation which may exacerbate bleeding complications. Hemolysis may occur with development of thrombus in the device or malposition of the pump. In rare cases, injury to the aortic valve and distal lower extremity ischemia may occur.

TandemHeart The TandemHeart VAD is an extracorporeal, centrifugal flow device that is capable of 5 l/min output. Left atrial access is obtained by venous cannulation that traverses the intra-atrial septum (Fig. 24.3). The blood is returned to the arterial circulation via a catheter placed in the contralateral femoral artery (Fig. 24.3). The relative instability of the system necessitates the patient be bed-bound during support as retraction of the inflow cannula into the right atrium results in recirculation of deoxygenated blood in the systemic arterial system. The device has been used in a variety of clinical settings including

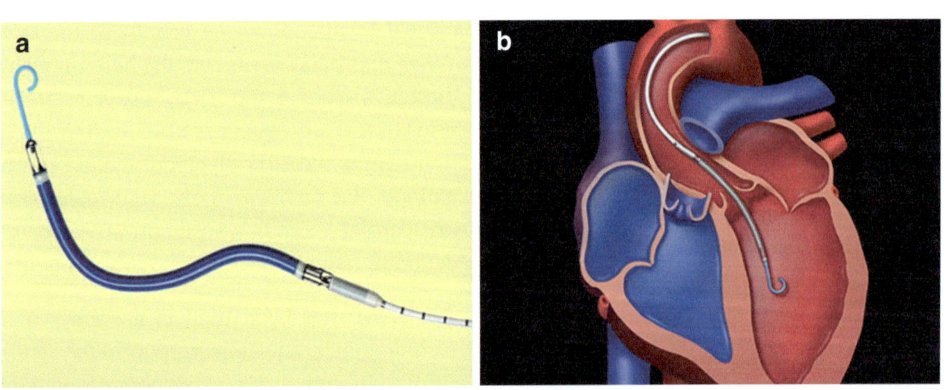

Fig. 24.2 Impella catheters. The Impella RP (**a**) is designed for insertion through the femoral venous system with the proximal inflow portion of the catheter positioned at the inferior vena cava-right atrial junction. The Impella 2.5 (**b**) is inserted via the femoral artery and traverses the aortic valve. The device draws blood from the left ventricle and delivers the blood into the aortic root. (Illustrations courtesy of Medscape)

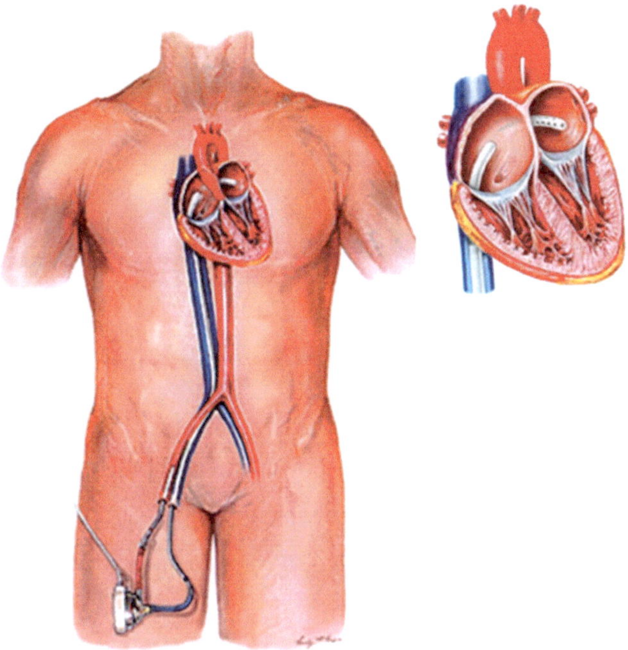

Fig. 24.3 The Tandem Heart is an extracorporeal centrifugal flow device that obtains inflow from the left atrium via a trans-septal catheter and blood is returned to the circulation via a femoral artery catheter. (Eur Heart J 2007;28:2057–63)

mechanically supported coronary interventions and treatment of cardiogenic shock. Kar and colleagues reported a series of 117 patients with cardiogenic shock treated with TandemHeart and demonstrated clinically meaningful improvements in hemodynamics and end-organ function in the cohort. Despite these improvements, the 30-day mortality rate was 40% [13]. In this setting, the TandemHeart should be viewed as a short term support device that will stabilize patients until recovery occurs or a more durable mechanical support approach is selected. Other complications of the TandemHeart include access site bleeding, hemolysis and distal lower extremity arterial occlusion. Recently, a new catheter has been developed that allows the TandemHeart pump to provide right heart support. The catheter is inserted in the right internal jugular vein, draws blood from the right atrium and delivers the blood back in to the pulmonary artery.

Surgically Implanted Temporary Pumps Several surgically-implanted devices are marketed for short-term support and are intended for rapid deployment in the setting of acute cardiogenic shock or inability to wean from cardiopulmonary bypass. The platforms have sufficient flexibility that allows support of either or both ventricles. The Centrimag (Abbott Medical, Lake Bluff, IL) and Rotaflow (Maquet, Rastatt, DE) devices are extracorporeal, centrifugal flow pumps that can be implanted with minimal trauma to the ventricular myocardium and are capable of up to 10 l/min flow although practically flow rates of 4–6 l/min are common. The cannulas may be tunneled transcutaneously allowing sternal closure and patient movement. Bleeding, thrombosis, hemolysis and infection are the most commonly reported complications of these devices.

ECMO Extracorporeal membrane oxygenation (ECMO) is a support strategy used with increasing frequency in advanced heart failure centers based upon rapid deployment capabilities, and the ability to support both the circulatory and respiratory systems. ECMO has been used to support high risk PCI but more commonly for the treatment of respiratory failure (veno-venous [V-V]) or cardiogenic shock (veno-arterial [V-A]) from a variety of causes including myocardial infarction with profound ventricular dysfunction or a mechanical complication such as a ventricular septal defect or rupture of a papillary muscle, refractory ventricular tachycardia, and cardiac arrest. The ECMO circuit consists of cannulae inserted either percutaneously via the femoral vasculature or centrally. Veno-venous ECMO is used for respiratory failure – blood is drawn from the right atrium and circulated through an oxygenator where there is passive exchange of O_2 and CO_2 prior to return of oxygenated blood to the right atrium Fig. 24.4). Success of V-V ECMO depends upon adequate function of the right ventricle. In V-A ECMO, blood is drawn from the right atrium and passed through the oxygenator prior to return to the arterial circulation. In the V-A configuration, the ECMO circuit is essentially functioning as a biventricular support device.

There are several important clinical considerations when using peripheral ECMO. First, return of oxygenated blood to the iliofemoral system may be insufficient to ensure adequate oxygenation of the head vessels and heart (Fig. 24.5). The oxygen saturation in the right arm is a good indicator of adequacy of central and cerebral oxygenation. Second, peripherally cannulated patients with profound left ventricular dysfunction may develop pulmonary edema resulting an elevated left ventricular pressure. Despite cannulation of the right heart, residual pulmonary circulation, thebesian vein drainage and aortic insufficiency all may contribute to LV volume loading. Daily chest radiographs should be performed to monitor the pulmonary volume status. If pulmonary edema is noted, additional venting of the LV is required to avoid permanent lung injury. Venting techniques include surgical placement of an LV apical drain, or further support with a percutaneous device such as IABP or Impella. Additional ECMO complications include insertion site bleeding, infections and vascular occlusion. In the case of peripheral ECMO, arterial occlusion from the large arterial cannula may result in lower extremity arterial insufficiency. An antegrade perfusion catheter may be prophylactically placed that provides oxygenated blood distally in the leg with arterial cannulation.

The outcomes with ECMO support are highly dependent upon the underlying etiology of the cardiopulmonary condition. V-A ECMO is intended for short-term (days) support

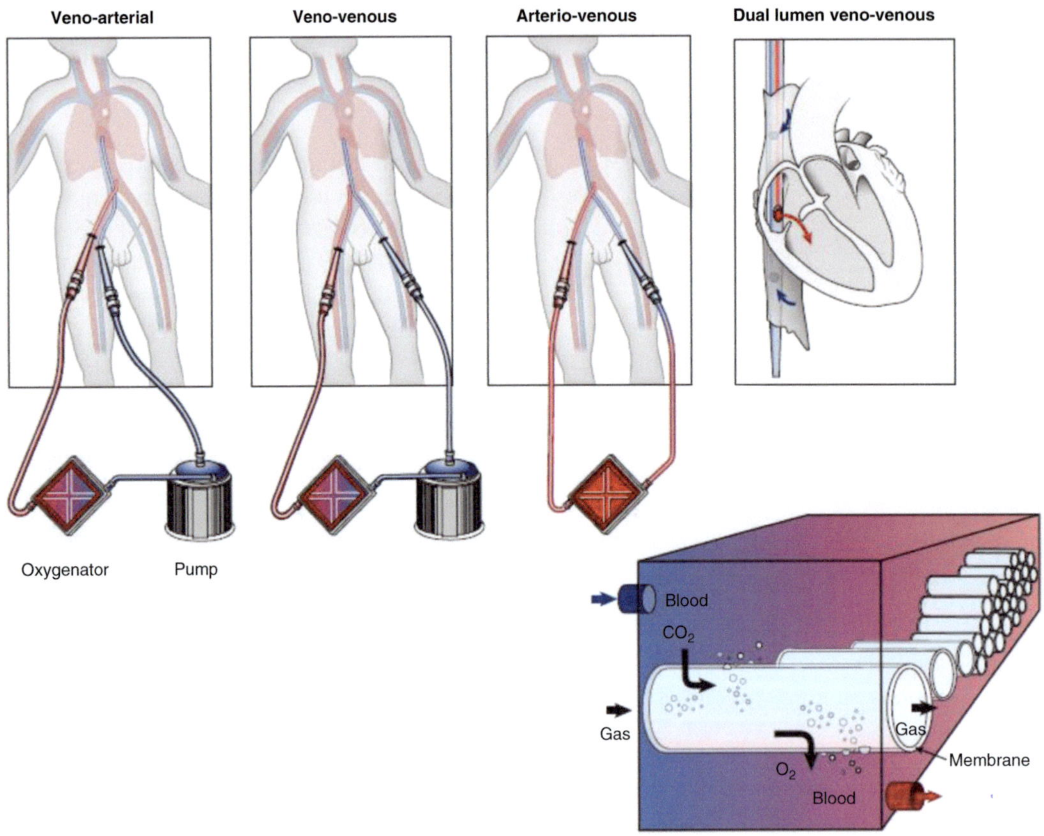

Fig. 24.4 Configuration of ECMO circuit. Blood is drawn from the venous circulation and passes through an oxygenator prior to return to the venous circulation (V-V ECMO) or the arterial circulation (V-A ECMO). A rotary blood pump is placed in the circuit to enhance the circulation

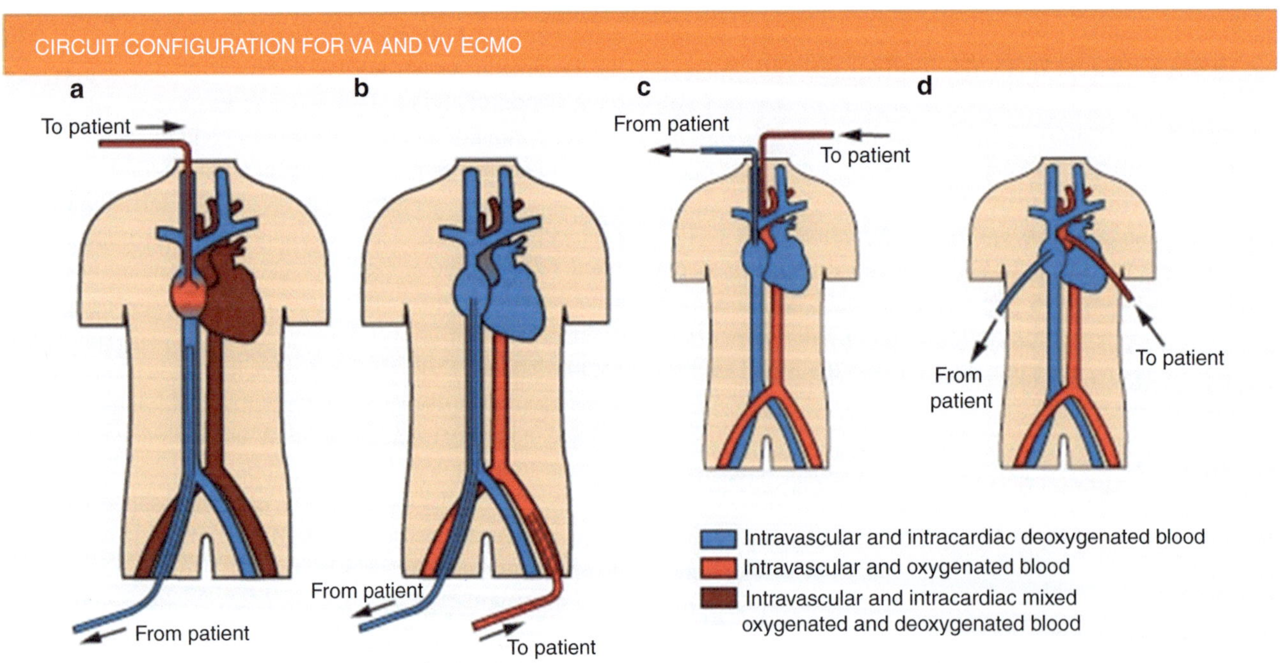

Fig. 24.5 Schematic representation of relative oxygen concentrations in the native circulation of patients supported with ECMO. Panel A is a patient supported with V-V ECMO. Blood is drawn from the IVC, oxygenated and returned to the right atrium. The patient must have a functional right ventricle for this support to be effective. Panel B demonstrates peripheral V-A ECMO. Blood is drawn from the right atrium and oxygenated prior to return to the femoral artery. Note the relative concentration of deoxygenated blood in the aortic arch and carotid circulation. Panels C (carotid cannulation) and D (thoracic cannulation) shows central cannulation for V-A ECMO. Oxygenated blood is returned to the proximal aorta improving end-organ oxygenation to heart and brain. (BMJ 2010; 341:982–86)

and is most effective in patients with a condition that is likely to recover such as myocarditis or transplant rejection. The worst ECMO outcomes are associated with patients supported following cardiac arrest [14, 15].

24.2 Chronic Support

The concept of using mechanical blood pumps to provide long-term circulatory support extends back more than 50 years. Original pumps were designed to function like the native heart, operated in a pulsatile mode, and had the capacity of a normal human stroke volume. The resultant devices were necessarily large, complex devices that required incorporation of either bioprosthetic or mechanical valves. The durability of these pumps was limited and they were fraught with mechanical failure. During the early 2000s, new devices were developed that provided continuous blood flow via an impeller actuated by electromagnets (Fig. 24.6). The relative simplicity of these pumps, ease of implant, and durability has resulted in a marked increase in utilization and acknowledgement from the clinical community of an alternative to cardiac transplantation. At present, there are two designs for continuous flow devices: (1) axial flow pumps in which the impeller is aligned in series with the left ventricle and (2) centrifugal flow pumps in which the rotor is aligned perpendicularly to the left ventricle. Contemporary understanding of these devices is that there are differences in management strategies, adverse event profiles, and patient outcomes.

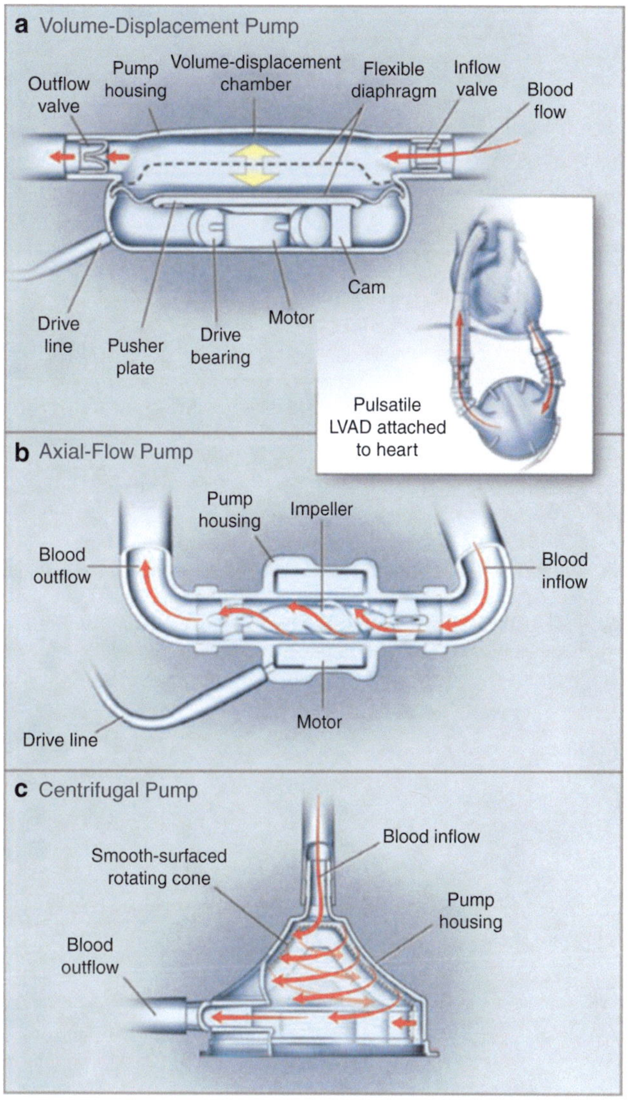

Fig. 24.6 Mechanisms of Durable Mechanical Circulatory Support Devices. Volume displacement pumps (panel A) contain a blood chamber that is displaced during "systole" of the device. The volume displacement pumps created pulsatile blood flow and required valved components to prevent regurgitation of flow during systole. Panels B and C represent axial and centrifugal flow devices, respectively. These devices move blood continuously rather than with a pulsatile mechanism. The impellar is actuated by electromagnets. This change allowed for miniaturization and elimination of the valves. (N Engl J Med 2007;357:846–9)

HeartMate II (Abbott Medical, Lake Bluff, IL) The HeartMate II is an axial flow pump that was the first continuous flow device approved in the US for bridge to transplant and destination therapy. The functional aspect of the device is an elongated impeller that is suspended in the blood stream by synthetic ruby bearings (Fig. 24.7). Clinically, the device operates between 8000–12,000 RPM and is capable of providing up to 10 l/min of output under optimized conditions.

HeartMate II was tested in a controlled clinical trial of patients awaiting cardiac transplantation and failing optimal medical therapy. The primary endpoint of this study was survival to 6 months, transplant or device removal for myocardial recovery. The study cohort consisted of 133 patients treated with inotropic support and a mean left ventricular ejection fraction of 16%. The primary outcome was successfully achieved in 75% of the patients [16]. Actuarial survival was 89% at 30-days and 68% at 12 months. Common adverse events with the HeartMate II included bleeding, ventricular arrhythmias and infection.

The HMII also underwent evaluation in transplant ineligible patients. Two hundred patients were randomized in a 2:1 allocation to receive either the HeartMate II or the Heartmate XVE pulsatile flow device. Baseline characteristics were similar to those enrolled in the bridge to transplant study but the patients were older. The primary endpoint of this trial was survival to 24 months without disabling stroke or the need to repair or replace the VAD. Treatment with the HeartMate II was associated with a four-fold higher likelihood of achieving the primary endpoint than those who received the HeartMate XVE. Component analysis of primary endpoint demonstrated significantly lower rates of mortality and re-operation with the HeartMate II whereas the stroke rate was statistically similar [17].

The final pivotal trial with HeartMate II was ROADMAP [18]. This trial enrolled 200 patients ineligible for transplant

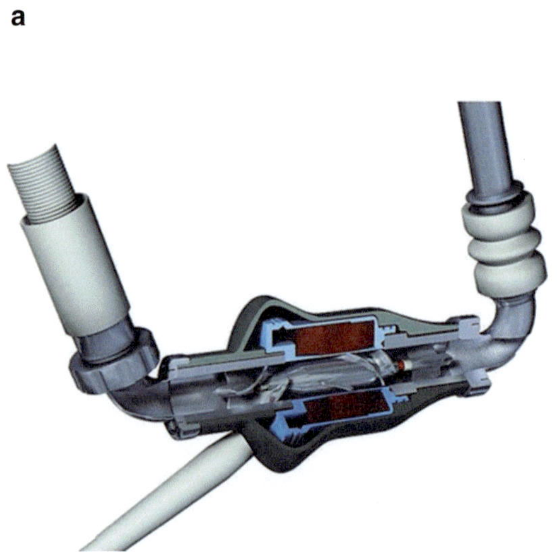

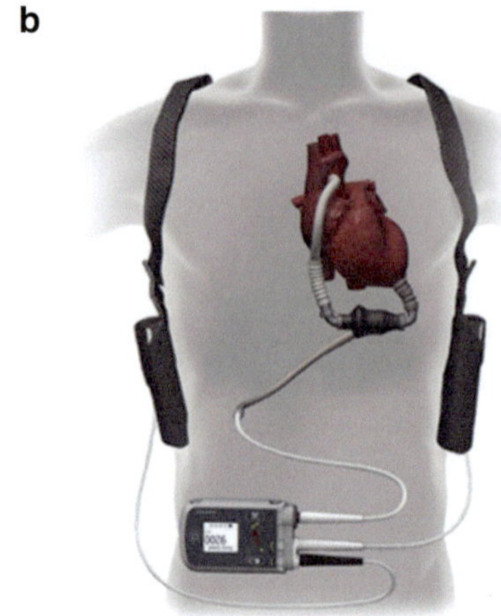

Fig. 24.7 The HeartMate II LVAD. Panel A demonstrates the inner aspects of the device. The impellar is suspended between two bearings. Panel B demonstrates the implantation configuration. The inflow cannula is surgically attached to the apex of the left ventricle and the outflow graft is sewn to the ascending aorta. An electrical driveline is tunneled subcutaneously from the device to the right abdomen. The driveline attaches to the controller that modulates pump speed and collects information about device performance. The controller is attached to two batteries that supply energy to the pump. (Figures courtesy of Thoratec)

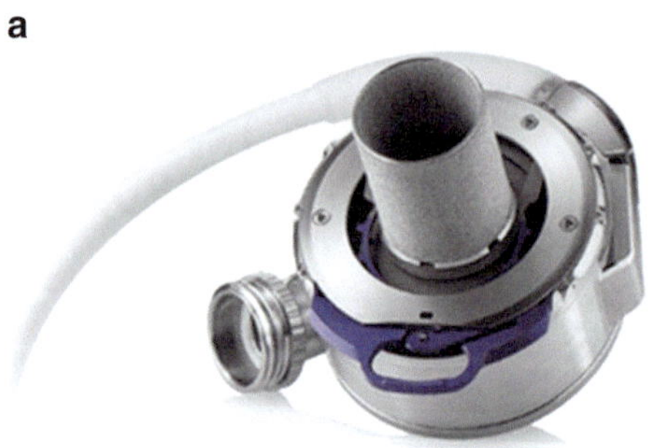

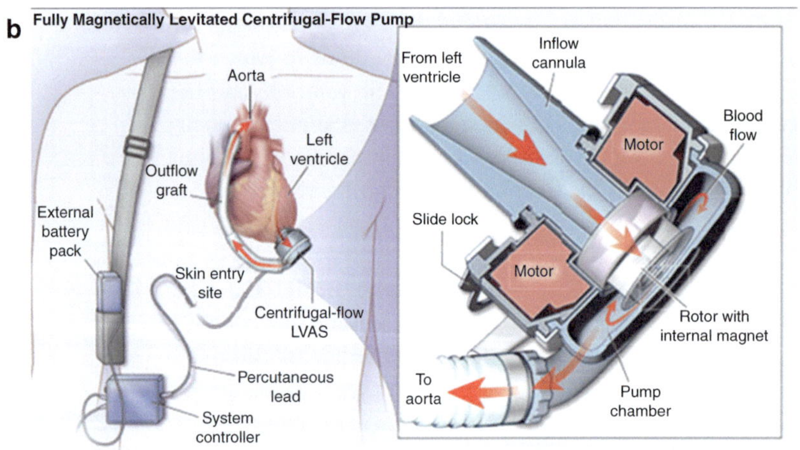

Fig. 24.8 The HeartMate III LVAD. The HeartMate III is a centrifugal flow LVAD that has a fully magnetically levitated rotor. The device (Panel A) is a small intra-pericardial pump with a maximal flow of 10 l/min. Panel B demonstrates the implantation configuration as well as a cut-away of the pump interior. (Figures courtesy of Thoratec and N Engl J Med 2016, ePub ahead of print)

but whose heart failure had not yet progressed to the need for inotropic support to test the hypothesis that an earlier implant strategy may improve outcomes. The trial was not randomized and patient were allowed to select the most desired treatment at enrollment. Of the 103 patients who opted for medical therapy as an initial treatment, 18 crossed over to VAD by 12 months. Importantly, the crossover cohort did not have a higher post-implant mortality. The primary endpoint of ROADMAP was also survival with increased 6-min walk distance of ≥75 m, an endpoint successfully achieved by 2.4x more LVAD patients than those staying on medical therapy. Event-free survival was better in the LVAD arm. The LVAD treated patients were also more likely to have a better improvement in 6-min walk distance, NYHA functional class, and depression and quality of life scores.

HeartMate III (Abbott Medical, Lake Bluff, IL) HeartMate III is a centrifugal flow device implanted in the pericardium that has a rotor suspended by an electromagnet. The device has no bearings and wider gaps between the rotor and the pump casing, design features anticipated to reduce the risks of pump thrombosis (Fig. 24.8). The HeartMate III has completed analysis in Europe and the US [19, 20]. The US clinical trial was designed to test short- (6 months) and long-term (24 months) support as opposed to prior studies that have examined support in transplant or transplant ineligible patients. The short-term trial randomized to HMII (n = 142) vs. HMIII (n = 152). The primary endpoint of survival without stroke or device failure met the primary non-inferiority endpoint for HeartMate III. In a pre-specified analysis in the case of non-inferiority, the HeartMate III was found to be statistically superior (86.2% vs. 76.8%, p = 0.04) for the composite primary endpoint, a finding driven mostly by a reduction in device failure. Patient quality of life and functionality were similar between study groups. The stroke rate with HMIII was 7.9% and there were no reported cases of device thrombosis.

HVAD (Medtronic, Minneapolis, MN) The HVAD is an intra-pericardial centrifugal flow pump capable of providing up to 10 l/min of flow under optimized physiological conditions but typically has flows of 4–5 l/min clinically (Fig. 24.9). The output of centrifugal flow devices is more sensitive to afterload than the axial flow pumps highlighting the importance of blood pressure control. The HVAD was studied in a 140 patient non-inferiority bridge to transplant trial that examined the impact of the device supporting the cohort for 180 days to transplant or to myocardial recovery with successful removal. The comparator was a concomitantly implanted cohort of patients who received a commercially available device enrolled in the Interagency Registry for Mechanically Assisted Circulatory Support (INTERMACS) registry [21]. The HVAD was non-inferior to the control population with HVAD actuarial survivals at 1-, and 12- months of 99%, and 86%, respectively. As was seen in other LVAD trials, there was a statistically meaningful improvement in submaximal exercise performance and quality of life following VAD implantation. Bleeding, ventricular arrhythmias, infection, stroke and right heart failure were common complications with HVAD.

This device was also studied in a randomized, controlled clinical trial of 446 patients ineligible for transplantation [22]. The comparator device was the HeartMate II. The primary endpoint was survival to 24 months, free from disabling stroke or the need to repair or replace the device. The HVAD successfully met the primary non-inferiority endpoint. Measures of patient functionality and quality of life were similar between devices but the adverse event profile differed with a nearly three-fold increase in the stroke risk with HVAD. A secondary analysis of data accumulated from the HVAD experience demonstrated that a low aspirin dose and concomitant atrial fibrillation were risk factors for ischemic stroke whereas INR > 3, low aspirin dose and a mean arterial blood pressure >90 mm Hg were risk factors for hemorrhagic stroke [23]. As a result, the trial was subsequently extended to prospectively test the hypothesis that appropriate anticoagulation and antiplatelet therapy in combination with improved blood pressure control would reduce the risk of stroke.

JARVIK 2000 The Jarvik 2000 is a small axial flow device implanted entirely in the left ventricle. This pump has several unique features including the ability to anastomose the outflow graft to the descending aorta, a driveline that can be tunneled to the posterior auricular area that may lower the risk of infection and a variable speed controller. The device is currently being studied in clinical trials.

Berlin Heart The Berlin Heart EXCOR VAD is an extracorporeal, pulsatile device designed to support either ventricle or for use as a biVAD in children. The device is commercially available with ventricular volumes of 5–60 ml (Fig. 24.10). The Berlin Heart was studied in children under the age of 16 weighing 3–60 Kg that had advanced heart failure and compared to an ECMO-supported cohort [24]. Children treated with the Berlin Heart had a statistically better survival rate relative to the ECMO-supported children. The most common adverse events associated with the Berlin Heart in this trial were bleeding, infection, stroke and systemic hypertension.

Reliant Heart The Reliant Heart aVAD is a small intracardiac axial flow device anticipated to enter US clinical trials in 2017 for short and long-term support. The device has CE mark approval.

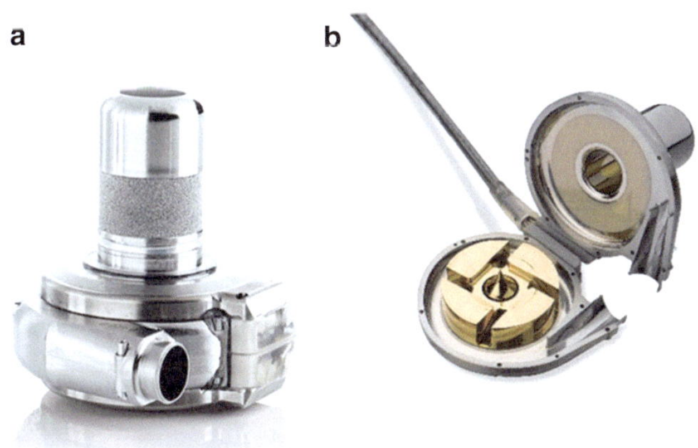

Fig. 24.9 The HeartWare HVAD. This device is a small intra-pericardial, centrifugal flow device. The inflow cannula of the pump is sintered to reduce thrombus formation (Panel A). The pump rotor (Panel B) is suspended by an electromagnet and a hydrodynamic bearing. (Figures courtesy of HeartWare)

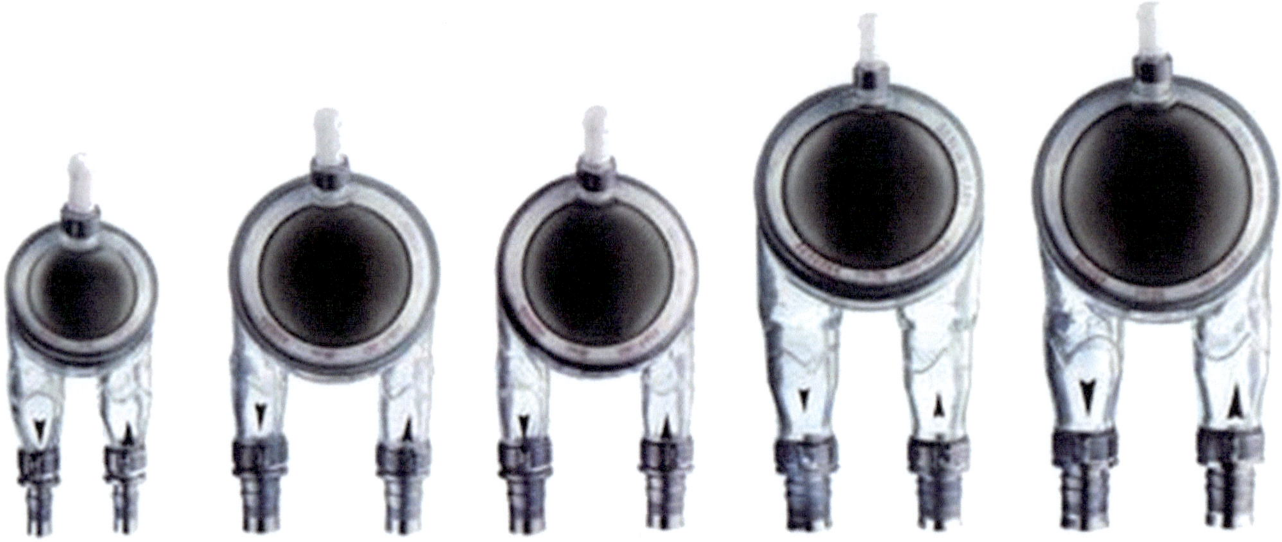

Fig. 24.10 The Berlin Heart Excor is a pneumatic, pulsatile device available in a range of sizes (10, 25, 30, 50, and 60 mL) to accommodate variable chest size and support requirements in children. (Figure courtesy of Medscape)

24.3 Total Artificial Heart

Some cardiac disorders are more effectively treated with replacement of both ventricles rather than single ventricular support. Myocardial infarction with ventriculoseptal defect, cardiac transplant rejection with severe biventricular dysfunction, refractory arrhythmias, and infiltrative diseases often require both LV and RV support. In these settings, a total artificial heart (TAH) that replaces the entire ventricular myocardium and the majority of the atrial myocardium may be a superior choice relative to the use of an LVAD or BiVADs.

SynCardia TAH (SynCardia, Tuscon, AZ) The SynCardia TAH is the oldest and best studied TAH. The device is now manufactured in two sizes (50 cc and 70 cc) to accommodate a greater number of patients (Fig. 24.11). The relatively large size requires careful sizing to avoid difficulty with chest closure. The device is pneumatically driven and requires the use of air compressors to actuate the pump. The compressor is housed in a relatively large console for hospital use but a smaller, portable driver is available for home use as well. The interior surface of the device is synthetic and the valves are mechanical. The SynCardia TAH is approved as a bridge to transplant based upon an 81 patient study that compared survival of TAH-supported patients to a historical control group treated primarily with IABP [25]. Enrollment criteria included NYHA class IV symptoms, a body surface area of 1.7–2.5 m^2, a cardiac index <2 $l/min/m^2$, and treatment with at inotropic drugs, IABP or cardiopulmonary bypass. Nearly 80% of the TAH patients survived to transplant compared to 46% of the control group. Complications of the device include bleeding, infection and stroke.

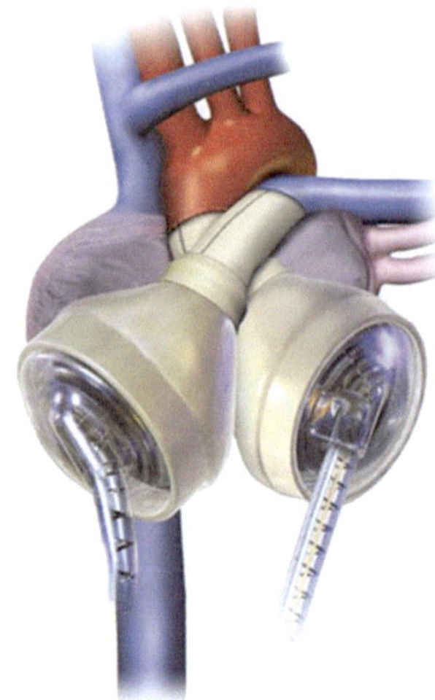

Fig. 24.11 The SynCardia TAH is a pneumatic support device manufactured in 50 cc and 70 cc sizes. Placement requires cardiectomy and the artificial ventricles are anastomosed to a cuff of atrial tissue. Outflow from the pump is to the great vessels. (Figure courtesy of SynCardia)

CARMAT (CARMAT, Velizy Villacoublay, FR) The CARMAT TAH has biological blood contacting surface made of bovine pericardium designed to enhance hemocompatibility (Fig. 24.12). The device also features an electrical drive system, has biological valves, and has a remote monitoring system [25]. The device has integrated sensors capable of balancing the pulmonary and systemic circulation and responding to alterations in preload and afterload. This TAH has been implanted in a limited number of European recipients with a cumulative 21 months of support and is entering a pivotal trial in Europe.

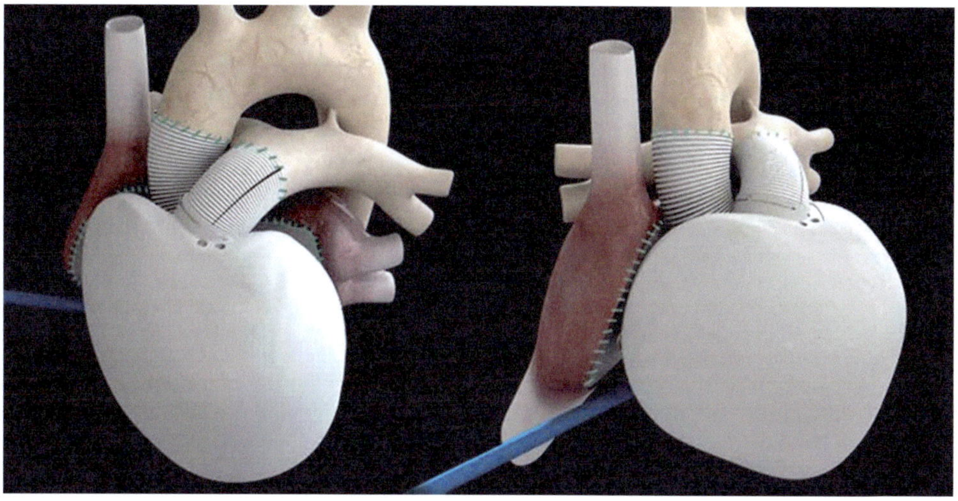

Fig. 24.12 The CARMAT total artificial heart has a similar implant configuration to other complete heart replacement strategies. This device has biological blood contacting surfaces that may reduce the risk of thrombus formation. (Figure courtesy of Carmat)

BIVACOR (BIVACOR, Houston, Tx) The BIVACOR TAH is a novel biventricular support device comprised of rotary pumps capable of providing up to 12 l of flow/min. The design may permit use in a broad range of patient sizes including a pediatric population. The rotors have the same theoretical advantage as the previously discussed LVAD technology with rotary flow pumps – simple design and magnetic suspension that should maximize durability [26]. The device has not yet entered clinical trials.

References

1. Trost JC, Hillis LD. Intra-aortic balloon counterpulsation. Am J Cardiol. 2006;97:1391–8.
2. Santa-Cruz RA, Cohen MG, Ohman EM. Aortic counterpulsation: a review of the hemodynamic effects and indications for use. Catheter Cardiovasc Interv. 2006;67:68–77.
3. Barron HV, Every NR, Parsons LS, Angeja B, Goldberg RJ, Gore JM, Chou TM. For the investigators in the National Registry of myocardial infarction 2. The use of intra-aortic balloon counterpulsation in patients with cardiogenic shock complication acute myocardial infarction: data from the National Registry of myocardial infarction 2. Am Heart J. 2001;141:933–9.
4. Stone GW, Marsalese D, Brodie BR, Griffin JJ, Donohue B, Costantini C, Balestrini C, Wharton T, Esenta P, Spain M, Moses J, Nobuyoshi M, Ayres M, Jones D, Mason D, Grines L, O'Neill WW, Grines C. A prospective, randomized evaluation of prophylactic intra-aortic balloon counterpulsation in high risk patients with acute myocardial infarction treated with primary angioplasty. J Am Coll Cardiol. 1997;29:1459–67.
5. Thiele H, Zeymer U, Neumann FJ, Ferenc M, Olbrich HG, Hausleiter J, Richardt G, Hennersdorf M, Empen K, Fuernau G, Desch S, Eitel I, Hambrecht R, Fuhrmann J, Bohm M, Ebelt H, Schneider S, Schuler G, Werdan K. Intraaortic balloon support for myocardial infarction with cardiogenic shock. N Engl J Med. 2012;367:1287–96.
6. Estep JD, Cordero-Reyes AM, Bhimaraj A, Trachtenberg B, Khalil N, Loebe M, Bruckner B, Orrego CM, Bismuth J, Kleiman NS, Torre-Amione G. Percutaneous placement of an intra-aortic balloon pump in the left axillary/subclavian position provides safe, ambulatory long-term support as bridge to heart transplantation. JACC Heart Fail. 2013;1:382–8.
7. Lima B, Kale P, Gonzalez-Stawinski GV, Kuiper JJ, Carey S, Hall S. Effectiveness and safety of the Impella 5.0 as a bridge to transplantation or durable left ventricular assist device. Am J Cardiol. 2016;117:1622–8.
8. O'Neill WW, Kleiman BS, Moses J, et al. A prospective randomized clinical trial of hemodynamic support with Impella 2.5 versus intra-aortic balloon pump in patients undergoing high-risk percutaneous coronary intervention. The PROTECT II study. Circulation. 2012;126:1717–27.
9. Ouweneel DM, Eriksen E, Sjauw KD, van Dongen IM, Hirsch A, Packer EJS, Vis MM, Wykrzkowska JJ, Koch KT, Baan J, de Winter RJ, Piek JJ, Lagrand WK, de Mol B, Tijssen JGP, Henriques JPS. Impella CP versus intra-aotic balloon pump in acute myocardial infarction complicated by cardiogenic shock: The IMPRESS trial. J Am Coll Cardiol. 2016; ePub ahead of print.
10. Ouweneel DM, Eriksen E, Seyfarth M, Henriques JPS. Impella versus intra-aortic balloon pump for the treatment of cardiogenic shock: a meta-analysis of randomized controlled trials. J Am Coll Cardiol. 2016; ePub ahead of print.
11. Griffith BP, Anderson MB, Samuels LE, et al. The RECOVER I: a multicenter prospective study of Impella 5.0/LD for postcardiotomy circulatory support. J Thorac Cardiovasc Surg. 2013;145:548–54.
12. Anderson MB, Goldstein J, Milano CA, Morris LD, Kormos RL, Bhama J, Kapur NK, Bansal A, Garcia J, Baker JN, Silvestry S, Holman WL, Douglas PS, O'Neill W. Benefits of a novel percutaneous ventricular assist device for the right heart: the prospective RECOVER RIGHT study of the IMPELLA RP device. J Heart Lung Transplant. 2015;34:1549–60.
13. Kar B, Gregoric ID, Basra SS, Idelchik GM, Loyalka P. The percutaneous ventricular assist device in severe refractory cardiogenic shock. J Am Coll Cardiol. 2011;57:688–96.
14. Allen S, Holena D, McCunn M, Kohl B, Sarani B. A review of the fundamental principles and evidence base in the use of extracorporeal membrane oxygenation (ECMO) in critically III adult patients. J Intensive Care Med. 2011;26:13–26.
15. Bougouin W, Aissaoui N, Combes A, Deye N, Lamhaut L, Jost D, Maupain C, Beganton F, Bougle A, Karam N, Dumas F, Marijon E, Jouven X, Cariou A, on behalf SDEC Investigators. Post-cardiac arrest shock treated with veno-arterial extracorporeal membrane oxygenation An observational study and propensity analysis. Resuscitation. 2017;110:126–32.
16. Miller LW, Pagani FD, Russell SD, John R, Boyle AJ, Aaroonson KD, Conte JV, Naka Y, Mancini D, Delgado RM, MacGillivray TE, Farrar DJ, Frazier OH. Use of a continuous-flow device in patients awaiting heart transplantation. N Engl J Med. 2007;357:885–96.

17. Slaughter MS, Rogers JG, Milano CA, Russell SD, Conte JV, Feldman D, Sun B, Tatooles AJ, Delgado RM, Long JW, Wozniak TC, Ghumman W, Farrar DJ, Frazier OH. Advanced heart failure treated with continuous-flow left ventricular assist device. N Engl J Med. 2009;361:2241–51.
18. Estep JD, Starling RC, Horstmanshof DA, Milano CA, Selman CH, Shah KB, Loebe M, Moazami N, Long JW, Stehlik J, Kasirijan V, Haas DC, O'Connell JB, Boyle AJ, Farrar DJ, Rogers JG. Risk assessment and comparative effectiveness of left ventricular assist device and medical management in ambulatory heart failure patients. J Am Coll Cardiol. 2015;66:1747–61.
19. Netuka I, Sood P, Pya Y ZD, Krabatsch T, Gaargade J, Rao V, Morshuis M, Marasco S, Beyersdorf J, Damme L, Schmitto JD. Fully magnetically levitated left ventricular assist system for treating advanced heart failure. J Am Coll Cardiol. 2015;66:2579–89.
20. Mehra MR, Naka Y, Uriel N, Goldstein DJ, Cleveland JC, Colombo PC, Walsh MN, Milarno CA, Patel CB, Jorde UP, Pagani FD, Aaronson KD, Dean DA, McCants K, Itoh A, Ewald GA, Horstmanshof D, Long JW, Salerno C. A fully magnetically levitated circulatory pump for advanced heart failure. N Engl J Med. 2016; ePub ahead of print.
21. Aaronson KD, Slaughter MS, Miller LW, McGee EC, Cotts WG, Acker MA, Jessup ML, Gregoric ID, Loyalka P, Frazier OH, Jeevanandam V, Anderson AS, Kormos RL, Teuteberg JJ, Levy WC, Naftel DC, Bittman RM, Pagani FD, Hathaway DR, Boyce SW, for the HeartWare Ventricular Assist Device (HVAD) Bridge to Transplant ADVANCE Trial Investigators. Use of an intrapericardial, continuous-flow, centrifugal pump in patients awaiting heart transplantation. Circulation. 2012;125:3191–200.
22. Rogers JG, Pagani FD, Tatooles AJ, Bhat G, Slaughter MS, Birks EJ, Boyce SW, Najjar SS, Jeevanandam V, Anderson AS, Gregoric ID, Mallidi H, Leadley K, Aaronson KD, Frazier OH, Milano CAIntra-pericardial left ventricular assist device for advanced heart failure. N Engl J Med. 2017;376:451–60.
23. Teuteberg JJ, Slaughter MS, Rogers JG, McGee EC, Pagani FD, Gordon R, Rame E, Acker M, Kormos RL, Salerno C, Schleeter TP, Goldstein DJ, Shin J, Starling RC, Wozniak T, Malik AS, Silvestry S, Ewald GA, Jorde UP, Naka Y, Birks E, Najarian KB, Hathaway DR, Aaronson KD, for the ADVANCE Investigators. The HVAD left ventricular assist device. Risk factors for neurological events and risk mitigation strategies. JACC Heart Fail. 2015;3:818–28.
24. Fraser CD, Jaquiss R, Rosenthal DN, Humpl T, Canter CE, Blackstone EH, Naftel DC, Ichord RN, Bomgaars L, Tweddell JS, Massicotte P, Turrentine MW, Cohen GA, Devaney EJ, Pearce FB, Carberry KE, Kroslowitz R, Almond CS, for the Berlin Heart Study Investigators. Prospective trial of a pediatric ventricular assist device. N Engl J Med. 2012;367:532–41.
25. Mohacsi P, Leprince P. The CARMAT total artificial heart. Eur J Cardiothorac Surg. 2014;46:933–4.
26. Goerlich CE, Frazier OH, Cohn WE. Previous challenges and current progress – the use of total artificial heart in patients with end-stage heart failure. Expert Rev Cardiovasc Ther. 2016;14:1095–8.

25

Veno-Arterial ECMO

P. Leprince and G. Lebreton

Throughout the last 10 years, Veino-Arterial (VA) ECMO (Extra-Corporeal Membrane Oxygenation) became the first line mechanical circulatory support (MCS) system to rescue dying patients experiencing acute heart failure. This initially happened mainly because technology evolution. However, more ECMO were used, more we were able to understand limits as well as potential of the system. With the raise in knowledge brought through the clinical experience, it became obvious that ECMO use can't be summarize in connecting patients to a centrifugal pump plus oxygenator. Thus it has to be pointed out that optimal use of ECMO requires a multidisciplinary, well trained medico-surgical team. In this chapter, only VA ECMO will be treated.

25.1 VA ECMO Principle and Physiology

The principle of VA ECMO is very simple: deoxygenated blood is drawn from the venous compartment, decarboxylated and oxygenated through an oxygenator and reinjected by a centrifugal pump into the systemic arterial compartment. Thus, ECMO is a circulatory support system more than a cardiac support system. Moreover, ECMO is a close circuit which makes it different from regular cardiopulmonary bypass. Of course, in a VA setting, ECMO replace not only the circulatory function but the pulmonary function as well.

Before to describe more in details oxygenator functioning, there are two very important principles to point out and understand.

Firstly, ECMO does unload very efficiently the venous compartment and right side heart cavities. However, wherever the oxygenated blood is reinjected (ie femoral, axillary or ascending aorta) the flow is always retrograde regarding the aortic valve. Thus, VA ECMO does not unload the left ventricle and even increase left ventricle afterload. There are hypothesis that more central cannulation (axillary or aortic) has a less deleterious effect on LV afterload by directing the flow antegradely, away from the aortic valve but there is no experimental or clinical data confirming it. Of course, the direct effect of that is an increase in LV pressure which lead to pulmonary capillary increasing pressure and thus to pulmonary edema. This assessment has to be balanced by the fact that mean arterial pressure on ecmo is usually lower than 80 mmHG and thus is physiologic. Despite this low pressure, left ventricular failure is sometime so bad that remaining contractility is not strong enough to open the aortic valve leading to volume accumulation. Secondly, the unloading of the right side decreases the transpulmonary flow and the pulmonary vascular bed perfusion pressure, which decrease lung perfusion and facilitate the development of pulmonary edema through ischemic mechanism. This secondary mechanism might explain occurrence of pulmonary complications even if there is remaining ejection.

25.2 Gas Exchange

In VA ECMO, the gas exchanges are carried out partly through the lungs by the persistent trans-pulmonary flow, and partly by the ECMO. Oxygen delivery (DO2) is therefore difficult to establish because it is the sum of the DO2 of the lungs and the DO2 of the ECMO. SvO2 is a reliable marker of total balance between DO2 and VO2, but a true SvO2 through pulmonary artery catheter cannot be measured, as it is divided between the native and ECMO circulation.

The oxygenator ensures the gas exchange (oxygenation and decarboxylation) of the blood pumped by the ECMO, but also the heat exchange. Oxygenators have a tubular membrane on which the gas / blood interface is made. In contrast to CPB oxygenators, it is currently non-microporous

P. Leprince (✉) · G. Lebreton
Sorbonne University, APHP, Groupe hospitalier Pitié Salpêtrière, Paris, France
e-mail: pascal.leprince@aphp.fr

D. S. Feldman, P. Mohacsi (eds.), *Heart Failure*, Cardiovascular Medicine, https://doi.org/10.1007/978-3-319-98184-0_25

polymethylpentene hollow fibers, combining the benefits of complete blood-air insulation, durability (up to 2 weeks) and excellent gas exchange. Although the gas exchange is a little less efficient than the usual microporous polypropylene membranes, the biocompatibility is better and the durability longer because there is no blood-air contact.

PaO2 is determined by ECLS flow, O2 fraction of the O2/air mixture administered and residual lung function. So, even in ECMO, the patient must be ventilated to prevent blood distributed to the coronary and brain from being non-oxygenated blood. Indeed, retrograde flow from the femoral artery does not ensure adequate perfusion of the root of the aorta, which is infused primarily by blood from the lungs and ejected by the left ventricle. The ventilator is then set to pressure-assisted mode (inspiratory pressure peak <25 cm H2O), with a tidal volume of 4–6 mL/kg, a FiO2 at 0.3–0.5, a PEEP at 10–15 cm H2O and a frequency of 6–10/min, to obtain a SaO2 > 90%. In veno-arterial ECMO, hypoxemia may be due to several factors: oxygenator failure (thrombosis, fibrin), low pump flow and/or fresh gas, increased metabolic demand (fever, sepsis), deterioration of pulmonary function, or low hemoglobin rate.

PaCO2 is mainly determined by the fresh gas flow and rather little by the pump flow. CO2 transfer being 10 times faster than that of O2, the CO2 removal by oxygenator is very efficient.

The pressure gradient across the oxygenator can vary from 30 to 150 mmHg. Its increase may be related to an increase in ECMO afterload (high blood pressure, plication or thrombosis of the arterial line, small cannula) or thrombosis of the oxygenator. Its continuous monitoring, provided by some devices, can be useful.

25.3 Devices

The ECMO circuit consists of tubing, cannulas, an oxygenator (with heat exchanger) and a centrifugal pump (Fig. 25.1). Each of these components is important and must be considered). The tubing, first of all, consists of 3/8 section PVC pipes. In order to improve the biocompatibility of these materials and to limit the consequences of the activation of coagulation and inflammation, the circuits are pre-heparinized to improve the endothelial hemocompatibility. Other non-heparinized surface treatments are used, offering an alternative in case of heparin-induced thrombocytopenia: hydrophilic polymers, phosphorylcholine, poly-2-methoxyethyl acrylate (PMEA).

Venous (inflow) and arterial (outflow) cannulas partly condition the flow of assistance and the efficiency of the technique. The pressure drops due to these cannulas depend

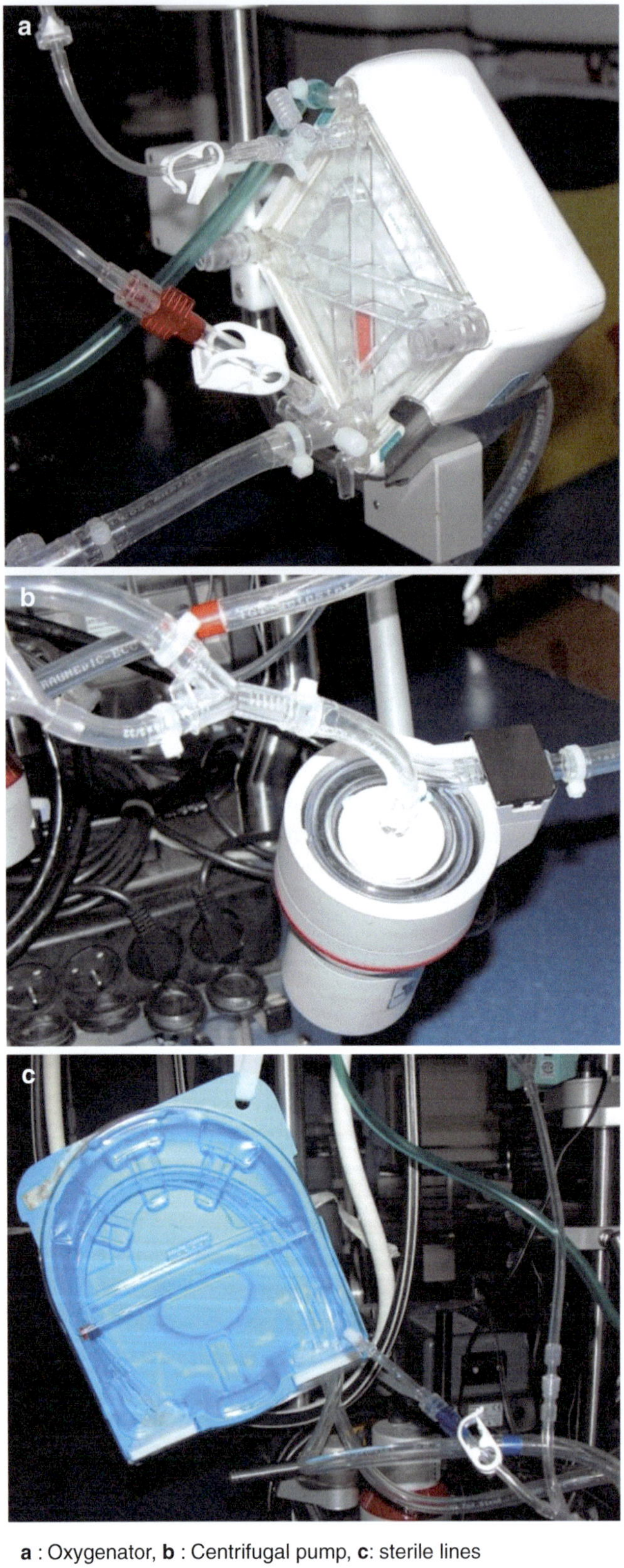

Fig. 25.1 ECMO circuit. (**a**) Oxygenator, (**b**) Centrifugal pump, (**c**) sterile lines

not only on their length but also on their diameter (Poiseuille's law). Thus, the longer the cannula, the smaller the diameter, the greater the pressure drop and the lower the assistance flow rate. Consequently, a compromise must be found between the largest possible diameter cannula and non-occlusion of the cannulated vessels. So, it should be known that the size of the cannulas, expressed in French (1/3 mm) corresponds to the outer diameter of the cannula and not to the inner diameter, which nevertheless conditions the pressure drops. The wall thicknesses of the cannulas can vary enormously from one model to another. Regarding the cannulas, it is important to choose the most suitable cannula in terms of size, but also length, coating, perforations, and profile (some cannulas, with a sharp extremity, are more suitable for a percutaneous insertion than others with a smooth one).

ECMO pumps are non-occlusive centrifugal pumps, so the flow rate depends on the speed of rotation but also load conditions. The pump head comprises either cones or fins (straight or curved), driven by a rotational movement transmitted by the console via a magnet. A Vortex effect is created inside the pump head, which draws blood into the center of the pump head and ejects it on the periphery, as happens in a cyclone. As they are not occlusive, they produce (for reasonable rotation speeds) little hemolysis but are sensitive to the afterload: their flow rate decreases if the resistance to ejection (arterial resistances, High blood pressure) increase. They produce an upstream suction effect which ensures the drainage of blood but makes them sensitive to hypovolemia: In case of hypovolemia or poor drainage, too high speed of rotation leads to a venous collapse which causes the flow rate to fall sharply. Moreover, since it's a non-occlusive pump, when a centrifugal pump is stopped, the blood flows back into the circuit (back-flow).

The console, by animating an electromagnet on which is positioned the pump head, sets the speed of rotation. These centrifugal pumps can provide a continuous non-pulsatile flow rate in the range of 4–6 L / min for rotational speeds of up to 4000–5500 rpm for most (Rotaflow ™ / CardiohelpTM Maquet, Biomedicus / Affinity CP ™ Medtronic, Revolution ™ Sorin, Levitronix ™ Centrimag) and 10,000 rpm for one of them (DeltastreamTM Medos). The consoles indicate the rotational speeds and the flow, measured on the reinjection line. Some consoles of last generation offer in addition a continuous monitoring of the pressures (inflow, outflow, oxygenator) and sometimes even biological parameters (SvO2, Hemoglobin, temperatures). Some consoles are specially designed (compact, advanced monitoring) to allow the transport of patients, and have an aeronautical approval for an air transfer.

25.4 Implantation Technique

Classically, VA ecmo is ran between the femoral vein and the femoral artery. The two homolateral vessels can be cannulated. Cannulating the artery on one side and the vein on the other side might help to decrease the risk of lower limb ischemia. Because arterial canula can be occlusive, superficial femoral artery should be reperfused through a small catheter (4–5 French) connected in parallel to the arterial line (Fig. 25.2). A good positioning of the reperfusion catheter is very important and even surgical insertion can be tricky. Particularly catheterizing the profound femoral artery should be avoided. Another option to avoid the risk of lower limb ischemia is to introduce the arterial cannula through a vascular prosthetic graft end-to-side anastomosed to the artery. Surgical and percutaneous methods both use Seldinger technic. Echography is very helpful for percutaneous method. The position of the tip of the venous cannula can be secondarily check through chest X-ray or echocardiography.

For peripheral ecmo, the other option for the venous canula is the right internal jugular vein which is rarely used but allows to easier mobilize the patients. Similarly, axillary artery (right or more preferred left) can be used for the arterial cannulation but require a surgical cut-down. Axillary artery cannulation can be performed directly using Seldinger technic or through a vascular prosthetic graft anastomosed to the artery.

Finally, ecmo can be inserted centrally between the right atria and the ascending aorta.

25.5 LV Unloading

Technical solutions to unload the left ventricle while on ecmo are still a matter of controversies. Preventing occurrence of left side cavities overloading and pulmonary edema is crucial because it is a life-threatening complication which reversal is difficult. Furthermore, diagnosis of pulmonary edema on ecmo is usually late, made on chest X-ray because ecmo assure an efficient oxygenation and thus there is no sign such as hypoxemia to alarm the clinician. Medical management with diuretics or dialysis and inotropes might be sufficient to prevent LV overloading. However, in situations such as decompensated heart failure or acute MI, medical prevention is usually not efficient enough. In our experience, we validated that the use of intra-aortic balloon pump with ecmo could efficiently prevent occurrence of pulmonary edema [1, 2]. More invasive treatment can be used to prevent or treat ongoing pulmonary edema: atrioseptostomie, left atria or left ventricle passive vent through a canula Y connected to the venous line, active LV

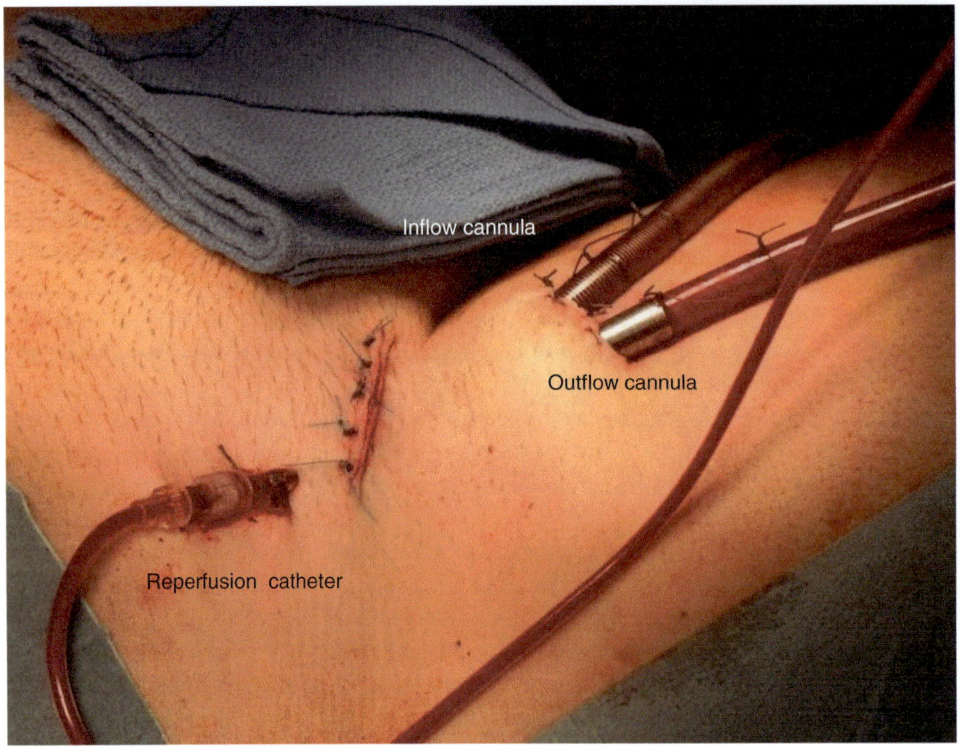

Fig. 25.2 Peripheral ECMO

venting with a percutaneous VAD like the impella. In the latter situation, the percutaneous vent can be used to try to wean the ecmo and thus assess the function of the right ventricle to move the patient toward a long term LVAD implantation. Up to now, there is no trial assessing the best option for LV unloading on ecmo. Thus, it is a matter of team experience and highly depends of heart failure etiology and severity of the clinical situation.

25.6 Complications Associated with Ecmo

Complications occurring while supported with ecmo are not only related to the device by itself but also to the patient clinical status. Moreover, because ecmo is a rescue system, complications are often considered as "normal" although a better insertion technic, a more experience team and a better patient selection should help to decrease the rate of complications.

In 2014, R Cheng et al. [3] published a meta-analysis specifically focused on ECMO related complications. They analyzed 20 studies regrouping 1, 866 patients. Table 25.1 summarized the ratio of reported complications.

Another complication which is not discussed in this paper is Harlequin syndrome. This occurs when recovering heart pulse the blood through non-functioning lungs. Thus the LV ejects non oxygenated blood toward the aorta, upper limbs and brain. The only solution is to switch VA ecmo to VV ecmo sometimes either directly or with an intermediary period of VAV ecmo.

Table 25.1 ECMO related complications [3]

	N studies	Pooled estimated rate (%)	% confidence interval
Lower limb ischemia	13	16.9	12.5–22.6%
Lower extremity fasciotomy	5	10.3	7.3–14.5%
Lower extremity amputation	5	4.7	2.3–9.3%
Stroke	3	5.9	4.2–8.3%
Neurologic complication	9	13.3	9.9–17.7%
Renal replacement therapy	15	46	36.7–45.5%
Major or significant bleeding	5	40.8	26.8–56.6%
Infection	10	34.8	30.4–44%
Retrograde aortic dissection	3	1.5	1.4–2.2%
Arterial thrombus	3	6.7	4.2–19%
Venous thrombus	4	3.6	1.1–17%
Intra cardiac clot	5	2.6	0.8–6.3%

25.7 Indications and Outcome

Use of ECMO should be undertaken in patients experiencing circulatory failure refractory to medical treatment. Even if ECMO is a rescue system, decision for implantation should be early enough to avoid irreversible organ damage. Of course, decision depends of severity, evolution and etiology of circulatory failure but also of team involvement in ECMO management, on site system availability…. It is recommended to contact a reference shock team managing ecmo patients and offering if necessary a spoke and hub service to discuss early enough the potential indication. Some would advocate that a clear therapeutic plan should be one of the criteria to undergo ecmo implantation in order to avoid situations in which patient survive on ecmo wih no cardiac function recovery and no other option such as ventricular assist device implantation or cardiac transplantation. Even if such a situation should be avoided, the threshold has to be high enough to avoid recusing patient by excess.

25.8 Refractory Cardiac Arrest

In this setting, we have to differentiate two situations whether the patients is in hospital or out of the hospital.

In the in-hospital situation, evaluation of the duration of now flow is more accurate and low flow can be shorter if there an on-site ecmo team. Sheng et al. showed in a retrospective series using propensity score that ECMO was associated with a significantly better survival in comparison to regular resuscitation [4]. At 1 year, the survival rate in the ecmo group was significantly better than in the conventional group: 18.6% vs 9.7%. It has to be pointed out that only witnessed cardiac arrests were included and that ecmo team was contacted as soon as cardiac arrest was longer than 10 min. Neurological outcome was similar in both groups showing that survival on ecmo was not associated with neurological sequels.

Out-of- hospital refractory cardiac arrest is a very different situation and futility of ECMO in such a situation has been and is still is questioned. There are two different ways of managing those patients: moving the patient to the ECMO team or moving the ecmo team to the patient. In the more current one, the patient under cardiopulmonary resuscitation (CPR) usually using automatic machine is transferred to the emergency room where ECMO is implanted. The Achilles' heel of this method is the long duration of low flow. On the other hand, this allows having a well-trained team available when the CPT patient reaches the emergency room. Our initial experience with this management was associated with 2–4%survival rate [5]. This is why as a working group we defined criteria in order to select patients who should undergo ECMO implantation for resuscitation and those who should be contra-indicated and eventually implanted for organ perfusion as Maastricht 1 organ donors [6] (Fig. 25.3). With a better selection we could reach a 12% survival rate at hospital discharge (non-published personal data). Fortunately, the rate of neurologic impairment in survivors was very low. In a non-randomized prospective observational trial, Sakamoto et al. [7] reported a significantly better neurological outcome in a group of 260 ECMO patients compared to 194 non ecmo patients at 1 month (12.3% vs 1.5%) and 6 months (11.2% vs 2.6%). This difference remained even in per-protocol analysis. Inclusion criteria in this trial were as follow: (1) VF/VT on the initial ECG, (2) cardiac arrest on hospital arrival with or without pre-hospital ROSC, (4) within 45 min from reception of the emergency call (119) or the onset of cardiac arrest

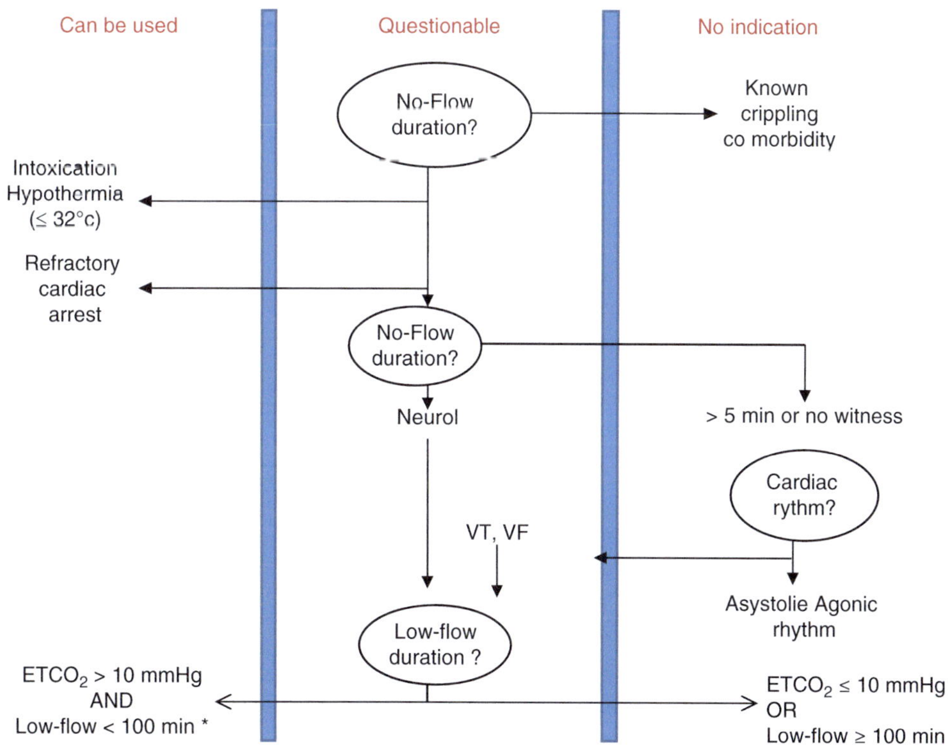

Fig. 25.3 Cardiac arrest decision algorithm. (From Riou et al. [6])

to the hospital arrival, and (6) no ROSC at least during the 15 min after hospital arrival (or after contact with a doctor) even though conventional CPR was performed.

The second solution for managing out-of-hospital refractory cardiac arrest patient is to move an ECMO team to the patient. This organization was tested by the Parisian emergency organization, ie. samu de Paris and is tested as well by the ECMO team from Regensburg, Germany. Up to now there is no published results showing superiority in comparison to the scoop and run organization but improvement in team training and material could help this management to reduce low flow duration and thus save few more lives. Of course, results will anyway be highly dependent of no flow duration appreciation and etiology of cardiac arrest. Furthermore, one should not forget the primary importance of citizen training in alarm call and CPR management.

Finally, due to the lack of randomized clear data, the 2015 AHA guidelines recommend using ECMO "in selected patients (Class IIb, level or proof C) [8] for whom the suspected etiology of cardiac arrest is potentially reversible". Proposed inclusion criteria for such a therapy are: "age 18 to 75, cardiac arrest of cardiac origin, after conventional CPR for at least 10 min with no return to spontaneous circulation". Of course, persistence of cardiogenic shock after return to spontaneous circulation should be discussed for ecmo support. It has to be pointed out that automated ecmo system like the controlled automated reperfusion for the whole body (CARL system) and controlled integrated resuscitation device (CIRD) are under clinical evaluation.

25.9 Acute Myocardial Infarction

Although percutaneous management of acute myocardial infarction dramatically decreased the rate of cardiogenic shock as low as 5–10%, its occurrence remains associated with an unacceptable rate of death as high as 40% and even up to 90% if cardiogenic shock becomes refractory to medical treatment. Despite randomized trial, clinical experience obviously shows a benefit in supporting with ecmo patients experiencing refractory shock related to myocardial infarction. It has to be pointed out that in such a situation ecmo is used again as a rescue therapy for lifesaving. Indeed, there is no real data exploring the role of ecmo in moderate shock in order to prevent aggravation or to facilitate myocardial recovery.

In several reported experiences, survival rate to hospital discharge in patients undergoing ecmo support for acute MI related cardiogenic shock is 30–50%. This might be judged as poor results if one does not take into account the severity of the shock. Unfortunately, there is no efficient score to stratify shock patients. In our first series of 77 patients experiencing acute MI SC and supported with a VA ecmo, we reported a 39% 30 days survival and 33.7% to hospital discharge [9]. Poor perfusion status was assessed by high lactate at the time of implantation: 8.4 ± 4. Moreover, SAPS2 score was 69.4%. The multivariate analysis showed 3 independent risk factors for death: pre-implantation cardiopulmonary resuscitation, lactate and serum creatinine level.

In a more recent paper, we demonstrated that outcome is very dependent of patient selection. We reported a series of 138 two-center patients who experience an acute MI related CS. Survival rate to ICU discharge and 6 months was 47% and 41% respectively. The mean duration of ecmo was 7 days (ranged from 4 to 9; survivors: 8 days from 5 to 12; non-survivors: 5 days from 3 to 9). Logistic multivariable regression analysis retained 7 criteria from which the predictive Encourage score was derived [10] (Table 25.2). We reported highly different ICU survival rate from 16% to 92% associated with different score. Again, high lactate was the most powerful predictor for death showing that ecmo implantation should not be postponed if patient shows rising lactate even if hemodynamic looks stable on inotropic support.

Although the usefulness of ecmo support in acute MI related refractory cardiogenic shock, there is no evidence that ecmo should be used in less severe shock (i.e.: low dose inotrope, slight alteration of ventricular function) in order to prevent shock worsening. Moreover, because ecmo does not unload the left ventricle, the role of ecmo in recovery is questioned particularly in comparison to percutaneous LVAD like

Table 25.2 Encourage score criteria [10]

Parameter	β Coefficient	OR (95% CI)	*P* value	ENCOURAGE component score
Age >60 years	0.966	2.63 (1.01–6.85)	0.048	5
Female	1.470	4.35 (1.29–14.72)	0.018	7
Body mass index >25 kg/m^2	1.131	3.10 (1.21–7.92)	0.018	6
Glasgow coma score <6	1.128	3.09 (1.19–8.05)	0.021	6
Creatinemia >150 μmol/L	0.957	2.60 (1.05–6.49)	0.040	5
Serum lactate				
< mmol/L	0	1		0
2–8 mmol/L	1.551	4.71 (1.31–17.01)	0.020	8
>8 mmol/L	2.165	8.71 (1.76–43.10)	0.004	11
Prothrombin activity <50 %	1.029	2.80 (1.01–7.77)	0.049	5

impella. There is no clinical neither experimental data to support the hypothesis that ecmo impairs LV recovery. In our clinical experience, ECMO does not seem to have a negative impact on recovery potential.

25.10 Fulminant Myocarditis

Acute myocarditis is probably the situation in which ecmo shows the highest benefit. Indeed, patients with acute myocarditis have a high risk of death if ongoing shock is only treated with inotropes. However, myocardial injury can show rapid and complete recovery after few days of circulatory support. Moreover, most of the acute myocarditis patients have little comorbidity and thus their potential for survival is high.

In a series of 33 acute fulminant myocarditis supported with an ecmo we reported a 69% rate of long term survival [11]. In this series, pre-implantation lactate was 5.3 ± 3.6 in survivors and 10.4 ± 9.0 in non-survivors. The mean duration of support was 16 ± 21 days. The 28 ICU hospital survivors had a median follow up-of 520 days and there was only one death due to suicide. Moreover, the quality of life as assessed with SF-36 questionnaire showed a good performance, close to control population, comparable to bridge to transplantation and better than patients who did recover from ARDS.

Because of good short term and long-term outcome of ecmo in this situation with such a potential for recovery, and due to the fact that with experience complication rate associated with ecmo had dramatically decreased, the threshold for ecmo implantation in acute myocarditis patients should be very low to avoid emergent implantation on or after CPR.

25.11 ECMO in Cardiogenic Shock Related to Decompensated Chronic Heart Failure and Bridge to Transplantation or VAD Therapy

The treatment of advanced heart failure is mainly cardiac transplantation or VAD/TAH therapy. However, decompensated chronic heart failure patients are usually too sick for cardiac transplantation and poor candidate for long term MCS. In this setting, VA ecmo might be the only option to stabilize hemodynamic, screen for neurologic status and transplantation or VAD contra-indication, and thus give a chance for those who will stabilize under ecmo to reach long term therapies.

The use of ecmo in this situation is poorly documented. In a recent paper, our group described the outcome of 105 patients who experienced chronic heart failure acutely decompensated and refractory to medical treatment [12]. In half of the patients, etiology of heart failure was idiopathic cardiomyopathy and mean delay between heart failure diagnosis and ecmo was 2.3 years with a wide range from 0 to 10 years. One-year survival rate was 42%. Among the 105 patients, three quarter (73) were kept on VA ecmo. Thirty-three of them were transplanted while still on ecmo. In our group patients on ECMO are considered for transplantation if they are awake and extubated (or "extubable"), with recovered kidney and liver function. One-year survival of these patients was 84%. Thirty-two patients were switched to either BIVAD levitronix (for the sickest, n = 20) or to LVAD (9) or TAH (7). In the former group, 9 were transplanted and 6 survived and in the latter, 3 died on device, 4 were still on device and 5 were transplanted all of them surviving to transplantation.

Multivariable analysis found that pre-ecmo organ failure assessment score greater than 11 (OR 3.3), duration of pre ecmo cardiac disease longer than 2 years (OR2.4) and pre ecmo lactate greater than 4 mmol/L (OR 2.6) were independent risk factors for 1-year mortality although idiopathic etiology was a protective factor with an OR at 0.4.

The French experience of cardiac transplantation in 80 patients who were on ECMO at the time of listing was recently reported in a retrospective study in which the outcome was compared to 866 non-ecmo patients [13]. One-year post transplant survival rate in the ecmo group was 70 and 81% in the non-ecmo group. At the time of transplantation, 46 patients were still on ECMO with a median duration of 9 days and 9 were switched to a long term MCS. For the 25 others, 18 had died on ecmo, 7 were delisted because of worsening in 3 and improvement toward recovery in 4. Even if transplantation outcome was poorer in the ECMO group, multivariate analysis showed that in this group, transplantation was associated with a significant benefit. Of course, these results have to be analyzed in the setting of French organ allocation which allows patients on EMO to be prioritized on the high emergency waiting list for 4 days.

25.12 ECMO and Post Cardiotomy Shock (Including Post-Transplantation)

In a recent meta-analysis, Biancari et al. [14] pooled 31 studies including 2986 patients supported with a VA ecmo for post-cardiotomy shock. The mean proportion of patients requiring ecmo support after cardiac surgery was 1.4%. ECMO was initiated at the time of surgery only in half of the patients (53.8%). Mean duration of ECMO was 5 days. Although the pooled weaning rate od ecmo was 59.1%, survival rate to hospital discharge was only 36.1% for a mean length of stay of 22.5 days. Finally, the 1-year survival was 30.9%. These results reflect very well the usual outcome of pot-cardiotomy ecmo patients. However, this paper requires several comments. Firstly, the rate of post-transplant ecmo was 11.6% and outcome in this population was significantly better (39.8% vs 31.2% survival to hospital discharge). Secondly, close to half of the ecmo were implanted secondly, out of the OR. Unfortunately, the authors were not able to differentiate the 2 group of patients although it is well known that delayed ecmo is associated with a worse outcome because patients are usually in a worse, uncontrolled situation and ecmo is emergently implanted bedside. Third, median duration of ecmo appears short which might explain the gap between rates of ecmo weaning and hospital survival.

Post cardiac transplantation is a very special situation which should not be mixed with post-cardiotomy. Primary graft failure is the main reason to use an ecmo after cardiac transplantation although, in our experience, pre-transplant pulmonary artery hypertension, combined kidney/cardiac transplantation, known technical difficulties for transplantation and the use of pre-transplant ecmo are other reasons. We reported our experience in 91 patients who required ecmo support because of graft failure [15]. Among those, 4% were implanted with an ecmo because of secondary graft failure occurring after a mean duration of 148 h. The global survival to hospital discharge was 46%. Survival at 1 and 5 years was significantly worse in the graft dysfunction group: 39% vs 78% and 34% vs 71% respectively. However, the patients who did survive graft dysfunction had the same outcome than non-dysfunction patients. In the most recent experience (manuscript in review) the survival of patients who required and ECMO post-transplant was similar to other patients: at 1 year: 90% if the patient was on ecmo prior to transplantation and 70% if not.

25.13 ECMO and Septic Shock

Although initial phase of septic shock is not a good indication for ecmo support because its main characteristic is vasodilation, ongoing severe bacterial septic shock can be associated with a profound myocardial dysfunction and thus become a good indication for circulatory support. Literature on this topic is very seldom except for case reports. We recently published our experience in 14 patients presenting a sepsis associated cardiac failure and supported with a VA ecmo [16]. The median time between shock onset and ecmo implantation was 24 h, the median SAPSIII score was 84 and median blood lactate 9. Two patients died on ecmo and two others after ecmo was removed. In the 10 survivors, the median duration for VA ecmo was 5.5 days (ranged from 2 to 12) but the median ICU stay duration was 17.5 days. Five patients were switched from VA to VV ecmo for a median duration of 5 days because of sustained respiratory failure. The ten ICU survivors were still alive after a mean follow-up of 13 months and reported a good health-related quality of life.

25.14 ECMO and Drug Poisoning

Acute heart failure related to drug poisoning is a very special issue, even more acute than fulminant myocarditis, with a high risk of sudden cardiac arrest, severe alteration of ventricular function but also full recovery if the patient survives to the acute phase. It would be a mistake to think those patients can be managed the same way than other acute cardiogenic patients. The best management of these patients requires an expertise in ECMO as well as in drug poisoning. Of course this expertise can be centralized in one single team or be the result of a collaboration.

Regarding the indication of ecmo implantation, one has to know that depending of the drug, some poor hemodynamic situations can be stabilized with IV medication although some other more stable situation will require a more emergent ecmo implantation. Thus, algorithm using predicting factors and based on the type of drug can be very useful [17]. Interestingly, even if in many cases the impact of drug poisoning on heart function is complete asystoly, it is rare that patients develop a cardiogenic edema probably due to the rapid resolution of the heart dysfunction. On the other hand, some drugs can induce lung lesion which can be associated to the cardiac dysfunction and be responsible of an harlequin syndrome requiring a veno-venous ECMO after cardiac recovery.

Of course there is no randomized trial showing the efficiency of VA ECMO in the specific situation of drug induce cardiac failure and only case report or short series are published and the severity and emergency of the situation make trial improbable.

25.15 Other Short Term Circulatory Support

The recent paper from Thiele et al. [18] excluded any benefit of IABP in acute myocardial infarction related cardiogenic shock. Of course there are many situations in which IABP might play a significant role for instance in post-cardiotomy cardiogenic shock, in bridging shock patients to ecmo or as described above associated with ECMO.

Impella pumps (Abiomed) are a series on axial micropump. There are 3 left side (2.5, CP and 5) and one right side (RP). We will focus in this paragraph only on left side impella. Pro and con regarding impella pumps in comparison to ECMO is summarized in Table 25.3.

There is probably no place for Impella 2.5 in cardiogenic shock. Although impella CP (3.5 L/min) is too weak for severe cardiogenic shock, it could be helpful to prevent aggravation toward cardiogenic shock after (or before) emergent PCI for acute MI. However, this remains to be proven. Impella CP is efficient as well to unload the left ventricle in patients who do experience a pulmonary edema

Table 25.3 Comparison of different short term circulatory support systems

	IABP	Impella 2.5 C-VAD	Impella 5.0	Tandem heart	Peripheral ECMO	BIVAD levitronix
Fast to implant	+	+	+/–	–	+	–
Easy to implant	+	+	+	–	+	–
Bed side	+ F–	+/– F+	– F+	– F+	+ F–	– F–
Cost effective	+	+/–	+/–	?	+	+
Efficient	–	+/–	+	+/–	+	++
Respiratory support	–	–	–	–	+	+
BiV support	–	–	–	–	+	++

F fluoroscopy required

on peripheral ecmo. Although this concept is still under investigation, one should make the difference between 2 different situations. On one hand some patients do develop a real cardiogenic pulmonary edema on ECMO because they have a bad left ventricular function but a remaining right ventricular function. In this situation the effectiveness of impella is obvious. There is on the other hand the situation in which patients on ECMO has biventricular failure and develops a lesioned pulmonary edema because of reduced transpulmonary flow and ischemic lungs. Of course, in this latter situation, Impella will not improve lung damage to the same extent than in the first one.

Impella 5.0 is more efficient and thus can be used in severe cardiogenic shock with isolated left ventricular dysfunction. Impella 5.0 can be used as well in patients already implanted with a peripheral ecmo [19] not only to unload the left ventricle (impella CP can do it efficiently) but also in an attempt to switch from ECMO to impella allowing an easier and more accurate evaluation of the right ventricular function and thus getting a better view for the chance of a safe LVAD implantation. The third indication for the impella 5.0 is after cardiac surgery in patients with a poor left ventricular function [20], particularly after valvular surgery in which ecmo is associated with high rate of complication. In these situations, implantation of an impella 5.0 can be schedule and performed before the CPB to be weaned if the attempt to wean it was unsuccessful.

Up to now, evidence based medicine related to impella remains poor and there is a need for registries and /or randomized trial to confirm the clinical feeling (it has to be pointed out that the evidence based medicine related to the use of ecmo in cardiogenic shock is very poor as well).

The tandem heart is a percutaneous LVAD. The inflow canula is inserted transeptal from the femoral vein into the left atrium and the outflow cannula into the femoral artery. Cannulas are connected to a centrifugal pump. The system can deliver up to 4 L/min. In a short trial (41 patients), Thiele et al. [21] randomly compared the efficiency of IABP and tandem heart. They showed that tandem heart was more efficient to restore flow. However, complication rate (ie. bleeding and lower limb ischemia) was significantly higher with this device and finally 30 days mortality was comparable in both groups.

The last short term device which can be used as circulatory support is BIVAD using centrifugal ecmo pump. This concept restore physiologic situation with a pump between the right atrium and the pulmonary artery (eventually associated with an oxygenator) and a second pump between the left ventricle and the aorta. In our experience, this is more efficient and associated with a lower rate of complication in comparison to simple central ecmo which, even it is associated with a left ventricular vent, does not restore transpulmonary flow.

The pump usually used for BIVAD is mainly levitronix (Abbot) for its midterm quality and easy management for biventricular support but literature is still very poor [22]. In our experience, we use this system in patients who are already on peripheral ecmo but too sick to be transplanted or implanted with a TAH. In this situation, the rate of death of BIVAD levitronix is very high but we were able to stabilize and then transplant 14 patients with a 1 year survival rate of 100%.

25.16 Conclusion

VA ecmo can be useful for several situations of cardiogenic shock in order to stabilize patient hemodynamic and improve organ perfusion. The force of ecmo is its easiness of use, efficiency and cost effectiveness. However, every step from patient selection to implantation and management requires multidisciplinary and specialized team in order to avoid as much as possible complication and thus give the better chance of survival to dying patients.

References

1. Bréchot N, Demondion P, Santi F, Lebreton G, Pham T, Dalakidis A, Gambotti L, Luyt CE, Schmidt M, Hekimian G, Cluzel P, Chastre J, Leprince P, Combes A. Intra-aortic balloon pump protects against hydrostatic pulmonary oedema during peripheral venoarterial-extracorporeal membrane oxygenation. Eur Heart J Acute Cardiovasc Care. 2018;7(1):62–9.

2. Petroni T, Harrois A, Amour J, Lebreton G, Brechot N, Tanaka S, Luyt CE, Trouillet JL, Chastre J, Leprince P, Duranteau J, Combes A. Intra-aortic balloon pump effects on macrocirculation and microcirculation in cardiogenic shock patients supported by veno-arterial extracorporeal membrane oxygenation*. Crit Care Med. 2014;42(9):2075–82.
3. Cheng R, Hachamovitch R, Kittleson M, Patel J, Arabia F, Moriguchi J, Esmailian F, Azarbal B. Complications of extracorporeal membrane oxygenation for treatment of cardiogenic shock and cardiac arrest: a meta-analysis of 1,866 adult patients. Ann Thorac Surg. 2014;97(2):610–6.
4. Chen YS, Lin JW, Yu HY, Ko WJ, Jerng JS, Chang WT, Chen WJ, Huang SC, Chi NH, Wang CH, Chen LC, Tsai PR, Wang SS, Hwang JJ, Lin FY. Cardiopulmonary resuscitation with assisted extracorporeal life-support versus conventional cardiopulmonary resuscitation in adults with in-hospital cardiac arrest: an observational study and propensity analysis. Lancet. 2008;372(9638):554–61.
5. Le Guen M, Nicolas-Robin A, Carreira S, Raux M, Leprince P, Riou B, Langeron O. Extracorporeal life support following out-of-hospital refractory cardiac arrest. Crit Care. 2011;15(1):R29.
6. Riou B, Adnet F, Baud F, Cariou A, Carli P, Combes A, Devictor D, Dubois-Randé JL, Gérard J-L, Gueugniaud P-Y, RicardHibon A, Langeron O, Leprince P, Longrois D, Pavie A, Pouard P, Rozé J-C, Trochu J-N, Vincentelli A. Recommandations sur les indications de l'assistance circulatoire dans le traitement des arrêts cardiaques réfractaires. Annales Françaises d'Anesthésie et de Réanimation. 2009;28:182–6.
7. Sakamoto T, Morimura N, Nagao K, Asai Y, Yokota H, Nara S, Hase M, Tahara Y, Atsumi T, SAVE-J Study Group. Extracorporeal cardiopulmonary resuscitation versus conventional cardiopulmonary resuscitation in adults with out-of-hospital cardiac arrest: a prospective observational study. Resuscitation. 2014;85(6):762–8.
8. Neumar RW, Shuster M, Callaway CW, Gent LM, Atkins DL, Bhanji F, Brooks SC, de Caen AR, Donnino MW, Ferrer JM, Kleinman ME, Kronick SL, Lavonas EJ, Link MS, Mancini ME, Morrison LJ, O'Connor RE, Samson RA, Schexnayder SM, Singletary EM, Sinz EH, Travers AH, Wyckoff MH, Hazinski MF. Part 1: executive summary: 2015 American Heart Association guidelines update for cardiopulmonary resuscitation and emergency cardiovascular care. Circulation. 2015;132(18 Suppl 2):S315–67.
9. Demondion P, Fournel L, Golmard JL, Niculescu M, Pavie A, Leprince P. Predictors of 30-day mortality and outcome in cases of myocardial infarction with cardiogenic shock treated by extracorporeal life support. Eur J Cardiothorac Surg. 2014;45(1):47–54.
10. Muller G, Flecher E, Lebreton G, Luyt CE, Trouillet JL, Bréchot N, Schmidt M, Mastroianni C, Chastre J, Leprince P, Anselmi A, Combes A. The ENCOURAGE mortality risk score and analysis of long-term outcomes after VA-ECMO for acute myocardial infarction with cardiogenic shock. Intensive Care Med. 2016;42(3):370–8.
11. Mirabel M, Luyt CE, Leprince P, Trouillet JL, Léger P, Pavie A, Chastre J, Combes A. Outcomes, long-term quality of life, and psychologic assessment of fulminant myocarditis patients rescued by mechanical circulatory support. Crit Care Med. 2011;39(5):1029–35.
12. Dangers L, Bréchot N, Schmidt M, Lebreton G, Hékimian G, Nieszkowska A, Besset S, Trouillet JL, Chastre J, Leprince P, Combes A, Luyt CE. Extracorporeal membrane oxygenation for acute decompensated heart failure. Crit Care Med. 2017;45(8):1359–66.
13. Jasseron C, Lebreton G, Cantrelle C, Legeai C, Leprince P, Flecher E, Sirinelli A, Bastien O, Dorent R. Impact of heart transplantation on survival in patients on venoarterial extracorporeal membrane oxygenation at listing in France. Transplantation. 2016;100(9):1979–87.
14. Biancari F, Perrotti A, Dalén M, Guerrieri M, Fiore A, Reichart D, Dell'Aquila AM, Gatti G, Ala-Kokko T, Kinnunen EM, Tauriainen T, Chocron S, Airaksinen JKE, Ruggieri VG, Brascia D. Meta-analysis of the outcome after postcardiotomy venoarterial extracorporeal membrane oxygenation in adult patients. J Cardiothorac Vasc Anesth. 2017.; pii: S1053-0770(17)30730-9.
15. D'Alessandro C, Golmard JL, Barreda E, Laali M, Makris R, Luyt CE, Leprince P, Pavie A. Predictive risk factors for primary graft failure requiring temporary extra-corporeal membrane oxygenation support after cardiac transplantation in adults. Eur J Cardiothorac Surg. 2011;40(4):962–9.
16. Bréchot N, Luyt CE, Schmidt M, Leprince P, Trouillet JL, Léger P, Pavie A, Chastre J, Combes A. Venoarterial extracorporeal membrane oxygenation support for refractory cardiovascular dysfunction during severe bacterial septic shock. Crit Care Med. 2013;41(7):1616–26.
17. Baud FJ, Megarbane B, Deye N, Leprince P. Clinical review: aggressive management and extracorporeal support for drug-induced cardiotoxicity. Crit Care. 2007;11(2):207. Review
18. Thiele H, Zeymer U, Neumann FJ, Ferenc M, Olbrich HG, Hausleiter J, de Waha A, Richardt G, Hennersdorf M, Empen K, Fuernau G, Desch S, Eitel I, Hambrecht R, Lauer B, Böhm M, Ebelt H, Schneider S, Werdan K, Schuler G. Intraaortic balloon pump in cardiogenic shock II (IABP-SHOCK II) trial investigators. Intra-aortic balloon counterpulsation in acute myocardial infarction complicated by cardiogenic shock (IABP-SHOCK II): final 12 month results of a randomised, open-label trial. Lancet. 2013;382(9905):1638–45.
19. Pappalardo F, Schulte C, Pieri M, Schrage B, Contri R, Soeffker G, Greco T, Lembo R, Müllerleile K, Colombo A, Sydow K, De Bonis M, Wagner F, Reichenspurner H, Blankenberg S, Zangrillo A, Westermann D. Concomitant implantation of Impella(®) on top of veno-arterial extracorporeal membrane oxygenation may improve survival of patients with cardiogenic shock. Eur J Heart Fail. 2017;23(3):404–12.
20. Mastroianni C, Bouabdallaoui N, Leprince P, Lebreton G. Short-term mechanical circulatory support with the Impella 5.0 device for cardiogenic shock at La Pitié-Salpêtrière. Eur Heart J Acute Cardiovasc Care. 2017;6(1):87–92.
21. Thiele H, Sick P, Boudriot E, Diederich KW, Hambrecht R, Niebauer J, Schuler G. Randomized comparison of intra-aortic balloon support with a percutaneous left ventricular assist device in patients with revascularized acute myocardial infarction complicated by cardiogenic shock. Eur Heart J. 2005;26(13):1276–83.

26 Bridge to Recovery (BTR)

Juliane K. Vierecke

Intermacs Defination for BTR The use of a durable device to allow recovery from chronic cardiac failure (at least 3 months in duration).

Mechanical circulatory support for heart failure (HF) is a life-saving procedure that is typically categorized as either a bridge to transplantation (BTT) or destination therapy (DT). However, failing hearts have often shown the ability to recover and there is also increasing evidence that in some of those patients heart can recover and turn into "bridge to myocardial recovery" allowing device removal.

26.1 Reverse Remodeling Is Not the Same as Recovery or Remission

Ventricular remodeling in patients with end-stage heart disease was thought to be largely irreversible. Observations of reversal of chronic ventricular dilation and improvement of LVEF in patients with end-stage cardiomyopathy after prolonged mechanical unloading with left ventricular support devices was first described in the mid 90s [1–4]. Based on regression of cellular hypertrophy, fiber architecture and ventricular geometry these changes were cumulatively called reverse remodeling.

26.1.1 Reverse Remodeling

Some reverse remodeling can be seen on cellular, extracellular, molecular and global levels in a majority of patients with LVAD support. Improvements in ventricular geometry, myocardial function, cellular hypertrophy, calcium cycling, beta-adrenergic signaling, metabolism, myocyte death, sympathetic innervation, endothelial function, microvasculature structure and function have all been documented and occur mostly during the first couple of month of support [4–11]. Another sign of recovery is that LVADs restore blood pressure and flow leading to secondary improvements of neurohormone and natriuretic peptides levels [12, 13]. These factors have been shown to be important mechanisms for reverse remodeling.

26.1.2 Recovery

Although LVAD induced reverse remodeling [9, 14–16] has been frequently observed after VAD implantation, the translation of these changes into functional recovery of the heart has been observed less frequently. Additionally, normalization of LV function and reversal of dilatation to the point where LVADs could be explanted has occurred even less frequently.

26.1.3 Remission

The early reports of LVAD explants were soon followed by reports of heart failure recurrence [3]. This led to the term remission, which was defined as "…the normalization of the molecular, cellular, myocardial, and LV geometric changes that provoke cardiac remodeling that are insufficient to prevent the recurrence of heart failure in the face of normal and/or perturbed hemodynamic loading conditions" [17].

Reverse remodeling	Recovery	Remission
Improvements at cellular, extracellular, molecular and global levels of the heart	Reverse remodeling that that lead to functional recovery of the heart allowing device removal	Reverse remodeling with functional recovery that is insufficient to prevent the recurrence of heart failure after VAD removal

J. K. Vierecke (✉)
Department of Internal Medicine, Division of Cardiovascular Health and Disease, Univesrity of Cincinnati, Cincinnati, OH, USA
e-mail: juliane.vierecke@uc.edu

D. S. Feldman, P. Mohacsi (eds.), *Heart Failure*, Cardiovascular Medicine, https://doi.org/10.1007/978-3-319-98184-0_26

26.2 Incidence of LVAD-Induced Recovery

In the mid 90s, the observed improvement in myocardial function in patients on LVAD support was first published by the Berlin and Texas group who began successfully explanting these devices [1, 2, 14, 18–25]. Since then, multiple single-center experiences on myocardial recovery reported wide ranges of rates of recovery. The recovery rate from nine different centers has ranged from 9% to 63% [26].

The lowest myocardial recovery rates occur in retrospective studies, and the highest are reported from studies prospectively aimed at inducing recovery with specific protocols.

Only 2 groups used a standardized aggressive drug protocol [27–31].

In 2006 [27] the Harefield group reported a high success rate of LVAD explantation. 73.3% of the patients with a pulsatile LVAD HeartMate XVE, (Thoratec, Pleasanton, California) and treated with clenbuterol. In 2011 they repeated their success with continuous flow devices, 12 of 20 patients were successfully explanted [28]. Of note, this cohort of patients consisted of young patients with a short duration of heart failure prior to LVAD implantation. Thereafter, A multicenter study was conducted in the United States (HARP; the results trended toward a favorable outcome but were not statistically significant, out of 13 patients only one met explantation criteria). Taken together, the Harefield results could not be really confirmed [30].

Compared with the prospective studies, the myocardial recovery rates were low in the retrospective studies [32, 33].

Retrospective data from INTERMACS (Interagency Registry for Mechanically Assisted Circulatory Support) confirms a low rate of myocardial recovery for the overall LVAD population (1.3%) [34]. The incidence of recovery was 11.2% (n = 14) in BTR compared with 1.2% (n = 178) in non-BTR patients ($p < 0.0001$).

A review of 13,454 adult patients showed that recovery to the point that explantation was possible occurred at a low rate defined as 0.9% at 1-year, 1.9% at 2-year, and 3.1% at 3-year follow-up [35].

These differences in weaning success may arise from

- differences in patient selection for VAD implantation
- devices used for ventricular support (pulsatile vs. continuous flow, axial vs. centrifugal pumps)
- differences in medical treatment strategies during mechanical unloading
- differences in explantation criteria
- consequent testing strategy (weaning protocol)
- duration of support [36]

The variability in incidence of recovery may also reflect the difficulty of decision-making of VAD removal, and suggests that the experience of the VAD center with recovery after LVAD support is essential to identify potential explant candidates.

26.3 Prediction of Recovery

Recovery appears to be related to the etiology of the heart failure and lengths of heart failure (HF) [37].

Patients with non-ischemic cardiomyopathy have higher likelihood of recovery during LVAD support [38]. Patients with myocarditis (7.7%), postpartum (4.4%) and adriamycin-induced cardiomyopathy (4.1%) showed higher recovery rates then dilated cardiomyopathies, particularly in the setting of optimal drug management [35, 39, 24, 40]. Chronic ischemic cardiomyopathy patients have nearly no recovery potential.

Patients more likely to recover during LVAD support are young with a relatively short duration of symptoms prior VAD implantation [41]. Interestingly, these characteristics overlap with those patients likely to recover with optimal medical therapy [39, 42].

The most recent cohort of patients evaluated for recovery, were coming from the UNOS registry: 594 patients were supported with a HeartMate II and 92 patients with a HeartWare HVAD. Five percent of these patients were explanted in the setting of LV recovery. The patients more likely to recover were younger, female, had a lower BMI, as well as a lower serum Creatinine.

91.2% of recovered patients had a non-ischemic cardiomyopathy.

Independent predictors of device explantation for recovery [35] were

Age < 50 years (OR 2.5)
Non-ischemic etiology (OR 5.4)
Time since initial diagnosis <2 years (OR 3.4)
Suboptimal HF therapy prior to implant (OR 2.2)
LVEDD <6.5 cm (OR 1.7)
Pulmonary systolic artery pressure < 50 mmHg (OR 2.0)
BUN <30 mg/dL (OR 3.3)
Axial-flow device (OR 7.6)
Absence of ICD (showing short duration of HF)
Creatinine ≤1.2 mg/dl

26.4 Pulsatile Vs. Continuous Flow

Several studies have investigated the effects of pulsatile and continuous-flow VADs on cardiac function, some studies showed that recovery with pulsatile devices is more likely [43].

The reasons for this disparity in recovery is not clear.

Based on the experience with different generations of LVADs, it looks like the degree of unloading provided by the device, influences reverse remodeling. Pulsatile LVAD seems to unload the left ventricle more efficient [44–46].

Other authors purpose that the more normal the pulsatility/pressure and flow in the arterial system may contribute to normalizing genomic signaling and ultimately lead to the observed phenotypic recovery [47, 48]. Data to support this hypothesis was shown in a study that revealed improved LV size, function and circulating levels of BNP with pulsatile devices [49].

More recently, studies performed in hearts of patients receiving partial support by a low flow continuous flow LVAD showed less reverse remodeling than those supported with a high flow device Continuous-flow LVAD [50].

26.5 Goals to Achieving a Strategy of Recovery

1. Optimal unloading

After LVAD implantation, it may be useful to change the RPMs of the pumps to optimize the unloading (increase the RPMs) [1, 5, 7, 51].

LVAD speed/flow should be set high enough to provide adequate cardiac output and ventricular unloading (while maintaining a (HMII) pulsatility index >3.5 and) a septum position in the middle whenever possible. (Pulsatility index is calculated through the following calculation: [(maximum pump flow – minimum pump flow)/average flow] × 10).

LVAD speed/flow should be set low enough to allow intermittent aortic valve opening with a ratio of at least 1:3. Optimized based on the patient's fluid status and clinical events (e.g. suction events).

Repeated echocardiograms should be performed after implantation to detect cardiac recovery. A suggested schedule would be 2 weeks preceding LVAD implantation, and then days after implantation, as well as at months 1, 3, 6, 9, and 12 after implantation. See Fig. 26.1.

2. Optimal medication during LV unloading

Few centers have standardized protocol for optimal medical management during LVAD support. But in general, during LV unloading, patients should be treated with β-blockers, angiotensin-converting enzyme inhibitors, aldosterone antagonists, diuretics, and to achieve the best possible reverse remodeling [13, 52].

Target doses used by the Harefield group are: lisinopril, 40 mg daily; carvedilol, 50 mg twice daily; spironolactone, 25 mg daily; and losartan, 100 mg daily [27].

Heart failure medication should be individually adapted to reduce heart rate toward 55–60 beats/min [53] and blood pressure to the lowest optimally tolerated pressures as well as to maintain optimal renal function (optimal MAP 65–85 mmHg). Sinus rhythm is favorable [54].

3. Timeline of recovery

Improvement in myocardial structure, systolic and diastolic function seems to be largely completed within 6–12 months (there are some outlying patients that may take years to recover). LV systolic function improves, LV end-diastolic and end-systolic volumes decrease as early as 30 days, with the greatest degree of improvement achieved by 6 months of mechanical unloading [7]. Hence we recommend assessment of recovery continuously during the first 1–12 month after VAD implantation.

26.6 Assessment of Recovery

One in every ten LVAD patients demonstrates partial or complete myocardial recovery and should be targeted for BTR [35]. Recovery and subsequent LVAD removal require careful assessment of myocardial function. The main diagnostic methods used to assess cardiac recovery is echocardiography and right heart catheterization while reducing mechanical support. Cardiopulmonary exercise testing is also increasingly used by some centers [4, 8].

In general patients with LVEDD <55–60 mm, LVEF >45% and normal filling pressure during right heart catheterization and normalized V02 with and without mechanical support are considered as candidates for VAD explantation [28, 32, 55–57].

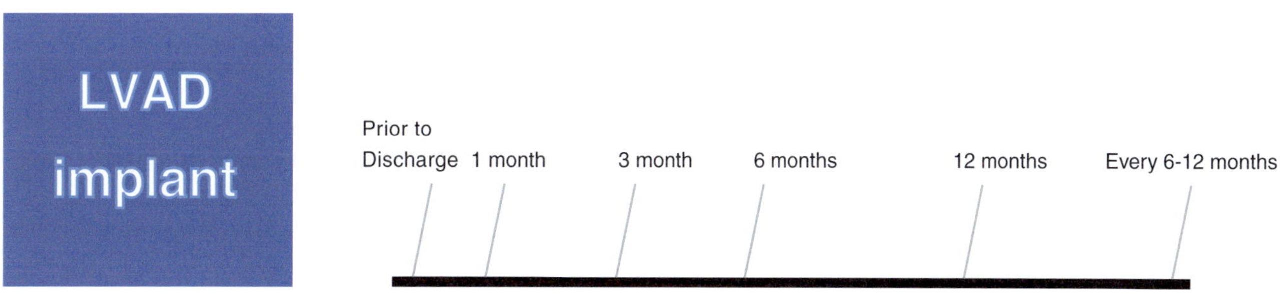

Fig. 26.1 Timeline for recovery TTE

Table 26.1 TTE: Signs for recovery [58]

Improved LVEF (>45%)
Decreased LVEDD (<60 mmHg)
Increased AV-opening duration or frequency
Improved functional MR
Improved TR
Decreased pulmonary hypertension [66]
Improved RVOT cardiac outputs
Improved native LVOT cardiac outputs LVAD: possible decrease in flows/watts
LVAD: Increase in flow/watts

Table 26.2 Speed setting of different cf. LVADs

	HVAD (centrifugal)	Heart mate II (axial)	Heart mate 3 (centrifugal)
Min –max. RPM	1800–4000	6000–15,000	3000–9000
Operating speeds (RPM)	2400–3200	8800–10,000	4800–6200
Lowest speed (RPM)	1800	6000	3000
Changes (RPM)	20–40	200–400	100–200

26.6.1 Recovery TTE

Ventricular recovery can be seen by improvements in LV systolic function, geometry, increase in AV- valve opening duration and frequency and improvement in functional valve regurgitations (see Table 26.1) at baseline and lower pump speeds. A greater portion of the cardiac output maybe pumped through the AV by the improved left ventricle what can lead to a decreased LVAD flow. The RVOT VTI cardiac output will be increased [58].

26.6.2 Turn Down Studies

Temporary reduction of the pump speed ("turn down studies) or temporary pump stops ("off-pump trials") are necessary to discover the native heart function without mechanical assist. This allows the assessment of the heart function with echocardiography or right heart catheterization under the same circumstances that will exist after VAD removal.

Pulsatile VADs allow optimal assessment of heart function during complete pump stops because there is no backflow or forward flow over the device during pump stop.

Complete stops of continuous flow pumps lead to a retrograde flow over the graft into the LV leading to additional volume loading of the heart, resulting in misinterpretation of myocardial recovery (according to acute AR). In continuous-flow LVADs, there is a diastolic backward flow of up to 2 liters/min when the pump is stopped [59]. Therefore most centers prefer to reduce the pump speed to achieve a flow of +/−0 (neutral- neither loading or unloading). An example of this has been achieved with speeds of the HeartMate II at 6000 rpm. There was no difference between 6000 rpm and lower speeds, suggesting that 6000 rpm is sufficient to assess native myocardial function [60].

Alternatively, the HVAD is a centrifugal pump, partial-magnetic levitated with hydrodynamic bearings. The lowest possible RPM is 1800 resulting still in a forward flow, complete pump stop result in a backflow making the assessment of the native heart function difficult. An approach to address this problem is to use a temporary balloon occlusion of the outflow graft during pump stop. This occlusion eliminates the backflow, resulting in proper assessment by echocardiography and right heart hemodynamics [61, 62].

The lowest possible speed of the Heart Mate 3 is 3000 RPM (Table 26.2).

26.6.3 Anticoagulation

The *turn-down* studies should only be performed with a therapeutic INR (international normalized ratio) 2.0–3.0. Turn-down echocardiographic studies should not be performed in patients with a history of stroke/transient ischemic attack, LVAD thrombosis, hemolysis, difficulties in achieving optimal anticoagulation, or during sub-therapeutic international normalized ratio [7].

To prevent thrombus formation inside the pump, intravenous heparin during pump stop or reduction should be considered [24, 40]. Duration of individuals "off-pump" or turn down trials may vary between 3 and 30 minutes, but may be even longer. With appropriate caution, the risk of speed reduction or interruption of unloading is low. These assessments needs be repeated to make the final decision regarding VAD explantation [54].

26.7 Protocol for BTR

1. Assess probability for BTR (bridge to recovery)
   High probability:

Non-ischemic Etiology of HF, Myocarditis, post-partum CMP, adriamycin-induced cardiomyopathy
Short duration of Heart Failure
Young age (<50y)

2. Optimal heart failure medication
3. Repeat baseline echocardiography
4. Speed adjustments (RAMP studies) to achieve optimal unloading
5. Turn down Echocardiography to assess recovery without LVAD
   (a) with full support of the LVAD
   (b) with reduced LVAD support

(c) without LVAD support (net LVAD flow +/− 0)/pump stop with ballon occlusion of outflow graft

	HVAD (centrifugal)	Heart mate II (axial)	Heart mate 3 (centrifugal)
Min –max. RPM	1800–4000	6000–15,000	3000–9000
Operating speeds (RPM)	2400–3200	8800–10,000	4800–6200
Lowest speed (RPM)	1800	6000	3000
Changes (RPM)	20–40	200–400	100

TTE: Explant criteria [54]

Stable LV ejection fraction ≥45%
LV end-diastolic dimension (LVEDD) <55 mm
No or less than grade II mitral and/or aortic valve regurgitation
No RV dilation (RVOT diameter < 35 mm, short−/long-axis ratio < 0.6)
No or maximum grade II tricuspid or pulmonary valve regurgitation

(e) Dobutamine Stress-echocardiography
   (i) Improvement in LVEF
6. Hemodynamic measurements, right heart catheterization
   (a) with full support of the LVAD
   (b) with reduced LVAD support
   (c) without LVAD support (net LVAD flow +/- 0/ pump stop and balloon occlusion of outflow graft)
   RHC: Explant criteria [54]

Pulmonary capillary wedge pressure (mean) <13 mm Hg
Cardiac index >2.6 L/min per m²
RA pressure < 10 mmHg
MAP >65 mmHg
SR, Heart rate< 90 beats/min, not more than 25% heart rate increase during off-pump trials

7. Exercise Test
   (i) CPET maximal oxygen consumption with exercise (mVO2) >16 mL/ kg/min, >65% predicted
   (ii) Normal 6 min walk test

Certain echocardiography parameters appeared highly predictive for long-term (≥5 years) post-weaning cardiac function and reliable for weaning decisions [24, 40, 54, 57, 63].

26.8 Survival After VAD Explantation and Heart Failure Recurrence

Despite all efforts, a significant number of patients show worsening of heart function after VAD removal long term [32, 64].

One-year survival after LVAD explantation, available in INTERMACS for 21 patients, was 86% [34]. The post VAD explantation survival is comparable with that of patients who recovered from acute myocarditis, non-coronary postcardiotomy HF and peripartum cardiomyopathy [54], 5 and 10-year survival, reaching 87.8 ± 5.3%and 82.6 ± 7.3%.

Comparison of outcome of patients BTR and BTT, the survival rate at 5 years after LVAD explantation was 73.9% [65].

The optimal method for assessment of recovery unknown and the prediction of long term stability after VAD explantation remains difficult. The largest published series to examine echocardiographic imaging parameters and cardiac stability included 45 patients with explanted LVADs, 27% had continuous-flow devices (INCOR or HM II). LV end-diastolic diameter < 55 mm and/or LVEF >45% before LVAD removal at off pump trial and a history of HF <5 years before LVAD implantation were major risk factors for early recurrence of HF. Patients without any of these 3 risk factors showed no HF recurrence during the first 3 years after VAD removal. Conversely, all of those with at least 2 of these 3 risk factors developed early recurrence of HF.

In those with long-term stable cardiac function, the LVEF after 6 month of VAD explantation was the same like before LVAD explantation [37].

10-year survival rates after LVAD removal reached 70.7 ± 9.2%. HF recurred in up to 37% of patients during 5 years. Less than 20% died after HF recurrence or non-cardiac complications related to left VAD explantation.

Comparison of patients with and without heart failure recurrence showed that stable patients were younger, with shorter history of HF and time of support. Left ventricular ejection fraction during the first 6 months post-weaning, appeared predictive for long-term stability. HF history >5 years and instability of cardiac improvement appeared predictive for HF recurrence [40].

References

1. Muller J, Wallukat G, Weng YG, Dandel M, Spiegelsberger S, Semrau S, et al. Weaning from mechanical cardiac support in patients with idiopathic dilated cardiomyopathy. Circulation. 1997;96(2):542–9.
2. Hetzer R, Muller J, Weng Y, Wallukat G, Spiegelsberger S, Loebe M. Cardiac recovery in dilated cardiomyopathy by unloading with a left ventricular assist device. Ann Thorac Surg. 1999;68(2):742–9.
3. Levin HR, Oz MC, Catanese KA, Rose EA, Burkhoff D. Transient normalization of systolic and diastolic function after support with a left ventricular assist device in a patient with dilated cardiomyopathy. J Heart Lung Transplant. 1996;15(8):840–2.
4. Levin HR, Oz MC, Chen JM, Packer M, Rose EA, Burkhoff D. Reversal of chronic ventricular dilation in patients with end-stage cardiomyopathy by prolonged mechanical unloading. Circulation. 1995;91(11):2717–20.
5. Burkhoff D, Klotz S, Mancini DM. LVAD-induced reverse remodeling: basic and clinical implications for myocardial recovery. J Card Fail. 2006;12(3):227–39.
6. Madigan JD, Barbone A, Choudhri AF, Morales DL, Cai B, Oz MC, et al. Time course of reverse remodeling of the left ventricle during support with a left ventricular assist device. J Thorac Cardiovasc Surg. 2001;121(5):902–8.

7. Drakos SG, Wever-Pinzon O, Selzman CH, Gilbert EM, Alharethi R, Reid BB, et al. Magnitude and time course of changes induced by continuous-flow left ventricular assist device unloading in chronic heart failure: insights into cardiac recovery. J Am Coll Cardiol. 2013;61(19):1985–94.
8. Birks EJ. Molecular changes after left ventricular assist device support for heart failure. Circ Res. 2013;113(6):777–91.
9. Hall JL, Fermin DR, Birks EJ, Barton PJ, Slaughter M, Eckman P, et al. Clinical, molecular, and genomic changes in response to a left ventricular assist device. J Am Coll Cardiol. 2011;57(6):641–52.
10. Akhter SA, D'Souza KM, Malhotra R, Staron ML, Valeroso TB, Fedson SE, et al. Reversal of impaired myocardial beta-adrenergic receptor signaling by continuous-flow left ventricular assist device support. J Heart Lung Transplant. 2010;29(6):603–9.
11. Ogletree ML, Sweet WE, Talerico C, Klecka ME, Young JB, Smedira NG, et al. Duration of left ventricular assist device support: effects on abnormal calcium cycling and functional recovery in the failing human heart. J Heart Lung Transplant. 2010;29(5):554–61.
12. Klotz S, Barbone A, Reiken S, Holmes JW, Naka Y, Oz MC, et al. Left ventricular assist device support normalizes left and right ventricular beta-adrenergic pathway properties. J Am Coll Cardiol. 2005;45(5):668–76.
13. Klotz S, Burkhoff D, Garrelds IM, Boomsma F, Danser AH. The impact of left ventricular assist device-induced left ventricular unloading on the myocardial renin-angiotensin-aldosterone system: therapeutic consequences? Eur Heart J. 2009;30(7):805–12.
14. Frazier OH, Benedict CR, Radovancevic B, Bick RJ, Capek P, Springer WE, et al. Improved left ventricular function after chronic left ventricular unloading. Ann Thorac Surg. 1996;62(3):675–81. discussion 81-2
15. Saito S, Matsumiya G, Sakaguchi T, Miyagawa S, Yamauchi T, Kuratani T, et al. Cardiac fibrosis and cellular hypertrophy decrease the degree of reverse remodeling and improvement in cardiac function during left ventricular assist. J Heart Lung Transplant. 2010;29(6):672–9.
16. Ambardekar AV, Walker JS, Walker LA, Cleveland JC Jr, Lowes BD, Buttrick PM. Incomplete recovery of myocyte contractile function despite improvement of myocardial architecture with left ventricular assist device support. Circ Heart Fail. 2011;4(4):425–32.
17. Mann DL, Barger PM, Burkhoff D. Myocardial recovery and the failing heart: myth, magic, or molecular target? J Am Coll Cardiol. 2012;60(24):2465–72.
18. Frazier OH, Myers TJ. Left ventricular assist system as a bridge to myocardial recovery. Ann Thorac Surg. 1999;68(2):734–41.
19. Komoda T, Komoda S, Dandel M, Weng Y, Hetzer R. Explantation of INCOR left ventricular assist device after myocardial recovery. J Card Surg. 2008;23(6):642–7.
20. Mueller J, Wallukat G, Weng Y, Dandel M, Ellinghaus P, Huetter J, et al. Predictive factors for weaning from a cardiac assist device. An analysis of clinical, gene expression, and protein data. J Heart Lung Transplant. 2001;20(2):202.
21. Loebe M, Weng Y, Muller J, Dandel M, Halfmann R, Spiegelsberger S, et al. Successful mechanical circulatory support for more than two years with a left ventricular assist device in a patient with dilated cardiomyopathy. J Heart Lung Transplant. 1997;16(11):1176–9.
22. Liang H, Lin H, Weng Y, Dandel M, Hetzer R. Prediction of cardiac function after weaning from ventricular assist devices. J Thorac Cardiovasc Surg. 2005;130(6):1555–60.
23. Hetzer R, Muller JH, Weng Y, Meyer R, Dandel M. Bridging-to-recovery. Ann Thorac Surg. 2001;71(3 Suppl):S109–13. discussion S14-5
24. Dandel M, Weng Y, Siniawski H, Stepanenko A, Krabatsch T, Potapov E, et al. Heart failure reversal by ventricular unloading in patients with chronic cardiomyopathy: criteria for weaning from ventricular assist devices. Eur Heart J. 2011;32(9):1148–60.
25. Estep JD, Chang SM, Bhimaraj A, Torre-Amione G, Zoghbi WA, Nagueh SF. Imaging for ventricular function and myocardial recovery on nonpulsatile ventricular assist devices. Circulation. 2012;125:2265–77.
26. Drakos SG, Mehra MR. Clinical myocardial recovery during long-term mechanical support in advanced heart failure: insights into moving the field forward. J Heart Lung Transplant. 2016;35(4):413–20.
27. Birks EJ, Tansley PD, Hardy J, George RS, Bowles CT, Burke M, et al. Left ventricular assist device and drug therapy for the reversal of heart failure. N Engl J Med. 2006;355(18):1873–84.
28. Birks EJ, George RS, Hedger M, Bahrami T, Wilton P, Bowles CT, et al. Reversal of severe heart failure with a continuous-flow left ventricular assist device and pharmacological therapy: a prospective study. Circulation. 2011;123(4):381–90.
29. Drakos SG, Terrovitis JV, Anastasiou-Nana MI, Nanas JN. Reverse remodeling during long-term mechanical unloading of the left ventricle. J Mol Cell Cardiol. 2007;43(3):231–42.
30. Aaronson KD, Pagani FD, Maybaum SW, Feldman DS, Bogaev RC, O'Connell JB, Boyce SW, McGee EW, Sun BC, Goldstein DJ, Frazier OH, Myles JD, Weatherwax KJ, Basobas L, McGowan L, Farrar DJ, Yacoub MH, Birks EJ, Miller LW. Combination therapy with pulsatile left ventricular assist device, heart failure medication and clenbuterol in chronic heart failure: results from HARPS. J Heart Lung Transplant. 2011;30:S8–9. abstract.
31. Patel SR, Saeed O, Murthy S, Bhatia V, Shin JJ, Wang D, et al. Combining neurohormonal blockade with continuous-flow left ventricular assist device support for myocardial recovery: a single-arm prospective study. J Heart Lung Transplant. 2013;32(3):305–12.
32. Mancini DM, Beniaminovitz A, Levin H, Catanese K, Flannery M, Ditullio M, et al. Low incidence of myocardial recovery after left ventricular assist device implantation in patients with chronic heart failure. Circulation. 1998;98(22):2383–9.
33. Farrar DJ, Holman WR, McBride LR, Kormos RL, Icenogle TB, Hendry PJ, et al. Long-term follow-up of Thoratec ventricular assist device bridge-to-recovery patients successfully removed from support after recovery of ventricular function. J Heart Lung Transplant. 2002;21(5):516–21.
34. Wever-Pinzon O, Drakos SG, McKellar SH, Horne BD, Caine WT, Kfoury AG, et al. Cardiac recovery during long-term left ventricular assist device support. J Am Coll Cardiol. 2016;68(14):1540–53.
35. Topkara VK, Garan AR, Fine B, Godier-Furnemont AF, Breskin A, Cagliostro B, et al. Myocardial recovery in patients receiving contemporary left ventricular assist devices: results from the interagency registry for mechanically assisted circulatory support (INTERMACS). Circ Heart Fail. 2016;9(7).
36. Drakos SG, Kfoury AG, Stehlik J, Selzman CH, Reid BB, Terrovitis JV, et al. Bridge to recovery: understanding the disconnect between clinical and biological outcomes. Circulation. 2012;126(2):230–41.
37. Dandel M, Weng Y, Siniawski H, Potapov E, Lehmkuhl HB, Hetzer R. Long-term results in patients with idiopathic dilated cardiomyopathy after weaning from left ventricular assist devices. Circulation. 2005;112(9 Suppl):I37–45.
38. Goldstein DJ, Maybaum S, MacGillivray TE, Moore SA, Bogaev R, Farrar DJ, et al. Young patients with nonischemic cardiomyopathy have higher likelihood of left ventricular recovery during left ventricular assist device support. J Card Fail. 2012;18(5):392–5.
39. Givertz MM, Mann DL. Epidemiology and natural history of recovery of left ventricular function in recent onset dilated cardiomyopathies. Curr Heart Fail Rep. 2013;10(4):321–30.
40. Dandel M, Weng Y, Siniawski H, Potapov E, Drews T, Lehmkuhl HB, et al. Prediction of cardiac stability after weaning from left ventricular assist devices in patients with idiopathic dilated cardiomyopathy. Circulation. 2008;118(14 Suppl):S94–105.
41. Pan S, Aksut B, Wever-Pinzon OE, Rao SD, Levin AP, Garan AR, et al. Incidence and predictors of myocardial recovery on long-

term left ventricular assist device support: results from the united network for organ sharing database. J Heart Lung Transplant. 2015;34(12):1624–9.
42. Basuray A, French B, Ky B, Vorovich E, Olt C, Sweitzer N, et al. Response to letter regarding article, "heart failure with recovered ejection fraction: clinical description, biomarkers, and outcomes". Circulation. 2015;131(6):e344.
43. Krabatsch T, Schweiger M, Dandel M, Stepanenko A, Drews T, Potapov E, et al. Is bridge to recovery more likely with pulsatile left ventricular assist devices than with nonpulsatile-flow systems? Ann Thorac Surg. 2011;91(5):1335–40.
44. Klotz S, Deng MC, Stypmann J, Roetker J, Wilhelm MJ, Hammel D, et al. Left ventricular pressure and volume unloading during pulsatile versus nonpulsatile left ventricular assist device support. Ann Thorac Surg. 2004;77(1):143–9. discussion 9-50
45. Thohan V, Stetson SJ, Nagueh SF, Rivas-Gotz C, Koerner MM, Lafuente JA, et al. Cellular and hemodynamics responses of failing myocardium to continuous flow mechanical circulatory support using the DeBakey-noon left ventricular assist device: a comparative analysis with pulsatile-type devices. J Heart Lung Transplant. 2005;24(5):566–75.
46. Haft J, Armstrong W, Dyke DB, Aaronson KD, Koelling TM, Farrar DJ, et al. Hemodynamic and exercise performance with pulsatile and continuous-flow left ventricular assist devices. Circulation. 2007;116(11 Suppl):I8–15.
47. John R, Boyle A, Pagani F, Miller L. Physiologic and pathologic changes in patients with continuous-flow ventricular assist devices. J Cardiovasc Transl Res. 2009;2(2):154–8.
48. Guan Y, Karkhanis T, Wang S, Rider A, Koenig SC, Slaughter MS, et al. Physiologic benefits of pulsatile perfusion during mechanical circulatory support for the treatment of acute and chronic heart failure in adults. Artif Organs. 2010;34(7):529–36.
49. Kato TS, Chokshi A, Singh P, Khawaja T, Cheema F, Akashi H, et al. Effects of continuous-flow versus pulsatile-flow left ventricular assist devices on myocardial unloading and remodeling. Circ Heart Fail. 2011;4(5):546–53.
50. Jacobs S, Geens J, Rega F, Burkhoff D, Meyns B. Continuous-flow left ventricular assist devices induce left ventricular reverse remodeling. J Heart Lung Transplant. 2013;32(4):466–8.
51. Feldman DS, Moazami N, Adamson PB, Vierecke J, Raval N, et al. The utility of a wireless implantable hemodynamic monitoring system in patients requiring mechanical circulatory support. ASAIO J. 2018;64(3):301–8.
52. Klotz S, Danser AH, Foronjy RF, Oz MC, Wang J, Mancini D, et al. The impact of angiotensin-converting enzyme inhibitor therapy on the extracellular collagen matrix during left ventricular assist device support in patients with end-stage heart failure. J Am Coll Cardiol. 2007;49(11):1166–74.
53. Feldman D, Elton TS, Menachemi DM, Wexler RK. Heart rate control with adrenergic blockade: clinical outcomes in cardiovascular medicine. Vasc Health Risk Manag. 2010;6:387–97.
54. Dandel M, Weng Y, Siniawski H, Potapov E, Krabatsch T, Lehmkuhl HB, et al. Pre-explant stability of unloading-promoted cardiac improvement predicts outcome after weaning from ventricular assist devices. Circulation. 2012;126(11 Suppl 1):S9–19.
55. Maybaum S, Mancini D, Xydas S, Starling RC, Aaronson K, Pagani FD, et al. Cardiac improvement during mechanical circulatory support: a prospective multicenter study of the LVAD working group. Circulation. 2007;115(19):2497–505.
56. Dandel M, Hetzer R. Echocardiographic strain and strain rate imaging--clinical applications. Int J Cardiol. 2009;132(1):11–24.
57. Dandel M, Hetzer R. Myocardial recovery during mechanical circulatory support: weaning and explantation criteria. Heart Lung Vessel. 2015;7(4):280–8.
58. Stainback RF, Estep JD, Agler DA et al. Echocardiography in the management of patients with left ventricular assist devices: recommendations from the American Society of Echocardiography. J Am Soc Echocardiogr. 2015;28(8):853–909. https://doi.org/10.1016/j.echo.2015.05.008.
59. Ando M, Nishimura T, Takewa Y, Ogawa D, Yamazaki K, Kashiwa K, et al. What is the ideal off-test trial for continuous-flow ventricular-assist-device explantation? Intracircuit back-flow analysis in a mock circulation model. J Artif Organs. 2011;14(1):70–3.
60. George RS, Sabharwal NK, Webb C, Yacoub MH, Bowles CT, Hedger M, et al. Echocardiographic assessment of flow across continuous-flow ventricular assist devices at low speeds. J Heart Lung Transplant. 2010;29(11):1245–52.
61. Potapov EV, Schweiger M, Krabatsch T. Percutaneous balloon occlusion of a left ventricular assist device outflow cannula to facilitate evaluation of myocardial recovery. J Heart Lung Transplant. 2011;30(11):1300–1.
62. Vierecke J, Hernanedes-Enriquez M, Dandel M, Muller M, Stawowy P, Dreysse S, et al. Percutaneous balloon occlusion of a left ventricular assist device outflow cannula during right heart catheterization with pumpstop as part of the evaluation of myocardial recovery. J Heart Lung Transplant. 2014;33(4):S156–S.
63. Dandel M, Knosalla C, Hetzer R. Contribution of ventricular assist devices to the recovery of failing hearts: a review and the berlin heart Center experience. Eur J Heart Fail. 2014;16(3):248–63.
64. Phan K, Huo YR, Zhao DF, Yan TD, Tchantchaleishvili V. Ventricular recovery and pump explantation in patients supported by left ventricular assist devices: a systematic review. ASAIO J. 2016;62(3):219–31.
65. Birks EJ, George RS, Firouzi A, Wright G, Bahrami T, Yacoub MH, et al. Long-term outcomes of patients bridged to recovery versus patients bridged to transplantation. J Thorac Cardiovasc Surg. 2012;144(1):190–6.
66. Schweiger M, Potapov E, Vierecke J, Stepanenko A, Hetzer R, Krabatsch T. Expeditious and less traumatic explantation of a heartware LVAD after myocardial recovery. ASAIO J. 58(5):542–4.

Mechanical Circulatory Support Part II; Management of Devices After Implantation, Incl. Complications

27

A. L. Meyer, I. Netuka, and M. S. Slaughter

27.1 RV Function

Post-operative right heart failure after LVAD implantation occurs in 9–20% [1] and is associated with high 30-days mortality [2]. Several options are given to optimize the post-operative right ventricular function. A pulmonary artery catheter is obligate for optimal hemodynamic and volume management. Recommended parameters are CVP < 15 mmHg and PCWP 15–20 mmHg with a mean artery pressure between 70 and 80 mmHg.

A reduction of the pulmonary vascular resistance can be achieved by administration of inhaled nitric oxide, Iloprost (prostaglandine) via inhaled nebulizer after extubation or Sildenfil (phosphodiesterase inhibitor) per oral in addition to adequate ventilation to reduce hypoxia, hypercapnia and acidosis [3].

An optimal speed adjustment is necessary to avoid a septal shift. RV contractility can be enhanced with inotropes. First line are Milrinone and Dobutamin due to only minimal effects to the pulmonary vascular resistance. To optimize right ventricular performance the heart rate should be adapted via CRTD or pacemaker.

In terms of severe right ventricular failure (CI <2.0 l/min/m^2 and CVP >20 mmHg with high dose inotropes and hypotension) the implantation of an RVAD is indispensable [4]. There are center specific strategies. Several temporal right ventricular support systems are approved by the FDA. Veno-arterial extracorporeal membrane oxygenation have the advantage of oxygenation in terms of hypoxia. Impella® (Abiomed, Inc. Danvers, MA, US) or TandemHeart® (Cardiac Assist, Inc., Pittsburgh, US) can be implanted percutaneously. The Thoratec®CentriMag® blood pump needs surgical implantation via pulmonary artery and femoral vein (percutaneous). A long-term approved devices is the pVAD (Thoratec, Pleasanton, US) for bridge to transplant.

27.2 Anticoagulation

Anticoagulation in LVAD patients needs to be individualized for each patient due to the different devices, platelet count, resistance against platelet inhibitors or accumulate bleeding complications. During implantation with the use of a cardiopulmonary bypass the administration of Heparin with an ACT >400 s is necessary with complete reversal of Heparin in the end of the implantation. In common continuous flow LVADs the post-operative anticoagulation starts on the first post-operative day with 10 IU/kg/h to a target PTT of 40–60 s. The heparin dose can be increased after 48 h, Table 27.1. The recommended long term oral anticoagulation regime for the cfLVAD is usually a combination of warfarin with a target INR of 2.0–2.5 and acetylsalicylic acid (ASA). In general, ASA should be started at a dose between 81 and 150 mg/day within 24 h after implant if there are no postoperative bleeding complications. A check for ASA resistance with a reliable tests is recommended. Patients with Aspirin intolerance, clopidogrel at dosis of 75–150 mg/day is a viable alternative [5].

In pulsatile devices like the PVAD (Thoratec®, Pleasanton, US) Heparin should be started after drainage is less than 50 ml/h with a 1.5 fold target PTT. Warfarin should be titrated to maintain an INR of 2.5–3.5 [6]. A higher INR (3.0–3.5) is required from the Excor in combination with Aspirin (75 mg daily) and Dipyridamol (150 mg daily) [7].

A. L. Meyer
University Department for Cardiac Surgery, Leipzig Heart Center, Leipzig, Germany
e-mail: Meyer@medizien.uni-leipzig.de

I. Netuka
Institute for Clinical and Experimental Medicine, Prague, Czech Republic
e-mail: ivne@medicon.cz

M. S. Slaughter (✉)
Department of Cardiovascular and Thoracic Surgery, University of Louisville, Louisville, KY, USA
e-mail: mark.slaughter@louisville.edu

D. S. Feldman, P. Mohacsi (eds.), *Heart Failure*, Cardiovascular Medicine, https://doi.org/10.1007/978-3-319-98184-0_27

Table 27.1 Anticoagulation protocol for HM III device implantation [8]

Timing	Action
Prior leaving the OR	Complete reversal of heparin
After 12–24 h	Begin IV heparin /chest tube drainage is less than 50 ml/h over a 2–3 h period: Initially titrate to a PTT of 45–50 for 24 h (1.2–1.4 times control)
After 24–48 h	IV heparin and titrate to PTT 50–60 (1.4–1.7 times control)
After 48–72 h	IV heparin and titrate to PTT 55–65 (1.5–1.8 times control)
POD 2–3	Initiate Aspirin 81–100 mg QD
POD 3–5	Once there is no evidence of bleeding and the chest tubes have been removed, begin Warfarin (overlapping with heparin). Discontinue heparin after obtaining an acceptable, stable INR. The INR should be maintained in the range of 2.0–3.0
Duration support	Maintain patient throughout support on Aspirin and Warfarin

Protocol for HM 3 CE Mark Trial
INR international normalized ratio, *IV* intravenous, *PTT* partial thromboplastin time

27.2.1 Acquired von Willebrand Syndrome

Please note that patients with a continuous flow LVAD develop an acquired von Willebrand syndrome. The high molecular weight multimers are missing due to shear stress. Therefore these patients have a disorder in the primary hemostasis [9].

27.2.2 Non-Cardiac Surgery

Warfarin and Aspirin should be switched to Heparin for elective non-cardiac surgeries in LVAD patients. Heparin can be paused during the intervention [10]. In emergency cases FFP, coagulation factors or platelet concentrates can be administered [11]. In uncomplex surgeries like tooth extraction the anticoagulation can be continued.

27.2.3 Non-Vitamin K Antagonist Oral Anticoagulants

The anticoagulation with non-vitamin K antagonist oral anticoagulants is not adequately studied. So far only a case series was published about Dabigatran. The rate of thromboembolic events, device thrombosis and major bleeding were similar with Dabigatran or vitamin K antagonist [12].

27.2.4 Anticoagulation in Term of Bleeding

In the US-Trace study was evaluated the safety of reduced anti-thrombotic therapy in patients with a HeartMate II in response to a bleeding event. Patients were treated only with Aspirin (28%), Warfarin (38%) or no antithrombotic agent (34%). Freedom from ischemic stroke at 1- year was 93.8 ± 2.5%, and freedom from device thrombosis was 92.7 ± 2.7%. Bleeding events occurred in 52% [13].

27.3 Timing for Transplant

After LVAD implantation a listing for heart transplantation can be performed after stabilization of the patient. The percentage of patients who were bridged with a mechanical circulatory support (MCS) increased every years. In 2013 almost 50% of the patients with adult heart transplant were bridge with a MCS (LVAD, RVAD, TAH, ECMO) [14].

Interestingly the survival after heart transplantation were similar comparing patients with and without an LVAD or inotropes before transplantation [14].

Reasons for high urgency listing for patients after LVAD implantation are listed in Table 27.2. In patients with a high pulmonary vascular resistance before LVAD implantation a current right heart catheter before listing should be repeated to exclude pulmonary hypertension. In patients with a fixed pulmonary hypertension a reduction of the pulmonary artery pressure was observed after 6 weeks [15].

27.4 Bleeding

Bleeding is a common and severe complication after continuous flow LVAD implantation. The incidence is described between 15 and 30% with an incidence per patient year between 0.27 and 0.45 [16–19]. Re-operation after LVAD implantation due to bleeding is described in 7–31% of the patients [20, 21]. Bleeding complications are defined in the INTERMACS definition as an episode of suspected internal or external bleeding that results in death, re-operation, hospitalization or transfusion of ≥4 U packed red blood cells (PRBC) within any 24 h period during first 7 days post implant or any transfusion of packed red blood cells (PRBC) after 7 days following implant.

Table 27.2 Indications for urgent listing for heart transplantation

Accepted indications for urgent listing for heart transplantation
Systemic LVAD infection
Arrhythmia
Psychological problems
Right heart failure
Intermittent bleeding complications
Intracranial bleeding without neurological limitations
Recurrent pump thrombosis
Non-optimal LVAD positioning with intermittent suction events

27.4.1 Gastrointestinal Bleeding

Especially gastro-intestinal bleeding (GIB) is a recurrent complication in LVAD patients. Patients with the most common assist devices show in around 34% a GIB with a frequency of events per patient year of 0.44 eppy (HM II) and 0.55 eppy (HVAD), respectively.

Most frequently the bleeding is located in the upper gastrointestinal tract 48% (until Treitz band), in 22% in the lower gastrointestinal tract [17]. The source of a GIB is offered in Table 27.3 [16]. Notably, a high percentage is caused by angiodysplasias.

The cause of bleeding is found in approximately 75% of the patients. In case of a suspicious upper GIB the best diagnostic tool is an upper endoscopy, for lower GIB a colonoscopy. If the upper or lower endoscopy is not successful, a capsule endoscopy is a less traumatic method. The diagnostic yield of capsule endoscopy has been superior in the diagnosis of small bowel disease compared to small bowel series, computerized tomography or push enteroscopy. The results of the capsule study may indicate the further need for therapeutic intervention by a double balloon endoscopy [22]. Importantly, patients with a continuous flow LVAD develop an acquired von Willebrand syndrome due to the shear stress of the pump, therefore they show a dysfunction of the primary hemostasis [23]. Additionally, an impaired platelet function was detected in these patients by Klovaite et al. [24]. Furthermore several risk factors were identified to influence the GIB like age and history of GIB [16, 18].

Table 27.3 Lesions identified as source of lower gastrointestinal bleeding in patients after LVAD implantation, modified from Draper et al. [17]

Source	Frequency (%)
Angiodysplasia	29
Gastritis	22
Ulcer	13
Diverticulitis	6
Polyp	5
Colitis	3
Other/Unkown	22

The therapy of a GIB primarily consists of the analysis of blood and coagulation parameter with subsequent correction of anemia and potential excessive anticoagulation. The administration of fresh frozen plasma and coagulation factors is recommended. Due to the chronic antiplatelets therapy, application of platelet concentrates should be considered. Secondly, detection of the source of bleeding with its possible elimination is of a paramount importance. An algorithm for the evaluation and treatment of GIB is provided by Suarez et al., Fig. 27.1 [25]. The anticoagulation should resume with Vitamin K antagonist. A platelet inhibitor may be paused.

The recurrence of a GIB was described in up to 43% of the patients with a GIB. Aggarwal et al. found, that 60% of

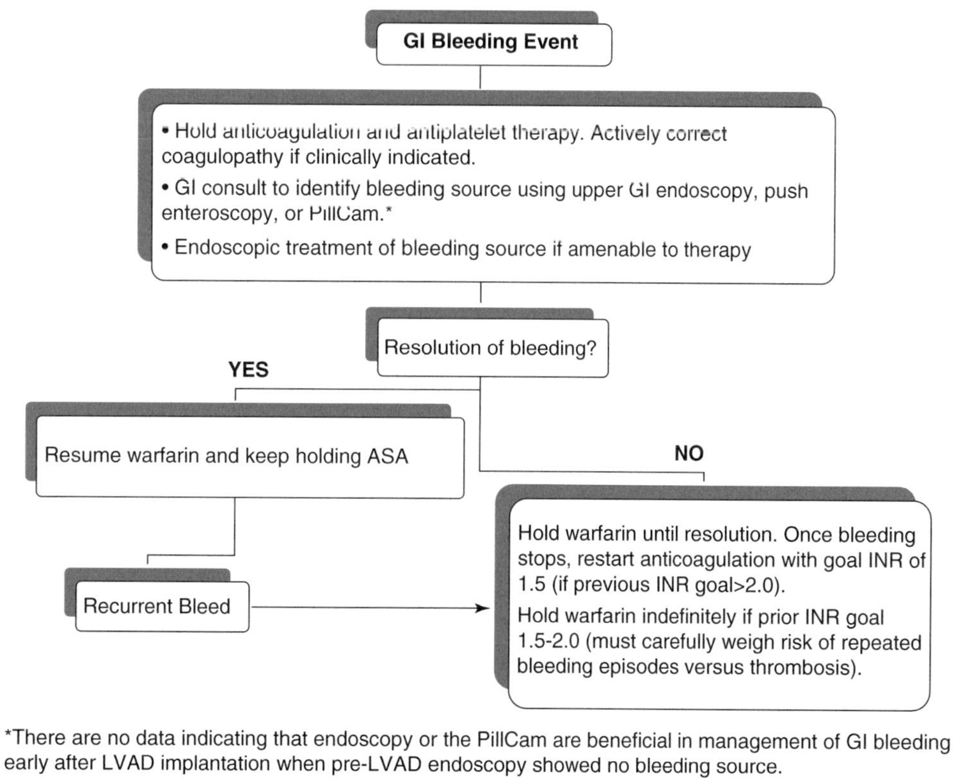

Fig. 27.1 Algorithm for gastrointestinal bleeding in LVAD patients [25]

the patients had a recurrence of the bleeding from the same anatomic site [26].

For medical management Octreotide can be considered as intramuscular (20 mg every 30 days) or subcutaneous (100 µg twice daily) administration [27].

27.5 Renal and Hepatic Considerations

A function of both parenchymatous organs is primarily influenced by a predisposing deleterious hemodynamic and humoral milieu, yet further worsened by a perioperative LVAD implant. However, a close attention must be devoted to discriminate other superimposing factors such as persistent RV failure, which may impair both antegrade flow and also decrease a microcirculation perfusion gradient. A potential impact of a pharmacological toxicity and infection needs to be adjudicated.

27.5.1 Renal Considerations

Given a typically predisposing cardiorenal syndrome and low cardiac output prior to LVAD, there is a common association with postoperative renal dysfunction. The enhanced hemodynamics on LVAD improves organ perfusion and thus renal function overtime [28]. Currently utilized continuous flow LVADs generate less physiologic flow pattern. Notably, despite several experimental signals [29], in most studies the association with adverse effect on kidneys was not revealed [28, 30, 31].

However a significant proportion of patients in an acute phase experience aggravation of a chronic renal insufficiency or an acute onset due to perioperative impetus as an acute kidney injury (AKI) (7–14%) [28, 32] with a need for a renal replacement therapy (RRT). AKI after LVAD placement is associated with a high mortality between 25% and 40% [28, 33], nonetheless it suggests being more a surrogate of an initial critical state rather than a primary trigger.

In an immediate postoperative care, RRT is initiated in a continuous fashion. Using CRRT; once stabilized without a meaningful recovery, a transition to intermittent hemodialysis or peritoneal dialysis typically occurs. There may be several advantages of peritoneal dialysis in a means of rarity of bacteremia associated to a peritoneal catheter likewise logistic burden of an LVAD patient in outpatient hemodialysis regimen. However the clear superiority of one over the other is yet to be determined. Nonetheless, in case of hemodialysis, it appears intuitive to timely transition the patient from a tunneled catheter towards a shunt to minimize the risk of infection.

27.5.2 Hepatic Considerations

Despite an impact of significantly elevated pre-implant total bilirubin on mortality, early and sustained improvement in hepatic function is consistently reported in LVAD patients. Primary adverse effects of hepatic dysfunction on early and late outcomes after continuous flow left ventricular assist are not yet understood in a full complexity.

Also the expansion of LVAD therapy to more specific patient populations, such as restrictive cardiomyopathy or grown up congenital hearts, should bring to a context presumed trajectory of hepatic dysfunction.

Previous study has shown a relationship between the perioperative MELD Score (a Model of End-Stage Liver Disease) and a risk of severe bleeding and deaths after an LVAD implant. This underscores of proactive postoperative bleeding management in the patients with underlying liver dysfunction.

27.6 Stroke

Cerebral ischemic stroke and hemorrhage are with an annual incidence exceeding 6% among the principal sources of morbidity and mortality in LVAD patients. Due to a prothrombotic nature of a device surface - blood interface, an appropriate guidelened/IFU based anticoagulation and anti-platelet therapy (see **Anticoagulation management**) remains a paramount in the prevention. Unless these complications are substantially eliminated by new technologies and enhanced therapeutical strategies, acceptance of LVADs to higher INTERMACS profiles will remain limited since a disabling stroke is one key obstacles to a meaningful survival benefit.

27.6.1 Ischemic Stroke

Systemic infection represents the most consistent risk factor, both by clear association with a device thrombosis and a potential of cerebral embolization [34]. A previous stroke and also mean arterial pressure >90 mmHg exhibit strong association with the event [35, 36]. Besides primary neurological deficit, an ischemic stroke may lead to a hemorrhagic cerebral transformation representing one of the most ominous complications with high rates of brain edema and stem herniation.

27.6.2 Hemorrhagic Stroke

Cerebral hemorrhage in LVAD patients should always rise a suspiciency of a mycotic aneurysm or septic arteritis. Other systemic causes as hypertension and excessive anticoagulation may play a role. These factors may also contribute to a spontaneous subarachnoid aneurysm rupture [37].

27.6.3 Clinical Evaluation and Imaging

The evaluation consists of a neurological assessment, importantly including determination of the duration of symptoms to quantify a therapeutic window for a vascular intervention and head CT scan (a combination of non-contrast CT and CT scan angiography). Standardized neurological examination scales of a deficit and level of consciousness (National Institutes of Health Stroke Scale; Glasgow Coma Scale) are instrumental to minimize a subjective bias. Due to the association of both events with infection, detailed screening including blood cultures should be mandatory.

27.6.4 Therapy

27.6.4.1 Ischemic Stroke

If clinically significant stroke is diagnosed within therapeutical window, timely reperfusion strategy should be utilized. In LVAD patients, systemic and to certain extent even selective intra-arterial thrombolysis are not recommended due to a high risk of hemorrhagic transformation in territorial infarctions due to likelihood of septic origin in a underlying setting of combined anticoagulation/anti-platelet therapy and acquired von Willebrand syndrome [38]. Mechanical desobliteration tends to be a preferred option to leverage on efficacy and minimizing of the risk of complications.

27.6.4.2 Hemorrhagic Stroke

The therapy is based on a control of blood pressure, and reversal of anticoagulation. The mean systemic blood pressure should be maintained <90 mm Hg [39]. The degree and speed of anticoagulation normalizing still remain contentious. Current guidelines of the American Stroke Association on reversing of vitamin K antagonists recommend fresh frozen plasma (FFP) or prothrombin complex concentrates without a specific INR target [40]. The latter should be preferred in LVAD patients based on less volume expansion, controlled dosage and avoidance of immunosensitization. A correction to the INR < 1.5 is reasonable. Recent report also recommend a use of platelet concentrates and desmopressin infusion [41]. A presumed potential risk of the pump thrombosis should be monitored by periodical lab evaluation of biomarkers of hemolysis.

In both strokes etiologies, a consult of a neurosurgeon should be obtained for a highly individualized assessment of decompressive hemicraniectomy benefit.

27.6.5 Resumption of Anticoagulation and Eligibility for Surgical Procedures

In ischemic strokes, the anticoagulation/antiplatelet therapy should not be discontinued without an evidence of the hemorrhagic transformation. Despite an absence of clear guidance on resuming a blood thinning therapy, it is desirable to defer it for a reasonable period while not compromising the pump operation. The same applies for full heparinization procedures such as a heart transplant to avoid secondary cerebral bleed. Timing should be subject to highly individualized multidisciplinary team decision given individual patient characteristics.

27.7 Hemolysis

Hemolysis is a known surrogate of LVADs attributed to a shear stress exerted on circulating red blood cells (RBCs). Contemporaneous durable assist devices exhibit very low levels of ambient hemolysis within standard pump setting. Recent reports suggest lower rates of hemolysis in favor of centrifugal compared to axial flow continuous flow LVADs [42–44].

Clinicaly significant hemolysis in LVAD patients manifests as hemoglobinuria and a drop in hemoglobin level. However, biomarkers of hemolysis, namely serum free hemoglobin (sfHg) and lactatse dehydrogenase (LDH) have been identified as sensitive harbingers of a pump thrombosis. Given their elevation, other standard causes have to be ruled out. Assessment of an aortic regurgitation is mandatory as it may inflict significant hemolysis [45]. Notably, as LVADs may contribute to increased oxidative stress, recent study has identified an association between glucose-6-phosphate dehydrogenase (G6PD) deficiency and increased hemolysis with. In the relative absence of NADPH in red blood cells, these may be subject to substantial injury by reactive oxygen species, which cannot be appropriately scavenged [46].

Based on the INTERMACS hemolysis definition [47] with a threshold of 40 mg/dl sfHg with signs of hemolysis, the registry analysis revealed freedom from hemolysis of 97% at 3 months, 94% at 1 year and 91% at 2 years. Mean time from implant to first hemolysis event was 7.4 months resulted in significantly higher incidence of thrombotic device malfunction, device exchange and mortality were all after hemolysis, with the greatest risk for each occurring within 6 months [48].

Numerous studies sought to determine discriminative association with other markers of hemolysis such as lactate dehydrogenase (LDH) with a proposed cut off 600 IU/liter (2.5-times the upper limit normal value). Indeed, several studies support the observation that LDH may provide an earlier diagnosis of adverse events compared to current INTERMACS definition of hemolysis [49, 50]. That said, both sfHg and serum LDH should be periodically monitored and an upstream trends closely followed with echocardiography and clinical diagnostics to proceed to timely treatment of the pump thrombosis.

27.8 Device Change-Out

Despite improvements in a technical reliability of a single moving part continuous flow devices compared to previous generation devices, there is an increasing era dependent trend in an occurrence of the pump exchange [51]. Importantly, significant decrement in survival is still reported in the INTERMACS for each additional pump exchange [52], despite controlled retrospective series of 57 pump exchange reported low early mortality of 3.5% [53].

Currently, out of three major causes of replacement, an indication due to hemolysis/pump thrombosis became the most frequent one followed by mechanical failure and infection. Despite satisfactory safety profile of the exchange, in a setting of pump thrombosis, the recurrence rate remains high at 31% [54].

Besides original full sternotomy device exchange, limited subcostal or anterolateral thoracotomy approach gained in popularity overtime. The procedure is then performed on a cardiopulmonary bypass inserted from a groin [55]. The strategy allows for sparing the outflow graft in place, likewise the inflow cannula segment in devices requiring a pump pocket [56]. In such techniques, a caution is required to verify that the primary issue of the failure is confined to a center piece segment of the pump only.

Based on a growing technical experience and thus popularity of a less invasive pump exchange, currently published data demonstrated far superior outcomes with the device exchange over watchful observation in patients with significant thrombosis related hemolysis [57].

An infection may urge for a preference of full device reimplantation, however the device removal, and if necessary a temporary support on ECMO, should be considered.

Since reasons for pump failure may be device specific, an exchange to alternative circulatory support system can be safely performed from limited access approach [58].

27.9 Device Malfunction

Based on the INTERMACS definition, device malfunction denotes a failure of one or more of the components of the cardiac assist device system which either directly causes or could potentially induce a state of inadequate circulatory support (low cardiac output state) or death (Table 27.4) [59]. These are not confined only to a mechanical failure, however include also software failures which typically equate to a controller malfunction.

Table 27.4 Device failure classification based on affected components

Device malfunction	Affected components
Pump failure	Blood contacting components of pump or a motor or other pump actuating mechanism that is housed with the blood contacting components The special situation of pump thrombosis, thrombus is documented to be present within the device or its conduits that result in or could potentially induce circulatory failure
Non-pump failure	External pneumatic drive unit Electric power supply unit Batteries Controller Interconnecting cable

A systematic review of retrospective observational studies has demonstrated a weighted incidence of device failure of 3.9% (range, 1–11.3%). The pump thrombosis was the most common cause of device failure (50.5%), followed by lead or cable damage (21.7%) and a mechanical pump failure (11.6). Long-term device failure rate at 24-months post-implantation was 6.5% [60].

The emergence of continuous flow LVADs posited the elimination of pulsatile device components deterioration such as biological valves or a bearing wear. Indeed, mechanical failure of pump components has dramatically decreased in recent years [61] however these have been replaced by substantially increased rates of thrombosis in newer generation devices [62–64]. These observations have been reflected in refinements of a patient-device interface management, technological improvements as well as a development of the next generation devices to allow for a broader expansion towards permanent therapy.

Late fractures of the driveline were reported as a significant cause of a device specific exchange, however a modification of HeartMate II cable significantly reduced incidence of serious device malfunctions [65].

Peripherals failure may be largely mitigated by a permanent presence of a back-up set with a patient to allow for urgent exchange. Dedicated techniques may facilitate a repair of external driveline cracks [66].

A significant caveat of a malfunction of continuous flow device represents a valveless design which incurs a retrograde flow through the outflow graft. This condition may substantially compromise a residual forward flow of the heart. Advisable solution may be emergency transfer to a local catheterization lab for immediate occlusion of the outflow graft with a device and then only transporting for a definitive procedure to a VAD center [67]. As subsequent device exchange in an emergent setting represents incremental risk factor [68], a circulatory and organ stabilization with an ECMO may represent a reasonable approach.

27.10 Infection

Major infection represents consistently one of key causes of both morbidity and mortality on LVAD [68]. Likewise, accounts for a third most frequent cause for readmission [69, 70]. Recent technological advancements towards CF-LVADs demonstrated a consistent decrease of infection complications [71], in a randomized trial the incidence was almost halved compared to pulsatile-flow LVAD [72]. However, multiple reports illustrate that implant era also importantly drives the association and thus may suggest a progress in indication and comprehensive treatment [73, 74].

Currently exist two generally recognized classifications of LVAD associated infection; INTERMACS criteria reported elsewhere [75] and more recent standardized consensus definition by ISHLT (Table 27.5) [76]. Subsequently, multicenter outcomes analysis strictly adherent to ISHLT formula yet emerge [77]. Notably, VAD infection, if actively treated and controlled, does not preclude heart transplantation and nor affect short and long term survival post transplant [78].

27.11 VAD-Specific Infections

VAD-specific infections represent particular therapeutical challenge due to a proclivity to form microbial biofilms on prosthetic surfaces limiting a probability of germs elimination by pharmacotherapy alone. To avoid contamination of the implantable hardware, all known sources should be eliminated prior to the implant followed by perioperative antibiotic prophylaxis.

27.11.1 Pump and Cannulas Infection

27.11.1.1 Perioperative Considerations and Prevention

Strict adherence to the basic principles of pre-, perioperative infection control guidelines [79] is of a paramount to minimize a risk of internal pump components surfaces. Active systemic infection should be resolved prior implant. The implant is recommended to postpone for patients with localized infections that can be effectively treated, if clinically feasible.

Table 27.5 ISHLT Infection working formula

Category of infection	Working formula
VAD-specific	related to device hardware which do not occur in non-VAD patients /pump and cannulas; pocket infections and driveline infections/
VAD-related	also occurring in patients without VAD, however may inflict unique considerations /infective endocarditis, bloodstream infection and mediastinitis/
non-VAD infections	occur within a general population

Always exercise caution in patients who are at increased risk of developing infection, such as patients with established or suspected infections, prolonged intubation, cutaneous lesions at surgical sites, or other co-morbidities, including multisystem organ dysfunction, immunosuppression, poorly controlled diabetes, renal failure, or malnutrition.

27.11.1.2 Complications Management

These are typically difficult to diagnose conclusively, the algorithm [76] stems in part from modified Duke's criteria [80]. Even despite negative TEE findings, these should be still considered in case of bloodstream infection persistent despite adequate antimicrobial therapy or in case of bloodstream infection relapse after a course of antibiotics.

Aggressive systemic targeted antibiotic therapy should last a minimum of 4 weeks, guided upon a blood stream infection and endocarditis recommendations [81, 82]. Device explant or/and exchange should be considered as an ultimate solution in gravely refractory course only. Transplant list prioritization may be also considered.

27.11.2 Pump Pocket Infection

27.11.2.1 Perioperative Considerations and Prevention

Strict asepsis, meticulous hemostasis and physiological operating technique are a paradigm to avoid pump pocket infection. In devices requiring pump pocket, this should be appropriately measured to avoid additional interspace for hematoma formation as well as along side connecting cannulas. For a drainage of fluid and blood, an appropriate chest tubes number and positioning. Eventually, deliberate pleural space opening and tube placement may be reasonable. To maintain patency, a use of active clearance drains is advisable. Rinsing of the operating field prior to the closure is probably recommended. Based on report demonstrating equal composite infection end-point compared to primary closure cohort [83], planned delayed sternal closure in case of serious coagulopathy to avoid hematomas around the pump may be reasonable.

27.11.2.2 Complications Diagnosis and Management

Pump pocket infection assessment is typically based on elevated inflammatory markers, echocardiogram, CT scan and labeled white blood cell scintigraphy. Pump exploration is performed through left subcostal or intercostal approach with debridment and abscess fluid drainage. Systemic targeted parenteral antibiotics and continuous irrigation or vacuum assisted drainage are indicated [84]. Once stabilized, with negative local cultures as well as blood stream infection, direct surgical closure or a use of muscle and omental flap [85] can be recommended.

Progression of local and systemic response despite adequate suppressive antibiotic and topical treatment may urge pump explantation (in case of functional recovery only) or complete pump exchange. Usefulness of provisional ECMO support to allow for aggressive antibiotic therapy prior to reimplantation is not well established. Even after pump exchange suppressive therapy is indicated to be continued as it is placed in presumably infection seeded ambience.

27.11.3 Percutaneous Driveline Infection

27.11.3.1 Perioperative Considerations and Prevention

Despite encouraging decrease of recently reported driveline infection event rates [86, 87], the complication remains a serious cause of morbidity and rehospitalization [69, 70]. Moreover, INTERMACS registry analysis revealed significantly better survival in patients on continuous flow VADs who did not develop this complication [88].

Contemporaneous drivelines consist of velour and silicon portion. Velour skin interface provides excellent tissue adhesion, however even a minor trauma poses irreversible disruption to the surrounding skin. By contrast, silicone skin interface (SSI) forms a sinus less susceptible to minor trauma. Moreover, low porosity silicon may prevent bacterial seeding. Multiple series have proven significant reduction of the driveline infection by using SSI externalization technique [89, 90].

Recently, a double tunnel technique as compared to conventional straight tunneling received attention. It provides virtually an extension of the exit site - pump distance. Tunneling of the driveline into the fascia of the musculus rectus abdominis results in a longer intrafascial run provides a better resistance against ascending infections. Further, this approach is supposed to eliminate inward pulling of the exit site by better distribution of tension forces once patient puts on weight. The results are encouraging however remain less plausible due to relatively small series [91, 92].

Minimizing of the exit site trauma represents a cornerstone of the driveline infection prevention. There is growing evidence that disposable anchoring device in combination with standardized dressing technique by a use of customized kits may further reduce this complication [93, 94].

Previous findings, also known as an obesity paradox, showed that obesity had no deleterious effect on overall VAD therapy outcome. Albeit, data suggest that obesity or continued weight gain over VAD support may increase a risk of driveline infection, thereby increased measures in prevention and treatment may be warranted in this subgroup [95].

27.11.3.2 Complications Management

Continuous patients education, training, showering instructing remains indispensible for the success of early stages driveline infection. Likewise, improved driveline stabilization plays a fundamental role.

Positive cultures should be subject to thoughtful evaluation due to frequent skin colonizers. Local progression characterized by a copious amount of drainage and tenderness may require hospitalization for parenteral antibiotics therapy based on the bacterial culture. Patients with blood stream infection, proven fungus or Gram-negative infection requires particularly aggressive antimicrobial treatment.

When exit site infection deteriorates towards fascia, surgical discision and debridement should be considered. Evaluation by ultrasonography, CT scan, and gallium scintigraphy is useful to verify the ascent of infection along the driveline. Depending on the extent of infection, the tunnel may need to be opened and treated with redressing and drained. Vacuum-assisted closure therapy by providing continuous drainage with germs and debris elimination is recommended. Once stabilized, the driveline may be a subject to contralateral transposition.

In patients with driveline infection caused by intractable multi-drug resistant pathogens, the pump exchange is probably recommended before pump pocket may get infected.

References

1. Strueber M, Larbalestier R, Jansz P, Zimpfer D, Fiane AE, Tsui S, Simon A, Schmitto JD, Khaghani A, Wieselthaler GM, et al. Results of the post-market registry to evaluate the HeartWare left ventricular assist system (ReVOLVE). J Heart Lung Transplant. 2014;33(5):486–91.
2. Kormos RL, Teuteberg JJ, Pagani FD, Russell SD, John R, Miller LW, Massey T, Milano CA, Moazami N, Sundareswaran KS, Farrar DJ. Right ventricular failure in patients with the HeartMate II continuous-flow left ventricular assist device: incidence, risk factors, and effect on outcomes. J Thorac Cardiovasc Surg. 2010;139(5):1316–24.
3. Tedford RJ, Hemnes AR, Russell SD, Wittstein IS, Mahmud M, Zaiman AL, Mathai SC, Thiemann DR, Hassoun PM, Girgis RE, et al. PDE5A inhibitor treatment of persistent pulmonary hypertension after mechanical circulatory support. Circ Heart Fail. 2008;1(4):213–9.
4. Patlolla B, Beygui R, Haddad F. Right-ventricular failure following left ventricle assist device implantation. Curr Opin Cardiol. 2013;28(2):223–33.
5. http://www.heartware.com/products-technology/patient-management
6. https://www.thoratec.com/_assets/download-tracker/15579_A.pdf
7. https://www.berlinheart.de/UserFiles/downloaddokumente/Medical_Professionals_Distributoren/Non_US/EXCOR_Parakorporales_Herzunterstuetzungssystem/Gebrauchsanweisungen/EXCOR_VAD_Ikus_Antrieb_Ikus_Rev_2_1_Software_3_40/Gebrau3.40AMRev80en.pdf
8. CE trial HM 3 anticoagulation study protocol.
9. Meyer AL, Malehsa D, Budde U, Bara C, Haverich A, Strueber M. Acquired von Willebrand syndrome in patients with a centrifugal or axial continuous flow left ventricular assist device. JACC Heart Fail. 2014;2(2):141–5.

10. Morgan JA, Paone G, Nemeh HW, Henry SE, Gerlach B, Williams CT, Lanfear DE, Tita C, Brewer RJ. Non-cardiac surgery in patients on long-term left ventricular assist device support. J Heart Lung Transplant. 2012;31(7):757–63.
11. Feldman D, Pamboukian SV, Teuteberg JJ, Birks E, Lietz K, Moore SA, Morgan JA, Arabia F, Bauman ME, Buchholz HW, et al. The 2013 International Society for Heart and Lung Transplantation guidelines for mechanical circulatory support: executive summary. J Heart Lung Tranplant. 2013;32(2):157–87.
12. Terrovitis JV, Ntalianis A, Kapelios CJ, Vakrou S, Diakos N, Katsaros L, Tsamatsoulis M, Kaldara E, Charitos C, Nanas JN. Dabigatran etexilate as second-line therapy in patients with a left ventricular assist device. Hell J Cardiol. 2015;56(1):20–5.
13. Katz JN, Adamson RM, John R, Tatooles A, Sundareswaran K, Kallel F, Farrar DJ, Jorde UP. Safety of reduced anti-thrombotic strategies in HeartMate II patients: a one-year analysis of the US-TRACE study. J Heart Lung Transplant. 2015;34(12):1542–8.
14. https://www.ishlt.org/registries/slides.asp?slides=heartLungRegis try
15. Riebandt J, Haberl T, Mahr S, Laufer G, Rajek A, Steinlechner B, Schima H, Zimpfer D. Preoperative patient optimization using extracorporeal life support improves outcomes of INTERMACS Level I patients receiving a permanent ventricular assist device. Eur J Cardiothorac Surg. 2014;46(3):486–92. discussion 492
16. Goldstein DJ, Aaronson KD, Tatooles AJ, Silvestry SC, Jeevanandam V, Gordon R, Hathaway DR, Najarian KB, Slaughter MS. Gastrointestinal bleeding in recipients of the HeartWare ventricular assist system. JACC Heart Fail. 2015;3(4):303–13.
17. Draper KV, Huang RJ, Gerson LB. GI bleeding in patients with continuous-flow left ventricular assist devices: a systematic review and meta-analysis. Gastrointest Endosc. 2014;80(3):435–46. e431
18. Wever-Pinzon O, Selzman CH, Drakos SG, Saidi A, Stoddard GJ, Gilbert EM, Labedi M, Reid BB, Davis ES, Kfoury AG, et al. Pulsatility and the risk of nonsurgical bleeding in patients supported with the continuous-flow left ventricular assist device HeartMate II. Circ Heart Fail. 2013;6(3):517–26.
19. Boyle AJ, Jorde UP, Sun B, Park SJ, Milano CA, Frazier OH, Sundareswaran KS, Farrar DJ, Russell SD. Pre-operative risk factors of bleeding and stroke during left ventricular assist device support: an analysis of more than 900 HeartMate II outpatients. J Am Coll Cardiol. 2014;63(9):880–8.
20. John R, Naka Y, Smedira NG, Starling R, Jorde U, Eckman P, Farrar DJ, Pagani FD. Continuous flow left ventricular assist device outcomes in commercial use compared with the prior clinical trial. Ann Thorac Surg. 2011;92(4):1406–13. discussion 1413
21. Miller LW, Pagani FD, Russell SD, John R, Boyle AJ, Aaronson KD, Conte JV, Naka Y, Mancini D, Delgado RM, et al. Use of a continuous-flow device in patients awaiting heart transplantation. N Engl J Med. 2007;357(9):885–96.
22. Adler SN, Bjarnason I, Metzger YC. New balloon-guided technique for deep small-intestine endoscopy using standard endoscopes. Endoscopy. 2008;40(6):502–5.
23. Meyer AL, Malehsa D, Budde U, Bara C, Haverich A, Strueber M. Acquired von Willebrand syndrome in patients with a centrifugal or axial continuous flow left ventricular assist device. JACC Heart Fail. 2014;2(2):141–5.
24. Klovaite J, Gustafsson F, Mortensen SA, Sander K, Nielsen LB. Severely impaired von Willebrand factor-dependent platelet aggregation in patients with a continuous-flow left ventricular assist device (HeartMate II). J Am Coll Cardiol. 2009;53(23):2162–7.
25. Suarez J, Patel CB, Felker GM, Becker R, Hernandez AF, Rogers JG. Mechanisms of bleeding and approach to patients with axial-flow left ventricular assist devices. Circ Heart Fail. 2011;4(6): 779–84.
26. Aggarwal A, Pant R, Kumar S, Sharma P, Gallagher C, Tatooles AJ, Pappas PS, Bhat G. Incidence and management of gastrointestinal bleeding with continuous flow assist devices. Ann Thorac Surg. 2012;93(5):1534–40.
27. Loyada-Rendon RY, Hashim T, Tallaj JA, Acharya D, Holman W, Kirklin J, Pamboukian SV. Octreotide in the management of recurrent gastrointestinal bleed in patients supported by continuous flow left ventricular assist devices. ASAIO J. 2015;61(1):107–9.
28. Hasin T, Topilsky Y, Schirger JA, Li Z, Zhao Y, Boilson BA, Clavell AL, Rodeheffer RJ, Frantz RP, Edwards BS, Pereira NL, Joyce L, Daly R, Park SJ, Kushwaha SS. Changes in renal function after implantation of continuous-flow left ventricular assist devices. J Am Coll Cardiol. 2012;59:26–36.
29. Ootaki C, Yamashita M, Ootaki Y, Kamohara K, Weber S, Klatte RS, Smith WA, Massiello AL, Emancipator SN, Golding LAR, Fukamachi KA. Reduced pulsatility induces periarteritis in kidney: role of the local renin-angiotensin system. J Thorac Cardiovasc Surg. 2008;136:150–8.
30. Slaughter MS, Rogers JG, Milano CA, Russell SD, Conte JV, Feldman D, Sun B, Tatooles AJ, Delgado RM 3rd, Long JW, Wozniak TC, Ghumman W, Farrar DJ, Frazier OH. HeartMate II investigators: advanced heart failure treated with continuous-flowleft ventricular assist device. N Engl J Med. 2009;361:2241–51.
31. Russell SD, Rogers JG, Milano CA, Dyke DB, Pagani FD, Aranda JM, Klodell CT Jr, Boyle AJ, John R, Chen L, Massey HT, Farrar DJ, Conte JV. HeartMate II clinical investigators: renal and hepatic function improve in advanced heart failure patients during continuous-flow support with the HeartMate II left ventricular assist device. Circulation. 2009;120:2352–7.
32. Yoshioka D, Sakaguchi T, Saito S, Miyagawa S, Nishi H, Yoshikawa Y, Fukushima S, Saito T, Daimon T, Ueno T, Kuratani T, Sawa Y. Predictor of early mortality for severe heart failure patients with left ventricular assist device implantation: significance of INTERMACS level and renal function. Circ J. 2012;76:1631–8.
33. Demirozu ZT, Etheridge WB, Radovancevic R, Frazier OH. Results of HeartMate II left ventricular assist device implantation on renal function in patients requiring post-implant renal replacement therapy. J Heart Lung Transplant. 2011;30:182–7.
34. Backes D, van den Bergh WM, van Duijn AL, et al. Cerebrovascular complications of left ventricular assist devices. Eur J Cardiothorac Surg. 2012;42:612–20.
35. Kato TS, Schulze PC, Yang J, et al. Pre-operative and post-operative risk factors associated with neurologic complications in patients with advanced heart failure supported by a left ventricular assist device. J Heart Lung Transplant. 2012;31:1–8.
36. Najjar SS, Slaughter MS, Pagani FD, et al. An analysis of pump thrombosis events in patients in the HeartWare ADVANCE bridge to transplant and continued access protocol. J Heart Lung Transplant. 2014;33:23–34.
37. Qureshi AI, Mendelow AD, Hanley DF. Intracerebral haemorrhage. Lancet. 2009;373:1632–44.
38. Willey JZ, Demmer RT, Takayama H, Colombo PC, Lazar RM. Cerebrovascular disease in the era of left ventricular assist devices with continuous flow: risk factors, diagnosis, and treatment. J Heart Lung Transplant. 2014;33(9):878–87.
39. Lampert BC, Eckert C, Weaver S, et al. Blood pressure control in continuous flow left ventricular assist devices: efficacy and impact on adverse events. Ann Thorac Surg. 2014;97:139–46.
40. Morgenstern LB, Hemphill JC 3rd, Anderson C, et al. Guidelines for the management of spontaneous intracerebral hemorrhage: a guideline for healthcare professionals from the American Heart Association/ American Stroke Association. Stroke. 2010;41:2108–29.
41. Willey JZ, Gavalas MV, Trinh PN, Yuzefpolskaya M, Reshad Garan A, Levin AP, Takeda K, Takayama H, Fried J, Naka Y, Topkara VK, Colombo PC. Outcomes after stroke complicating left ventricular assist device. J Heart Lung Transplant. 2016.; pii:S1053–2498(16)30067–5

42. Shah P, Mehta VM, Cowger JA, Aaronson KD, Pagani FD. Diagnosis of hemolysis and device thrombosis with lactate dehydrogenase during left ventricular assist device support. J Heart Lung Transplant. 2014;33:102–4.
43. Birschmann I, Dittrich M, Eller T, Wiegmann B, Reininger AJ, Budde U, Strüber M. Ambient hemolysis and activation of coagulation is different between HeartMate II and HeartWare left ventricular assist devices. J Heart Lung Transplant. 2014;33(1):80–7.
44. Netuka I, Sood P, Pya Y, Zimpfer D, Krabatsch T, Garbade J, Rao V, Morshuis M, Marasco S, Beyersdorf F, Damme L, Schmitto JD. Fully magnetically levitated left ventricular assist system for treating advanced HF: a multicenter study. J Am Coll Cardiol. 2015;66(23):2579–89.
45. Gopalan RS, Arabia FA, Noel P, Chandrasekaran K. Hemolysis from aortic regurgitation mimicking pump thrombosis in a patient with a HeartMate II left ventricular assist device: a case report. ASAIO J. 2012;58(3):278–80.
46. Alhosaini H, Jensen BC, Chang PP, Sheridan BC, Katz JN. A novel link between G6PD deficiency and hemolysis in patients with continuous-flow left ventricular assist devices. J Heart Lung Transplant. 2014;33(1):116–7.
47. Interagency Registry for Mechanically Assisted Circulatory Support, National Heart Lung and Blood Institute.Adverse event definitions. Contract Award HHSN268201100025C. Available at: http://www.uab.edu/medicine/intermacs/manual-of-operations/manual-of-operations-dropdown3/appendix-a-adverse-event definitions. Accessed 12 Dec 2013.
48. Katz JN, Jensen BC, Chang PP, Myers SL, Pagani FD, Kirklin JK. A multicenter analysis of clinical hemolysis in patients supported with durable, long-term left ventricular assist device therapy. J Heart Lung Transplant. 2015;34(5):701–9.
49. Shah P, Mehta VM, Cowger JA, Haft JW, Romano MA, Aaronson KD, Pagani FD. Lactate dehydrogenase is superior to serum free hemoglobin as a marker of pump thrombosis in left ventricular assist devices. J Heart Lung Transplant. 2013;32:S37.
50. Cowger JA, Romano MA, Shah P, Shah N, Mehta V, Haft JW, Aaronson KD, Pagani FD. Hemolysis: a harbinger of adverse outcome after left ventricular assist device implant. J Heart Lung Transplant. 2014;33:35–43.
51. McCarthy FH, Kobrin D, Rame JE, Groeneveld PW, McDermott KM, Atluri P, Acker MA, Desai ND. Increasing frequency of left ventricular assist device exchanges in the United States. Ann Thorac Surg. 2015;100(5):1660–4. discussion 1665
52. Kirklin JK, Naftel DC, Pagani FD, Kormos RL, Stevenson LW, Blume ED, Myers SL, Miller MA, Baldwin JT, Young JB. Seventh INTERMACS annual report: 15,000 patient sand counting. J Heart Lung Transplant. 2015;34(12):1495-1504. Ota T, Yerebakan H, Akashi H, Takayama H, Uriel N, Colombo PC, Jorde UP, Naka Y. Continuous-flow left ventricular assist device ex- change: clinical outcomes. J Heart Lung Transplant 2014;33: 65–70.
53. Stulak JM, Cowger J, Haft JW, Romano MA, Aaronson KD, Pagani FD. Device exchange after primary left ventricular assist device implanta- tion: indications and outcomes. Ann Thorac Surg. 2013;95:1262–7. discussion 1267
54. Levin AP, Uriel N, Takayama H, Mody KP, Ota T, Yuzefpolskaya M, Colombo PC, Garan AR, Dionizovik-Dimanovski M, Sladen RN, Naka Y, Jorde UP. Device exchange in HeartMate II recipients: long-term out- comes and risk of thrombosis recurrence. ASAIO J. 2015;61:144–9.
55. Soleimani B, Stephenson ER, Price LC, El-Banayosy A, Pae WE. Clinical experience with sternotomy versus subcostal approach for exchange of HeartMate II left ventricular assist device. Ann Thorac Surg. 2015;100(5):1577–80.
56. Ota T, Yerebakan H, Akashi H, Takayama H, Uriel N, Colombo PC, Jorde UP, Naka Y. Continuous-flow left ventricular assist device exchange: clinical outcomes. J Heart Lung Transplant. 2014;33(1):65–70.7.
57. Levin AP, Saeed O, Willey JZ, Levin CJ, Fried JA, Patel SR, Sims DB, Nguyen JD, Shin JJ, Topkara VK, Colombo PC, Goldstein DJ, Naka Y, Takayama H, Uriel N, Jorde UP. Watchful waiting in continuous-flow left ventricular assist device patients with ongoing hemolysis is associated with an increased risk for cerebrovascular accident or death. Circ Heart Fail. 2016;9(5). pii: e002896
58. Hanke JS, Haverich A, Schmitto JD. Exchange of a HeartMate II left ventricular assist device with a HeartMate 3 pump. J Heart Lung Transplant. 2016. pii: S1053–2498(16)30066–3.
59. http://www.uab.edu/medicine/intermacs/appendices-4-0/appendix-a-4-0
60. Xie A, Phan K, Yan TD. Durability of continuous-flow left ventricular assist devices: a systematic review. Ann Cardiothorac Surg. 2014;3(6):547–56.
61. Slaughter MS, Rogers JG, Milano CA, et al. Advanced heart failure treated with continuous-flow left ventricular assist device. N Engl J Med. 2009;361:2241–51.
62. Starling RC, Moazami N, Silvestry SC, et al. Unexpected abrupt increase in left ventricular assist device thrombosis. N Engl J Med. 2014;370:33–40.
63. Najjar SS, Slaughter MS, Pagani FD, et al. An analysis of pump thrombosis events in patients in the HeartWare ADVANCE bridge to transplant and continued access protocol. J Heart Lung Transplant. 2014;33:23–34.
64. Mehra MR, Stewart GC, Uber PA. The vexing problem of thrombosis in long-term mechanical circulatory support. J Heart Lung Transplant. 2014;33:1–11.
65. Soltani S, Kaufmann F, Vierecke J, Kretzschmar A, Hennig E, Stein J, Hetzer R, Krabatsch T, Potapov EV. Design changes in continuous-flow left ventricular assist devices and life-threatening pump malfunctions. Eur J Cardiothorac Surg. 2015;47(6):984–9.
66. Schima H, Stoiber M, Schlöglhofer T, Hartner Z, Haberl T, Zimpfer D. Repair of left ventricular assist device driveline damage directly at the transcutaneous exit site. Artif Organs. 2014;38(5):422–5.
67. Chrysant GS, Horstmanshof DA, Snyder T, Chaffin JS, Elkins CC, Kanaly PJ, Long JW. Successful percutaneous management of acute left ventricular assist device stoppage. ASAIO J. 2010;56(5):483–5.
68. Kirklin JK, Naftel DC, Pagani FD, Kormos RL, Stevenson LW, Blume ED, Myers SL, Miller MA, Baldwin JT, Young JB. Seventh INTERMACS annual report: 15,000 patients and counting. J Heart Lung Transplant. 2015;34(12):1495–504.
69. Hasin T, Marmor Y, Kremers W, Topilsky Y, Severson CJ, Schirger JA, Boilson BA, Clavell AL, Rodeheffer RJ, Frantz RP, Edwards BS, Pereira NL, Stulak JM, Joyce L, Daly R, Park SJ, Kushwaha SS. Readmissions after implantation of axial flow left ventricular assist device. J Am Coll Cardiol. 2013;61(2):153–63.
70. Akhter SA, Badami A, Murray M, Kohmoto T, Lozonschi L, Osaki S, Lushaj EB. Hospital readmissions after continuous-flow left ventricular assist device implantation: incidence, causes, and cost analysis. Ann Thorac Surg. 2015;100:884–9.
71. Stulak JM, Davis ME, Haglund N, Dunlay S, Cowger J, Shah P, Pagani FD, Aaronson KD, Maltais S. Adverse events in contemporary continuous-flow left ventricular assist devices: a multi-institutional comparison shows significant differences. J Thorac Cardiovasc Surg. 2016;151(1):177–89.
72. Slaughter MS, Rogers JG, Milano CA, Russell SD, Conte JV, Feldman D, Sun B, Tatooles AJ, Delgado RM 3rd, Long JW, Wozniak TC, Ghumman W, Farrar DJ, Frazier OH. HeartMate II investigators. Advanced heart failure treated with continuous-flow left ventricular assist device. N Engl J Med. 2009;361(23):2241–51.
73. Kirklin JK, Naftel DC, Pagani FD, Kormos RL, Stevenson LW, Blume ED, Miller MA, Timothy Baldwin J, Young JB. Sixth INTERMACS annual report: a 10,000-patient database. J Heart Lung Transplant. 2014;33(6):555–64.

74. Schaffer JM, Allen JG, Weiss ES, Arnaoutakis GJ, Patel ND, Russell SD, Shah AS, Conte JV. Infectious complications after pulsatile-flow and continuous-flow left ventricular assist device implantation. J Heart Lung Transplant. 2011;30(2):164–74.
75. http://www.uab.edu/medicine/intermacs/appendices-4-0/appendix-a-4-0
76. Hannan MM, Husain S, Mattner F, Danziger-Isakov L, Drew RJ, Corey GR, Schueler S, Holman WL, Lawler LP, Gordon SM, Mahon NG, Herre JM, Gould K, Montoya JG, Padera RF, Kormos RL, Conte JV, Mooney ML. International Society for Heart and Lung Transplantation. Working formulation for the standardization of definitions of infections in patients using ventricular assist devices. J Heart Lung Transplant. 2011;30(4):375–84.
77. Nienaber JJ, Kusne S, Riaz T, Walker RC, Baddour LM, Wright AJ, Park SJ, Vikram HR, Keating MR, Arabia FA, Lahr BD, Sohail MR. Mayo cardiovascular infections study group. Clinical manifestations and management of left ventricular assist device-associated infections. Clin Infect Dis. 2013;57(10): 1438–48.
78. Tong MZ, Smedira NG, Soltesz EG, Starling RC, Koval CE, Porepa L, Moazami N. Outcomes of heart transplant after left ventricular assist device specific and related infection. Ann Thorac Surg. 2015;100(4):1292–7.
79. Chinn R, Dembitsky W, Eaton L, Chillcott S, Stahovich M, Rasmusson B, Pagani F. Multicenter experience: prevention and management of left ventricular assist device infections. ASAIO J. 2005;51(4):461–70.
80. Li JS, Sexton DJ, Mick N, Nettles R, Fowler VG Jr, Ryan T, Bashore T, Corey GR. Proposed modifications to the Duke criteria for the diagnosis of infective endocarditis. Clin Infect Dis. 2000;30(4):633–8.
81. Mermel LA, Allon M, Bouza E, Craven DE, Flynn P, O'Grady NP, Raad II, Rijnders BJ, Sherertz RJ, Warren DK. Clinical practice guidelines for the diagnosis and management of intravascular catheter-related infection: 2009 update by the Infectious Diseases Society of America. Clin Infect Dis. 2009;49(1):1–45.
82. Baddour LM, Wilson WR, Bayer AS, Fowler VG Jr, Tleyjeh IM, Rybak MJ, Barsic B, Lockhart PB, Gewitz MH, Levison ME, Bolger AF, Steckelberg JM, Baltimore RS, Fink AM, O'Gara P, Taubert KA. American Heart Association Committee on Rheumatic Fever, Endocarditis, and Kawasaki Disease of the Council on Cardiovascular Disease in the Young, Council on Clinical Cardiology, Council on Cardiovascular Surgery and Anesthesia, and Stroke Council. Infective endocarditis in adults: diagnosis, antimicrobial therapy, and management of complications: a scientific statement for healthcare professionals from the American Heart Association. Circulation. 2015;132(15):1435–86.
83. Stulak JM, Romans T, Cowger J, Romano MA, Haft JW, Aaronson KD, Pagani FD. Delayed sternal closure does not increase late infection risk in patients undergoing left ventricular assist device implantation. J Heart Lung Transplant. 2012;31(10):1115–9.
84. Kimura M, Nishimura T, Kinoshita O, Okada S, Inafuku H, Kyo S, Ono M. Successful treatment of pump pocket infection after left ventricular assist device implantation by negative pressure wound therapy and omental transposition. Ann Thorac Cardiovasc Surg. 2014;20(Suppl):842–5.
85. Shafii AE, Chamogeorgakis TP, Gonzalez-Stawinski G. Omental flap transposition with intra-abdominal relocation for LVAD pump-pocket infection. J Heart Lung Transplant. 2011;30(12):1421–2.
86. Park SJ, Milano CA, Tatooles AJ, Rogers JG, Adamson RM, Steidley DE, Ewald GA, Sundareswaran KS, Farrar DJ, Slaughter MS. HeartMate II clinical investigators. Outcomes in advanced heart failure patients with left ventricular assist devices for destination therapy. Circ Heart Fail. 2012;5(2):241–8.
87. John R, Aaronson KD, Pae WE, Acker MA, Hathaway DR, Najarian KB, Slaughter MS, HeartWare Bridge to Transplant ADVANCE Trial Investigators. Drive-line infections and sepsis in patients receiving the HVAD system as a left ventricular assist device. J Heart Lung Transplant. 2014;33(10):1066–73.
88. Goldstein DJ, Naftel D, Holman W, Bellumkonda L, Pamboukian SV, Pagani FD, Kirklin J. Continuous-flow devices and percutaneous site infections: clinical outcomes. J Heart Lung Transplant. 2012;31(11):1151–7.
89. Dean D, Kallel F, Ewald GA, Tatooles A, Sheridan BC, Brewer RJ, Caldeira C, Farrar DJ, Akhter SA, SSI Registry Investigators. Reduction in driveline infection rates: results from the HeartMate II Multicenter Driveline Silicone Skin Interface (SSI) Registry. J Heart Lung Transplant. 2015;34(6):781–9.
90. Singh A, Russo MJ, Valeroso TB, Anderson AS, Rich JD, Jeevanandam V, Akhter SA. Modified HeartMate II driveline externalization technique significantly decreases incidence of infection and improves long-term survival. ASAIO J. 2014;60(6):613–6.
91. Schibilsky D, Benk C, Haller C, Berchtold-Herz M, Siepe M, Beyersdorf F, Schlensak C. Double tunnel technique for the LVAD driveline: improved management regarding driveline infections. J Artif Organs. 2012;15(1):44–8.
92. Fleissner F, Avsar M, Malehsa D, Strueber M, Haverich A, Schmitto JD. Reduction of driveline infections through doubled driveline tunneling of left ventricular assist devices. Artif Organs. 2013;37(1):102–7.
93. Baronetto A, Centofanti P, Attisani M, Ricci D, Mussa B, Devotini R, Simonato E, Rinaldi M. A simple device to secure ventricular assist device driveline and prevent exit-site infection. Interact Cardiovasc Thorac Surg. 2014;18(4):415–7.
94. Cagliostro B, Levin AP, Fried J, Stewart S, Parkis G, Mody KP, Garan AR, Topkara V, Takayama H, Naka Y, Jorde UP, Uriel N. Continuous flow left ventricular assist devices and usefulness of a standardized strategy to reduce drive-line infections. J Heart Lung Transplant 2015. S1053–2498(15)01309-1.
95. Raymond AL, Kfoury AG, Bishop CJ, Davis ES, Goebel KM, Stoker S, Selzman CH, Clayson SE, Smith H, Cowley CG, Alharethi R, Budge D, Reid BB. Obesity and left ventricular assist device driveline exit site infection. ASAIO J. 2010;56(1):57–60.

Correction to: Immunosuppression, Including Drug Toxicity, Interactions, New Immunosuppressants in the Pipeline

Denise Wang, Bruno Meiser, Howard J. Eisen, and Sandra Eifert

Correction to:
Chapter 19 in: D. S. Feldman, P. Mohacsi (eds.), *Heart Failure*, Cardiovascular Medicine,
https://doi.org/10.1007/978-3-319-98184-0_19

The original version of this chapter was revised. This chapter was inadvertently published with incorrect author name "Denise Wanga" instead of "Denise Wang".

The updated online version of this chapter can be found at
https://doi.org/10.1007/978-3-319-98184-0_19

D. S. Feldman, P. Mohacsi (eds.), *Heart Failure*, Cardiovascular Medicine, https://doi.org/10.1007/978-3-319-98184-0_28

Index

D. S. Feldman, P. Mohacsi (eds.), *Heart Failure*, Cardiovascular Medicine, https://doi.org/10.1007/978-3-319-98184-0

L

M

N

MIX
Papier aus verantwortungsvollen Quellen
Paper from responsible sources
FSC® C105338

If you have any concerns about our products,
you can contact us on
ProductSafety@springernature.com

In case Publisher is established outside the EU,
the EU authorized representative is:
Springer Nature Customer Service Center GmbH
Europaplatz 3, 69115 Heidelberg, Germany

Printed by Libri Plureos GmbH
in Hamburg, Germany